THE ENTRY LEVEL

Occupational Therapy
Doctorate Capstone

A Framework for The Experience and Project

THE ENTRY LEVEL

Occupational Therapy Doctorate Capstone

A Framework for The Experience and Project

Editors

Elizabeth D. DeIuliis, OTD, MOT, OTR/L, CLA

Clinical Associate Professor
Assistant Department Chair
Academic Fieldwork Coordinator
John G. Rangos Sr. School of Health Sciences
Department of Occupational Therapy
Duquesne University
Pittsburgh, Pennsylvania

Julie A. Bednarski, OTD, MHS, OTR

Clinical Associate Professor
Associate Program Director
School of Health & Human Sciences
Department of Occupational Therapy
Indiana University
Indianapolis, Indiana

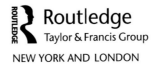

Routledge
Taylor & Francis Group

NEW YORK AND LONDON

First published in 2020 by SLACK Incorporated

Published in 2024 by Routledge
605 Third Avenue, New York, NY 10158

and by Routledge
4 Park Square, Milton Park, Abingdon, Oxon, OX14 4RN

Routledge is an imprint of the Taylor & Francis Group, an informa business

Cover Artist: Lori Shields

Library of Congress Cataloging-in-Publication Data

Names: DeIuliis, Elizabeth D., 1981- editor. | Bednarski, Julie A., editor.

Title: The entry level occupational therapy doctorate capstone : a
  framework for the experience and project / editors, Elizabeth D
  DeIuliis, Julie A Bednarski.
Description: Thorofare, NJ : SLACK Incorporated, 2019. | Includes
  bibliographical references and index.
Identifiers: LCCN 2019029172 (print) | ISBN 9781630916114 (paperback)
Subjects: MESH: Occupational Therapy--education | Curriculum | Education,
  Graduate | Clinical Competence--standards | Educational
  Measurement--methods
Classification: LCC RM735.42 (print) | NLM WB 18
  | DDC 615.8/515071--dc23
LC record available at https://lccn.loc.gov/2019029172

ISBN: 9781630916114 (pbk)
ISBN: 9781003523970 (ebk)

DOI: 10.4324/9781003523970

DEDICATION

For the future of the Occupational Therapy profession—

Be curious, Observe. Show empathy. Ideate. Do. Embrace risk. Refine.
Fail forward.

"Be so good that they can't ignore you."
—Steve Martin

CONTENTS

ACKNOWLEDGMENTS

I express sincere gratitude to my family, colleagues, and the students who contributed to this project. I thank my husband, Alessio, for his unconditional support of my "wild-hair" ideas and professional endeavors. I also thank my amazing faculty team and "occupational therapy family" at Duquesne University, including Department Chair Dr. Jaime Muñoz, Dr. Elena V. Donoso Brown, Dr. Kim Szucs, Dr. Jeryl Benson, Dr. Ann B. Cook, Dr. Ann Stuart, Dr. Meghan Blaskowitz, Dr. Amy M. Mattila, Dr. Rich Simpson, Professor Retta Martin, and our incredible administrative duo, Adriana Pearson and Jennifer Maselli, for their wisdom, encouragement, and inspiration.

A special note of consideration given to the contributing authors, who provided their valuable input and expertise across several important topics. A number of students/alumni at Duquesne University also deserve special recognition, including Graduate Student, Alex Raymond, for her attention to detail and superb organizational skills and Drs. Abbey Moonis, Anna Olexsovich, Justin McTish, Nikki Yeckel, and Cayla Leichtenberger for their willingness to share their own personal experiences and reflections from their capstone experience and project.

—Elizabeth D. DeIuliis, OTD, MOT, OTR/L, CLA

I thank my husband, James, and son, Connor, for their patience, love, and understanding throughout this entire process. I also thank my sister, Pam, and my parents, John and JoAnn, for their encouragement and support.

A special thanks to my students, who inspire me each day, and to the site mentors who are willing to embrace this capstone journey. I especially want to thank my students and alumni who offered their insights and reflections. For giving me the inspiration to look through the lens of human-centered design, I thank Dr. Penelope A. Moyers.

I began this journey at the University of Indianapolis (UIndy) and want to thank; Dr. Kate DeCleene Huber and Dr. Becky Barton, who laid the curricular groundwork for the capstone experience and project at UIndy; and Dr. Lori Breeden, Dr. Lucinda Dale, Dr. Jenny Fogo, Dr. Brenda Howard, Dr. Taylor McGann, Dr. Alison Nichols, Dr. Erin Peterson, Dr. Katie Polo, Dr. Beth Ann Walker, Mr. Jayson Zeigler, and Nicole Vicars. I thank you all for creating such a collaborative work environment and the friendship and support shown each day while I was at UIndy.

Finally, I thank my new colleagues at Indiana University (IU) with whom I am just beginning a new chapter in my work life. I am grateful to Dr. Terry Petrenchik, Chair of the Department of Occupational Therapy at Indiana University, Dr. Victoria Wilburn, Dr. Sally Wasmuth, and all of the IU faculty for supporting me and welcoming me to IU OT!

—Julie A. Bednarski, OTD, MHS, OTR

ABOUT THE EDITORS

Elizabeth D. DeIuliis is a Clinical Associate Professor and the Assistant Department Chair, Director of Community/ Clinical Education and Academic Fieldwork Coordinator at Duquesne University, which maintains dual-entry occupational therapy programs at the entry level masters and doctoral degree level in Pittsburgh, Pennsylvania. Dr. DeIuliis attended Duquesne University and graduated with a master's degree in occupational therapy in 2004. In December 2009, she completed a post-professional doctorate of occupational therapy degree at Chatham University in Pittsburgh, Pennsylvania. She continues to practice clinically on a per diem basis at UPMC Shadyside Hospital within Centers of Rehab Services. Dr. DeIuliis is an active member of the American Occupational Therapy Association and Pennsylvania Occupational Therapy Association, and a long-standing volunteer for the National Board for Certification in Occupational Therapy (NBCOT). Dr. DeIuliis completed the AOTA Academic Leadership Institute and earned the credential Certified Academic Leader (CLA) in 2018.

Julie A. Bednarski is currently a Clinical Associate Professor and the Associate Program Director in the Department of Occupational Therapy at Indiana University in Indianapolis, Indiana. Prior to joining the faculty at Indiana University, she was an Associate Professor, the Doctoral Capstone Coordinator, and Assistant Director of the School of Occupational Therapy at the University of Indianapolis. Dr. Bednarski graduated from Boston University in 1986 with her Bachelor of Science in Occupational Therapy. She went on to receive her master's in health science at the University of Indianapolis in 1996. In December 2010, she received her post-professional doctorate in Occupational Therapy at Chatham University in Pittsburgh, Pennsylvania. Dr. Bednarski has more than 30 years of clinical experience. She is an active volunteer for the NBCOT. It was through committee work at NBCOT that Dr. Bednarski and Dr. DeIuliis became friends and colleagues and began this book collaboration. Dr. Bednarski has presented at state and national conferences on topics including occupational justice, teaching methodologies, and community practice, among others. Dr. Bednarski is passionate about the doctoral capstone and the positive impact this experience has on students, clients, sites, and the profession.

CONTRIBUTING AUTHORS

Rebecca Barton, DHS, OTR, FAOTA (Chapter 4)
School of Occupational Therapy
University of Indianapolis
Indianapolis, Indiana

Alison Bell, OTD, OTR/L (Chapter 3)
Department of Occupational Therapy
College of Rehabilitation Sciences
Thomas Jefferson University
Philadelphia, Pennsylvania

Meghan Blaskowitz, DrPH, MOT, OTR/L (Chapter 8)
Department of Occupational Therapy
John G. Rangos Sr. School of Health Sciences
Duquesne University
Pittsburgh, Pennsylvania

Ann B. Cook, OTD, OTR/L (Chapter 10)
Department of Occupational Therapy
John G. Rangos Sr. School of Health Sciences
Duquesne University
Pittsburgh, Pennsylvania

Elena V. Donoso Brown, PhD, OTR/L (Chapter 8)
Department of Occupational Therapy
John G. Rangos Sr. School of Health Sciences
Duquesne University
Pittsburgh, Pennsylvania

Tina DeAngelis, EdD, OTR/L (Chapter 3)
Department of Occupational Therapy
College of Rehabilitation Sciences
Thomas Jefferson University
Philadelphia, Pennsylvania

Amy M. Mattila, PhD, OTR/L (Chapters 5 & 8)
Department of Occupational Therapy
John G. Rangos Sr. School of Health Sciences
Duquesne University
Pittsburgh, Pennsylvania

Katie M. Polo, DHS, OTR, CLT-LANA (Chapter 11)
School of Occupational Therapy
University of Indianapolis
Indianapolis, Indiana

Sally Wasmuth, PhD, OTR (Chapter 11)
Department of Occupational Therapy
School of Health & Human Sciences
Indiana University
Indianapolis, Indiana

INTRODUCTION:
AN OVERVIEW OF THE CAPSTONE

The purpose of this textbook is to provide a step-by-step guide and recommendations for the development, planning, implementation, and dissemination of the entry level occupational therapy doctoral (OTD) capstone experience and project (formerly known as the doctoral experiential component). This textbook is intended for a variety of audiences, including the doctoral capstone student, doctoral capstone coordinator, and occupational therapy faculty and site mentors. The Accreditation Council for Occupational Therapy Education (ACOTE) sets educational standards that must be met and maintained for accreditation for occupational therapy educational programs. The standards established by ACOTE are to serve as the minimum level of expectations for occupational therapy assistant programs, master's level occupational therapy programs, and entry level occupational therapy doctorate programs. The curricular standards go through a review, update, and adoption process approximately every 5 years in response to changes in health care, national educational trends, and other higher education accrediting bodies. The first entry level doctorate program was established in 1999 by Creighton University. Although ACOTE has been regulating entry level OTD education since 2006, there is a paucity of occupational therapy resources to guide faculty, prepare students, and socialize mentors to the capstone experience and project. This textbook is the first of its kind to serve as a manual to provide recommendations to guide the OTD capstone experience and project.

A universal requirement for OTD programs is the successful completion of a capstone experience and capstone project (ACOTE, 2018). A capstone (or comprehensive project) is a requirement of many doctoral degree programs. A capstone traditionally represents a culmination of one's doctoral studies with an evidenced-based, scholarly project. It is an opportunity for doctoral students to translate their acquired knowledge (usually reflecting a specialization or area of interest) into practice and potentially laying the groundwork for future scholarship. Although specific requirements will vary among institutions, a capstone typically requires the doctoral student to engage in a self-directed practice experience, with faculty or external advisors/mentors support (or a combination of these), as appropriate. Differing from a dissertation, which tends to require a doctoral candidate to produce new knowledge and is heavily focused on research and science, a capstone emphasizes the application of knowledge and dissemination of evidence into (clinical) practice.

The minimum standards for the capstone curricula in OTD programs are delineated in the D standards. ACOTE (2018) indicates that:

> the doctoral capstone shall be an integral part of the program's curriculum design. The goal of the doctoral capstone is to provide an in-depth exposure to one or more of the following focus areas: clinical practice skills, research skills, administration, leadership, program and policy development, advocacy, education, or theory development. (p. 43)

Chapter 2 explores these focus areas in greater detail. ACOTE further defines the doctoral capstone as consisting of two distinct parts: the capstone **project** and the capstone **experience**.

The capstone project is directly aligned with the capstone experience and should be designed to help the doctoral student synthesize and apply knowledge gained through the capstone experience. In prerequisite curriculum, the OTD student will develop and showcase many talents specific to competencies that help prepare the student for the capstone and related focus areas, including but not limited to the following (ACOTE, 2018):

- Explain to consumers, potential employers, colleagues, third-party payers, regulatory boards, policymakers, and the general public the distinct nature of occupation and the evidence that occupation supports performance, participation, health, and well-being (Standard. B.3.3).
- Identify, analyze, and evaluate the contextual factors; current policy issues; and socioeconomic, political, geographic, and demographic factors on the delivery of occupational therapy services for persons, groups, and populations to promote policy development and social systems as they relate to the practice of occupational therapy (Standard B.5.1).
- Implement a scholarly study that aligns with current research priorities and advances knowledge translation, professional practice, service delivery, or professional issues (e.g., Scholarship of Integration, Scholarship of Application, Scholarship of Teaching and Learning) (Standard B.6.1).
- Create scholarly reports appropriate for presentation or for publication in a peer-reviewed journal that support skills of clinical practice. The reports must be made available to professional or public audiences (Standard B. 6.3).
- Demonstrate an understanding of the process of locating and securing grants and how grants can serve as a fiscal resource for scholarly activities (Standard B.6.4).
- Demonstrate an understanding of how to design a scholarly proposal in regard to ethical policies and procedures necessary to conduct human-subject research, educational research, or research related to population health (Standard. B.6.5).
- Promote occupational therapy by educating other professionals, service providers, consumers, third-party payers, regulatory bodies, and the public (Standard B.7.3).

The doctoral capstone experience is an in-depth mentored and student-driven (or learner-centered) experience. In contrast to Level II fieldwork expectations, the capstone experience requires the student to be mentored, rather than supervised, by an individual with documented expertise, aligned with the focus of the capstone student's project. Mentoring is defined as "a relationship between two people in which one person (the mentor) is dedicated to the personal and professional growth of the other (the mentee)," and the mentor has more experience and knowledge than the mentee (ACOTE, 2018, p. 50). The planning and execution of a capstone student's experience will require successful collaboration among several individuals to ensure integrity with the academic institution's curriculum philosophy and the capstone student's individualized objectives for the doctoral capstone experience. This textbook provides an overview of the roles, responsibilities, and expectations for all individuals involved within the doctoral capstone process. Therefore, the audience for this text includes OTD students, occupational therapy faculty, doctoral capstone coordinators, and individuals who will serve as mentors to OTD students.

The goal of the capstone is to provide OTD students with in-depth exposure to a specific area of focus, demonstrate synthesis and application of knowledge gained, and disseminate results (ACOTE, 2018). This textbook examines a variety of types of capstone projects using the ACOTE focus areas of clinical practice skills, research skills, administration, leadership, program and policy development, advocacy, education, and/or theory development (ACOTE, 2018). Capstone projects may take a number of forms and should ultimately mutually benefit the capstone student and the site where the capstone takes place. Examples of how to structure capstone project proposals, including recommendations for structure and formatting of the final written document, additional scholarly products derived from the project, and other scholarly deliverables including formats for professional presentations and submissible papers are provided here.

This textbook utilizes human-centered design as a conceptual framework to intentionally thread content within the development, planning, implementation, and dissemination of the capstone. Human-centered design is a framework designed to help individuals develop a mindset to creatively think through key aspects of innovation, problem-solving, and viability (IDEO.org, 2015). This human-centered mindset is frequently used in the startup and technology global market, such as industry located in Silicon Valley, to unlock the creative potential in people and organizations to innovate routinely. This unique framework can be a useful strategy to increase the understanding of all stakeholders involved in the capstone process.

Similar to occupational therapy, human-centered design uses a holistic process that includes three phases: inspiration, ideation, and implementation (IDEO.org, n.d.). The inspiration phase is about "learning on the fly," opening up to creative possibilities, building empathy, and trusting that your ideas will evolve into a creative solution. In the ideation phase, individuals come up with ideas, brainstorm possibilities, and refine and improve ideas to build a simple "prototype" that is something tangible. This phase involves getting feedback from those who will benefit from the prototype and integrating their feedback to make it a more client-, group-, and population-centered product (or program). During the implementation phase, individuals are building partnerships and getting their idea, product, or prototype into the world. The philosophy of human-centered design complements occupational therapy nicely because it suggests that to build a truly innovative and useful product (or program), one needs to focus on the needs, contexts, behaviors, and emotions of the people that the solutions (program) will serve. Viewing the capstone experience and project through this lens can provide a helpful framework to motivate occupational therapy doctorate students, facilitate engagement with the capstone experience, and enable meaningful collaboration with the capstone coordinator and site mentor. See Figure 1 for a schematic illustrating human-centered design as a framework for the doctoral capstone and project.

The content in this textbook supports AOTA's Vision 2025, which challenges the profession to expand our reach and impact, prepare and develop the profession, and advance quality and recognition of occupational therapy practice (AOTA, 2017). In conclusion, this textbook is an essential resource for current, developing, and new OTD programs.

CHAPTERS AT A GLANCE

The concept of critical reflection has been identified as an important part of doctoral education (Brookfield, 2015). To initiate the process and sustain innovation and momentum throughout the capstone experience and project, each chapter begins with reflective questions for the capstone student that have been intentionally designed to anticipate your learning and stimulate the formation of thoughts and ideas regarding the developmental stage of the capstone process. The conceptual model, human-centered design, is also infused throughout this book as a theoretical framework.

Part I of this text (Chapters 1 through 4) is the inspiration phase, focusing on the development stage of the capstone process. Building a solid foundational understanding for the overall capstone process is the first focus here, and understanding the ACOTE areas of focus to allow for the brainstorming process of the capstone ideas is the second major focus. The importance of searching the literature to support and develop the purpose for the capstone experience and project is examined next. Finally, the intricacies of building site relationships with current fieldwork sites and role emerging sites and developing communication skills important for this self-directed experience is also explored.

Part II of this text (Chapters 5 and 6) provides an overview of the planning stage (or ideation phase) of the capstone process. These chapters explore strategies for developing practice-ready and self-regulation skills for the capstone student and the essential collaboration relationship among the occupational therapy doctoral student, faculty, capstone coordinator, and site mentor. Developing a memorandum of understanding (MOU) including determining individualized goals and objectives for the capstone project and experience is an important aspect of the planning stage that is explored. Finally, recommendations for supervision requirements, a plan for mentorship, proposal planning, and developing a project timeline are discussed.

Part III of this text (Chapters 7 through 9) discusses the implementation stage, which includes the doctoral capstone experience. Project management is the first major focus of the implementation phase. Evaluation of the impact and outcomes of the project is examined next. Finally, the importance of a sustainability plan is explored, as is the overall importance of student evaluations and site evaluations.

Finally, Part IV (Chapters 10 and 11) discuss the dissemination stage of the capstone process. This final phase, involves production and dissemination of the capstone project. Examples of how to prepare (format) and present scholarly deliverables (such as submissible papers and presentations) and their impact are explored.

Each chapter provides sample resources and useful documents appropriate for use with OTD students, faculty, doctoral capstone coordinators, and site mentors. Supplemental materials including learning activities and resources to enhance teaching and learning regarding the various topics discussed in this text are also provided.

REFERENCES

Accreditation Council for Occupational Therapy Education. (2018). *Standards and interpretive guide* [PDF]. Retrieved from https://www.aota.org/~/media/Corporate/Files/EducationCareers/Accredit/StandardsReview/2018-ACOTE-Standards-Interpretive-Guide.pdf

American Occupational Therapy Association. (2017). Vision 2025. *American Journal of Occupational Therapy, 71*(3), 710342001. doi:10.5014/ajot.2017.713002

Brookfield, S. (2015). Critical reflection as doctoral education. *New Directions for Adult and Continuing Education, 147*, 15–23.

IDEO. (2015). *The field guide to human-centered design.* San Francisco, CA: Ideo.org.

IDEO. (n.d). *About IDEO.* Retrieved from https://www.ideo.com/about

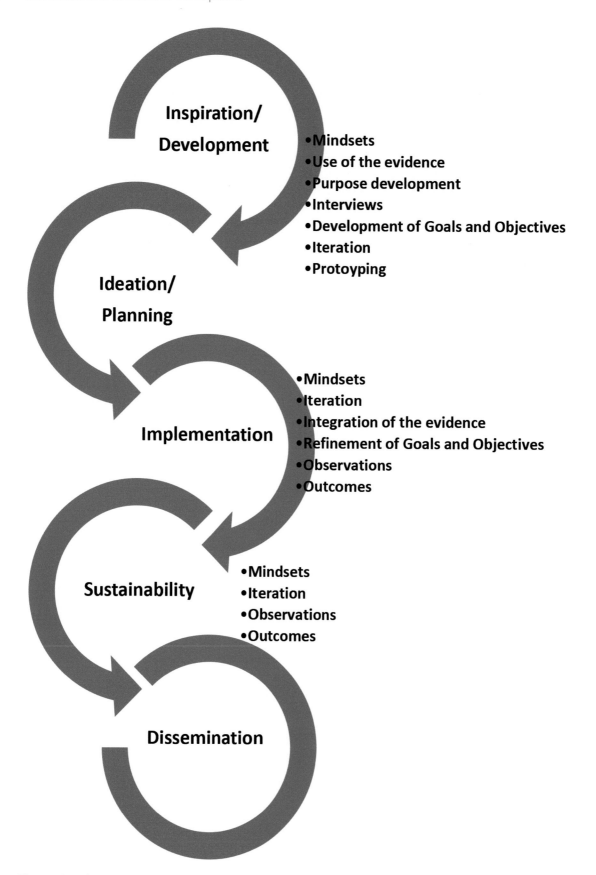

Figure 1. Using human-centered design as a framework for the doctoral capstone project. (Adapted from IDEO. [2015]. *The field guide to human-centered design*. San Francisco, CA: Ideo.org.)

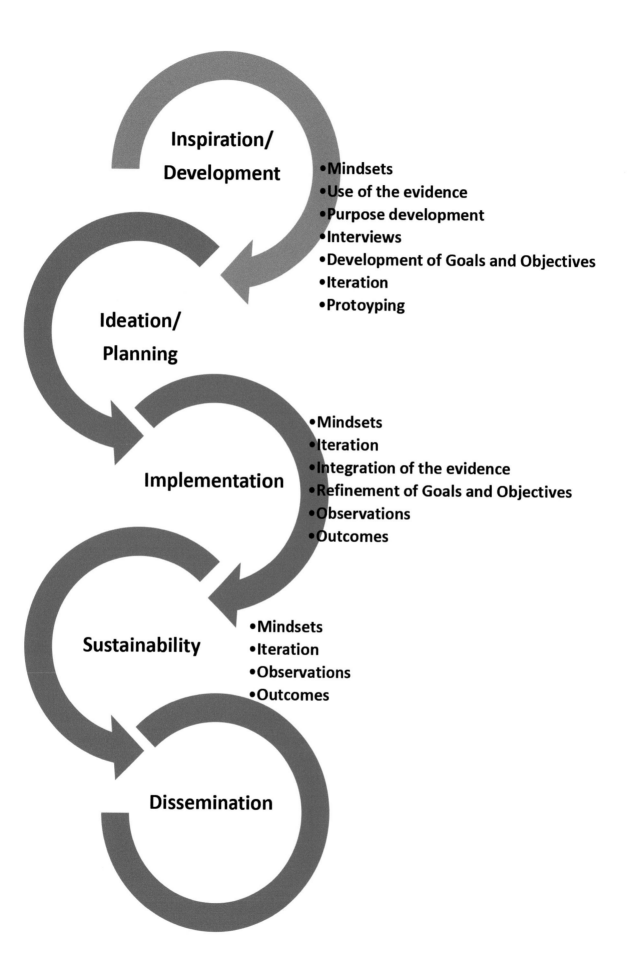

Inspiration/
Development

- Mindsets
- Use of the evidence
- Purpose development
- Interviews
- Development of Goals and Objectives
- Iteration
- Protoyping

Ideation/
Planning

Implementation

- Mindsets
- Iteration
- Integration of the evidence
- Refinement of Goals and Objectives
- Observations
- Outcomes

Sustainability

- Mindsets
- Iteration
- Observations
- Outcomes

Dissemination

Part I. Development

The first step is **development** of the capstone experience and project, which aligns with the **inspiration** process of human-centered design. This preparatory phase involves knowledge and skill-building. During the inspiration phase, brainstorming is required to begin the initial development of the capstone experience. Once the inspiration phase has begun, capstone students will use evidence, interview potential people that their experience will affect, and frame their design challenge to refine their capstone experience purpose. Goals and objectives are developed to allow for iteration and prototyping to ensure a client-centered approach to the experience.

CHAPTER 1

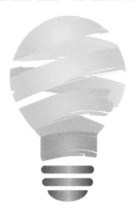

Roles, Responsibilities, and Expectations for the Capstone

Elizabeth D. Deluliis, OTD, MOT, OTR/L, CLA
Julie A. Bednarski, OTD, MHS, OTR

Human-Centered Design Mindsets for the Doctoral Students

The human-centered design mindset concepts of optimism and empathy are important for doctoral students to embrace as they begin the initial understanding of the overall capstone experience and project and the roles and responsibilities of the team members.

Optimism: "Optimism is the thing that drives you forward" (John Bielenberg, Founder, Future Partners, IDEO.org, 2015, p. 24). The doctoral capstone requires you to take on a big challenge, and by remaining optimistic, you are able to embrace the possibility of finding solutions to these challenges. Keep your sense of optimism as you begin this initial stage of development. Optimism will **drive you forward** at a time when you may feel overwhelmed. Optimism will drive you toward solutions, keep you creative, and encourage you to keep moving forward even when things get tough.

Empathy: "Empathy is the capacity to step into other people's shoes, to understand their lives, and start to solve problems from their perspectives" (Emi Kolawole, 2015, IDEO.org, 2015, p. 22). The concept of empathy will be at the forefront of your mind throughout your capstone experience and project. You are designing innovative solutions to problems, but to solve the problems, you must understand your client.

INTRODUCTION

It takes a village! This well-known proverb is a good metaphor to describe the development, planning, and implementation of the doctoral capstone experience (DCE) and project. Not unlike fieldwork education, successful completion of the doctoral capstone requires a sophisticated collaboration among various individuals, both inside and outside the educational program. The capstone is distinct from fieldwork because it is a major aspect of the final preparation of the capstone student for entry-level practice. The capstone student, occupational therapy faculty, doctoral capstone coordinator, academic fieldwork coordinator, and site mentor each have a significant role and unique responsibilities and expectations for the capstone. This chapter serves as an introduction to the *capstone team*, which includes the doctoral capstone coordinator, capstone student, and faculty and site mentors. It provides a comparison (and contrast) of fieldwork education

Deluliis ED, Bednarski JA.
The Entry Level Occupational Therapy Doctorate Capstone:
A Framework for The Experience and Project (pp 3-19).
© 2020 Taylor & Francis Group.

and the capstone experience and provides a description of the roles and responsibilities of each team member.

Capstone Student Reflective Questions

During the development phase of the doctoral capstone, the occupational therapy student may find it helpful to reflect on the following questions:

1. Describe how you feel the roles and expectations of being a capstone student differ from fieldwork.
2. How might the relationship with your site mentor differ from a traditional fieldwork educator?
3. What initial thoughts do you have about your capstone experience?
4. How do you embrace ambiguity?
5. What plan can you set in motion to keep an optimistic attitude throughout this process?

Learning Objectives

After reading this chapter and completing the learning activities, the reader should be able to:

1. Compare and contrast the curricula and outcomes of occupational therapy fieldwork education and the capstone.
2. Explain the unique expectations of occupational therapy fieldwork students and occupational therapy doctoral (OTD) students in the capstone.
3. Distinguish roles and responsibilities of the doctoral capstone student, occupational therapy faculty, doctoral capstone coordinator, and the site mentor.

FIELDWORK EDUCATION VERSUS CAPSTONE

Experiential learning is not unfamiliar to the occupational therapy profession. Like other health care professions, occupational therapy education requires the component of practical application in the curriculum. Other professions use various terminologies to describe this experiential learning, such as clinical education, residencies, externships, or internships. Historically, the occupational therapy profession has primarily identified it as *fieldwork education*. Fieldwork education is often described as a bridge that connects the theoretical didactic classroom instruction to real-world clinical practice and is argued to be the most integral piece of the occupational therapy education process (Aikens, Menaker, & Barsky, 2001; Brandenburger-Shasby et al., 1998; Haynes, 2011). Fieldwork is integrated with occupational therapy coursework to apply core values (including professionalism) and curricular threads in practice with mentorship from occupational therapy faculty and fieldwork educators. In occupational therapy education, there are currently two levels of fieldwork education intended to provide students with

this opportunity: Level I fieldwork and Level II fieldwork. In addition, the curriculum for the entry level doctorate degree requires an in-depth practicum called the capstone (Accreditation Council for Occupational Therapy Education [ACOTE], 2018). Before we take a deep dive into various members of the capstone team, it is important to compare and contrast the capstone with fieldwork.

Level I Fieldwork

According to the 2018 ACOTE Standards, the goal of Level I fieldwork is "to introduce students to fieldwork, apply knowledge to practice, and develop understanding of the needs of clients" (p. 40). Standard C.1.9 states that Level I fieldwork should "enrich didactic coursework through directed observation and participation in selected aspects of the occupational therapy process" (ACOTE, 2018, p. 40). Compared with Level II fieldwork, Level I fieldwork can be viewed as an introductory clinical learning experience. However, it is still "fieldwork," the first official experiential learning for occupational therapy students and a major steppingstone in the building of their professional identities and clinical skill development. Supervision of a Level I fieldwork student requires a qualified professional who may or may not be an occupational therapy practitioner. Examples may include, but are not limited to, currently licensed or otherwise regulated occupational therapists and occupational therapy assistants (OTAs), psychologists, physician assistants, teachers, social workers, nurses, and physical therapists. The American Occupational Therapy Association (AOTA) has recently put forth competencies to guide Level I fieldwork, which are discussed in more detail in Chapter 9.

Level II Fieldwork

The goal of Level II fieldwork is "to develop competent, entry-level, generalist occupational therapists," to promote clinical reasoning and reflective practice, to transmit the values and beliefs that enable ethical practice, and to develop professionalism and competence in career responsibilities (ACOTE, 2018, p. 41).

TEXT BOX 1-1

Generalist skills can include the following:
- Therapeutic use of self
- Clinical reasoning
- Professional behaviors
- Safety/judgment
- Evidence-Based practice
- Evaluations/interventions/discharge planning (AOTA, 2002)

Level II fieldwork is more highly regulated by ACOTE than Level I. ACOTE states that 16 weeks of Level II fieldwork are required for occupational therapy assistant (OTA) educational programs and 24 weeks for occupational therapy programs. The outcome of Level II fieldwork student learning is traditionally evaluated by the AOTA Fieldwork Performance Evaluation of the Level II Student (AOTA, 2002). Level II fieldwork students are required to be supervised by a currently licensed or otherwise regulated occupational therapist or, for OTA programs, OTA (under the supervision of an occupational therapist) who has a minimum of 1 year full time (or its equivalent) of practice experience subsequent to initial certification and who is adequately prepared to serve as a fieldwork educator. The supervising therapist may be engaged by the fieldwork site or by the educational program (ACOTE, 2018; AOTA, 2012).

> ### TEXT BOX 1-2
>
> New interpretive language provided by ACOTE requires occupational therapy programs to verify the qualifications and preparation of Level II fieldwork educators **PRIOR TO** the start of the experience (ACOTE, 2018). Some occupational therapy educational programs are requiring their Level II fieldwork educator to provide verification of their credentials and evidence of preparation to serve as fieldwork educator by requesting their resume or a list of continuing education and professional development units.
>
> Completion of the *AOTA Fieldwork Educator Certificate Workshop* is another strategy to demonstrate preparation to serve as a fieldwork educator.

The Level II fieldwork educator is responsible for evaluating if the student's performance demonstrates entry-level competency based on Level II fieldwork objectives and a formal evaluation process at the end of the Level II fieldwork experience (ACOTE, 2018).

Doctoral Capstone Experience

The entry level occupational therapy doctorate curriculum differs from the master's level in many ways. One of the most significant differences is the addition of the 14-week capstone experience. This experiential learning requirement for the occupational therapy educational programs is in addition to the existing Levels I and II fieldwork education requirements. The goal of the capstone is to provide in-depth exposure to an area of focus (ACOTE, 2018). The DCE "shall be an integral part of the program's curriculum design, and shall include an in-depth experience in one or more of the following: clinical practice skills, research skills, administration, leadership, program and policy development, advocacy, education, or theory development" (ACOTE, 2018, p. 43). These areas of focus for the capstone outlined by ACOTE are discussed in greater detail in Chapter 2. The capstone student must successfully complete all coursework, Level II fieldwork, and completion of preparatory activities (which

include a literature review, needs assessment, goals and objectives, and an evaluation plan) before the commencement of the capstone (ACOTE, 2018). To meet the ACOTE Standards, the capstone student must have a unique set of skills and abilities. Chapter 5 clearly outlines specific "practice-ready" skills that are necessary for the success of the capstone experience and recommendations for occupational therapy programs to facilitate environments or tasks that foster growth in this area.

In contrast to fieldwork educators during fieldwork, the supervising individual during the capstone experience is called a *mentor*. According to the ACOTE Standard D.1.6, the doctoral capstone coordinator will ensure documentation and "verify that the capstone student is being mentored by an individual with expertise consistent with the student's area of focus prior to" the initiation of the doctoral capstone (ACOTE, 2018, p. 45). Mentoring is defined as "a relationship between two people in which one person (the mentor) is dedicated to the personal and professional growth of the other (the mentee)" (ACOTE, 2018, p. 50). A mentor can be defined as an individual having more experience and knowledge than the mentee. An OTD student will most likely have several "mentors" throughout the capstone, which may include faculty at the occupational therapy program, individuals who work at their capstone site, or external mentors who may have subject matter expertise aligned with the doctoral student's focus area. ACOTE Standard D.1.4 states that the doctoral capstone coordinator is responsible for ensuring that there is a memorandum of understanding (MOU) that, at a minimum, includes individualized specific objectives, plans for supervision or mentoring and responsibilities of all parties (ACOTE, 2018, p. 44). The MOU and process to develop the individualized learning objectives are discussed in greater detail in Chapter 6. Depending on the capstone focus or emphasis, the student may have more than one site/facility mentor, but this should be outlined in the student's learning plan or the MOU. (See Table 1-1 for a snapshot of the similarities and differences among Level I fieldwork, Level II fieldwork, and the DCE.)

To ensure a successful collaboration, it is important that all stakeholders involved in the capstone are familiar with one another's roles, responsibilities, and expectations. Now that we have contrasted the different levels of fieldwork education with the capstone experience, let's identify and discuss the key individuals who are involved throughout the planning, execution, and evaluation of the capstone. These individuals include the capstone student, occupational therapy faculty, doctoral capstone coordinator, and site mentor; we refer to this collective group as the *capstone team* throughout this text. Although not directly involved with the capstone, roles, responsibilities, and expectations of the academic fieldwork coordinator are also introduced.

Table 1-1. Similarities and Differences Among Level I Fieldwork, Level II Fieldwork, and Capstone

LEVEL I	**Length:** Not prescribed by ACOTE. **Supervision Requirement:** "Ensure that personnel who supervise Level I fieldwork are informed of the curriculum and program design and affirm their ability to support the fieldwork experience. Examples include, but are not limited to, currently licensed or otherwise regulated occupational therapists and OTAs, psychologists, physician assistants, teachers, social workers, physicians, speech language pathologists, nurses, and physical therapists" (ACOTE, 2018, p. 40). **Supervision Type:** Not prescribed by ACOTE. **Purpose/Goal:** "To introduce students to fieldwork, apply knowledge to practice, and develop understanding of the needs of clients" (ACOTE, 2018, p. 40).
LEVEL II	**Length:** A minimum of 24 weeks of full-time Level II fieldwork. This may be completed on a part-time basis, as defined by the fieldwork placement in accordance with the fieldwork placement. **Supervision Requirement:** Traditional setting: A minimum of 1 year full-time (or its equivalent) practice experience as a licensed or otherwise regulated occupational therapist before the onset of the Level II fieldwork experience (ACOTE, 2018). Role-Emerging setting: "Document and verify that supervision provided in a setting where no occupational therapy services exist includes a documented plan for provision of occupational therapy services and supervision by a currently licensed otherwise regulated occupational therapist with at least 3 years' full-time or its equivalent of professional experience prior to the Level II fieldwork experience. Supervision must include a minimum of 8 hours of direct supervision each week of the fieldwork experience. An occupational therapy supervisor must be available, via a variety of contact measures, to the student during all working hours. An on-site supervisor designee of another profession must be assigned while the occupational therapy supervisor is off-site" (ACOTE, 2018, p. 42). International: Supervised by an occupational therapist who graduated from a program approved by the World Federation of Occupational Therapists and has at least 1 year of experience in practice. **Supervision Type:** "Ensure that Level II fieldwork supervision is direct and then decreases to less direct supervision as appropriate for the setting, the severity of the client's condition, and the ability of the student to support progression towards entry-level competence" (ACOTE, 2018, p. 42). **Purpose/Goal:** Develop into competent entry-level generalist occupational therapy practitioners (ACOTE, 2018).
DOCTORAL CAPSTONE EXPERIENCE	**Length:** Must be started upon completion of all coursework and Level II fieldwork and completion of preparatory activities. Fourteen weeks (560 hours). This may be completed on a part-time basis and must be consistent with the individualized specific objectives and capstone project. No more than 20% of the 560 hours can be completed off-site from the mentored practice setting(s) to ensure a concentrated experience in the designated area of interest. Time spent off-site may include independent study activities such as research and writing. Prior fieldwork or work experience may not be substituted for this DCE. **Supervision Requirement:** Student is mentored by an individual with expertise consistent with the student's area of focus prior to the initiation onset of the DCE. The mentor does not have to be an occupational therapist. **Supervision Type:** Not prescribed by ACOTE. **Purpose/Goal:** To provide in-depth exposure to one or more of the following: clinical practice skills, research skills, administration, leadership, program and policy development, advocacy, education, or theory development (ACOTE, 2018, p. 43).

THE OCCUPATIONAL THERAPY DOCTORAL CAPSTONE STUDENT

It is important that the capstone student play an active role throughout the development, planning, implementation, and evaluation stages of the capstone. The focus and expectations of the capstone differ from fieldwork education. Therefore, the responsibilities and skill set required for the capstone also stand apart. Chapter 5 goes into greater detail regarding recommended skills, attitudes, and behaviors that a capstone student should embrace to be successful and effective throughout the capstone process. The following list provides an overview of both general and specific tasks and actions a capstone student can take to ensure preparation and success on the capstone experience and project.

> **TEACHING TIP 1:** Expectations from individual OTD programs, faculty, and doctoral capstone coordinators may vary, yet the information in this chapter can provide a model of how to help a capstone student understand various components of their role.

1. Understand and abide by the academic program policies and procedures relative to the capstone. (This may include a capstone manual or course syllabi.)
2. Identify personal goals, interests, and appropriate outcomes as a basis for planning the capstone experience and project.
3. Collaborate to develop and plan his or her capstone experience with the doctoral capstone coordinator, and other faculty as appropriate, including possible settings and populations for the capstone. (This may include a capstone proposal, which will be discussed in Chapter 6.)
4. Collaboratively develop the MOU with site mentor and doctoral capstone coordinator; this includes individualized specific objectives, plan for supervisor/mentoring, responsibilities of all parties and authorship; obtain appropriate signatures.
5. Obtain evidence of "expertise," aligned with the focus area, of the site mentor and submit to the doctoral capstone coordinator when required.
6. Synthesize knowledge from preparatory coursework in the occupational therapy curriculum to support the development of a capstone project which may include creating a scholarly question, conducting a needs assessment, identifying a guiding theoretical perspective, developing a research question, appraising the literature proposal, and designing a project methodology. (Types of capstone projects and strategies to disseminate are discussed in Chapters 10 and 11.)

7. Complete the 14-week capstone experience, with no more than 20% of the time completed outside the mentored practice setting. Students are responsible to ensure that missed hours are made up appropriately, at discretion of their site mentor and capstone coordinator. (Examples of how to negotiate and structure the weekly schedule are presented in Chapter 6.)
8. Complete tasks* assigned by the site mentor to ensure success of the experience, alignment with chosen focus area(s) and outcome of capstone.

TEXT BOX 1-3

*This may include assigned readings, attending meetings or workshops, and interviewing or meeting with other individuals within the capstone site to support the development of in-depth knowledge and achievement of the individualized objectives.

9. Take initiative to communicate with the site mentor, occupational therapy faculty, and doctoral capstone coordinator when expected to do so or as needed to ensure success.
10. Demonstrate respectful interaction and communication with the student cohort, faculty, mentors, doctoral capstone coordinator, and other individuals who may be a part of the capstone. For example, this may include an individual who is responsible for the institutional review board (IRB) process at the academic institution or capstone site.
11. Develop and maintain a structure for working with the capstone team to conduct and complete the capstone experience and project. This should be included in the MOU and include clearly delineated responsibilities and timelines, both individual and group.
12. Provide appropriate feedback to the site (and mentor) at the formal midterm and final evaluation to enhance the experience. (Although there is not a formal endorsed tool like the AOTA Fieldwork Performance Evaluation to evaluate the capstone, Chapter 9 provides examples of ways to structure evaluation of the capstone site and the student.)
13. Utilize constructive feedback from faculty, site mentor, and doctoral capstone coordinator for personal and professional growth.
14. Take responsibility for one's own skills and professional development. (This can include professional writing skills and knowledge of IRB application process, for example.)

15. Collect, manage, and analyze data for capstone project as proposed.

16. Demonstrate a professional approach to the capstone, including demonstrating effective and appropriate intrinsic and extrinsic aspects of professionalism (DeIuliis, 2017) including but not limited to time management, observing deadlines, initiating, and reading and responding to communications from the capstone team; regular and thorough communication regarding updates/progress with all members of the team is critical.

17. Complete and submit evaluation of the capstone experience form, per capstone policy manual or the deadline indicated on course syllabus.

18. Be **self-directed** throughout the capstone process, including in developing, planning, and completing the capstone experience and project. (Strategies to foster self-directedness and practice-ready skills are discussed in Chapter 5.)

19. Take initiative to finalize all documentation with the site mentor, faculty mentor (chair), or doctoral capstone coordinator. (This may include release of consent forms, IRB requirements, signature for use in academic library's electronic theses and dissertation system, and additional medical/legal documents, for example.)

20. Complete and disseminate a culminating capstone project in a format and forum, within the time frame determined by the academic program.

DOCTORAL CAPSTONE COORDINATOR

The doctoral capstone coordinator is a full-time core faculty member as defined by ACOTE and is specifically responsible for the occupational therapy program's compliance with the capstone requirements listed in Standards Section D (ACOTE Standard A.2.5). Although the specific responsibilities of the doctoral capstone coordinator may vary by program, the general role of the capstone coordinator is to provide students with the structure and information to begin the development of their capstone experiences and oversee each phase of the capstone from development to completion and dissemination. (See Table 1-2 for a brief overview of the capstone project.)

The doctoral capstone coordinator will ensure the capstone experience is unique and does not duplicate or interfere with the capstone student's previous fieldwork experiences. Although the doctoral capstone coordinator is typically the primary faculty member responsible for the overall capstone experience, it can be helpful to have a model where other faculty serve as faculty mentors (or chairs) of doctoral students' capstone projects. The doctoral capstone coordinator should not be assumed to be the faculty mentor for each student. In a program with a large student cohort, this would not be possible. Figures 1-1 and 1-2 allow the reader to visualize a structure for the capstone roles.

The doctoral capstone coordinator may take the lead, possibly working with the program director or department chair, to organize the match process for capstone students and faculty mentors (or capstone chair) and ensure good fit and appropriate mentorship. Depending on the program or school curriculum design and based on the capstone student's goals, interests, and planned focus areas, the doctoral capstone coordinator or assigned faculty mentor will work with each student individually to identify and confirm each doctoral site for the capstone experience and project. The doctoral capstone coordinator will also assist the faculty mentors and site mentors, as needed through the planning and execution of the DCEs. The following list provides an overview of both general and specific tasks and actions the doctoral capstone coordinator can take to ensure preparation and success on the capstone.

Table 1-2. Brief Overview of the Capstone Process

PHASE I: DEVELOPMENT	PHASE II: PLANNING PHASE	PHASE III: IMPLEMENTATION PHASE	PHASE IV: DISSEMINATION PHASE
• Understand ACOTE requirements • Determine ACOTE Area of Focus for the capstone project and experience • Complete review of the literature to support project idea • Define purpose • Determine potential capstone site and site mentor • Develop initial goals and objectives	• Visit with potential sites/site mentors • Complete capstone project proposal • Determine whether IRB is required; complete IRB if needed • Finalize site and site mentor and meet with site mentor to complete MOU • Complete literature review and needs assessment to support project • Develop timeline	• Complete site requirements • Update literature review needs assessment • Finalize MOU with updated goals and objectives • Implement capstone project and experience • Evaluate impact/outcome • Develop sustainability plan	• Plan for dissemination • Disseminate results to site • Disseminate results to university/peers • Disseminate to community as appropriate • Disseminate to the field of occupational therapy • Determine future plans

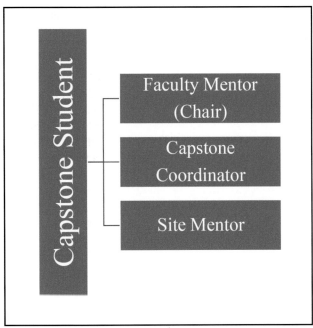

Figure 1-1. Members of the capstone team.

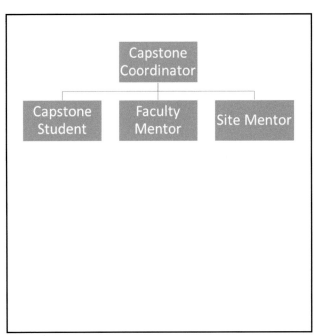

Figure 1-2. Example of an organization chart for the capstone team.

1. Verify that the capstone student has successfully completed coursework, prior fieldwork experiences, and required preparatory activities defined in ACOTE Standard D.1.3.

2. Ensure that the DCE and project is consistent with the program's curricular design.

3. Instruct students regarding the capstone processes and expectations. (This may include orientation sessions, individualized counseling sessions, creation and use of a capstone manual, and course syllabi. See Appendix 1-A for a sample table of contents for a policy manual.)

4. Collaborate with the capstone student and academic fieldwork coordinator to identify their goals and interests and to ensure no overlap with fieldwork education experiences.

5. Educate the capstone students and site mentors on the ACOTE focus areas.

6. Advise capstone students in determining site preferences and project focus.

7. Identify and correspond with potential capstone sites and potential site mentors/supervisors, establish affiliation agreements, and confirm capstone experience placements.

8. Ensure that all policies and procedures are followed according to the academic institution and ACOTE.

9. Obtain and disseminate necessary capstone student and site information (including but not limited to confirmation letters, student data form, and student health/security clearances, for example.)

10. Maintain adequate records of capstone site information and allow student access.

11. Ensure that the student will be mentored by an individual with expertise consistent with the student's area of focus.

TEACHING TIP 2: One strategy to verify that the site mentor's expertise is consistent with the student's area of focus is for the doctoral capstone coordinator to request that the capstone student obtain the site mentor's current resume, curriculum vitae, or list of credentials and verify credentials via public domain databases (which may include state licensure board and/or National Board for Certification in Occupational Therapy certification).

12. Collaborate with the capstone team and assign faculty mentors (chairs). This can be based on alignment of focus areas, faculty expertise and training, and so on.

13. Ensure and verify length and hours of the experience (14 weeks, 560 hours) and that no more than 20% of the time is completed outside the mentored practice setting.

14. Ensure all sites have signed an MOU, which must include individualized specific objectives, plan for supervisor/mentoring, and responsibilities of all parties; ensure that the student obtains appropriate collaboration and signatures. The MOU must be completed before the commencement of the capstone experience and according to the standards and regulations of all regulating bodies.

15. Correspond professionally with capstone student and site mentor via electronic communication, phone calls, and site visits, as appropriate.

16. Support capstone student progress and provide remediation as needed. (Refer to Appendix 9-D in Chapter 9 for a sample remediation plan.)

17. Ensure that an objective formal evaluation of the student's performance is completed during the capstone experience. (This may include a midterm and a final evaluation. Chapter 9 provides different strategies to structure and design an evaluation of the doctoral occupational therapy student and evaluation of the capstone experience.)

18. Be available as a resource and consultant to the capstone student, site mentor, and faculty mentor during the DCE.

19. Evaluate (including data collection and analysis) the capstone experience to ensure that the program complies with ACOTE D standards and meets academic institution specific student outcomes and goals. (Examples of evaluations are presented in Chapter 9.)

20. Record and assign grades for the capstone experience. (The capstone coordinator or faculty mentor could assign grade for the capstone project.)

21. Ensure that formal letters or certificates are provided to site mentors after completion of the DCE, acknowledging the mentorship provided.

TEACHING TIP 3: The formal letter for the site mentor provided by the occupational therapy program must include the dates of mentorship. Per National Board for Certification in Occupational Therapy guidelines, each week of mentorship is worth one professional development unit. See sample template in Appendix 1-B.

22. Collaborate or coordinate the capstone dissemination/defense and invite various stakeholders.

ACOTE (2018) standards (Standard A.2.10) indicate that the doctoral capstone coordinator should have adequate clerical support. Tasks that could be delegated to a clerical team or administrative assistant could include:
- Create and manage capstone site correspondence using letter template(s)
- Collate and store doctoral capstone site information
- Assist doctoral capstone coordinator in deploying program evaluation measures such as an exit survey (see Chapter 9)
- Create mentorship certificates to recognize site mentors
- Manage capstone site database

ACADEMIC FIELDWORK COORDINATOR

Depending on the faculty infrastructure at the educational program, the academic fieldwork coordinator can be an important support system for the doctoral capstone coordinator. The academic fieldwork coordinator can review student capstone proposals and provide appropriate feedback, as warranted. This level of review by the academic fieldwork coordinator can ensure that the proposed capstone experience is above and beyond the doctoral student's fieldwork experiences and does not duplicate or conflict with any fieldwork experiences. Prior fieldwork or work experience may not substitute for the capstone.

More specific resources related to the academic fieldwork coordinator role and fieldwork education can be found on the AOTA website under "Fieldwork" or by accessing these resources:
- Costa, D. M. (2004). *The essential guide to occupational therapy fieldwork education: Resources for today's educators and practitioners.* Bethesda, MD: American Occupational Therapy Association.
- Costa, D. M. (2015). *The essential guide to occupational therapy fieldwork education: Resources for educators and practitioners* (2nd ed.). Bethesda, MD: AOTA Press.
- Deluliis, E. D. (2017). What is fieldwork education? In E. F. Deluliis (Ed.), *Professionalism across occupational therapy* (pp. 163-200). Thorofare, NJ: SLACK Incorporated.

- Deluliis, E. D. (2017). Professionalism and fieldwork education. In E. D. Deluliis (Ed.), *Professionalism across occupational therapy* (pp. 201-222). Thorofare, NJ: SLACK Incorporated.
- Deluliis, E. D. (2017). Clinical vignettes: Common fieldwork professional behavior. In E. D. Deluliis (Ed.), *Professionalism across occupational Therapy* (pp. 223-228). Thorofare, NJ: SLACK Incorporated.

ROLE OF OCCUPATIONAL THERAPY FACULTY MENTOR (CAPSTONE CHAIR)

Although the doctoral capstone coordinator is identified by ACOTE as being the primary faculty member responsible for the program's compliance with the capstone requirements of Standards Section D.1.0, other faculty in the OTD program can play an important role on the capstone team. ACOTE Standards indicate that the capstone coordinator must have sufficient release time and support to ensure that the needs of the capstone program are being met. In addition to administrative staff to assist with clerical tasks, other occupational therapy faculty members can serve as a faculty mentor or capstone chair to OTD student's capstone projects.

TEACHING TIP 4: Determining the workload of the faculty mentors will be specific to each program and dependent on several factors, such as the number of students in the program. Students can be assigned to a faculty member to "chair" or "mentor" capstone students throughout the DCE or capstone project. One recommendation for division of workload is to have one faculty member assigned to four or five capstone students during their capstone experience and project. Therefore, if the class size is composed of 30 students, at least six faculty members would need to be assigned load credit for taking a group of four to five students each.

The doctoral capstone coordinator is responsible for the overall capstone experience; however, they could also take on the role of faculty mentor with a small group of students if their workload and release time allows this. The program or school curriculum structure will determine when the faculty mentors are assigned and how much load credit is given (Figure 1-3).

The faculty mentor (chair) assumes primary responsibility for ensuring that the capstone project meets university and program standards. The following list provides an overview of both general and specific tasks and actions of how an

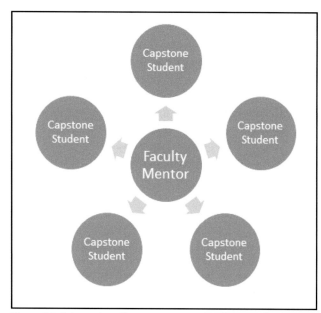

Figure 1-3. Schematic to illustrate an occupational therapy faculty member as capstone chair.

occupational therapy faculty member can be used to ensure success of the capstone project.

1. Collaborate with the capstone student on individualized specific objectives for the experience that coincide with their chosen focus area(s).

2. Collaborate with the site mentor as needed.

3. Be available to the capstone student as a resource and consultant (this may include providing feedback on capstone project drafts and assisting through the IRB process, for example).

4. Notify doctoral capstone coordinator if problems arise, and collaborate with the student, capstone coordinator, and site mentor on an action or remediation plan.

5. Provide meaningful feedback on drafts of the capstone project, as appropriate.

SITE MENTOR

ACOTE (2018) standards define that the individual directly working with the capstone student during the capstone as "a mentor" (p. 50). An important quality of the site mentor is to ensure a concentrated experience in the designed area of interest or focus area. Therefore, the site mentor should have expertise consistent with the capstone student's area of focus (ACOTE, 2018). Many professionals are qualified to "mentor" capstone students as they learn and carry out in-depth skills in one or more of the eight focus areas specific to their doctoral pursuit. Furthermore, the mentor does not have to be an occupational therapist, which affords the opportunity for interprofessional mentorship. The mentor does not have to have a doctoral degree. The primary requirement

for mentors is the foundation of the expertise they can provide capstone students, which coincides with their focus area(s) and capstone project. Table 1-3 depicts examples of types of site mentors at various settings and sites.

The site mentor is typically the on-site person who will provide instruction, support, supervision (if needed), and mentorship to the capstone student in applying knowledge to practical situations, developing problem-solving skills, and learning practical competencies within the chosen focus area(s). The level and type of supervision is customized to the type of setting, the capstone student's learning objectives, and the focus of the capstone. The doctoral capstone coordinator will collaborate with the site mentor and the capstone student to declare supervision responsibilities and mentorship plan in the MOU before the beginning of the capstone. **Direct clinical practice activities performed by the capstone student should be supervised by a qualified professional who meets the state and national requirements to perform the area of practice.** See Table 1-4 for an overview of formal supervision levels.

The following list provides an overview of both general and specific tasks and actions the site mentor can take to ensure preparation and success on the capstone:

1. Instruct and orient the capstone student as needed to perform specific negotiated learning activities consistent with the student's learning objectives.

2. Demonstrate willingness and the ability to provide evidence of expertise. This could include documented evidence of terminal degree, current curriculum vitae or resume, verification of completed specialty training, and certification or advanced trainings, for example.

3. Collaborate with capstone team to delineate mentorship responsibility.

4. Provide supervision or mentorship throughout the duration of the capstone, according to the agreed-on MOU.

5. Develop (in collaboration with the doctoral capstone coordinator) and maintain a system for documenting capstone students' experiential hours on site and the tasks and activities accomplished during those hours (as identified in the MOU). See Appendix 1-C for a sample time log template.

6. Provide orientation to the site, other personnel, and stakeholders.

7. Collaborate with the faculty mentor to guide the capstone student through the needs assessment component of the project proposal.

8. Provide guidance on the logistics of completing the capstone at the site, which could include greater detail on workflow at site, general hours of operation, and access to work spaces.

9. Proactively correspond with capstone team regarding any potential concerns.

Table 1-3. Examples of Types of Site Mentors

FOCUS AREA	TYPE OF SETTING/SITE	EXAMPLE OF SITE MENTOR
Clinical practice skills	Medical setting	Any individual with expertise aligned with the capstone focus (e.g., nurse, physician, respiratory therapist)
Clinical practice skills	School setting	Teacher, director of special education
Program development	Not-for-profit agency	Executive director Director of programming
Program development	Medical setting	Unit manager, corporate compliance officer
Leadership	Professional association (e.g., AOTA, state organization, National Board for Certification in Occupational Therapy)	Executive director Conference committee staff
Policy development	State or local office	Councilman, legislator, individual on a political action committee (PAC)
Administration	Private practice	Owner/sole proprietor, finance officer, department head or director
Research	Health care or academic setting	Principal investigator
Theory development	Health care or academic setting	Academician, researcher theorist
Education	Academia (higher education)	Occupational therapist or OTA faculty member Center of teaching excellence faculty or staff
	Publishing company	Academic publisher Senior editor
Advocacy	National or local association (e.g., local chapter for cystic fibrosis)	Executive director, fundraising chair, volunteer organizer

Table 1-4. Overview of Supervision Levels

TYPES OF FORMAL SUPERVISION LEVELS	DESCRIPTION
Close	Daily, direct contact
Routine	Direct contact at least every 2 weeks Interim supervision by other methods (phone/written)
General	At least monthly direct contact Supervision available as needed by other methods
Minimal	Only on as-needed basis

Adapted from American Occupational Therapy Association. (1993). Occupational therapy roles. *American Journal of Occupational Therapy, 47,* 1087-1099.

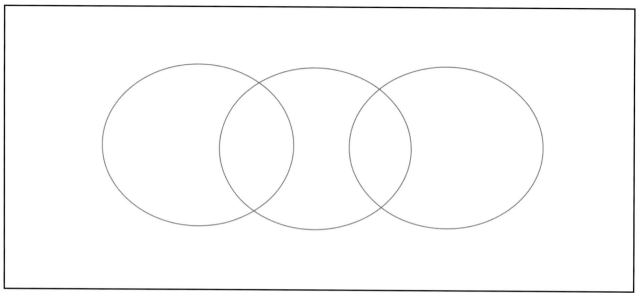

Figure 1-4. Venn diagram.

10. Evaluate the capstone student's performance formally (may include a midterm and final formal evaluation).

11. Actively participate in regular communication with the capstone team in person, virtually (Skype, Adobe Connect, etc.), by email, or through other means, including giving both verbal and written feedback on implementation and documentation.

12. Provide meaningful feedback on drafts of the capstone project, as appropriate.

CHAPTER SUMMARY

It is evident that the capstone differs from fieldwork education in many ways. Because of this, expectations of the capstone student, occupational therapy faculty, and the individual "mentoring" the capstone student are also distinctive. This chapter has provided recommendations of tasks, actions, and responsibilities of the entire capstone team. The concept of mentorship (vs fieldwork supervision) was also described. Ensuring that the capstone team members understand their role throughout the duration of the capstone process is also critical.

The capstone promotes a fundamental philosophy of occupation: doing beyond knowing (Rowles, 1991). This "doing" is accomplished by the application of evidence-based theory to practice and a focused synthesis of advanced knowledge in a practice focus area through completion of a culminating project. Recommendations of sample policies and other procedures to clarify, initiate, and promote the "doing" of the capstone are provided in Appendices B and C.

Learning Activities

1. A Venn diagram is a diagram that shows all possible logical relations between variables (See illustration in Figure 1-4). Review Table 1-1 in this chapter. Create a Venn diagram comparing and contrasting the capstone and fieldwork education.

2. Think about your current (or previous) fieldwork educators. Identify one quality or area of expertise that this individual has that could align with one of the ACOTE focus areas.

3. Create a list of your responsibilities for the doctoral capstone.

4. Brainstorm members of your occupational therapy faculty who could serve as your capstone chair based on your initial interests and focus area.

REFERENCES

Accreditation Council for Occupational Therapy Education. (2018). *Standards and interpretive guide* [PDF]. Retrieved from https://www.aota.org/~/media/Corporate/Files/EducationCareers/Accredit/StandardsReview/2018-ACOTE-Standards-Interpretive-Guide.pdf

Aikens, F., Menaker, L., & Barsky, L. (2001). Fieldwork education: the future of Occupational therapy depends on it. *Occupational Therapy International, 8*(2), 86-95.

American Occupational Therapy Association. (1993). Occupational therapy roles. *American Journal of Occupational Therapy, 47*, 1087-1099.

Brandenburger-Shasby, S., Hills, L., Huie, C., Jansen, K., Johnson, L., & Josey-Lamont, (1998). Fieldwork: The critical link. *Education Special Interest Section Quarterly, 8*(3), 1-3.

DeIuliis, E.D. (2017). *Professionalism across Occupational Therapy Clinical Practice.* Thorofare, NJ: SLACK Incorporated.

IDEO. (2015). *The field guide to human-centered design.* San Francisco, CA: Ideo.org.

Haynes, C. J. (2011). Active participation in fieldwork level I: Fieldwork educator and student perceptions. *Occupational Therapy in Health Care, 25*, 257-269. doi:10.3109/07380577.2011.595477

Rowles, G. D. (1991). Beyond performance: Being in place as a component of occupational therapy. *American Journal of Occupational Therapy, 45*, 265-271. doi:10.5014/ajot.45.3.265

Appendix 1-A

SAMPLE FIELDWORK AND DOCTORAL CAPSTONE EXPERIENCE POLICY MANUAL TABLE OF CONTENTS

CONFLICT OF INTEREST
STUDENT HEALTH REPORTS/CLEARANCES
    CRIMINAL BACKGROUND CHECK
    FBI FINGERPRINTING
    DRUG TESTING
PROFESSIONAL BEHAVIOR EXPECTATIONS
    CELL PHONE AND ELECTRONIC DEVICE USE
    COMPUTER USE SOCIAL MEDIA & NETWORKING
    USE OF PHOTO OR VIDEO
    DRESS CODE
    TARDINESS/ABSENTEEISM
        HOLIDAYS
        INCLEMENT WEATHER
    CONFIDENTIALITY, PRIVACY & HIPAA
AFWC AND CAPSTONE COORDINATOR MONITORING & SITE VISITS
POST-GRADUATION INFORMATION
REQUESTING PROFESSIONAL REFERENCE
    FACULTY
    FIELDWORK EDUCATOR
    SITE MENTOR
GUIDELINES FOR NATIONAL AND STATE CREDENTIALING

Appendix 1-B

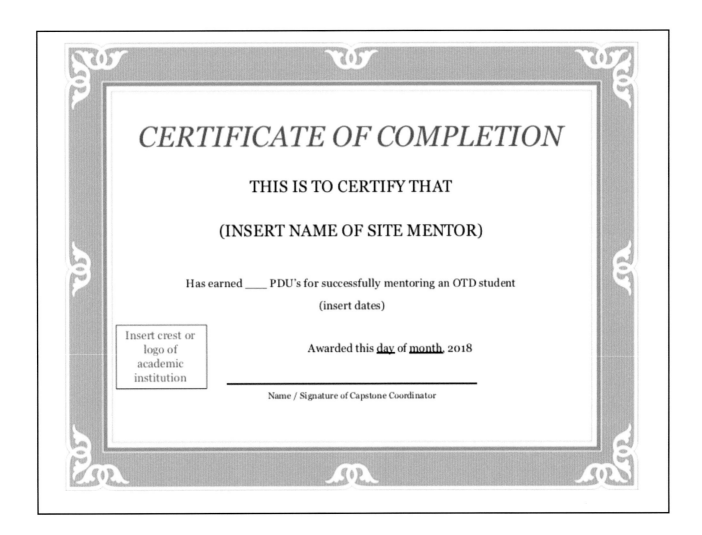

CERTIFICATE OF COMPLETION

THIS IS TO CERTIFY THAT

(INSERT NAME OF SITE MENTOR)

Has earned _____ PDU's for successfully mentoring an OTD student

(insert dates)

Insert crest or logo of academic institution

Awarded this day of month, 2018

_____

Name / Signature of Capstone Coordinator

Appendix 1-C

Appendix C Sample Template for Time Long

DCE Log of Hours

Overall total hours must equal 560 hours with at least 80% occurring on-site. Periodic site mentor signature required.

Week 1	On Site	Off Site	Accomplished
Sunday			
Monday			
Tuesday			
Wednesday			
Thursday			
Friday			
Saturday			
Total			
Site Mentor Signature			

Week 2	On Site	Off Site	Accomplished
Sunday			
Monday			
Tuesday			
Wednesday			
Thursday			
Friday			
Saturday			
Total			
Site Mentor Signature			

Week 3	On Site	Off Site	Accomplished
Sunday			
Monday			
Tuesday			
Wednesday			
Thursday			
Friday			
Saturday			
Total			
Site Mentor Signature			

Week 4	On Site	Off Site	Accomplished
Sunday			
Monday			
Tuesday			
Wednesday			
Thursday			
Friday			
Saturday			
Total			
Site Mentor Signature			

Week 9	On Site	Off Site	Accomplished
Sunday			
Monday			
Tuesday			
Wednesday			
Thursday			
Friday			
Saturday			
Total			
Site Mentor Signature			

Week 10	On Site	Off Site	Accomplished
Sunday			
Monday			
Tuesday			
Wednesday			
Thursday			
Friday			
Saturday			
Total			
Site Mentor Signature			

Week 11	On Site	Off Site	Accomplished
Sunday			
Monday			
Tuesday			
Wednesday			
Thursday			
Friday			
Saturday			
Total			
Site Mentor Signature			

Week 12	On Site	Off Site	Accomplished
Sunday			
Monday			
Tuesday			
Wednesday			
Thursday			
Friday			
Saturday			
Total			
Site Mentor Signature			

Week 5	On Site	Off Site	Accomplished
Sunday			
Monday			
Tuesday			
Wednesday			
Thursday			
Friday			
Saturday			
Total			
Site Mentor Signature			

Week 6	On Site	Off Site	Accomplished
Sunday			
Monday			
Tuesday			
Wednesday			
Thursday			
Friday			
Saturday			
Total			
Site Mentor Signature			

Week 7	On Site	Off Site	Accomplished
Sunday			
Monday			
Tuesday			
Wednesday			
Thursday			
Friday			
Saturday			
Total			
Site Mentor Signature			

Week 8	On Site	Off Site	Accomplished
Sunday			
Monday			
Tuesday			
Wednesday			
Thursday			
Friday			
Saturday			
Total			
Site Mentor Signature			

Week 13	On Site	Off Site	Accomplished
Sunday			
Monday			
Tuesday			
Wednesday			
Thursday			
Friday			
Saturday			
Total			
Site Mentor Signature			

Week 14	On Site	Off Site	Accomplished
Sunday			
Monday			
Tuesday			
Wednesday			
Thursday			
Friday			
Saturday			
Total			
Site Mentor Signature			

Overall Total	On Site	Off Site

CHAPTER 2

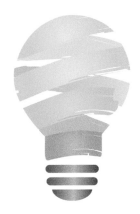

Understanding the ACOTE Areas of Focus for the Capstone

Elizabeth D. DeIuliis, OTD, MOT, OTR/L, CLA

Julie A. Bednarski, OTD, MHS, OTR

Human-Centered Design Mindsets for the Doctoral Students

Human-centered design mindset concepts of creative confidence, embracing ambiguity, and optimism are important for the doctoral student to adopt as they begin to explore and develop their capstone area of focus.

Creative Confidence: "Creative confidence is the belief that everyone is creative, and that creativity isn't the capacity to draw or compose or sculpt, but a way of understanding the world" (IDEO.org, 2015, p. 19). This is a time to learn, understand, and digest the areas of potential focus for your capstone and begin to think creatively about problems in these areas and problems you might want to solve.

Embrace Ambiguity: Remember ambiguity can lead to creativity. The process of the capstone experience and project is not linear. It is a fluid process and will continue to be so. Take the time to explore and embrace the ambiguity!

Optimism: This will continue to be an important mindset throughout your capstone experience and project. Your journey is in the initial stages; be patient, stay positive, and enjoy the learning!

INTRODUCTION

As the initial process of inspiration and development begins, it is important to understand the Accreditation Council for Occupational Therapy Education (ACOTE) areas of focus and how these areas will guide the development of the doctoral capstone experience (DCE) and project. ACOTE Standards continue to emphasize "consultation skills, care coordination, and advocacy roles" (Case-Smith, Page, Darragh, Rybski, & Cleary, 2014, p. e55) which directly correlate to the ACOTE areas of focus. This chapter defines and describes the ACOTE areas of focus for the DCE and assist the reader to brainstorm (become inspired) potential populations, potential settings or sites for the 14-week capstone experience and potential ideas for the type of capstone project.

DeIuliis ED, Bednarski JA.
The Entry Level Occupational Therapy Doctorate Capstone:
A Framework for The Experience and Project (pp 21-39).
© 2020 Taylor & Francis Group.

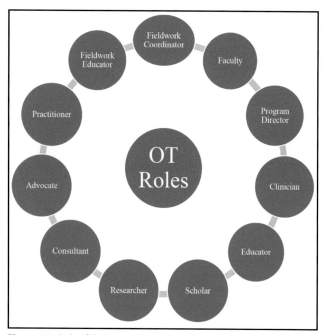

Figure 2-1. Role of the occupational therapist.

Capstone Student Reflective Questions

When developing the doctoral capstone, the occupational therapy student may find it helpful to reflect on the following questions:

1. What area of focus is most important to you as you think about your capstone?

2. What is your inspiration for your capstone?

3. How does your plan for your capstone compare or contrast with your planned or completed fieldwork experiences?

4. What type of sites are you interested in exploring that fit your planned focus area?

5. What type of individuals can you see yourself being mentored by, based on your planned focus area?

Chapter Objectives

By the end of reading this chapter and completing the learning activities, the reader should be able to:

1. Describe each of the ACOTE areas of focus.

2. Compare and contrast the areas of focus across different types of settings.

3. Formulate general ideas for a capstone project within each of the areas of focus.

ROLES AND FUNCTIONS OF AN OCCUPATIONAL THERAPY PRACTITIONER

The ACOTE focus areas for the capstone provide a framework to propel occupational therapy students to develop and synthesize in-depth knowledge. Depending on the focus area, this could (potentially) move the doctoral student beyond a generalist level in a concentrated area. In layperson terms, a generalist can be described as a "Jack-of-All-Trades, a Master of None." Occupational therapy generalists are expected to have comprehensive skills and knowledge from a set of core knowledge that is essential for all occupational therapy practitioners (established by ACOTE) and deliver care across a spectrum of ages, conditions, and practice settings. The role of an occupational therapy practitioner has long been referred to as multifaceted (see Figure 2-1) even at the generalist level and demands a vast set of responsibilities, functions and performance areas (American Occupational Therapy Association [AOTA], 1993). In contrast, specialists acquire a deeper understanding of specific areas of practice, a particular aspect of occupational therapy, or knowledge of particular impairments (Foto, 1996).

Reviewing these basic role descriptors in Table 2-1 can help a capstone student become further inspired as they begin to think about their capstone experience and potential individuals to serve as mentors.

The ACOTE Standards indicate that the capstone student must demonstrate and synthesize in-depth knowledge through an in-depth experience, where occupational therapy is currently practiced or settings where it is emerging. In-depth practice gives capstone students a greater opportunity to immerse themselves in evidence-based practice and include data collection for interventions (Case-Smith et al., 2014). The capstone must include one or more of the following focus areas: clinical practice skills, research skills, administration, leadership, program and policy development, advocacy, education, or theory development (ACOTE, 2018). Guided by these focus areas, the doctoral capstone will help occupational therapy students address the complexity of client diagnoses, requirements to collect and analyze clinical data, use evidence-based practice, emphasize health promotion programs, and strengthen interprofessional relationships (Case-Smith et al., 2014). The capstone requires students to seek in-depth competencies in practice and service delivery models and helps future occupational therapy practitioners to assume advanced roles in practice settings, such as a direct care provider, consultant, educator, manager, leader, researcher, and advocate. Although the glossary in the ACOTE Standards does not specifically define the connotation of in-depth, *Merriam-Webster's Dictionary* defines *in-depth* as being a stage or condition beyond introductory; being exposed to detailed and extensive; comprehensive and thorough (https://www.merriam-webster.com/dictionary/in-depth).

Table 2-1. Occupational Therapist Roles and Functions

OCCUPATIONAL THERAPIST ROLE	MAJOR FUNCTION
Practitioner	Provide assessment, intervention, and program planning and implement discharge planning
Educator	Develop and provide educational offerings and trainings
Fieldwork Educator	Manage Level I or Level II fieldwork in practice setting while providing opportunities for students to fulfill practitioner competencies
Supervisor	Manage overall daily operations of occupational therapy services
Administrator	Manage department, program, services, or agency providing occupational therapy services
Researcher/Scholar	Examine, develop, refine, and evaluate the profession's body of knowledge and theoretical and philosophical foundations

Adapted from American Occupational Therapy Association. (1993). Occupational therapy roles. *American Journal of Occupational Therapy, 47,* 1087-1099. doi:10.5014/ajot.47.12.1087.

To further understand experience and competence continuums, it can be helpful to look towards the Dreyfus and Dreyfus Skill Acquisition Model (Dreyfus & Dreyfus, 1980) and the Benner Stages of Clinical Competence (Benner, 1984). Dreyfus and Dreyfus (1980) developed a framework of skill acquisition that provides developmental stages of competency for the mental processing, logic, and principles that guide reasoning as one advances through the various stages of skill attainment. Dreyfus and Dreyfus propose four stages: (a) novice, (b) competence, (c) proficiency, and (d) expertise (Table 2-2).

Patricia Benner, a nursing-scholar and theorist, reworked the model created by Dreyfus and Dreyfus (1980) and presented the novice to expert continuum to describe the process through which nurses develop skills and understanding, as well as experience, over time. Benner's (1984) model, which appeared in *From Novice to Expert: Promoting Excellence and Power in Clinical Nursing Practice* also frames skill acquisition as moving through various stages, yet in a more suggestive manner. The five stages are (1) novice, (2) advanced beginner, (3) competency, (4) proficiency, and (5) expert (Table 2-3).

A commonality of these frameworks is that feedback and self-monitoring decrease over time and with experience. An individual develops competency, proficiency, and expertise by knowing "how," not knowing "what." This provides a useful lens to view the progression of the capstone student.

Occupational therapy educators can use these research-based frameworks in the preparation of capstone students. According to Benner (1984), an expert has a deep connection and understanding of the situation. Although the language used by ACOTE to describe the capstone does not include expert, experience (in conjunction with reflection) is depicted as having a significant impact on the development of professional growth and innovative change and is a prerequisite for expertise. The combination of higher level learning didactic requirements and in-depth practice and experience (such as the 14-week capstone) can allow the capstone student to move along the continuum of skill development and help better discern the capstone student moving beyond the generalist and developing increased professional maturity in a chosen focus area.

We can look to other clinical doctorate degrees for guidance in how they describe practice beyond a generalist or introductory stage. For example, the International Council of Nursing defines advanced practice as the demonstration of skills that reflect an expert knowledge base, complex decision-making skills and clinical competencies for expanded practice, the characteristics of which are shaped by the context in which services are being provided (ICN Nurse Practitioner/Advanced Practice Nursing Network, 2018). Physical therapy organizations in the United Kingdom use the term *advanced practice physiotherapy* (APP) to describe a clinician with advanced skills, knowledge, and attitudes together with the core set of physiotherapy skills and knowledge, tailored to individual patients and local environments (Chartered Society of Physiotherapy, 2018). Although a different degree level, the American Physical Therapy Association (2017) has an Advanced Proficiency Pathway for physical therapist assistants, which is curricula that include a group of didactic courses and mentored clinical experiences. Pharmacy educational programs are also adopting similar language, such as the advanced practice pharmacist. For example, the University of Southern California's School of Pharmacy offers an advanced practice pharmacy curriculum, which requires a residency-training program and at least 1,500 hours of direct patient care services. These examples support the combination of didactic and mentored-experiential learning.

Table 2-2. Dreyfus and Dreyfus Skill Levels

STAGE	DEFINITION	APPLICATION TO THE PROGRESSION OF THE CAPSTONE
Novice	In this stage, a person follows rules that are context-free and feels no responsibility for anything other than following the rules.	Rules determine action. The novice considers every idea as possibility.
Competence	This stage develops after an individual has considerable experience. The individual can troubleshoot.	Guidelines determine action.
Proficiency	This stage is shown in individuals who use intuition in decision-making and develop their own rules to formulate plans.	Individuals anticipate deviations from their plan. Individuals are able to self-correct.
Expertise	This stage is characterized by a fluid performance that happens unconsciously and automatically and no longer depends on explicit knowledge.	Individuals with expertise respond to situations by intuition. At this stage, individuals establish a relevant focus.

Adapted from Deluliis, E.D. (2017). *Professionalism across Occupational Therapy Clinical Practice.* Thorofare, NJ: SLACK Incorporated and Dreyfus, H., & Dreyfus, S. (1980). *A five-stage model of mental activities involved in directed skill acquisition.* Berkeley, CA: Operations Research Center, University of California, Berkeley.

Table 2-3. Benner's Model of Skill Development

STAGE	DESCRIPTION	APPLICATION TO THE CAPSTONE
Novice	Beginner with no experience, taught general rules to help perform tasks, e.g., "Tell me what to do, and I'll do it"; learners focus on learning the rules of a particular skill.	Needs constant guidance. Seeks affirmation regularly.
Advanced Beginner	Demonstrates acceptable performance, has gained prior experience in actual situations to recognize recurring components, principles are based more on experience. Learners focus on applying the rules of a skill in specific situations that become increasingly dependent on the particular context of the situation.	Begins to apply knowledge and skills.
Competence	More aware of long-term goals, gains perspective from planning own actions based on conscious, abstract, and analytical thinking and helps to achieve greater efficiency and organization. Learners see actions in terms of long-range goals or plans.	Consciously aware of their skills.
Proficiency	More holistic understanding, improved decision-making. Learns from experiences what to expect in certain situations and how to modify plans.	Perceives situations as "wholes" rather than "aspects," and performance is guided by intuitive behavior.
Expert	No longer relies on principles, rules, or guidance to connect situations and determine actions. Has an intuitive grasp of situations. Learners integrate mastered skills with their own personal styles (Driscoll, 2002; Leach, 2002).	Performance is now fluid, flexible and highly proficient (within their focus area).

Adapted from Benner, P. (1984). *From novice to expert: Excellence and power in clinical nursing practice.* Menlo Park, CA: Addison-Wesley and Deluliis, E.D. (2017). *Professionalism across Occupational Therapy Clinical Practice.* Thorofare, NJ: SLACK Incorporated.

Common themes among the description of clinical or professional doctorates and advanced practice include the following:

- Expertise based on significant experience and training
- Focus on interpersonal competence
- Formal education beyond entry level
- Involvement in leadership, research, teaching, and mentoring
- Activities performed may be outside of the traditional scope of practice

Research has demonstrated that it takes time to gain expertise. The capstone is not designed to develop practitioners with expert-level skills, but instead to develop an in-depth knowledge and skill set in a focused area that is developed under mentorship over 14 weeks. The ACOTE focus areas provide opportunities for occupational therapy students to learn outside of the traditional scope of practice and develop an in-depth skill(s) and knowledge in the focused area of study.

FRAMING THE ACOTE FOCUS AREAS

With mentorship from their faculty and doctoral capstone coordinator, capstone students need to have a clear understanding of what the focus areas are and how they complement their previous fieldwork experiences and professional development plan. The DCE and project should be directly aligned with one or a combination of focus areas. Although this list is not exhaustive, this chapter illustrates examples and strategies of how to help capstone students and potential site mentors increase their understanding of the focus areas. Although ACOTE indicates that the capstone should be designed and administered by faculty and provided in setting(s) consistent with the program's curriculum design, the capstone should be a mutual benefit for the student and the site.

Evolving Compliance for Accreditation of Health Care Institutions

One vantage point within the brainstorming process can be to increase one's awareness of the needs, expectations and requirements of potential sites. Changes to health care service delivery models, reimbursement systems, and compliance agencies are challenging community and clinical sites to measure outcomes and improve quality. The Joint Commission (TJC) and the Commission on Accreditation of Rehabilitation Facilities (CARF) are just two examples of regulatory bodies that require their certificants to collect and analyze data on specific performance measures and operationalize clinical practice guidelines to ensure evidence-based and quality care.

TJC (2018a; 2018b) accredits and certifies nearly 21,000 health care organizations and programs in the United States. Accreditation and certification is recognized nationwide as a symbol of quality that reflects an organization's commitment to meeting certain performance standards. Accreditation can be earned by an entire health care organization (e.g., hospitals, nursing homes, ambulatory care centers, office-based surgery practices, home care providers, and laboratories). Certification is earned by programs or services that may be based within or associated with a health care organization (TJC, 2018b). For example, a TJC-accredited medical center can have TJC-certified programs or services for diabetes or heart disease care. These programs could be within the medical center or in the community.

Similar to ACOTE, which has educational standards, TJC has "National Patient Safety Goals," which are specific areas that accredited facilities need to address in regard to patient safety (TJC, 2018a). For hospital facilities, these include things such as correctly identifying patients, using medicine correctly, using alarms safely, preventing infection, identifying patient safety risks (such as falls or suicide risk), and preventing mistakes in surgery (TJC, 2018a). Various work units within the facility are responsible for creating a process, tracking data, and analyzing outcomes to improve patient safety. In regard to reduction of falls, a capstone student could be involved in various aspects of this quality initiative, such as creating staff education on best practices in fall prevention, reviewing retrospective data to look for trends among falls, and designing and measuring the impact of activities or interventions to reduce the rate of falls. For instance, outcome measures such as the Berg Balance Scale (Berg, Wood-Dauphinne, Williams, & Gayton, 1989), Functional Reach Test (Duncan, Weiner, Chandler, & Studenski, 1990), Physical Performance Test (Delbaere et al., 2006), and Timed Up and Go (Podsiadlo & Richardson, 1991) can be used to measure fall risk. When fall risk is high, occupation-based intervention activities to address aspects of dynamic balance can be developed, and these tools can then be used to show improvement during the clients stay and a reduction in the overall fall rate.

For TJC, reporting requirements include nonstandardized measures (Stage I) and standardized measures (Stage II). These performance measurements require collection of monthly data points as an indication of the organization's performance in relation to a specific process or outcome. Table 2-4 provides an overview of the types of performance measures.

CARF is an independent, international, nonprofit accreditor of health and human services in the following areas: aging services, behavioral health, child and youth services, employment and community services, vision rehabilitation, medical rehabilitation, among others. CARF accredits more than 50,000 programs and services at 25,000 locations. It is a voluntary accreditation that demonstrates accountability to funding sources and referral agencies (CARF, 2018). The criteria foci for CARF accreditation are similar to TJC, and include the following:

- Reducing risk
- Addressing health and safety concerns

Table 2-4. Overview of Performance Measures

CATEGORY	EVALUATE PROCESSES OR OUTCOMES OF CARE	CAPSTONE PROJECT EXAMPLE
Administrative/financial	Address organizational structure for coordinating and integrating services, functions, and activities	Develop and evaluate facility workflow using a contingency diagram to determine worker efficiency and productivity
Perception of care/service	Patient/customer satisfaction	Create, implement, and evaluate a model for concierge care to proactively address client concerns
Participants' health status	Examples: falls, vent-associated pneumonias, urinary tract infection rate, central-line infections, restraint use, and medication errors	Create and implement staff training modules based on current evidence regarding fall prevention

- Respecting cultural and individual preferences
- Providing the best possible quality of care

Like TJC, CARF is committed to improving service outcomes, satisfaction of the individuals served, and quality of the services delivered.

TEXT BOX 2-1

Receiving fewer deficiency citations is directly linked to better perception of patient and resident safety culture (Wagner, McDonald, & Castle, 2012).

Specific aspects that CARF certification require facilities to demonstrate compliance with accreditation requirements, including but not limited to competency of personnel, that services delivered are person-centered and individualized, and that service delivery and communication are based on acceptable field practice. A capstone student could create competencies or staff training to ensure that employees in a CARF-accredited setting have the knowledge and skills to work with patients of a specific age-group (e.g., neonatal intensive care unit [NICU]), specific skills involved in using specific equipment in performance of job duties (e.g., the use of the ArmeoSpring technology in an inpatient rehabilitation unit) or competencies related to specific skill or procedure (e.g., manual lymph drainage and complete decongestive therapy for lymphedema management).

Learning and understanding these two international health care compliance organizations is just one perspective of how the doctoral capstone coordinator and student can think about existing mechanisms in traditional health care settings that require data collection, outcome measurement, and quality improvement.

TEXT BOX 2-2

Other compliance organizations that may be relevant to explore the integration of a capstone may include
- Department of Health
- Department of Education
- Occupational Safety and Health Administration

A capstone student has a skill set to support these data collection and interpretation initiatives. ACOTE (2018) requires entry level occupational therapy doctoral students to learn how to collect, analyze, and report data in a systematic manner for evaluation of client and practice outcomes. Because the outcome and expectations of the capstone differ from fieldwork (as discussed in Chapter 1), it is important for the doctoral capstone coordinator and the capstone student to educate the site mentor.

Evolving Dynamic of Our Consumers

Another critical vantage point to consider when planning and developing the capstone is the dynamic of our consumers, whether at the level of an individual client, groups, communities, or populations (AOTA, 2014). At the individual client level, current health care consumers are more sophisticated, educated, technologically savvy, and socially connected (Bachman, n.d.). Some literature labels these individuals as empowered health care consumers rather than patients, placing government agencies, insurance companies, employers, and private companies under greater scrutiny to collect, analyze, and publish data about their facility (McNamara, 2012) and to develop care models that personalize service. Readily available data on patient engagement, care outcomes, and quality measurement are in the hands of consumers, which challenge health systems to be at the top of their game with high-quality outcomes and strong patient satisfaction. Contemporary examples of consumer-driven health care are depicted using a concierge model, which provides a higher level of personal interaction to the patient. Measures of patient satisfaction (such as the Press Ganey Satisfaction Survey) and other patient-oriented report cards will assume increasing importance in the industry.

TEXT BOX 2-3

Press Ganey is a leading provider of patient experience measurement for health care organizations across the continuum of care (Press Ganey, 2018). The survey aims to address controllable factors that contribute to the patient experience. This could include:
- Friendliness/courtesy of the care provider
- Degree to which the care provider talked with the patient using words that the patient could understand
- Patient's confidence in the care provider (Press Ganey, 2018).

Occupational therapy doctoral students could work directly with a site to develop their capstone project and improve the patient experience, based on outcomes of a satisfaction survey such as Press Ganey (2018). For example, after interpreting feedback received from a Press-Ganey Survey, a site may desire to improve its process in integrating the client and family into a care plan. Capstone students could immerse themselves in the literature surrounding improving the patient experience, interview various health care providers, clients, and family members, then develop, pilot, and measure the impact of a new procedure to increase client and family involvement in care planning.

Health Care Industry Adopting Person-Centered and Team-Based Culture

Although certainly not new to the occupational therapy profession, we are in an era of health systems adopting patient-centeredness, which provides a clear opportunity for occupational therapy practitioners, who have long proclaimed a commitment to embracing a person-centered approach (Law, Baptiste, & Mills, 1995; Tickle-Degnen, 2002). Primary care has become a buzzword among the health care industry, legislation and policy, and service delivery models. An important aspect of primary care is the integration (and collaboration) of the health care team and a consumer-centered model. Team-based care is defined by the National Academy of Medicine (formerly known as the Institute of Medicine) as:

the provision of health services to individuals, families, and/or their communities by at least two health providers who work collaboratively with patients and their caregivers—to the extent preferred by each patient—to accomplish shared goals within and across settings to achieve coordinated, high-quality care. (Babiker et al., 2014, p. 9)

Interprofessional education, interprofessional collaboration, and interprofessional practice are now well-known terms used in health science education to better prepare allied health care students for the evolving demands of the industry.

Across the globe, health care systems are adopting a person-centered culture and putting importance in the delivery of care that is whole-person oriented, coordinated, and personal (Saha, Beach, & Cooper, 2008). A specific aspect of the Patient Protection and Affordable Care Act of 2010, the patient-centered medical home, is just one approach designed to facilitate higher quality care because it is more integrated and personalized. This shift in culture provides unique and novel opportunities for the discipline of occupational therapy (Dahl-Popolizio & Rogers, 2017), which is rooted in holism, person-centeredness, and inclusion. On behalf of the AOTA, Roberts, Farmer, Lam, Muir, and Siebert (2014) outlined the unique role that the occupational therapy profession plays in primary care. Metzler, Hartmann, and Lowenthal (2012) also discuss implications for the profession in primary care and identified that "developing sustained relationships" is an important aspect of person-centered care that occupational therapy should fully adopt and use. These papers can provide inspiration for both the coordinator and student on ideas for the DCE and project.

An important element of the capstone is that it is a clear win-win situation—both for the capstone student's learning and the growth and sustainability of the capstone site. Increasing quality measures and available evidence will demonstrate a capstone site's commitment to high standards of practice and provide a more competitive edge in the current health care arena. It is beneficial for the capstone student and doctoral capstone coordinator to be aware of setting or site compliance initiatives and strategic goals during the developing process of the capstone. Appendix 2-A provides a framework of how to brainstorm capstone fit and focus area alignment with sites. More on this is discussed in Chapters 4 and 6. Our professional organization, AOTA, also provides some guidance to help understand the rationale of the focus areas.

Vision 2025

A vision statement is a public way in which an organization indicates who or what they want to become. It indicates transformation, direction, and growth. Vision 2025 is the transformational roadmap for the future of the AOTA

As an inclusive profession, occupational therapy maximizes health, well-being, and quality of life for all people, populations, and communities through effective solutions that facilitate participation in everyday living. (AOTA, 2018)

The AOTA further narrows the scope of the organization's future vision by articulating five pillars. Vision 2025 and these five pillars (see Table 2-5) can be used to help explain and understand the value, purpose and rationale for the purpose of the capstone and more specifically the focus areas.

Table 2-5. The Five Pillars

PILLAR	DESCRIPTORS/RATIONALE
Effective	• Evidenced-based • Client-centered • Profitable or cost-effective • Capstone focus area example: research, clinical practice, administration
Leaders	• Influential • Change agent • Catalysts • Capstone focus area example: leadership, advocacy
Collaborative	• Teamwork • Systems approach • Outcome-oriented • Capstone focus area example: administration, program development
Accessible	• Responsive • Customized • Capstone focus area example: program development, advocacy, policy
Equity, Inclusion, and Diversity	• Inclusive • Equitable • Capstone focus area example: advocacy, policy, education

Advocating and articulating the distinct value of occupational therapy has been a prominent message from the AOTA. Through the implementation of a well-designed and mentored capstone, occupational therapy students can create and deliver compelling, targeted messages to various audiences including clients, other health care professionals, third-party payers, and policy makers about the distinct value of occupational therapy to help make Vision 2025 a reality and not just a company tagline.

As part of the capstone development process, the doctoral capstone coordinator and faculty need to empower the capstone student (who is also the next generation of practitioners) to see themselves as leaders and agents of change. The capstone experience provides additional learning opportunities to nurture leadership, communication, and systems skills, which society and our consumers are demanding. Now that we have discussed overarching influences on the ACOTE focus areas, and systems and organizations that could be used as inspirational guides for the development of the capstone, let's review the ACOTE focus areas, and recommendations for potential sites, and projects and within each area.

CLINICAL PRACTICE SKILLS

Description

A DCE that involves identification of a site or setting where more advanced (or a narrower focus of) occupational therapy interventions are utilized. Capstone students who choose clinical practice as a focus area could also satisfy components of their experience by pursuing and completing continuing education courses, advanced trainings, certificates, and so on. For example, capstone students interested in advancing their knowledge and skill set (beyond the generalist level) on sensory integration as a clinical practice focus area could pursue getting formally trained to administer the Sensory Integration and Praxis Test (SIPT) as a portion of their capstone experience. In contrast, capstone students who want to become competent in lymphedema management to deepen their knowledge may enroll in formal training courses (such as the Norton School or Academy of Lymphatic Studies) to develop an in-depth skill area in managing this chronic state of edema as a component of their capstone experience.

Types of Sites and Settings

A starting inspiration point to brainstorm DCE sites within this focus area could be to review the six AOTA Practice Areas: children and youth; health and wellness; mental health; productive aging; rehabilitation, disability, and participation; and work and industry (AOTA, 2018). Based on the type of specialty practice or the site chosen, examples could include an in-depth hand therapy clinic, specialty practice areas such as a low-vision center, a NICU, community-based programs including drivers rehabilitation or hippotherapy, work rehabilitation, or sites that offer a specialty services or programs in areas such as dysphagia or incontinence.

TEACHING TIP 1: Doctoral capstone coordinators: As discussed in Chapter 1, it is essential to collaborate with the academic fieldwork coordinator during the development and planning phase. During their preparation for Level II fieldwork, students often have specific ideas or interests that they originally intend to pursue for fieldwork yet do not provide them the generalist training that that is required. Settings or sites that offer very narrow, more specialized training most likely are not appropriate for Level II fieldwork, yet offer a great potential capstone experience (more on this collaboration is discussed in Chapter 6).

Examples of Capstone Projects

The capstone project can take many forms depending on the clinical practice area. Examples include the following:

- A case study
- A scoping literature review of an emerging practice focus
- A critically appraised topic
- A meta-analysis of evidence regarding a specific intervention or approach
- Creation (or refining) of a practice guideline, pathway, clinical protocol or best evidence statement (Case-Smith et al., 2014).

For example, a capstone student could develop and implement an evidenced-based bowel-bladder management protocol for individuals with neurodegenerative disorders, refine the critical pathway used in a NICU that triggers a lactation consultant for premature babies, or develop and implement an evidenced-based clinical practice care guideline to assist in assessing driver readiness amongst novice drivers with an autism spectrum disorder (ASD). Each of these examples provide the opportunity for the capstone student to be mentored by an individual inside or outside the field of occupational therapy. Further, using the previous example regarding a focus on developing in-depth skills in sensory

integration, and getting SIPT trained, the capstone project could involve helping a pediatric site develop an intense multi-sensory (IMS) stimulation program or a formalized non-invasive stimulation program. Other innovative ideas for a capstone project designed to advance in-depth clinical skills are depicted in Table 2-6.

TEACHING TIP 2: If the capstone experience requires any direct-care or service delivery, it is important for the doctoral capstone coordinator to vet supervision requirements per the site and/or state regulatory board and communicate proactively with the capstone student and site mentor.

RESEARCH

Description

A capstone focus area in research is an experience that involves participating, collaborating and learning from recognized individuals who are actively engaged in projects that include research design and planning, data collection, analyzing and affecting evidence-based practice, and disseminating results. Although the B standards in ACOTE do stipulate required learning objectives in this realm, a capstone experience would involve an in-depth exposure to the researcher role.

TEACHING TIP 3: Many occupational therapy programs already have a model in their curriculum that includes faculty-student research opportunities in which students have the opportunity to serve as an apprentice to a faculty member. A capstone focus in research could involve a continuation of this project yet with greater responsibilities and expectations for the student.

The researcher role responsibilities consist of examining, developing, refining, and evaluating the profession's body of knowledge along with theoretical and philosophical foundations (AOTA, 1993).

Types of Sites and Settings

A focus area in research could take place anywhere: in the clinic, in the community, or within academia.

Examples of Capstone Projects

A capstone project with a focus area of research can take many forms. Examples include the following:

- An outcome study (e.g., determining the outcome of smartphone training and use as an intervention and

Table 2-6. Examples of Practice Areas

AOTA PRACTICE AREA	DCE AND CAPSTONE PROJECT EXAMPLES
Children and Youth	Exploring the impact of hippotherapy on children with ASDs
Health and Wellness	Understanding the benefits of a kangaroo-care protocol in the NICU
Mental Health	Develop competency with a modality such as AlphaStim (a cranial electrotherapy stimulation device) to address posttraumatic stress disorder among veterans (Alpha-Stim, 2018)
Productive Aging	Understanding how sensory stimulation programs can be used with elderly adults with dementia
Rehabilitation, Disability, and Participation	Create a practice guideline to address sexuality with individuals who have a spinal cord injury
Work and Industry	Create a clinical pathway rooted in the biopsychosocial model to address chronic pain among individuals who have sustained a work-related injury

cognitive aide for individuals with mild traumatic brain injury).

- A systematic review of evidence related to an occupational therapy program or intervention of interest (e.g. systematic review of literature pertaining to a sensory integration intervention for children with ASD).
- Retrospective research study, such as looking at how many children with intensive feeding issues had NICU stays as infants. What can be done to improve current treatment in an outpatient setting with these children?

ADMINISTRATION

Description

A capstone student who chooses an administration focus area is responsible for developing in-depth knowledge and skills in systems of practice, administrative, or management function in traditional or role-emerging sites.

TEXT BOX 2-4

Aspects of an administration focus area may include a deeper understanding of systems theory to develop system-thinking skills such as a focus on interactions, relationships and adaptation (Mele, Pels, & Polese, 2010). The importance of occupational therapy educators to use systems theory as a structure or framework for learning was noted by occupational therapy pioneer and scholar Mary Reilly (Schemm, Corcoran, Kolodner, & Schaaf, 1993).

Types of Sites and Settings

Examples can include working with distinguished, expert administrators, entrepreneurs, managers and supervisors who may or may not be an occupational therapy practitioner. Settings could include private practices, managed care organizations, health systems, and community sites.

Examples of Capstone Projects

An administrative capstone project requires active skill building and collaboration in administration, management, and supervision, outside of the generalist expectations that be found in ACOTE Standard B. 5.3. Examples could include the following:

- Conduct a financial analysis to compare care models and potential cost savings or return on investment (ROI).
- Develop and/or evaluate care models or service delivery models (e.g., implement and evaluate the effectiveness of an evidence-based teamwork program such as TeamSTEPPS 2.0 [Agency for Healthcare Research and Quality, 2018]).
- Complete a workflow analysis on the use of transport in a health care facility and evaluate the impact on employee productivity.
- Write a strategic business plan to initiate a new program or entrepreneur effort.
- Write a grant proposal to secure funding for an occupational therapist 8 hours per week at an adult day center to provide consultative services.
- Develop a system based on evidence for a program evaluation process for merit and promotion of employees.
- Revamp the administrative onboarding process for occupational therapy fieldwork students at a clinical site.
- Create a system-wide approach for the adoption and integration of an electronic medical record.
- Create an evidence-based proposal to increase the retention of occupational therapy personnel.

- Evaluate and refine processes and systems to measure client satisfaction.
- Measuring the impact of "xyz" variables on reducing readmission rates.

TEXT BOX 2-5

A study published in *Medical Care Research and Review* found that "occupational therapy is the only spending category where additional hospital spending has a statistically significant association with lower readmission rates" for the three health conditions studied: heart failure, pneumonia, and acute myocardial infarction (Rogers, Bai, Lavin, & Anderson, 2016, p. 668).

How can this monumental research study provide inspiration for the capstone to demonstrate the distinct value of occupation from an administrative lens (e.g., reduce costs, lower readmission rates, improve client outcomes, and increase consumer satisfaction)?

LEADERSHIP

Description

A capstone focus area of leadership can involve working and collaborating with recognized individuals who are involved in exercising influence and representing different areas of the profession regionally, nationally, and internationally. This may involve capstone students to step out of their "comfort zone" to engage in effective and meaningful collaboration with clients, other professionals and key stakeholders; and not only to adapt and adjust to changing systems and practices but to become transformational in their leadership outcomes. Individualized learning objectives within this focus area may include exploration of personal styles of leadership, reexamination of leadership theories, and thorough assessment and critique of a leadership project.

TEXT BOX 2-6

Examples of leadership theories that may be beneficial for a capstone student to engage in a self-study to support in-depth learning and exposure to this focus area could include completion of the Six Sigma Leadership certifications (Atmaca & Girenes, 2011).

Types of Sites and Settings

Examples include a mentored experience at the World Health Organization, National Institutes of Health, other national volunteer organizations such as the AOTA, the National Board Certification for Occupational Therapy, state organizations, and other not-for-profit organizations.

TEXT BOX 2-7

Occupational Therapy Leaders and Legacies Society is a member organization that is made up of a community of occupational therapy leaders who have demonstrated expertise in leadership abilities and skills. Members of the society design and lead projects that honor occupational therapy history and social contributions as well as recognize and engage those individuals whose contributions have sustained and enriched the profession (Kolodner, 2018).

Doctoral capstone coordinators and doctoral students can explore existing leadership projects and/or promote the idea of a leadership project with Occupational Therapy Leaders and Legacies Society to support a focus area in leadership for the capstone.

Examples of Capstone Projects

The capstone project with a leadership focus area can take many forms. Examples include the following:

- Create and implement a leadership development project, such as leadership training, with your state occupational therapy association or licensure board related to occupational therapy practice and policy.
- Create and implement a leadership project within a Student Occupational Therapy Association.
- Create and implement a leadership initiative within your state organization to increase membership.
- Create and implement staff instruction and training to create a culture of safety through education by teaching other disciplines about patient handling (Copolillo, Shepherd, Anzalone, & Lane, 2010).

PROGRAM DEVELOPMENT

Description

Program development refers to the systematic process of identifying the needs of a group of individuals, community, or organization and designing evidence-based programs to meet the needs that have been identified (Centers for Disease Control and Prevention, 2013). A capstone with this focus would include approaches, principles, and methods for developing and evaluating occupation-based programs and interventions for individuals and groups. An essential component of this process is to evaluate the effectiveness and outcomes of the program once it has been implemented. This type of capstone project may address needs assessment, program planning, proposal writing, and measurement of program outcomes. Program development could take place in clinical and/or community (role-emerging) settings. Furthermore, as health care policy is continually evolving, greater emphasis is being placed on chronic disease management, care coordination, wellness, and prevention, which provide opportunities for program development for the capstone student. Although the focus areas stipulated by ACOTE do not specifically distinguish program development into clinical and community settings, recommendations for both are provided separately in these next sections.

CLINICAL PROGRAM DEVELOPMENT

Developing and testing outcomes of occupational therapy programs in clinical settings. This could include inpatient or outpatient rehabilitation, medical, or mental health facilities.

Types of Sites and Settings

Examples include hand therapy, geriatrics, pediatrics, mental health, rehabilitation, and school-based occupational therapy among others.

Examples of Capstone Projects

The capstone project with a program development focus can take many forms. A few examples include the following:

- Development of and implementation of a sensory diet for children with ASD in a school setting
- Creation of a cognitive rehabilitation program for adults with chemotherapy cognitive-induced impairment in an acute care hospital
- Development of an aquatic therapy program for children who have ASD
- Creation of a Snoezelen room or space in a dementia-care unit (Berkheimer, Qian, & Malmstrom, 2017)
- Development of a therapeutic garden to increase participation on an inpatient rehabilitation unit
- Creation of a reverse activities of daily living program on an inpatient rehabilitation unit to address sleep routine and sleep hygiene

COMMUNITY PROGRAM DEVELOPMENT

Program development focus areas could also occur in the community at role-emerging sites. Capstone students who choose this focus area can be responsible for developing a program or product idea and operationalize it based on specific need in the community, site, or population. Depending on the needs, this may also entail seeking grant funding or completing a program evaluation.

Types of Sites and Settings

Examples of sites can include homeless shelters, programs for at-risk youth, long-term structured residence (LTSR), veterans programs, inner-city outreach programs, criminal justice settings, foster care, adult day care facilities, or psychosocial clubhouse, to name a few possibilities.

Examples of Capstone Projects

The capstone project with a focus on program development can also include the following examples of capstone projects:

- Development of and implementation of a community wellness program for individuals who have a history of polysubstance use in a halfway house
- Development of and implementation of a sleep hygiene program in a day program for veterans with posttraumatic stress disorder
- Creation of sensory-friendly programs at a museum (Fletcher, Blake, & Shelffo, 2018) or other public spaces, such as a zoo
- Implementation of an evidence-based program for self-management of chronic disease (e.g., diabetes mellitus) in a primary care setting
- Development of and implementation of a medication management program for individuals with intellectual disabilities in an adult day program

*Although not an explicit ACOTE focus area, program development capstones can also be rooted in quality improvement-like projects.

TEXT BOX 2-8

Quality improvement includes the design and implementation of systematic, data-driven activities that are intended to bring about immediate improvements in the delivery and outcomes of services in a clinical/community setting. A capstone project can be rooted in quality improvement aimed to develop, improve, pilot, or evaluate the effectiveness of a new tool, program, or workflow at a clinical or community site.

POLICY DEVELOPMENT

Description

A policy development focus area for a capstone could include working and collaborating with recognized individuals who are engaged at federal or state legislative levels to develop and implement innovative programs or to create evidence-based health and social policy.

A capstone student can seek to further explore the distinct value of occupational therapy and health care reform. Lamb and Metzler (2014) provide a useful framework to inspire capstone projects that may align with initiatives from Center for Medicare and Medicaid or Primary Care. *Primary care* is defined as care provided by physicians trained for comprehensive first contact that is the patient's first entry into the health care system. Primary care is performed by a physician who often collaborates with other health care professionals to provide sufficient patient advocacy (American Academy of Family Physicians, 2016).

Types of Sites and Settings

Examples include primary care settings, state or local legislative office, state associations, state or national political action committees (e.g., AOTPAC).

AOTPAC is a voluntary, nonprofit, nonpartisan, unincorporated committee of members of AOTA. The purpose of AOTPAC is to further the legislative aims of the Association by influencing or attempting to influence the selection, nomination, election, or appointment of any individual to any Federal public office, and of any occupational therapist, occupational therapy assistant, or occupational therapy student member of AOTA seeking election to public office at any level.

Examples of Capstone Projects

The capstone project with a focus on policy can take many forms. Examples include, but are not limited to, the following:

- Analyze a local, state, or national health care policy and propose a change in the policy and implementation of the policy.
- Work with a legislator to propose policy changes related to access to and reimbursement for occupational therapy.
- Create and implement a professional development plan indicating that you will run for an elected position related to advocacy and legislation.
- Seek out and engage in lobbying efforts with national interest groups such as the Disability and Rehabilitation Research Coalition (DRRC) as it urges Congress to fully support disability, independent living, and rehabilitation research through a variety of federal agencies.
- Build and participate in a campaign with an elected official that aligns with important issues that matter to the occupational therapy profession.

ADVOCACY

Description

A focus area in advocacy could include working and collaborating with recognized individuals that are engaged at the federal and state legislative levels regarding issues that affect our practice (such as reimbursement and scope of practice guidelines).

Types of Sites and Settings

Examples can include community organizations, state and national organizations, and offices of legislators.

Examples of Capstone Projects

The capstone project with a focus on advocacy can take many forms. Some examples include the following:

- Develop and test a program that improves consumers' abilities to navigate health systems to improve access to, delivery of, or outcomes of health care.
- Create a referral pathway for occupational therapy in primary care.
- Create and implement an advocacy project to help promote CarFit with local offices such as the American Automobile Association (AAA) and the American Association for Retired Persons (AARP) (2018).
- Plan and implement an advocacy project such as AOTA's Capitol Hill Day.
- Create and implement a community occupational therapy advocacy project such as backpack awareness in a public school district or fall prevention initiative in a retirement community.
- Complete an in-depth analysis and policy statement regarding a particular practice issue.
- Work with an advocacy special interest group within a state organization to lobby for critical scope of practice issues such as encroachment.

For example, in the State of Pennsylvania there has been recent, ongoing advocacy initiated by the Board of Directors of the Pennsylvania Occupational Therapy Association and the Pennsylvania Occupational Therapy Political Action Committee (PAC) as the discipline of recreational therapy has ought Pennsylvania state licensure. Language in the proposed scope of practice from recreational therapy directly encroaches on the existing Pennsylvania Practice Act of Occupational Therapy. A capstone student could be mentored by an individual on the PAC or the state licensing board to build an awareness campaign and launch a statewide initiative.

EDUCATION

Description

A focus area in education would explore the role of the occupational therapist as educator, which could include various communities of learners such as clients, staff, and students in community, clinical and classroom settings. Understanding adult learning theory, comparing and contrasting pedagogy and andragogy, creating a teaching philosophy statement, addressing learning styles and other essential aspects of being an educator such as student assessment and curriculum development are examples of individualized learning objectives that may be used to guide a capstone student to engage in in-depth learning in a focus area of education. Collaborating and working with individuals who are actively pursuing an academic career or who have expertise in education, which can also include individuals that may have expertise in developing continuing education modules, programs, or academic publishers. Examples include understanding academic institution culture and policies; attending academic meetings, performing literature reviews to learn more about pedagogy, andragogy, and curriculum design; and assisting in teaching and mentoring students.

Types of Sites and Settings

Examples can include school systems, higher education settings including occupational therapy assistant and occupational therapy degree levels, and other sites that have employees/staff who require annual training/learning.

Examples of Capstone Projects

The capstone project with an education focus area can take many forms depending on the student's interest. Examples include, but are not limited to the following:

- Academic course development
- Curricular development and testing of learning outcomes of coursework in traditional and/or online educational environments with occupational therapy or occupational therapy assistant students
- Development and implementation of a hybrid (face-to-face and online) occupational therapy course
- Development and implementation of a continuing education course or webinar
- Client/family education program
- Curricular development and testing of learning outcomes of coursework in traditional and/or online educational environments with clients and/or their families and caregivers
- Development of a family program at a local pool geared towards promoting water safety among the ASD population
- Staff development program
- Creating a staff development training program at a local recreation center on best practice approaches to work with children with disabilities
- Development of a training module for staff in a disaster relief organization (such as American Red Cross, FEMA, and UNICEF) on cultural awareness
- Development of training modules for staff in a hospice facility on end-of-care occupational engagement
- Consultation with a school-system bus service to create an evidenced-based child-passenger safety protocol
- Textbook or instructional technology development
- Development of publishable teaching materials or instructional technology designed for occupational therapy or other health professional, non-health professionals, consumer or family audiences.
- Development of a systematic review of best practice guidelines and an outcome product such as clinical guidelines, a tool kit, or a video that can be used for educational purposes, manuscript for children's book on disabilities awareness, resource manual for parents of children with special needs

THEORY DEVELOPMENT

Description

The body of literature within the occupational therapy profession consists of numerous theories, models of practice, and frames of reference, which have been developed to serve as comprehensive frameworks, such as the Model of Human Occupation, or others have been intended for specific target populations, such as Sensory Integration or Biomechanical frames of reference. See Table 2-7 for a snapshot of commonly used theories, models, and frames of references by occupational therapy practitioners.

In her Eleanor Clarke Slagle lectureship, Dr. Anne Henderson (1988) disseminated that theory promotes the development of knowledge and practice for occupational therapy. A theory is a collection of ideas or concepts that guides action. Theories are a way of explaining or understanding phenomena. Theory building is a concept that occupational therapy practitioners need to engage in and accept the responsibility to contribute to developing theories (Henderson, 1988). Occupational therapy literature documents that practitioners in the field often have difficulty articulating theory that supports our interventions (Ikiugu & Smallfield, 2015). This provides an important opportunity for a capstone student to help fill this gap.

TEXT BOX 2-12

Importance of Theory
- Supports our need for professional knowledge base
- Shapes and guides practice (provides scientific support for practice and tests the effectiveness of occupational therapy interventions)
- Provides a foundation for professional paradigm
- Assists in professional reasoning

Table 2-7. Common Theories, Models, and Frames of Reference

COMMON THEORIES *(Cole, 2018)*	• Erikson's developmental stages • Piaget's intellectual development • Kohlberg's moral reasoning • Levinson' life stages • Laslett's age theory
MODELS OF PRACTICE *(Cole, 2018; Hinojosa, Kramer & Royeen, 2017)*	• MOHO (Model of Human Occupation) • EHP (Ecology of Human Performance) • PEO (Person Occupation Environment) • OA (Occupational Adaptation) • PEOP (Person Environment Occupation Performance)
FRAMES OF REFERENCE *(Cole, 2018; Reed & Sanderson, 1999)*	• Psychodynamic • Behavioral cognitive • Allen levels • Biomechanical • Sensory Integration

A capstone focus area in theory development could include a dynamic process of knowledge development by the capstone student collaborating with individuals who are developing and testing models that relate to the practice of occupational therapy.

Types of Sites and Settings

Examples include working with recognized researchers and centers of excellence where specialized models of intervention are being tested and utilized.

TEXT BOX 2-13

For example, the University of Southern California is known for its creation and continued work with Lifestyle Redesign (Clark, 2015), and the University of Illinois-Chicago continues to build on the late Dr. Gary Kielhofner's (2002) internationally acclaimed Model of Human Occupation (Kielhofner, 2002) and the Intentional Relationship Model (Taylor, 2008), created by occupational therapy theorist and clinical psychological Dr. Renee Taylor (2008).

Examples of Capstone Project

The capstone project with a focus on theory development can take many forms. Examples include the following:

• Explore a mindfulness theory to use for mindful eating among individuals who are struggling with obesity.
• Integrate the use of Growth Mindset among professional identity development of occupational therapy students (Duckworth, 2016).

• Investigate a new theory to guide clinical reasoning during fieldwork education.
• Develop a gender-as-occupation-based model for individuals who are transgender or gender nonconforming (Annie DeRolf, OTD, OTR, Class of 2018, University of Indianapolis).

TEXT BOX 2-14

After reviewing the focus areas, you may still wonder how the capstone differs from Level II fieldwork because it is possible for a Level II fieldwork to occur in a specialized setting, such as hand therapy. They key to developing and fostering an in-depth experience in the focus area is the **individualized learning objectives**, which are developed in collaboration among the occupational therapy doctoral student, the site mentor and the doctoral capstone coordinator. These objectives are where the mentor (expert) provides direction on the **in-depth** areas to explore. More on how to develop individualized learning objectives is discussed in Chapters 6 and 7.

CHAPTER SUMMARY

Vision 2025 and other influences in health care, community practice, and society are all sculpting the occupational therapy profession to pursue advanced roles in diverse settings. The growing focus on the provision of high-quality health care has significantly altered occupational therapy service delivery in the spectrum of health care settings. The occupational therapy profession continues to make the necessary adaptations in response to these challenges. Through the focus areas and doctorate capstone experience, occupational therapy doctoral students can develop knowledge and refine skills in practice areas such as consultant, educator, manager, leader, researcher, and advocate for the profession and the consumer to meet the unique demands of the time (Molitor & Nissen, 2018). The capstone creates meaningful opportunities that can have a positive impact on individuals, groups, and populations, and at the same time offer the capstone student opportunities for professional growth in an identified focus area. It is because of this that the capstone should be viewed (and marketed to potential DCE sites) as a win-win scenario. The capstone allows the development of forward-thinking students who, through mentorship, have the opportunity to design, evaluate, educate, and lead. A critical element to support success of the development of the capstone is rooting the capstone in evidence and collaboration and communication among the capstone team. The authors build on this foundation in subsequent chapters.

Learning Activities

1. After learning about some of the compliance and quality initiatives from accreditors such as TJC and CARF, list two or three initiatives that could be explored by a capstone at your planned fieldwork sites.

2. List two or three potential populations with which you would be interested in gaining in-depth knowledge.

   a. For each population, identify an occupational therapy-related outcome (using the Occupational Therapy Practice Framework: Domain and Process—Third Edition; AOTA, 2014) that you will want to help the participants achieve. (Also think about how you will measure this outcome—more on that topic is featured in Chapter 11.)

3. List two or three potential settings where you would be interested in gaining in-depth knowledge.

   a. Are these traditional or role-emerging settings?

   b. How do they complement your planned fieldwork experiences?

REFERENCES

Accreditation Council for Occupational Therapy Education. (2018). *Standards and interpretive guide* [PDF]. Retrieved from https://www.aota.org/~/media/Corporate/Files/EducationCareers/Accredit/StandardsReview/2018-ACOTE-Standards-Interpretive-Guide.pdf

Agency for Healthcare Research and Quality. (2018). TeamSTEPPS 2.0. Retrieved from https://www.ahrq.gov/teamstepps/instructor/index.html

Alpha-Stim. (2018). *What is Alpha-Stim?* Retrieved from https://www.alpha-stim.com/alpha-stim-technology/anxiety

American Academy of Family Physicians. (2016). Primary care. Retrieved from https://www.aafp.org/about/policies/all/primary-care.html

American Association of Retired Persons, American Automobile Association, & American Occupational Therapy Association. (2018). *CarFit: Helping mature drivers find their safest fit.* Retrieved from: https://www.car-fit.org/

American Occupational Therapy Association. (1993). Occupational therapy roles. *American Journal of Occupational Therapy, 47,* 1087-1099. doi:10.5014/ajot.47.12.1087

American Occupational Therapy Association. (2018). Vision 2025. Retrieved from https://www.aota.org/Publications-News/AOTANews/2018/AOTA-Board-Expands-Vision-2025.aspx

American Occupational Therapy Association. (2018). *Practice.* Retrieved from https://www.aota.org/Practice.aspx

American Physical Therapy Association. (2017). *About the PTA advanced proficiency pathways (APP) program.* Retrieved from http://www.apta.org/APP/About

Atmaca, E., & Girenes, S. S. (2011). Lean six sigma methodology and application. *Quality & Quantity, 47,* 2107-2127.

Babiker, A., El Husseini, M., Al Nemri, A., Al Frayh, A., Al Juryyan, N., Faki, M. O., ... & Al Zamil, F. (2014). Health care professional development: Working as a team to improve patient care. *Sudanese Journal of Paediatrics, 14*(2), 9-16.

Bachman, R. E. (n.d.) The future of healthcare consumerism: empowering consumers through new medical delivery models. Retrieved from http://www.theihcc.com/en/communities/health_access_alternatives/the-future-of-health-care-consumerism--empowering-htln3omt.html

Benner, P. (1984). *From novice to expert: Excellence and power in clinical nursing practice.* Menlo Park, CA: Addison-Wesley.

Berg, K., Wood-Dauphinee, S., Williams, J. I., & Gayton, D. (1989). Measuring balance in the elderly: Preliminary development of an instrument. *Physiotherapy, 41,* 304-311. https://doi.org/10.3138/ptc.41.6.304

Berkheimer, S. D., Qian, C., & Malmstrom, T. K. (2017). Snoezelen therapy as an intervention to reduce agitation in nursing home patients with dementia: A pilot study. *Journal of American Medical Directors Association, 18,* 1089-1091.

Case-Smith, J., Page, S. J., Darragh, A., Rybski, M., & Cleary, D. (2014). The professional occupational therapy doctoral degree: Why do it? *American Journal of Occupational Therapy, 68,* e55-e60. doi:10.5014/ajot.2014.008805

Centers for Disease Control and Prevention. (2013). *Community needs assessment.* Retrieved from https://www.cdc.gov/globalhealth/healthprotection/fetp/training_modules/15/community-needs_pw_final_9252013.pdf

Chartered Society of Physiotherapy. (2018). *Advanced practice in physiotherapy.* Retrieved from http://www.csp.org.uk/publications/advanced-practice-physiotherapy

Clark, F. A. (2015). *Lifestyle redesign: The intervention tested in the USC well elderly studies* (2nd ed.). Bethesda, MD: AOTA Press.

Cole, M. (2018). *Group dynamics in occupational therapy: The theoretical basis and practice application of group treatment* (5th ed.), Thorofare, NJ: SLACK Incorporated.

Commission on Accreditation of Rehabilitation Facilities. (2018). *Who we are.* Retrieved from http://www.carf.org/About/WhoWeAre

Copolillo, A., Shepherd, J., Anzalone, M., & Lane, S. J. (2010). Taking on the challenge of the centennial vision: Transforming the passion for occupational therapy into a passion for leadership. *Occupational Therapy in Health Care, 24,* 7-22. doi:10.3109/07380570903304209

Dahl-Popolizio, S., & Rogers, O. (2017). Interprofessional primary care: The value of occupational therapy. *Open Journal of Occupational Therapy, 5*(11), 1-10. doi:10.15453/2168-6408.1363

DeIuliis, E.D. (2017). *Professionalism across Occupational Therapy Clinical Practice.* Thorofare, NJ: SLACK Incorporated.

Delbaere, K., Van den Noortgate, N., Bourgois, J., Vanderstraeten, G., Tine, W., & Cambier, D. (2006). The physical performance test as a predictor of frequent fallers: A prospective community-based cohort study. *Clinical Rehabilitation, 20,* 83-90. doi:10.1191/0269215506cr885oa

Dreyfus, H., & Dreyfus, S. (1980). *A five-stage model of mental activities involved in directed skill acquisition.* Berkeley, CA: Operations Research Center, University of California, Berkeley.

Ducan, P.W., Weiner, D.K, Chandler, J. & Studenski, S. (1990). Function reach: A new clinical measure of balance. *Journal of Gerontology, 45*(6), 192-197.

Duckworth, A. (2016). Hope. In A. Duckworth (Ed.), Grit: *The power of passion and perseverance* (pp.180-186). New York, NY: Scribner.

Fletcher, T. S., Blake, A. B., & Shelffo, K. E. (2018). Can sensory gallery guides for children with sensory processing challenges improve their museum experience? *Journal of Museum Education, 43*, 66-77. https://doi.org/10.1080/10598650.2017.1407915

Foto, M. (1996). Generalist versus specialist occupational therapists. *American Journal of Occupational Therapy, 50*, 771-774. doi:10.5014/ajot.50.10.771

Henderson, A. (1988). Occupational therapy knowledge: From practice to theory. *American Journal of Occupational Therapy, 42*, 567-576. doi:10.5014/ajot.42.9.567

Hinojosa, J., Kramer, P., & Royeen, C. (2017) *Perspectives on human occupation: Theories underlying practice* (2nd ed.). Philadelphia, PA: F.A. Davis.

ICN Nurse Practitioner/Advanced Practice Nursing Network. (2018). *Definition and characteristics of the role.* Retrieved from https://international.aanp.org/Practice/APNRoles

IDEO. (2015). *The field guide to human-centered design.* San Francisco, CA: Ideo.org.

Ikiugu, M. N., & Smallfield, S. (2015). Instructing occupational therapy students in use of theory to guide practice. *Occupational Therapy In Health Care, 29*, 165-177. doi:10.3109/07380577.2015.1017787

Kielhofner, G. (2002). *A model of human occupation: Theory and application.* Baltimore, MD: Lippincott Williams & Wilkins.

Kolodner, E. (2018). *OT Leaders & Legacies Society.* Retrieved from http://www.otleaders.org/

Lamb, A. J., & Metzler, C. A. (2014). Defining the value of occupational therapy: A health policy lens on research and practice. *American Journal of Occupational Therapy, 6*, 9-14. doi:10.5014/ajot.2014.681001

Law, M., Baptiste, S., & Mills, J. (1995). Client-centred practice: What does it mean and does it make a difference? *Canadian Journal of Occupational Therapy, 62*, 250-257.

McNamara, S. A. (2012). Hospital report cards: what nurses need to know. *AORN Journal, 95*(3), 395-399. doi:http://dx.doi.org/10.1016/j.aorn.2011.12.016

Mele, C., Pels, J., & Polese, F. (2010). A brief review of system theories and their managerial applications. *Service Science, 2*, 126-135.

Metzler, C. A., Hartmann, K. D., & Lowenthal, L. A. (2012). Defining primary care: Envisioning the roles of occupational therapy. *American Journal of Occupational Therapy, 66*, 266-270. http://dx.doi.org/10.5014/ajot.2010.663001

Molitor, W. L., & Nissen, R. (2018). Clinician, educator and student perceptions of entry-level academic degree requirements in occupational therapy education. *Journal of Occupational Therapy Education, 2*, 1-23.

Podsiadlo, D., & Richardson, S. (1991). The timed "Up & Go": A test of basic functional mobility for frail elderly persons. *Journal of the American Geriatrics Society, 39*, 142-148. doi:10.1111/j.1532-5415.1991.tb01616.x

Press Ganey. (2018). *About the Press Ganey survey.* Retrieved from http://www.pressganey.com/solutions/patient-experience/consumerism-transparency/about-the-press-ganey-survey

Reed, K. L., & Sanderson, S. N. (1999). *Concepts of occupational therapy.* Philadelphia, PA: Lippincott Williams & Wilkins.

Roberts, P., Farmer, M. E., Lamb, A. J., Muir, S., & Siebert, C. (2014). The role of occupational therapy in primary care. *American Journal of Occupational Therapy, 68*(3), S25-S33. doi:10.5014/ajot.2014.686S06

Rogers, A. T., Bai, G., Lavin, R. A., & Anderson, G. F. (2016). Higher hospital spending on occupational therapy is associated with lower readmission rates. *Medical Care Research and Review, 74*, 668-686. doi:10.1177/1077558716666981

Saha, S., Beach, M. C., & Cooper, L. A. (2008). Patient centeredness, cultural competence and healthcare quality. *Journal of the National Medical Association, 100*, 1275-1285.

Schemm, R. L., Corcoran, M., Kolodner, E., & Schaaf, R. (1993). A curriculum based on systems theory. *American Journal of Occupational Therapy, 47*(7), 625-634. doi:10.5014/ajot.47.7.625

Taylor, R. R. (2008). *The intentional relationship: Occupational therapy and use of self.* Philadelphia, PA: F.A. Davis.

The Joint Commission. (2018a). *National patient safety goals.* Retrieved from https://www.jointcommission.org/standards_information/npsgs.aspx

The Joint Commission. (2018b). *What is certification?* Retrieved from https://www.jointcommission.org/certification/certification_main.aspx

Tickle-Degnen, L. (2002). Client centered practice, therapeutic relationships and the use of research evidence. *American Journal of Occupational Therapy, 56*(4), 470-474.

Wagner, L. M., McDonald, S. M., & Castle, N. G. (2012). Joint Commission accreditation and quality measures in U.S. nursing homes. *Policy, Politics, & Nursing Practice, 1*, 8-16. doi:10.1177/1527154412443990

Appendix 2-A

Framework to Help Guide Brainstorming of Doctoral Capstone Experience Fit at a Site

Type of site:

Review accreditations/certifications/outcome measures tracked/measured:

LTG of Department/Work Unit: (3 to 5 years)
1.
2.
3.

STG of Department/Work Unit: (6 months to 3 years)
1.
2.
3.
4.
5.

Individuals with specialty training/expertise (in and outside of your department/work unit)
1.
2.
3.
4.

Brainstorm an idea for a DCE experience/project using the focus areas below:

clinical practice skills

research skills

administration

leadership

program development

policy development

advocacy

education/teaching/staff training

theory development

CHAPTER 3

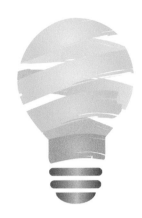

Synthesizing the Evidence
A Process to Determine a Course of Action for the Capstone

Alison Bell, OTD, OTR/L
Tina DeAngelis, EdD, OTR/L

Human-Centered Design Mindsets for the Doctoral Students

Human-centered design mindset concepts of starting out simple to learn and make your ideas real, giving yourself permission to explore a lot of ideas, and having optimism to drive yourself forward is the vision of this chapter.

Make It: It is important to brainstorm ideas for the capstone experience and project and get those ideas down on paper … what are you most passionate about, what is needed in the community, think about how what you want to do is within the scope of occupational therapy and what would be the link to occupation.

Embrace Ambiguity: You do not know the answer to your problem, and that is okay; be okay with the ambiguity. It will allow you to be more creative as you begin to research your interest area and define your purpose. Be fine with changing direction as you move into the literature. This ambiguity actually allows you to innovate and create. Looking for a gap or need is important in development of your problem statement.

Optimism: You do not know the answer yet, and that is fine—staying optimistic that you will find a solution to the problem will lead to the purpose of your capstone. You have a long journey. Stay optimistic—optimism will keep you on track as you move through the process.

INTRODUCTION

The development of a meaningful and robust capstone experience and project requires demonstration of need coupled with an area of passion for the doctoral candidate. In keeping with accreditation standards, the occupational therapy doctoral capstone project must be consistent with the educational program's curriculum design and reflects the ability of the doctoral student to synthesize knowledge

in one area of practice, such as clinical practice skills, research skills, administration, leadership, program and policy development, advocacy, education, or theory development (Accreditation Council for Occupational Therapy Education. [ACOTE], 2018). Ultimately, the doctoral capstone project must have evidence to support the need and use evidence to develop methods to achieve the desired outcome(s). The capstone process mirrors the American Occupational Therapy Association's (AOTA; 2018) Vision 2025 call to produce

- 41 -

Deluliis ED, Bednarski JA.
The Entry Level Occupational Therapy Doctorate Capstone:
A Framework for The Experience and Project (pp 41-59).
© 2020 Taylor & Francis Group.

effective occupational therapy practitioners who can collaborate with others to yield effective outcomes to better demonstrate the distinct value of occupation.

The excitement for the doctoral project was ignited in capstone students' curriculum as they were gradually socialized to the skills and competencies expected of a doctoral level occupational therapy practitioner—first through coursework, Level I and Level II fieldwork and now the capstone. The capstone experience is an exciting process. It is a systematic yet iterative journey that has the potential to impact *persons*, *communities*, *populations*, and *organizations*. The detailed steps that build to the eventual outcome are similar to putting together the small pieces of an intricate puzzle. The pieces must be placed just so to have the right fit for the final product. In this chapter, the process of searching and locating evidence from the literature to develop a problem statement and demonstrate the need for the doctoral capstone experience (DCE) and project is examined. This process of synthesis will develop professional skills and competencies necessary to assume a variety of roles beyond graduation.

Capstone Student Reflective Questions

When developing the doctoral capstone, the occupational therapy student may find it helpful to reflect on the following questions:

1. What initial ideas do I have for my capstone project?
2. What is my initial problem statement for my capstone and what is my inspiration?
3. Why is my idea important? (to me, the profession, individuals, groups/populations)
4. What individualized specific objectives have I identified before embarking on the capstone experience?

Keywords

- **Gap problem analysis**—A thoughtful analysis that contrasts what is occurring with what is desired (Davis-Ajami, Costa & Kulik, 2014)
- **PICO question**—An interdisciplinary approach to translate a clinical question into searchable terms (Cochrane Linked Data, 2018)
- **Rapid review**—A systematic process of reviewing the literature, with a narrow focus to ensure rapid use of the available evidence (Tricco et al., 2015)

Chapter Objectives

By the end of reading this chapter and completing the learning activities, the reader should be able to:

1. Determine how to search the literature to provide evidence to support ideas for the capstone project.
2. Identify the need and gap for the establishment of the capstone project.

3. Design an initial problem statement for the capstone experience and project.
4. Develop a strong rationale and purpose for the capstone experience and project.
5. Connect the ACOTE areas of focus with Boyer's (1990) types of scholarship.

BEFORE SEARCHING THE LITERATURE

All doctoral capstone projects begin with a literature search. This section details the processes of developing targeted clinical and/or doctoral capstone specific based questions that result in efficient and effective literature searches. Synthesizing the results of the search supports the development of a gap analysis statement in which the capstone project can be constructed.

Developing a Focused Question

The first step in a literature review is the development of a focused clinical question to support an efficient search. This essential initial step paves the way for an effective search strategy. Formulating a focused question will assist the capstone student in determining whether evidence is relevant to the capstone project. One challenge for the evidenced-based practitioner is the volume of research evidence.

TEXT BOX 3-1

A review of publications found that there are 75 randomized controlled trials and 11 systematic reviews published every day (Bastian, Glasziou, & Chalmers, 2010).

The pace of publication is daunting, and as an evidenced-based practitioner, it can be challenging to keep up with the research evidence that accumulates daily. A benefit of a well-developed clinical question is a focused search strategy that yields evidence that directly answers the question.

The PICO (patient/population/problem, intervention, comparison, and outcome) approach is well described in the interdisciplinary literature (Cochrane Linked Data, 2018). The PICO format transforms the clinical question into a searchable format with narrow search terms. The greater detail and focus the question has, the better the search terms—and therefore, the greater the likelihood of retrieving the evidence that is relevant to the question.

TEXT BOX 3-2

What is a **PICO**?
A model that helps break a search into small pieces. The PICO framework is used to create a well-built clinical question into a searchable question to

Table 3-1. Building a Better PICO Question

START	BETTER	BEST
1. In stroke, what treatment is most effective for hemiplegia?	For a woman with chronic hemiplegia, is CIMT or Bobath treatment more effective?	For a woman with chronic stroke, is CIMT or Bobath more effective for improvement of quality of life?
2. For people experiencing homelessness, what intervention is best for reducing substance use?	For lesbian, gay, bisexual, transgender, questioning/queer, intersex (LGBTQI) teens experiencing homelessness, what interventions are most effective to reduce substance use?	For LGBTQI teens experiencing homelessness, is harm reduction or cognitive-behavioral therapy approach most effective for reducing substance use?
3. What assessment is best to measure pain in people with multiple sclerosis?	For relapsing remitting multiple sclerosis, what assessment is best to measure pain?	For relapsing remitting multiple sclerosis, what assessment of pain is most sensitive to change after occupational therapy interventions?
4. Is group or individual treatment more effective for children with ASD?	For school-aged children with ASD, is group or individual treatment more effective?	For children in high school with ASD, is group or individual training more effective for the development of friendship?
5. What is the experience of caregivers engaged in a support group?	For informal caregivers, what is their experience when engaged in support groups?	For spouses of people with Alzheimer's disease, what is their experience when engaged in community support groups
6. Is anxiety common after concussion?	What is the likelihood of developing anxiety for athletes with postconcussive syndrome?	What is the likelihood of developing anxiety for female high school athletes with postconcussive syndrome?

ASD = autism spectrum disorder; CIMT = constraint-induced movement therapy.

TEXT BOX 3-2 (continued)

develop literature search strategies for evidence-based practice (Kloda & Bartlett, 2014):

P—patient, problem or population

I—intervention, program

C—comparison, control

O—outcome

For the capstone project, a PICO can guide the creation and development of the scholarly project.

Defining a population includes identifying characteristics that are relevant. This may include not only a diagnosis but also variables such as age and chronicity. The PICO format does not simply explore interventions in a traditional sense. Interventions may be a type of treatments (cognitive-behavioral therapy, for example) but can also explore a diagnostic test or prognosis (#3 and #6 in Table 3-1 provide examples). An example of this may be a capstone student whose doctoral experience and capstone project takes place in an academic setting, with a focus area of education with a need to identify outcome measures related to the efficacy of an active teaching methodology such as simulation.

Not every PICO question requires a comparison. The decision to compare two interventions will be based on the needs of the site and type of project. Finally, a specific outcome is an important last step. Just as goals of occupational therapy treatment are client-centered, so should an outcome of a PICO question. It is not enough to ask what is better; instead, identify what is the meaningful outcome of interest and define it.

Questions that are best answered by qualitative/naturalistic inquiry use a different format (Stern, Jordan, & McArthur, 2014). The clinical question is framed as Population/Problem/Interest/Context (PICo) question. The process of identifying the population or problem is the same as quantitative research; however, a clearly defined population and context is vital because qualitative research does not aim for results to generalize to a larger population or different context (Howlett, Rogo, & Shelton, 2013). Qualitative research does not introduce a treatment or manipulate variables but instead attempts to develop a deep understanding of a phenomenon. In qualitative research, the "lived experiences of individuals, groups, or cultures that reveal meaning and significance of phenomena" (Howlett et al., 2013, p. 32). The qualitative perspective typically views "the world through a lens of openness and complexity ... methods typically include gaining some type of word data, as opposed to numeric data" and explores information on knowledge, beliefs, and attitudes (Bonnel & Smith, 2018, p. 159). Whether the capstone project focus is qualitative, quantitative, or mixed methods in approach, the ability to construct a robust clinical question (see Table 3-1) will inform the literature search process.

> **TEACHING TIP 1**: Occupational therapy educators and students can refer to other prominent resources for evidence-based practice and research by referring to the following texts that are rated as most frequently used, according to the National Board for Certification in Occupational Therapy's (NBCOT) *OTR Curriculum Textbook and Peer-Reviewed Journal Report* (most recent version retrieved from https://www.nbcot.org/-/media/NBCOT/PDFs/2018_Textbook_Report_OTR.ashx?la=en).
>
> - DePoy, E., & Gitlin, L. N. (2016). *Introduction to research: Understanding and applying multiple strategies* (5th ed.). St. Louis, MO: Mosby Elsevier.
> - Kielhofner, G. (2006). *Research in occupational therapy: Methods of inquiry for enhancing practice*. Philadelphia, PA: F.A. Davis.
> - Law, M., & MacDermid, J. (Eds.). (2014). *Evidence-based rehabilitation: A guide to practice* (3rd ed.). Thorofare, NJ: SLACK Incorporated.

Selecting a Database

With a solid PICO question, selection of databases begins. Conducting a literature search involves the use of web-based search engines and electronic research databases. Electronic bibliographic databases collect and index publications in a focus area. Table 3-2 describes common databases relevant to occupational therapy. To find the right database(s), explore what material it covers, and develop knowledge of the search features in the database. It is best practice to search multiple databases that are relevant to the content area. Similar search strategies on different databases yield different results, highlighting the importance of searching multiple databases results (Wu, Aylward, Roberts, & Evans, 2012).

Typically, a database will permit a search or query by subject, journal, and/or author. After entering the query, results tend to be presented in summary format. Display settings also permit the user to manage and refine the information further (if desired). Some databases also include full-text articles and links to other institutions (Ecker & Skelly, 2010).

Developing Search Terms and Strategy

Search terms are based on the PICO/PICo question; however, each database has different methods to index publications, requiring different search terms for each database selected. The academic librarian can be helpful to tailor search terms to the selected databases. As seen from the PICO examples in Table 3-1, a well-built clinical question supports

more specific search terms. These search terms are words or phrases that described the key aspects of the PICO question. Individual databases use different search terminologies. For example, MedLine developed Medical Subject Heading (MeSH) terms. MeSH terms are a system to organize and categorize terms developed by librarians (Lipscomb, 2000). MeSH terms are a common vocabulary to ensure retrieval of relevant literature. To explain the thinking of a controlled vocabulary, think of searching for a topic or service on the Internet. An individual desiring to locate a facility to get a haircut may initially search the term haircut; however, the ultimate term to obtain the exact match for desired services may, in actuality, be Salon Services. "Using MeSH in a search focuses the results on more relevant evidence" (Howlett et al., 2013, p. 95).

Each database has different logic for search terms, and not all use MeSH terms. The common vocabulary set in the Cumulative Index to Nursing and Allied Health (CINAHL) is CINAHL subject headings, and EMBASE uses Emtree. This presents another opportunity to collaborate with a librarian to identify relevant databases and tailor search terms to the individual databases. Appendix 3-B provides examples, specific to MedLine, of using MeSH terms to develop a search strategy. Both CINHAL and EMBASE would be appropriate databases to search for the PICO question, requiring adjustments to the search terms.

Finally, consider other terms that may describe a similar concept to ensure a complete search. For example, spelling differences in the English language, based on region (e.g., orthopedic/orthopaedic) outdated terms such as *Asperger's syndrome* or *Pervasive Developmental Disorder* when searching for literature on autism spectrum disorder (ASD). Table 3-3 and Appendix 3-C, provide examples on terms that should be considered, based on outdated terms and terminology that is used interchangeably.

After identification of search terms, Boolean Operators, truncation, wildcards, and limits will support the efficient search. Boolean Operators connect and define the relationship between search terms. These include the words **AND**, **OR**, and **NOT**. Using AND to link search terms will yield results that include both terms. OR will yield results that include at least one of the terms. NOT will exclude results based on the search term (Howlett et al., 2013). Appendix 3-A provides a format to move a PICO question into search terms and strategies. Appendix 3-B is a completed example, using MeSH terms and Boolean Operators.

Truncation is a strategy to broaden a search, based on variation of word endings. A search with truncation for the root word "child" would search for terms that include child, children, and childhood. Most databases, but not all, denote truncation with an asterisk (e.g., child*). Here is another example of the need for collaboration with the academic librarian.

A wildcard character replaces a single character in a search term. For example, womAn and womEn. This may denoted with a question mark (e.g., wom?n or orthop?edic);

Table 3-2. Relevant Databases

NAME	AREA OF FOCUS	NOTES
MEDLINE, accessed for free via PubMed	Wide range of literature, including medicine, nursing, rehabilitation therapy, allied health, dentistry, veterinary medicine, health care system and preclinical sciences (National Institutes of Health United States National Library of Medicine, 2018)	
EMBASE	Wide range of biomedical literature. European database (Elsevier, n.d.)	Similar coverage to MEDLINE, but greater coverage of non-English and European journals
CINAHL	Nursing and allied health literature (including occupational therapy; EBSCOhealth, n.d.)	
Cochrane library	Independent review of clinical effectiveness to inform health care decision-making (Cochrane Library, n.d.)	
Educational Resource Information Center (ERIC)	Education-related research (Educational Resource Information Center, n.d.)	
PsycINFO	Literature from social and behavioral sciences (PsycINFO, n.d.)	
Google Scholar	Free web-based search engine that indexes citations and full-text articles from a wide range of disciplines (Google Scholar, n.d.)	Results from the searches will typically show the most cited articles, not the most relevant to the search term. The capstone student may find this a resource to discover or browse, *but this is not a systematic approach to a search*
Occupational Therapy Systematic Evaluation of Evidence (OTseeker)	Critical appraisals of literature relevant to occupational therapy; last updated in 2016 (OT Seeker, n.d.).	The critical appraisals may support understanding of a research article; however, they are not a substitution of obtaining and critically evaluating the research considering the clinical question and the context of the DCE site.
Physiotherapy Evidence Database (PEDro)	Critical appraisals of literature relevant to physical therapy. No longer updated (PEDro, n.d.).	
Psychological Database for Brain Impairment Treatment Efficacy (PsycBITE)	Critical appraisals of literature relevant to cognitive, behavioral, and other treatments for psychological problems and issues for people with acquired brain injuries (PsycBITE, n.d.)	
REHAB+	Critical appraisals of literature relevant to occupational and physical therapy (McMaster University, n.d.)	

Table 3-3. PICO Search Terms

P	I	C	O
• Stroke • Cerebral vascular accident (CVA) • Cerebrovascular accident	• Constraint-induced movement therapy (CIMT) • Constraint-induced therapy	• Bobath • Neurodevelopmental treatment	• Quality of life

however, there is not a common character across databases, compelling the support and expertise of a librarian.

Most databases also allow the user to limit searches based on characteristics of the article or study such as language, methodology, age of participants, and publication dates. These filters may help to better target the population of interest, such as age of participants or may be necessary to ensure rapid utilization of the literature, such as limits to English language. However, these necessary exclusions, to ensure a rapid review, can introduce bias.

The process used to search and select literature should be systematic, although unlikely to be a systematic review. Most doctoral capstone projects will undergo the process of a rapid review of the literature. Although standard features of a rapid review still need to be defined, a rapid review and a systematic review have similarities in that there is a focused question and a systematic search strategy (Tricco et al., 2015). Fundamental differences are that rapid reviews have narrow search criteria to answer a policy or practice issue compared to systematic reviews with expansive search criteria to answer a broad question (Tricco et al., 2015). A well-developed PICO question will narrow the search criteria and lead to inclusion and exclusion criteria. In keeping with the stroke example, an example of inclusion criteria would be studies with a population with first stroke greater than 6 months before study.

> **TEACHING TIP 2:** The PICO Terms Worksheet (Appendix 3-A) and the example in Appendix 3-B are helpful exercises to develop a search strategy and articulate inclusion and exclusion criteria.

START THE LITERATURE SEARCH

The work to develop clear search terms and inclusion and exclusion criteria is designed to limit the results to the most relevant. However, retrieval of irrelevant results will occur. The process to systematically identify the most pertinent information is the next step in the literature review process.

Selecting the Literature

After completing the searches, review the outcome of the scholarly inquiry. Capstone students should engage in a systematic review of the literature that is critical and consistent,

requiring that they to read and analyze a large amount of literature. Screening results for relevance can reduce the volume of literature to only what is relevant.

An initial step in the appraisal process can be a title screen. Some of the articles may be deemed irrelevant to the clinical question based on the title alone. Articles that are considered to be relevant or cannot be excluded based on the title alone move to the next step, an abstract screen, based on the review of the journal abstract (Mateen, Oh, Tergas, Bhayani, & Kamdar, 2013). If the content is not relevant to your PICO question, eliminate the article. Articles that are relevant or cannot be removed based on abstract alone must undergo a more critical review of the content. This final step is a full-text screen. In this step, obtain the full-text articles and review for relevance.

One system to consider using to guide the critical reading of the results derived from the literature search is the Preview, Question, Read, and Summarize (PQRS) model described by Cohen (1990). The method has been shown to improve readers' understanding and their ability to recall information (Ulu & Akyol, 2016). In other words, readers are more likely to learn, and to learn more, of the material they are reading.

Preview—Acquire an overview of the article through a quick scan or skim. Do the main points of the text align with your capstone? Is the article worth a closer read?

Question—Ask questions about what you are reading. Does the article relate to your capstone? What are you learning from the article scan?

Read—Read the article. Now, read the article again. What information is in the article and how does it relate to your capstone?

Summarize—Write notes to summarize or paraphrase what you read. Can you summarize how the content of the article helps support your capstone or focus area?

> **TEACHING TIP 3:** Another tip that can assist with the often-cumbersome title and abstract screening process is through the use of Screen2Go via a smartphone. It is suggested that the use of an app can expedite the screening process because it permits the user to examine small groups of citations at one time (Huckvale, van Velthoven, & Car, 2011).

Managing the Outcome of the Literature Review

In a doctoral project, it is essential to detail the search strategy, as well as the process and results of obtaining the final articles for review. An external reviewer should be able to evaluate the quality of the literature review through examination of the search strategy.

Table 3-4 is a tool to report the databases, search strategy, and describe the number of articles obtained and defend the rationale for excluding some. On the basis of the inclusion and exclusion criteria, articles may be excluded based on study design. Evidence level refers to a hierarchal categorization of study design, with higher level of evidence representing designs that have a lower probability of bias (see Table 3-5). The final column in Table 3-4 provides a preliminary assessment of the literature in relation to the proposed project. This process can be organized by labeling an article title and/or abstract as "highly relevant to not relevant … determining relevance helps you narrow the reading task so that it is manageable and productive" (DePoy & Gitlin, 2016, p. 76).

TEXT BOX 3-3

Did you know many bibliographic databases allow users to sign up for email alerts for new publications relevant to a search strategy?

The Preferred Reporting Items for Systematic Reviews and Meta-Analyses (PRISMA) is an evidence-based minimum set of items for reporting in systematic reviews and meta-analyses. In this minimum set, a recommended diagram depicts how many articles were screened and the process to remove (Moher, Liberati, Tetzlaff, Altman, & PRISMA Group, 2009). Although the capstone student will most likely not be completing a systematic review, the PRISMA Flow Diagram is a powerful tool to display the literature review process (Appendix 3-C).

EFFECTIVELY MANAGING THE EVIDENCE

Using reference management software will become a necessity throughout the capstone experience. Reference managers are an electronic space to organize, sort, and reference literature when writing. Most software systems will organize references by project, save notes on the citation, share with collaborators, develop a reference list in multiple citation formats (e.g., American Psychological Association, 6th ed., Vancouver Style) and accurately develop in-text citations. These programs insert cited sources into a written capstone paper or assist in the manuscript preparation process for a journal (see further discussion in Chapters 10 and 11 of this text). The academic library may offer access to reference managers. There are numerous vendors available, each with different features. Table 3-6 provides details on key features on programs used by health sciences scholars. However, it is

not exhaustive. Developers continually update products, so check with the vendors for the most up-to-date information.

TEXT BOX 3-4

Did you know that the NBCOT offers complementary access to ProQuest RefWorks to all current certificants? One of the many reasons to maintain and renew your NBCOT registration!

Finally, recognize that search strategies are iterative; when new terms are revealed through article reviews or work is found through citations of reviewed articles, there is a need to return to the databases. Literature searches are time-intensive. The capstone student may need references to which the library does not have access. Most academic or professional libraries have a process for an interlibrary loan. Work with the librarian to order what is not available at your institution; however, understand that the time to receive articles may take weeks. As discussed, developing rapport with the academic librarian is a must. Evidence is the foundation of a well-designed project. Developing clear search terms and strategies to manage the evidence will support continued work as a doctoral student.

EVALUATING THE LITERATURE

The capstone focus is informed by dozens of individual articles, so the capstone student must have a strategy to organize what is read. An evidence table is a good place to start (Table 3-7). This table should include the American Psychological Association citation, the research design, threats to internal validity of the study and how the study aligns with the specific practice context (external validity) and focus area. This would include similarity and differences between the setting and subjects to the doctoral capstone setting. The AOTA's Evidence-Based Review Project provides a coding framework to describe the research design, sample, internal validity and external validity (Lieberman & Scheer, 2002). Including this coding framework will give a quick snapshot of the relevance of the citation to the population and DCE site.

WRITING THE LITERATURE SYNTHESIS

After the critical appraisal, reflect on the available literature to make broad statements. A synthesis will compare and contrast the articles in a narrative format and is different from the literature review chart. (The chart can be useful because it lists the articles in a procedural manner, however.)

The first step in writing the synthesis is to review and understand the evidence table (see Table 3-7) and look for themes. For example, is there a frequently used outcome tool across many studies? Describe how work is both similar and different. Interpret the evidence considering both internal and

Table 3-4. Organizer Table for Tracking Search Strategies

RESOURCE	DATE OF SEARCH	KEYWORDS, MESH, OR SUBJECT HEADINGS	LIMIT SETS (PUBLICATION DATES OR TYPES)	ALERT INITIATED?	TITLE	LEVEL OF EVIDENCE (SEE TABLE 3-5)	SIGNIFICANCE TO QUESTION RANKING (SCALE 1-3)
PubMed MeSH							
Cochrane library							
CINAHL							
Governmental websites							
Other (e.g., open access; peer-reviewed scholarly journals)							

Adapted from Howlett, B., Rogo, E., & Shelton, T. G. (2013). *Evidence-based practice for health professionals. An interprofessional approach.* Burlington, MA: Jones and Bartlett Learning.

Table 3-5. Levels of Evidence

LEVEL I	Systematic reviews, meta-analyses, randomized controlled trials
LEVEL II	Two groups, nonrandomized studies (e.g., cohort, case control)
LEVEL III	One group, nonrandomized (e.g., before and after, pretest/posttest)
LEVEL IV	Descriptive studies that include analysis of outcomes (single subject design, case series)
LEVEL V	Case reports and expert opinion that include narrative literature reviews and consensus statements

Adapted from Sackett, D. L., Rosenberg, W. M., Gray, J. M., Haynes, R. B., & Richardson, W. S. (1996). Evidence based medicine: What it is and what it isn't. *BMJ, 312*, 71-72.

Table 3-6. Common Reference Management Programs

PRODUCT	MICROSOFT PLUG-IN TO DEVELOP THE BIBLIOGRAPHY AND IN-TEXT CITATION	GOOGLE DOC PLUG-IN TO DEVELOP THE BIBLIOGRAPHY AND IN-TEXT CITATION	PROJECT SHARING WITH COLLABORATORS	OPEN ACCESS	SAVE PDFS
F1000 https://f1000.com/	X	X	X		X
ProQuest RefWorks https://refworks.proquest.com	X		X		X
EndNote https://endnote.com/	X	X	X	Basic is free of charge, with limited features	X
Zotero https://www.zotero.org/	X	X	X	X	X
Mendeley https://www.mendeley.com/	X	X	X	X	X

Table 3-7. Evidence Table

CITATION	SUBJECTS	STUDY DESIGN	OUTCOME	COMMENTS ON INTERNAL VALIDITY	APPLICATION TO DCE SITE (EXTERNAL VALIDITY)	COMMENTS	AOTA CODING (I.E., IIA2A; LIEBERMAN & SCHEER, 2002)*

*Outcome research only.

external validity. A synthesis is not a list; rather it is a skilled assessment of the state of the relevant evidence. It is through the synthesis that broad statements from the literature become the foundation to create a problem statement and gap analysis, which further builds the capstone project.

DETERMINING A PROBLEM STATEMENT AND GAP ANALYSIS FOR THE CAPSTONE

Through a synthesis of the literature, with a focus on the DCE context, gaps in practice (or knowledge) will become evident. A gap is a difference between what is happening and what should be happening. Gaps exist in all areas, including research, clinical practice, and education. The "what should be happening" can be found in peer-reviewed publications such as research articles, but also includes clinical practice guidelines and standards of practice from accrediting agencies. Stating the gap is the first step in developing a robust capstone proposal. It is not enough to identify what is and what should be; students must be able to articulate what the actual gap is by describing what is happening and contrasting this to the desired action (Davis-Ajami et al., 2014). This is a gap analysis statement.

For example, constraint-induced movement therapy (CIMT) is one of the most well-studied and effective treatments of hemiplegia after stroke. There is a large body of work, with clinical trials and systematic reviews, that support the intervention; however, CIMT is not widely applied in practice (Morris & Taub, 2014). This is an example of where what should be happening is not the same as what is happening, and the gap is the use of less supported interventions to address hemiplegia, rather than the implementation of a CIMT protocol.

Gaps exist for a variety of reasons. A capstone project should use literature to understand both what the gap is, and then look for reasons, specific to the setting that is addressed. These include gaps in research, education, and practice. Boyer's Model of Scholarship (1990) has been proposed as a framework to describe the work of occupational therapists (AOTA, 2009) and to provide a useful framework for the development of the capstone project.

Boyer's (1990) model describes four areas of scholarship. Research and publication is most closely aligned with the scholarship of discovery. This type of scholarship describes the generation of new knowledge (Boyer, 1990). The scholarship of integration refers to the interpretation and synthesis of new knowledge and information (Boyer, 1990). It requires interdisciplinary study and work to coordinate knowledge from multiple arenas (Boyer, 1990). The scholarship of application looks to take new knowledge and develop ways to apply to specific settings or areas (Boyer, 1990). The scholarship of teaching goes beyond providing information. It occurs through carefully planned and evaluated pedagogical procedures, delivered by experts in the content area (Boyer,

1990). Table 3-8 provides a snapshot of how to align Boyer's model with the ACOTE focus areas.

Table 3-9 provides examples of how to contextualize the development of a capstone project through the lens of Boyer (1990).

After identifying the gap, is it important to complete another systematic process to understand why the gap is occurring. Gaps exist within a context and involve many stakeholders. A thoughtful examination of why a gap exists, through examination of work flow at the DCE site or interview and observation of the stakeholders, will provide insight into the gap (Davis-Ajami et al., 2014). Chapter 7 discusses the needs assessment process in detail. The literature may also provide insight into the reason for the gap. The clearly articulated reason for why a gap occurs is the problem statement. The problem statement is the foundation on which the capstone proposal is developed. Drawing from the CIMT example earlier in this chapter, the reason for the gap is multifaceted, requiring different problem statements (Table 3-10).

Literature must guide how to address the problem, resulting in a new literature search. The problem statement and the area of focus may lead to another clinical question. For example, if looking to address the problem in education, searches should explore evidence about how to provide education to experienced clinicians, rather than just a general search on education. For example "Are journal clubs (I) or didactic education sessions (C) more effective to increase therapist (P) competency with novel interventions (O)?"

Real-world problems are often multifaceted. A capstone project is unlikely to address all aspects during the DCE and may only focus on one problem area. The design of the DCE is to give students an in-depth experience in one or more of the focus areas: clinical practice skills, research skills, administration, leadership, program and policy development, advocacy, education, and theory development (discussed in detail in Chapter 2). Appendix 3-D provides inspiration of example PICO questions aligned with the focus areas.

Table 3-11 provides examples of how gaps and problem statements aligned with the ACOTE focus areas.

ROOTING SCHOLARLY INQUIRY AND CAPSTONE IN THEORY

Finally, capstone projects are grounded in theory. Theory is a proposed explanation, or a generalized statement aimed to explain a certain phenomenon. Frameworks are overall structures that help us organize the elements of the reality we are observing (Cole & Tufano, 2008). The theory and framework chosen will provide the scaffolding to address the stated problem. For example, learning theories, such as adult learning theory (Knowles, 1978) or situated learning (Lave, Wenger, & Wenger, 1991), provide a way to understand how adults (professionals) will access learning and benefit from education.

Table 3-8. ACOTE Focus Areas Aligned with Boyer's Model

CAPSTONE FOCUS AREAS	SCHOLARSHIP OF DISCOVERY: DESCRIPTIONS
Research	Participating in an ongoing study or creating a study. Includes research design and planning, data collection, analyzing data, and summarizing and disseminating results.
Theory development	Collaborating with individuals who are developing and testing models that relate to the practice of occupational therapy. Examples include working with recognized researchers and centers of excellence where specialized models of intervention are being tested and utilized.
	SCHOLARSHIP OF TEACHING: DESCRIPTIONS
Education (academic course development)	Curricular development and testing of learning outcomes of coursework with occupational therapy or occupational therapy assistant students.
Education (client/family education program)	Curricular development and testing of learning outcomes of coursework with clients and/or their families and caregivers.
Education (staff development program)	Curricular development and testing of learning outcomes of coursework with non–occupational therapy personnel.
Education (textbook or technology development)	Development of publishable teaching materials or teaching technology designed for occupational therapy or other health professional, non–health professional, consumer, or family audiences.
	SCHOLARSHIP OF APPLICATION: DESCRIPTIONS
Administration	Actively participating in the management of occupational therapy departments and/or specialized sites. Examples include working with experienced occupational therapists managing private practices and/or occupational therapy departments in various settings.
Advocacy	Development and testing of a program to consumers' abilities to navigate health systems to improve access to, delivery of, or outcomes of health care.
Program development (clinical)	Developing and testing outcomes of occupational therapy programs in traditional clinical settings (e.g., hand therapy, geriatrics, pediatrics, mental health, rehabilitation, school-based occupational therapy).
Program development (community)	Developing and testing outcomes of occupational therapy programs in role-emerging and community-based settings (e.g., homeless shelters, nonprofit health facilities, criminal justice settings, foster care, adult day care).
Leadership	Collaborating with leaders involved in exercising influence and representing different areas of the occupational therapy profession regionally, nationally and/or internationally.
Policy analysis	Meeting individualized learning objectives while collaborating with recognized individuals who are implementing innovative programs and/or developing health and social policy. Collaborating with recognized individuals who are engaged at the federal and state legislative levels regarding issues that affect our practice, what you are paid, whether you practice at all.
	SCHOLARSHIP OF INTEGRATION: DESCRIPTIONS
Any of the above	Scholarship that creates new relationships between two or more disciplines. Any of the mediums for scholarship listed above (discovery, teaching, application) can be used to study the interface between two disciplines.

Table 3-9. Boyer's (1990) Model of Scholarship Aligned With Potential Occupational Therapy Doctorate Capstone Projects

	SCHOLARSHIP OF DISCOVERY	SCHOLARSHIP OF INTEGRATION	SCHOLARSHIP OF APPLICATION	SCHOLARSHIP OF TEACHING AND LEARNING
TYPES OF CAPSTONE PROJECTS	Projects that may advance the knowledge base of a discipline (testing theories, generating knowledge)	Projects that may cross disciplines to create new ideas and/or perspectives	Projects that strive to connect theory to clinical practice; information is identified and applied	Projects that examine the teaching-learning process; facilitation of assisting students to understand and apply information
EXAMPLES OF CAPSTONE PROJECTS	Exploration of the impact of a novel, occupation-based group intervention to improve health and wellness in people with serious mental illness guided by cognitive-behavioral therapy	Interprofessional care planning across disciplines; nursing and occupational therapy collaborating on the impact of medication on falls/patient safety in a nursing home	Development of guidelines to establish a center of excellence in upper extremity rehabilitation	Classroom-based research such as the impact of standardized patient encounters on students perceived sense of clinical efficacy

Table 3-10. Problem Statement Examples

AREA OF SCHOLARSHIP	EVIDENCE	PROBLEM
Discovery	The first multicenter randomized controlled trial of CIMT recruited 222 subjects. However, only 6% of screened participants met the inclusion criteria (Wolf et al., 2008).	Subjects in research are not reflective of the population with whom most occupational therapists work. There is a gap in the knowledge on the impact of CIMT on populations that are reflective of typical practice.
Teaching	Only 2.7% of clinicians used all components of CIMT (Pedlow, Lennon, & Wilson, 2014).	Only a small percentage of clinicians (2.7%) are applying CIMT as the protocol describes. There appears to be a lack of knowledge of the protocol.
Application	75% of occupational therapy/physical therapy participants thought the implementation would be very difficult (Daniel, Howard, Braun, & Page, 2012).	Practical barriers toward implementation of best practice exist.
Integration	Use of interdisciplinary framework on knowledge to address any of the above problems is an example of the scholarship of integration.	

Table 3-11. Example Capstone Focuses

FOCUS AREA	METHOD	GAP	PROBLEM STATEMENT
Clinical practice	Develop advanced skills in the use of CIMT in multiple populations.	A large body of work, with clinical trials and systematic reviews, supports the intervention; however, CIMT is not widely applied in practice (Morris & Taub, 2014).	Only a small percentage of clinicians (2.7%) are applying CIMT as the protocol describes.
Research skills	Develop and deploy feasibility study of CIMT to include subjects that are representative of the context of DCE.		Subjects in research are not reflective of the population with which most occupational therapists work. There is a gap in the knowledge on the impact of CIMT on populations that are reflective of typical practice.
Administration	Develop workflow procedures to ensure clients who meet inclusion criteria for CIMT are offered service.		Practical barriers toward implementation of best practice exist.
Program and policy development	How can CIMT protocol be introduced with fidelity in current DCE environment?		
Advocacy	Engage with third-party payers to support reimbursement for hours of CIMT needed to provide protocol with fidelity.		
Education	Develop and implement training for staff at DCE on CIMT protocols.		Only a small percentage of clinicians (2.7%) are applying CIMT as the protocol describes. There appears to be a lack of knowledge of the protocol.
Theory development	Describe and assess the relationship between a particular non–occupational therapy-based perspective in alignment with one domain of occupational therapy.		Explore the use of the Transtheoretical Model (TTM) to guide occupation-based interventions based on stages of change for people in recovery.

The theory used to guide the capstone project does not need to be an occupational therapy theory. The integration of interdisciplinary knowledge will strengthen the project. The authors of this chapter use and have mentored students who have used theories from psychology, leadership, motor learning, education, and nursing. For example, Dmytryk and DeAngelis (2017) utilized the structure of clinical informatics (computer literacy) as well as a nursing-based TIGER (Technology Informatics Guiding Educational Reform) initiative to guide a descriptive study regarding electronic health record education in Occupational Therapy/Occupational Therapy Assistants curricula across the United States. In another project, a pilot study used the framework of an adult learning theory, (Mezirow's transformative learning) in higher education to inform the teaching of evidence-based practice in occupational therapy curricula (Daly & DeAngelis, 2017). These are just a few examples of non–occupational therapy theoretical perspectives that can guide the development of a capstone project. Chapter 8 builds on this notion of using theory and describes how concept maps can be a useful strategy to organize information and depict relationships between concepts, particularly in regard to measuring outcomes and impact of the capstone project.

The process to develop a capstone project also shares a lot with the field of knowledge translation (KT)—that is, moving what is learned in research to clinical practice (Sudsawad,

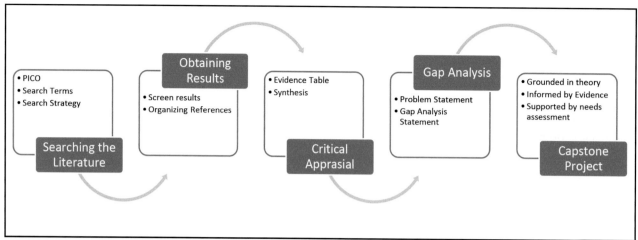

Figure 3-1. A schematic of the literature search and scholarly inquiry process.

2007). KT acknowledges that real-world applications of research-generated knowledge requires a systematic process, implemented by unique stakeholders, in individual contexts. The process of using literature to understand gaps, needs assessment and literature to illuminate why these gaps occur, and evidence and theory to develop real-world solutions, is an example of KT. The capstone project can have meaningful impact on the use of evidence at the DCE site. Both KT and the capstone project require the evaluation of outcomes. Through careful identification of meaningful outcomes and a systematic process to measure and report the outcomes, the distinct meaning and value of the work are seen.

Chapter Summary

This chapter presented recommendations to guide the process of scholarly inquiry for the capstone. Specific steps were presented to develop a course of action to build the capstone project. The capstone project is built out of a gap, defined by the problem identified by the capstone student, and guided in the application by theory (see Figure 3-1).

Equally important to the capstone being rooted in evidence, the capstone should relate to an area of strong interest and passion of the student. The ideal project should reflect capstone students' interests and help to develop skills that will support a professional trajectory. After completion of the DCE and project, graduates may be employed in a different area; however, the skill development of the DCE can enhance professional practice and support individual career trajectories throughout your career.

Learning Activities

1. Reflect on previous work experience or fieldwork experiences.
    a. Identify what was happening and what ideally should be happening.
    b. State the gap.

c. Describe the influence of knowledge, practice, and research on the gap.
    d. Develop a problem statement.
2. Select from the journal articles you retrieved during a recent literature search. Use the PQRS Model to complete the review. Reflect on how you completed each of the four steps:
    P
    Q
    R
    S

References

Accreditation Council for Occupational Therapy Education. (2018). *Standards and interpretive guide.* Retrieved from https://www.aota.org/~/media/Corporate/Files/EducationCareers/Accredit/StandardsReview/2018-ACOTE-Standards-Interpretive-Guide.pdf

American Occupational Therapy Association. (2009). Scholarship in occupational therapy. *American Journal of Occupational Therapy, 63,* 790-796. doi:10.5014/ajot.63-6.790

American Occupational Therapy Association. (2018). Vision 2025. Retrieved from https://www.aota.org/Publications-News/AOTANews/2018/AOTA-Board-Expands-Vision-2025.aspx

Bastian, H., Glasziou, P., & Chalmers, I. (2010). Seventy-five trials and eleven systematic reviews a day: How will we ever keep up? *PLoS Medicine, 7*(9), e1000326. doi:10.1371/journal.pmed.1000326-

Bonnel, W., & Smith, K. (2018). *Proposal writing for clinical nursing and dnp projects* (2nd ed.). New York, NY: books.google.com.

Boyer, E. L. (1990). *Scholarship revisited: Priorities of the professorate.* New York, NY: The Carnegie Foundation.

Cochrane Library. (n.d.). *About the Cochrane Library.* Retrieved from http://www.cochranelibrary.com/about/about-the-cochrane-library.html

Cochrane Linked Data. (2018). *PICO ontology.* Retrieved from http://linkeddata.cochrane.org/pico-ontology

Cohen, G. (1990). Memory. In I. Roth (Ed.), *The Open University's introduction to psychology* (Vol. 2, pp. 570-620). Milton Keynes, England: Erlbaum..

Cole, M. B., & Tufano, R. (2008). *Applied Theories in Occupational Therapy: A Practical Approach* (illustrated.). Thorofare, NJ: SLACK Incorporated.

Daniel, L., Howard, W., Braun, D., & Page, S. J. (2012). Opinions of constraint-induced movement therapy among therapists in southwestern Ohio. *Topics in Stroke Rehabilitation, 19,* 268-275. doi:10.1310/tsr1903-268

Davis-Ajami, M. L., Costa, L., & Kulik, S. (2014). Gap analysis: Synergies and opportunities for effective nursing leadership. *Nursing Economics, 32*(1), 17.

DePoy, E., & Gitlin, L. N. (2016). Introduction to research. *Understanding and applying multiple strategies* (5th ed.). St. Louis, MO: Elsevier.

Daly, M. M., & DeAngelis, T. (2017). Teaching evidence-based practice across curricula—An overview of a professional development course for occupational therapy educators. *Occupational Therapy in Healthcare, 31,* 102-109. doi:http://dx.doi.org/10.1080/07380577.2016.1227892

Dmytryk, L. F., & DeAngelis, T. (2017). Awareness and use of electronic health records in entry-level occupational therapy and occupational therapy assistant curricula. *The Open Journal of Occupational Therapy, 5*(2). doi:http://scholarworks.wmich.edu/ojot/vol5/iss2/11/

EBSCOhealth. (n.d). *CINHAL database.* Retrieved from https://health.ebsco.com/products/the-cinahl-database

Ecker, E. D., & Skelly, A. C. (2010). Conducting a winning literature search. *Evidence-Based Spine-Care Journal, 1,* 9-14. doi:10.1055/s-0028-1100887

Educational Resource Information Center. (n.d.). Frequently Asked Questions. Retrieved from https://eric.ed.gov/?faq

Elsevier. (n.d.). *Embase content.* Retrieved from https://www.elsevier.com/solutions/embase-biomedical-research/embase-coverage-and-content

Google Scholar. (n.d.). Retrieved from https://scholar.google.com/intl/us/scholar/about.html

Howlett, B., Rogo, E., & Shelton, T. G. (2013). *Evidence-based practice for health professionals. An interprofessional approach.* Burlington, MA: Jones and Bartlett Learning.

Huckvale, K., van Velthoven, M., & Car, J. (2011, October). *Screen2Go: A pilot smartphone app for citation screening.* Abstracts of the 19th Cochrane Colloquium, Madrid, Spain. Retrieved from https://www.cochranelibrary.com/cdsr/doi/10.1002/14651858.CD000003/full

Kloda, L. A., & Bartlett, J. C. (2014). A characterization of clinical questions asked by rehabilitation therapists. *Journal of the Medical Library Association, 102,* 69-77. doi:10.3163/1536-5050.102.2.002

Knowles, M. S. (1978). Andragogy: Adult learning theory in perspective. *Community College Review, 5,* 9-20. doi:10.1177/009155217800500302

Lave, J., Wenger, E., & Wenger, E. (1991). *Situated learning: Legitimate peripheral participation.* Cambridge, England: Cambridge University Press.

Lieberman, D., & Scheer, J. (2002). AOTA's evidence-based literature review project: An overview. *American Journal of Occupational Therapy, 56,* 344-349.

Lipscomb, C. E. (2000). Medical subject headings (MeSH). *Bulletin of the Medical Library Association, 88,* 265-266.

Mateen, F. J., Oh, J., Tergas, A. I., Bhayani, N. H., & Kamdar, B. B. (2013). Titles versus titles and abstracts for initial screening of articles for systematic reviews. *Clinical Epidemiology, 5,* 89-95. doi:10.2147/CLEP.S43118

McMaster University. (n.d.). REHAB+. *About this site.* Retrieved from https://plus.mcmaster.ca/rehab/Pages/About

Moher, D., Liberati, A., Tetzlaff, J., Altman, D. G., & PRISMA Group. (2009). Preferred reporting items for systematic reviews and meta-analyses: The PRISMA statement. *PLoS Medicine, 6,* e1000097. doi:10.1371/journal.pmed.1000097

Morris, D. M., & Taub, E. (2014). Training model for promoting translation from research to clinical settings: University of Alabama at Birmingham training for constraint-induced movement therapy. *Journal of Rehabilitation Research and Development, 51,* xi-ivii.

National Institutes of Health U.S. National Library of Medicine. (2018). *PubMed: MEDLINE® Retrieval on the World Wide Web.* Retrieved from https://www.nlm.nih.gov/bsd/pubmed.html

OT Seeker. (n.d.). Retrieved from http://www.otseeker.com

Pedlow, K., Lennon, S., & Wilson, C. (2014). Application of constraint-induced movement therapy in clinical practice: an online survey. *Archives of Physical Medicine and Rehabilitation, 95,* 276-282. doi:10.1016/j.apmr.2013.08.240

PEDro. (n.d.). *Welcome to PEDro.* Retrieved from https://www.pedro.org.au/

PsycBITE. (n.d.). Retrieved from http://psycbite.com/web/cms/content/home

PsycINFO. (n.d.). Retrieved from http://www.apa.org/pubs/databases/psycinfo/

Sackett, D. L., Rosenberg, W. M., Gray, J. M., Haynes, R. B., & Richardson, W. S. (1996). Evidence based medicine: What it is and what it isn't. *BMJ, 312,* 71-72.

Stern, C., Jordan, Z., & McArthur, A. (2014). Developing the review question and inclusion criteria. *The American Journal of Nursing, 114,* 53-56. doi:10.1097/01.NAJ.0000445689.67800.86

Sudsawad, P. (2007). Knowledge translation: Introduction to models, strategies and measures.

Tricco, A. C., Antony, J., Zarin, W., Strifler, L., Ghassemi, M., Ivory, J., … Straus, S. E. (2015). A scoping review of rapid review methods. *BMC Medicine, 13,* 224. doi:10.1186/s12916-015-0465-6

Ulu, H., & Akyol, H. (2016). The effects of repetitive reading and PQRS strategy in the development of reading skill. *Eurasian Journal of Educational Research, 63,* 225-242. http://dx.doi.org/ 10.14689/ejer.2016.63-13

Wolf, S. L., Winstein, C. J., Miller, J. P., Thompson, P. A., Taub, E., Uswatte, G., … Clark, P. C. (2008). Retention of upper limb function in stroke survivors who have received constraint-induced movement therapy: The EXCITE randomised trial. *Lancet Neurology, 7,* 33-40. doi:10.1016/S1474-4422(07)70294-6

Wu, Y. P., Aylward, B. S., Roberts, M. C., & Evans, S. C. (2012). Searching the scientific literature: Implications for quantitative and qualitative reviews. *Clinical Psychology Review, 32,* 553-557.

<u>Appendix 3-A</u>

PICO TERMS LIST WORKSHEET

PICO Question:

Databases Searched:

Inclusion and Exclusion Criteria:

- Patient characteristics:
- Study types: systematic reviews_____meta-analyses_____randomized controlled trials_____ Cohort_____case controlled_____other_____
- Date of publication (years):
- Languages:

P	AND	I	AND	C	AND	O
or		or		or		or
or		or		or		or
or		or		or		or
or		or		or		or
or		or		or		or

Appendix 3-B

PICO Terms List Worksheet

PICO Question: How does occupational therapy impact a patient's quality of life in the treatment of relapsing-remitting multiple sclerosis?

Database Searched: PubMed

Potential Search Terms - Concepts

P			I			C			O
relapsing-remitting multiple sclerosis	A		occupational therapy OR **"Occupational Therapy"[Mesh]**	A		comparison omitted for this PICO question	A		quality of life OR **"Quality of Life"[Mesh]**
OR	N		OR	N		OR	N		OR
"Multiple Sclerosis, Relapsing-Remitting"[Mesh]	D		diet management OR "Nutrition Therapy"[Mesh]	D			D		"Patient Reported Outcome Measures"[Mesh] OR "Treatment Outcome"[Mesh]
OR			OR			OR			OR
multiple sclerosis OR "Multiple Sclerosis"[Mesh]			energy conservation OR "Energy Metabolism"[Mesh] OR **fatigue management**						"Outcome Assessment (Health Care)"[Mesh] OR **"Activities of Daily Living"[Mesh]**
OR			OR			OR			OR
			"Exercise Therapy"[Mesh] OR "Resistance Training"[Mesh]						**"Mobility Limitation"[Mesh]** OR "Patient Outcome Assessment"[Mesh]
OR			OR			OR			OR
			assistive devices OR **"Self-Help Devices"[Mesh]**						**"Range of Motion, Articular"[Mesh]**
OR			OR			OR			OR
			"Pain Management"[Mesh]						

PubMed Search = 36 results

((((relapsing remitting multiple sclerosis) OR "Multiple Sclerosis, Relapsing-Remitting"[Mesh])) AND ((((("Occupational Therapy"[Mesh]) OR "Exercise Therapy"[Mesh]) OR "Self-Help Devices"[Mesh])) OR ((fatigue management) OR assistive devices))) AND ((((("Quality of Life"[Mesh]) OR "Activities of Daily Living"[Mesh]) OR "Mobility Limitation"[Mesh]) OR "Range of Motion, Articular"[Mesh])

Appendix 3-C
PRISMA

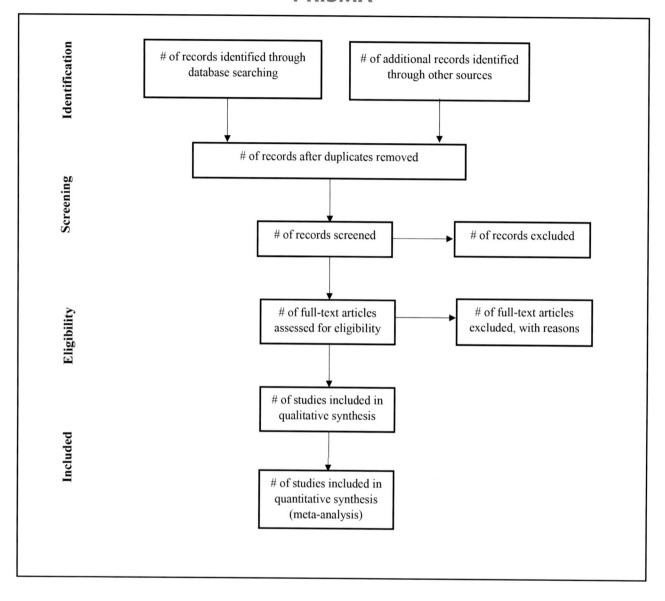

Appendix 3-D

Sample PICOs Using Focus Areas

FOCUS AREA	SAMPLE PICO(S)
Clinical Practice	• What is the effect of equine-facilitated wellness therapy on the quality of life for adults with substance use disorders? • Do classroom-level interventions for elementary students with emotional disturbances reduce maladaptive behaviors and improve academic performance?
Research	• Are sensory based strategies effective at reducing negative behaviors in long term care facilities? • For surgeons, what is the likelihood that occupational therapy ergonomic interventions to decrease work-related musculoskeletal disorders (MSDs)? • Are individuals with a history of opioid addiction who are prescribed Suboxone alone more likely to report relapse than those individuals who utilize cognitive behavioral strategies along with Suboxone?
Administration	• What is the impact of participation in occupational, physical and speech therapy on hospital admission after discharge for skilled nursing facilities? • What is the effect of mechanical lifting equipment on work related injuries for occupational therapists, when compared to traditional manual lifting for patient care?
Leadership	• In occupational therapy leaders, how does participating in an evidence-based leadership curriculum vs not participating affect staff retention, staff satisfaction and quality of care? • How does transformational/complexity leadership style compare to transactional leadership style affect occupational therapy practitioner retention and satisfaction?
Program Development	**Clinical** • Does community transition programing during inpatient rehabilitation improve community mobility and social participation once discharged to home? • What is the effectiveness of mindfulness practice on people with chronic pain for work-related outcomes? **Community** • What falls prevention programming is most effective for use with community-dwelling older adults in an adult day center? • What is the effect of occupational therapy in addressing the transition from school to work with individuals with an intellectual or developmental delay?
Policy	• What is this impact of an education program for occupational therapists on occupational justice on the well-being and quality of life of those residing in long-term care facilities? • How will policy development and education to occupational practitioners on issues of sexuality and the importance of addressing the sexuality needs of rehabilitation patients affect patient quality of life?
Advocacy	• For children with disabilities, do peer-mentored programs facilitate participation in 4-H (a nonprofit organization for youth)? • For refugee families from Somalia, how can occupational therapy have a positive effect on their occupational performance as they begin the process of resettlement?
Education	• Among OTD students, does taking the NBCOT certification exam within two months of graduating result in higher pass rates compared to taking the exam later? • Should health professionals' education and training institutions use simulation methods to support successful completion of clinical rotations?
Theory Development	• Will a gender-as-occupation model improve occupational therapy practice for transgender and gender non-conforming individuals?

CHAPTER 4

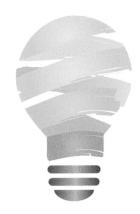

Capstone Site Development and Communication

Julie A. Bednarski, OTD, MHS, OTR
Rebecca Barton, DHS, OTR, FAOTA

Human-Centered Design Mindsets for the Doctoral Students

Human-centered design mindset concepts of learning from failure and continuing to embrace ambiguity are important for doctoral students to embrace as they embark on planning for a site and finding a site mentor for the capstone experience and project.

Learning From Failure: It takes time to determine a potential site for your experience and project, and not all initial ideas will be successful. Do not give up! Keep on communicating and reaching out to sites with your ideas, and you will find a site that needs help solving a problem. The first site you meet with may not be a good fit, but learn from the first site meeting and continue on to find another site, which may end up being the perfect fit. By meeting with people, you will continue to grow your doctoral capstone experience and project.

Embrace Ambiguity: Remember ambiguity allows you to be creative, and new ideas are formed from embracing ambiguity. You do not know the answers before you begin communicating with sites, and that is okay. You want the sites to communicate to you their specific needs and problems for you to assist in seeking solutions.

INTRODUCTION

The final phase in the development of the doctoral capstone experience (DCE) and project is site development. Development of sites for the capstone student is important and involves exceptional communication and education. Capstone placements tend to have more ambiguity than fieldwork placements because the DCE is a newer concept—not only to occupational therapy programs but also to fieldwork sites and community partners. Many occupational therapy programs are now developing their DCE frameworks while simultaneously educating and communicating with current sites while developing new sites (Evenson & Connor, 2015). Developing the DCE requires communication and collaboration with the occupational therapy student and potential sitessite mentor and is often a process of communication different from that of fieldwork. The differences between fieldwork and capstone experience placements are explored in this chapter. The DCE and project process is unknown to many sites, and there are often misconceptions about what

Deluliis ED, Bednarski JA.
The Entry Level Occupational Therapy Doctorate Capstone:
A Framework for The Experience and Project (pp 61-74).

the capstone is and what it is not. As the capstone development and inspiration continues, it is important to establish communication with both traditional and role-emerging areas of practice sites. This chapter assists the reader in exploring potential capstone sites, relationship development, and the importance of initial communication.

Capstone Student Reflective Questions

During the final steps of the development phase of the doctoral capstone, the occupational therapy student may find it helpful to reflect on the following questions:

1. What potential sites or populations do you have in mind for your DCE?

2. Think about your surrounding (or home) community. Are there unmet needs? If so, what are they?

3. Are you familiar with a specific site through Level I and Level II fieldwork or other means that might be of interest to you? If so, what are the sites?

4. What is your occupational therapy program's policy and expectations regarding communication with potential capstone sites?

Chapter Objectives

By the end of this chapter and completing the learning activities, the reader should be able to:

1. Compare and contrast site procurement for the fieldwork experience and the DCE.

2. Articulate a flow of communication to the DCE sites.

3. Determine a plan for site development in both the traditional roles and role-emerging areas of practice.

4. Assess how different rules and regulations may influence the DCE plan.

ROLES OVERVIEW

Chapter 1 explored the similarities and differences in the overall definitions of fieldwork Level I, Level II, and the DCE and project. This chapter begins by broadly exploring the roles of the academic fieldwork coordinator vs the capstone coordinator to give a foundation for the discussion of site communication and procurement. The academic fieldwork coordinator is responsible for the fieldwork curriculum and must ensure that fieldwork not only meets the Accreditation Council for Occupational Therapy Education (ACOTE) requirements but also is integrated within the academic program curricular threads and goals. The doctoral capstone coordinator is responsible for the capstone experience and project and also must adhere to the ACOTE requirements and "ensure that the doctoral capstone is designed through collaboration of the faculty and student, and provided in setting(s) consistent with the program's curriculum design" (ACOTE, 2018, p. 44). Both the doctoral capstone

coordinator and the academic fieldwork coordinator have multifaceted responsibilities, including education to faculty and administration, student education and preparation, and site development and oversight. Table 4-1 gives the reader a comparison of the roles and responsibilities of the academic fieldwork coordinator and the capstone coordinator.

Education to Faculty and Administration

Education to faculty and administration at the academic institution on the overall program, whether fieldwork or capstone, is often the first task of both the academic fieldwork coordinator and the doctoral capstone coordinator. Once faculty and administration have an understanding of each program, moving on to educating potential sites and site personnel is important. Throughout this educational process, the academic fieldwork coordinator and doctoral capstone coordinator are ensuring compliance of ACOTE Standards and establishing the legal agreements between the site and the academic institution.

Student Education and Preparation

Student education and preparation is another important role taken on by both the academic fieldwork educator and capstone coordinator. In preparation for both fieldwork and the DCE, professionalism is important to address with students. The academic fieldwork coordinator and doctoral capstone coordinator are educators and role models to the doctoral students for professional behaviors needed for fieldwork and the DCE (DeIuliis, 2017). Professional (practice-ready) behaviors and the importance of professional communications for the capstone student is an area addressed in Chapter 5. Determining fieldwork sites vs capstone sites is a different process, and students need to be aware of this early in their academic program. Education to students on the processes and expectations of fieldwork and DCEs is a role of both the academic fieldwork educator and doctoral capstone coordinator. This leads into the role of site development and oversight, which is another responsibility of the academic fieldwork coordinator and doctoral capstone coordinator.

Establishing and Developing New Sites

The academic fieldwork coordinator and doctoral capstone coordinator each have a significant role in establishing and developing fieldwork and DCE sites that will serve as an educational experience for students. From a fieldwork perspective, initiation of new sites often occurs when students are wanting to complete Level I or Level II fieldwork at a location where the fieldwork program does not have a current relationship. This same process will occur for initiation of a DCE site. Both the academic fieldwork coordinator and doctoral capstone coordinator are responsible for developing relationships with new sites that will meet the needs of the fieldwork and DCE programs. Both programs should be

Table 4-1. Role Comparison Between Academic Fieldwork and Doctoral Capstone Coordinators

ACADEMIC FIELDWORK COORDINATOR	DOCTORAL CAPSTONE COORDINATOR
Faculty and Administrative Education	
• Education of faculty and administration on the FW program • Assurance of compliance of ACOTE FW standards • Facilitation of legal agreements with FW sites • Education to students, sites, FW educators on all aspects of FW	• Overall education to faculty and administration on the capstone experience and project • Assurance of compliance of ACOTE DCE standards • Facilitation of legal agreements with DCE sites • Education to faculty mentors, site mentors, and students
Student Education and Preparation	
• Model and reinforce professional behaviors • Provide guidance to student in order to best match the student to the FW site • Integrate classroom learning with application to the FW setting • Provide education about the FW settings and expectations • Provide feedback on FW performance	• Model and reinforce professional behaviors • Collaborate with student on site identification • Integrate classroom learning for application to DCE setting • Provide education on self-directed learning and expectations of the DCE • Provide feedback on DCE performance
Site Development and Oversite	
• Develop new FW sites • Provide education regarding FW best practice • Mentor existing FW educators • Complete ongoing program evaluation	• Establish and develop new DCE sites and build relationships • Mentor and collaborate with current DCE sites • Determine which current FW sites may be appropriate DCE sites • Complete ongoing program evaluation
FW=fieldwork.	

congruent with the academic program and with accreditation standards (ACOTE, 2018).

Once a site is established, it is important to continue to build on the relationship and keep fieldwork/DCE site personnel up to date on new policies or ACOTE Standard changes, as well as occupational therapy curriculum information. For example, if students are completing Level I fieldwork, it is important that the fieldwork site and personnel understand the curriculum sequence and courses the students have completed. Students are encouraged to share their current knowledge of best practice learned within the classroom. Students can share with the fieldwork educators their course content and learning activities that they have completed before fieldwork or what they will be doing in future coursework. This reciprocal education between the fieldwork educator and the fieldwork students can be a rich experience. In addition, the role of the academic fieldwork coordinator can be "professionally rewarding and (involves) factors contributing to perceptions of professional reward" (Stutz-Tanenbaum, Greene, Hanson, & Koski, 2017, p. 20).

As sites are developed and relationships are established, students begin their site exploration for both fieldwork and the capstone experience. These are different processes and require different communication.

FIELDWORK SITE EXPLORATION

When first exploring fieldwork sites, students should consider the various settings in which practice occurs and the populations that would benefit from the distinct value of occupational therapy. This process may actually start informally before students enter the academic program through exploration of the occupational therapy profession as a possible career. As students continue this exploration during their courses, the exploration process deepens as they start to think about what lies ahead with their fieldwork placements. Investigating the fieldwork sites with whom the academic program has a relationship is a first step in exploring where the student would like to go for Level I and Level II fieldwork. The American Occupational Therapy Association

(AOTA) Fieldwork Data Form (FDF) is one tool that can facilitate student exploration of potential sites (AOTA, 2017). Occupational therapy faculty should have access to the AOTA FDF if this information has been provided to the academic fieldwork coordinator by the site.

In addition, students should be encouraged to research areas of practice and specific practice sites and settings used by the academic program to have a better understanding of the occupational therapy generalist. Students often come to the academic program with ideas for occupational therapy fieldwork placements based on previous shadowing experiences. More ideas will surface as the students continue to learn about the practice of occupational therapy in their didactic courses. The academic fieldwork coordinator will also facilitate this exploration during the education and planning phase and the fieldwork selection process.

Exploration of potential doctoral capstone sites begins in the development stage of the capstone as students are exposed to potential sites through in-class site presentations, previous doctoral student experiences, student contacts within their community, fieldwork placements, and community contacts through the school. Exploration of capstone sites is discussed later in this chapter.

FIELDWORK COMMUNICATION

The role of the academic fieldwork coordinator is to facilitate communication with the various fieldwork sites via fieldwork educators and, when applicable, the clinical coordinator of fieldwork (Hanson & DeIuliis, 2015). It is essential that there is congruence between the fieldwork site and the academic program (ACOTE, 2018). Does the fieldwork site embrace and exemplify the goals and objectives of the academic curriculum? Is best practice at the fieldwork site current with regard to evidence and accreditation standards? Do both the students and the fieldwork educators know what is expected of them?

It is important for students and their fieldwork educators to understand the policies and procedures of fieldwork and the importance of professional communication. With regard to fieldwork, most academic settings have procedures regarding communication between potential fieldwork sites and fieldwork educators. Traditionally, the academic fieldwork coordinator will be the point person in developing appropriate fieldwork sites including making initial contact with the fieldwork site regarding a student placement for Level I or Level II fieldwork. In addition, the academic fieldwork coordinator may be interviewing the fieldwork site clinical coordinator or potential individual fieldwork educators. The following are potential questions an academic fieldwork coordinator may ask when meeting with a potential fieldwork site.

TEXT BOX 4-1

The interview may consist of inquiring about what type of practice settings are available:

- Is this site a large hospital with many areas of practice?
- What is the age range of clients, and what type of occupational therapy programming is currently being used? Does the site currently host students from other schools for fieldwork?
- Are there existing goals and objectives for fieldwork from the site perspective?
- What is the supervision process at the fieldwork setting, and does this process meet ACOTE accreditation standards?
- Have the occupational therapy practitioners been provided with resources and training for their role as fieldwork educators?
- Does this potential fieldwork site have the resources and desire to provide an appropriate educational experience for Level I or Level II fieldwork?
- What is the supervision model for students?

In planning formal fieldwork experiences, most academic programs and traditional fieldwork sites prefer that the initial contact from the school come from the academic fieldwork coordinator rather than from individual students because of the administrative and educational questions noted in the preceding text box. In addition, some sites receive numerous requests and have organizational guidelines that are best addressed first by the academic fieldwork coordinator and the clinical coordinator at the fieldwork site. That being said, some sites require a face-to-face or phone interview, and those that do not may still appreciate the personal outreach.

In some areas of practice, students must shadow for a day to ascertain whether this is a good match for the student, the fieldwork educator, and the population. For instance, if a student wants to complete a fieldwork rotation in an area such as burns and wound care, it may be a fieldwork site requirement for that student to spend time with an occupational therapy practitioner working in this area of practice before being considered for placement.

FIELDWORK GOALS AND OBJECTIVES

Through guided learning, students will inevitably experience emotions and some ambiguity, especially at the beginning of the fieldwork rotation. For that matter, fieldwork educators may experience the same thing as they embark on training students. It is important to have clearly established goals and objectives for the student to reduce ambiguity (AOTA, 2009; Dickerson, 2006). Establishing goals and objectives is also needed for the DCE; however, it is a different process and is discussed later in this chapter. In contrast to the DCE site, the fieldwork site develops goals and objectives specific to that site before taking students. To facilitate this process, it is necessary for supervising personnel to have good interpersonal skills that can be modeled for students during fieldwork. These behavioral goals are developed in collaboration with the site and the academic fieldwork coordinator based on entry-level expectations for that specific site so that students are clear on what is expected of them (ACOTE, 2018). Even with these established goals and objectives, there will be times of ambiguity, and there are many multifaceted factors to consider in fieldwork, including the client's areas of concern, the family, the other disciplines involved, different approaches to practice, and many more. Learning to negotiate and analyze these factors that do not always follow the "protocol" or "what I learned in a textbook" creates ambiguity and may ultimately disrupt the student's plan. Some might call this a failure, but really, it is an opportunity for growth and improvement as noted in human-centered design.

DOCTORAL CAPSTONE SITE COMMUNICATION

Collaboration between the academic fieldwork coordinator and the doctoral capstone coordinator is a key aspect of developing capstone sites. At the start, it is important for the academic fieldwork coordinator and the doctoral capstone coordinator to educate the current fieldwork sites and community sites to the capstone experience and process. This preemptive communication will allow questions to be asked and misconceptions eliminated. The earlier in the process these educational meetings can take place, the better. The goals of these meetings reach beyond education and information gathering. These meetings often lead to discussion of site needs and how a capstone student may be able to assist in filling a need at the site. During the meetings, the capstone coordinator can also be determining congruence between the capstone experience site and the academic program.

TEACHING TIP 1: If the occupational therapy doctoral (OTD) program is new or has transitioned from a master's to a doctoral program, it is recommended that meetings with the doctoral capstone coordinator and the academic fieldwork coordinator are set up with fieldwork sites, especially larger hospitals, to discuss how the DCE is different from fieldwork. The goal of these meetings should be to educate the sites on the new ACOTE Standards for the capstone experience and project, discuss your school's process of the doctoral capstone, and describe the differences between fieldwork and the capstone. These meetings can also lead to brainstorming ideas for projects at the sites.

TEACHING TIP 2: *In my role as the capstone coordinator at the University of Indianapolis, I was able to meet with the therapy managers of a large local hospital to explain our program's transition to the OTD degree and the addition of the DCE and project. During this educational meeting, the managers identified potential program development needs, clinical skills areas, leadership areas, and research opportunities for the students. This led to one of the managers visiting class and describing to the students her ideas for potential capstone experiences and projects at the hospital as they were in the development phase. This in turn led to three students completing their capstones at that hospital system in 2018.*

—Julie A. Bednarski, OTD, MHS, OTR
Clinical Associate Professor
Associate Program Director
School of Health & Human Sciences
Department of Occupational Therapy
Indiana University
Indianapolis, Indiana

When meeting with sites to discuss the doctoral capstone process, the questions that are asked may be different from those that are asked to potential fieldwork sites. Plan ahead for these meetings and prepare questions. Table 4-2 identifies potential questions a doctoral capstone coordinator may ask when meeting with a potential capstone experience sites that are community or role-emerging sites.

Throughout the conversation at the site, think about your program's curricular threads (e.g., evidence based, occupation based, professionalism) and design. Determine if there is a link between the site and your program. For example, the site may be an adult day center and use a person-centered approach. The site director states that the "person" is central to all aspects of care and provides training to all staff on the person-centered approach. The site director is involved in the community and stays up to date on literature and legislation related to older adults and adult day centers. This philosophy is in congruence with the school's philosophy and this site appears to be a good fit.

TEXT BOX 4-2

In my role as the capstone coordinator at the University of Indianapolis, I found myself meeting with all types of people from a variety of organizations. Oftentimes I was reaching out and meeting with personal or professional connections I had, or people my colleagues, friends, and/or family members connected me with.

Table 4-2. Questions for Potential Community and/or Role-Emerging Sites

- What is the mission of your organization? (This will allow the doctoral capstone coordinator to determine whether there is a link between the organization and your program's mission.)
- Who are the clients you serve?
- What is the organizational structure?
- What types of professionals serve the clients, and are there any occupational therapists within the organization?
- Do you have personnel whom you feel may want to be a site mentors, and what are their educational backgrounds?
- Do you have students from other disciplines that serve your organization?
- What are your funding sources?
- What types of services do you provide?

TEXT BOX 4-2 (continued)

I love going out to sites to explain the doctoral capstone process and finding a link with an organization—finding the win-win connection. I have been meeting some wonderful people doing amazing things to improve the lives of others. Seeing the "light bulb" moment when they realize how occupational therapy can contribute to their mission is the start of a great partnership and how capstone projects begin.

—Julie A. Bednarski, OTD, MHS, OTR
Clinical Associate Professor
Associate Program Director
School of Health & Human Sciences
Department of Occupational Therapy
Indiana University
Indianapolis, Indiana

Questions that the doctoral capstone coordinator may ask when visiting traditional sites or that already have an established relationship with the program through fieldwork will be different from those discussed in Table 4-2. Table 4-3 give examples of potential questions for traditional sites or those with an established relationship through fieldwork.

Again, throughout the conversation, think about the link of the site to your program's curriculum design. Is there a link, and if so, what is it? Does the site provide services to an underserved, marginalized population? Does it practice an evidence-based approach to care? If social justice or occupational justice are central to your program design and the site is a public, urban hospital that serves all regardless of payer source, this may be a good collaboration.

There may be times the capstone student is making the first contact with a site, and the capstone coordinator may become involved in education after the initial communication. An example of when a capstone student may meet with a new site before the capstone coordinator is if the student already has a well-established relationship with the site. It is important, however, to discuss how site communication and

exploration will take place within your individual programs. Establishing a policy for communication will be helpful and is discussed later in the chapter. One-on-one meetings between the capstone coordinator and capstone student is important as site exploration begins. Some students may have well-established community connections and ideas for a site and project secondary to prior experiences.

TEXT BOX 4-3

From elementary to high school, I was a competitive cheerleader and always had a passion to start a cheerleading team for those with special needs in my hometown. As I went through school to one day become an occupational therapist, I thought those dreams would be put on the back burner. Little did I know the opportunities that the DCE would bring me. I am bringing my past passions into my future schooling, allowing the process to be easier and allowing my passion to guide me. In 2020, with the opportunity given by the doctoral capstone class, I will be starting a cheerleading program for special needs in my hometown, and I cannot wait! This cheerleading program for individuals with special needs will allow for so many opportunities that most people in this population do not have access to in my hometown. They will have the opportunity to learn basic cheerleading and tumbling skills, engage in social interactions, have a peer mentorship experience, and potentially increase their quality of life!

—Megan Kraft
Doctoral Occupational Therapy Student
Class of 2020
School of Occupational Therapy
University of Indianapolis
Indianapolis, Indiana

Table 4-3. Potential Questions for Traditional Fieldwork Sites

- Are you familiar with the DCE?
- Have you had any previous DCE students?
- Where do you see a fit for a DCE student?
- What types of clients do you serve?
- What types of services do you offer?
- What programming do you currently have at the site, and do you have program development needs?
- Are you doing research, and if so, do you have student involvement?
- What new initiatives has your organization identified?

Communication and Site Exploration Process for the Doctoral Capstone Experience

As we have noted, the academic fieldwork coordinator takes the lead on the fieldwork site procurement and development in most programs; however, this is not always the case for the capstone. For the DCE, the student may take the lead, working in collaboration with the capstone coordinator to identify a site that is a good match. Figure 4-1 gives the reader a visual of the site communication process for the DCE.

Initiating Communication With Proposed Sites

As students begin the development phase for their DCEs, first the students need to spend time brainstorming potential sites based on their proposed idea or focus area of interest. One way to do this is for the doctoral capstone coordinator (or occupational therapy faculty) to invite site personnel to the class when the OTD students begin the development phase of their capstones. This provides an excellent way to exchange ideas. It is a time for the sites to discuss their needs and ideas and for the student to get inspired about ideas for potential sites that might welcome them and their project purpose. Jirikowic et al. (2015) recommends having community and clinic sites present proposals on potential projects they would like to have master's level capstone students complete. The faculty members determine which proposals will move forward to the students, and the students rank their choices for capstone experiences and projects based on the proposals the site has outlined. This model could also be used for DCEs.

Throughout this process, it is important for the student to reflect back on the mindset of embracing ambiguity in human-centered design. Identifying a site is a process, and there is not a cookie-cutter or perfected method for securing the site that matches the student's doctoral capstone project purpose. Not all sites will be a good match for students and their idea, and not all sites will agree to take a capstone student. This can be frustrating to students because things may not "fall into place" as they would like. Students are driving the process and need to make decisions relative to site identification based on their project purpose and persevere until a site is mutually agreed on. The process of identifying and securing a DCE site has many ambiguities, and if the student can embrace this, it will be a more positive experience.

Although it can be done several ways, a determination needs to be made as to the process for securing capstone experience placements. Who will make the initial contact? Will the student be the one to reach out to the site, or will the doctoral capstone coordinator reach out first? A well-established policy is required if students are to understand their role in site procurement. Because this is a self-directed experience, it is important for students to take the lead in initiating site contacts when possible.

TEACHING TIP 3: Developing a policy for the initial communication with a potential site mentor is an important first step, and it is recommended that a policy be developed so that all parties understand responsibility. One recommendation may be to have this policy in the DCE and project section of the OTD program's student handbook. A simple statement could be as follows:

Sample Policy: Capstone students must FIRST identify whether the site they are interested in for their capstone is currently a fieldwork site for the program. If the site IS a current fieldwork site, the capstone coordinator will contact the site FIRST to establish the initial interest in taking a capstone student. If the site IS NOT a current fieldwork site, the capstone student may reach out to the potential site FIRST to describe the capstone experience and project, but the capstone coordinator must be notified that this conversation is taking place.

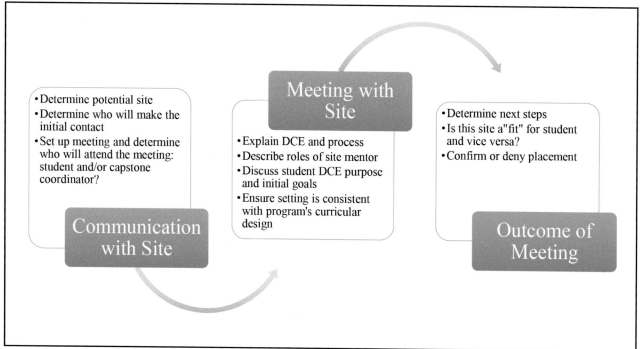

Figure 4-1. DCE flow of site communication.

Communication via email is often one of the first modes of communication to potential sites. Establishing email templates for the capstone student and doctoral capstone coordinator will be helpful in ensuring professionalism with the capstone student and reducing time for the capstone coordinator. Appendix 4-A at the end of the chapter provides examples for email communications for both the capstone student and doctoral capstone coordinator.

Communication with sites will be much more fluid than that for fieldwork Level I and Level II because students may be reaching out to make initial contact. Table 4-4 illustrates the differences in the type of communications between fieldwork sites and DCE sites.

Meetings With Sites

Once a determination is made as to who will make the initial contact with the site, individual meetings with sites may be an appropriate next step. This can take place over the phone, in person, or in an introductory email. This is important especially if; the OTD program is new in the state, or if the program is transitioning from the master of occupational therapy degree to an OTD degree, or if the transition has already occurred. The sites that OTD programs already have established relationships need to be provided education on the DCE and project process.

TEXT BOX 4-4

The DCE and project was a new concept for us, and we had never taken a capstone student, so we were not sure how it was all going to work. We had some initial meetings with the capstone coordinator at the school and were educated on the process, which was helpful and allowed us to spend time formulating ideas for potential projects. After these initial educational meetings, we were able to come into a doctoral capstone planning course and discussed needs we had in our hospital system with the students. Students who were interested interviewed and discussed goals and objectives before being accepted at our site as a capstone student. These interviews proved to be very beneficial to ensure we felt students would be successful with their project plan and that students felt comfortable in the setting. We feel the interview sets the student up for success and will continue this process as we move forward.

—Angela K. Palicki, OTR
Manager
Outpatient Rehabilitation Services
Eskenazi Health
Indianapolis, Indiana

—Hannah Porterfield, MOT, OTR, CSRS
Center Coordinator of Clinical Education
Rehabilitation Services
Eskenazi Health
Indianapolis, Indiana

—Theresa Rexroat, MS, OTR, NTMTC
Occupational Therapy—NICU
Eskenazi Health
Indianapolis, Indiana

Table 4-4. Site Communication: Fieldwork Versus Doctoral Capstone Experience

FIELDWORK SITES	DOCTORAL CAPSTONE EXPERIENCE SITES
Initial contact communication: directed by the academic fieldwork coordinator	Initial contact communication: either student or doctoral capstone coordinator depending on: • The relationship the site has with the school (often the doctoral capstone coordinator will reach out to a site that is already a fieldwork site) • The relationship the site has with the student • The relationship the site has with the doctoral capstone coordinator • The type of site • The policy established by the program
Site procurement: academic fieldwork coordinator	Site procurement: student or doctoral capstone coordinator
Verification of student at site and contract procurement: academic fieldwork coordinator	Verification of student at site and contract procurement: doctoral capstone coordinator

It is important for these sites to understand the differences in expectations, supervision (mentorship), and outcomes between the Level I or Level II fieldwork student and the doctoral capstone student. Identifying sites can be done through the following:

- Current sites that have established contracts with the school, including both medical sites (e.g., hospitals, outpatient centers) and community sites
- Sites with which the student has connections that are new to the academic institution (both traditional and role-emerging sites)
- Community sites that have reached out to the academic institution in the past for collaboration

The purpose of the initial site meeting should be to first explain the DCE to the site and have students clearly articulate their DCE project purpose and goals. This will help the site determine whether they are able to meet students' needs. During this meeting, the student and/or capstone coordinator needs to determine whether the site/mentor will be a good fit and vice versa and then begin establishing potential goals and objectives. A second purpose is to determine whether the site can provide an experience that aligns with the occupational therapy program's curriculum design (ACOTE, 2018). Who needs to attend the meeting depends on the site. If the student meets with a site first, the capstone coordinator will also need to meet with the site to determine whether it will be able to meet the planned capstone design and to be consistent with the program's curriculum design. The process of establishing the initial site meeting is different for each site, and there is no one right or wrong way to proceed with the initial meeting. Here is how one capstone student explains initiating communication with her site:

TEXT BOX 4-5

During the planning stages, I emailed the site I was interested in and provided them with a description of the DCE. I asked if I could meet in person to discuss any ideas they had, along with ideas I had developed. After, I met with the management team to discuss the requirements of the DCE. During that meeting, the topic for my DCE was solidified in that I would be working alongside the outcomes committee to improve the evaluation process. During this planning stage, the outcomes committee also did some planning before the start of my DCE. As a team, they identified assessments they thought would add value to their evaluations and helped complete the needs assessment for the site.
—Sarah Humbird, OTD, OTR
Class of 2018
School of Occupational Therapy
University of Indianapolis
Indianapolis, Indiana

Outcome of Site Meeting

Once the meeting takes place, it is important to determine the next steps. Will this be a good match for the student? Does the site agree to take the student for the capstone experience? Does the site feel it is not a good fit and they will not be able to meet the students needs? An outcome needs to be determined. The site may say yes or no to taking the student, or may need more information.

Common Misconceptions

Recent evidence indicates decreased awareness of the benefits of the entry level occupational therapy degree (Molitor & Nissen, 2018), which includes the capstone. A frequently heard misconception is that the capstone is an additional Level II fieldwork placement. Education to sites is an important first step in placing a capstone student at a site for the experience. Along with the sites understanding the differences, it is also important that the doctoral student to be able to articulate the differences.

TEACHING TIP 4: Fieldwork sites need to understand that DCE students are expected to be self-directed. Often, the prospective mentors at the site worry about how they will fill the students time. Management of time and projects are the student's responsibility. The mentors need to understand the benefits of having a capstone student. For example, the student can meet the needs of an occupational therapy department by providing program development, which often cannot be done by the staff occupational therapy practitioners due to productivity standards.

Benefits and Incentives of Taking a Doctoral Student

Evenson and Connor (2015) discussed improving professional development, creative program development, and strengthening the link between academia and practice as benefits to the site taking a capstone student. The fieldwork relationship has the potential for students to share new knowledge gained in evidence-based curricula, in addition to new technological ways of doing practice. A definite reciprocal learning experience occurs between the fieldwork educator and their students. The students learn from the many years of experience that the fieldwork educators have to offer and how organizations work. They learn the actual "doing" of what they read on the pages of their occupational therapy textbooks. In turn, the fieldwork educators learn new evidence and occupation-based ideas from their students (Hanson, 2012). In addition, fieldwork educators are allowed to use fieldwork education as professional development for state and national continuing education requirements. As stated in the National Board for Certification in Occupational Therapy (NBCOT) Certification Renewal Activities Chart, NBCOT accepts supervision of entry-level or postdoctoral advanced fieldwork direct supervision for renewal certification. This reciprocal learning process is a win-win because it enriches the whole profession. Likewise, it is anticipated that this same enrichment will continue through the DCE and maybe to an even greater degree as the circle of influence is broadened. The opportunity for students to work not only with occupational therapy practitioners but with a myriad of other professionals who are experts in their fields will allow future clinicians to practice with a deeper understanding of their role in health care. The academic fieldwork coordinator and capstone coordinator will frequently have discussions with fieldwork educators and site mentors about

the need for more resources, and innovations. These discussions allow for a creative exchange of potential program development needs and solving problems through both fieldwork and capstone students setting goals and objectives to meet site project needs. Following are examples of how a capstone student could be beneficial to the site.

TEXT BOX 4-6

Mentoring and hosting a doctoral capstone student allowed for the opportunity to complete research and develop programming for the implementation of a NICU (neonatal intensive care unit) follow-up clinic within our hospital system. The value of having a high-level student who could dedicate all of her time to the project to ensure complete thoroughness, with appropriate and safe research, is priceless and absolutely needed in our profession. The working rehab world expects, as it should, high productivity and best patient care, which most days does not allow a clinic therapist to pursue goals for program development without it taking a copious amount of time beyond scheduled working hours. The implementation of capstone students has opened a gateway for integrating programming and opportunities in the field that would otherwise be lost. I have a greater understanding, and now support, of the benefit that the doctoral program has for students. It was a great honor to have a student who accepted the lofty challenge and expectations I had to bring a much need program to fruition.

—Terri Cupp, MOT, OTR

TEXT BOX 4-7

We found that having capstone students allowed us to develop needed programming in three areas of our hospital system. These program development needs were on the back burner secondary to our focus needing to be on our primary roles involving direct patient care. The capstone students came in with knowledge of the literature and used the most up-to-date research to create innovative programming. The three students who came to our hospital had three unique mentoring experiences. One student worked with an OTR on the NICU in a traditional medical setting, one worked with a medical doctor in the transgender clinic, and the third student worked with an OTR who recently took on a new role as a clinical manager of outpatient services. It was wonderful to see these students grow, be self-directed, develop autonomy, and learn how to communicate, effectively and professionally, with doctors, nursing staff, social workers, and others to achieve program goals. The students learned from us, and we learned from the students—it was a win-win for all.

The students at the level they came into the capstone were at the point that they seemed like colleagues coming to work on projects that we just could not possibility get done but were all ideas and innovations that were swirling in our heads. In other words, having capstone students has been awesome, and we continue to work in partnership with the school of occupational therapy—we have two more capstone students for 2019 and are working on (finding) capstone students for 2020."

—Angela K. Palicki, OTR
Manager
Outpatient Rehabilitation Services
Eskenazi Health
Indianapolis, Indiana

—Hannah Porterfield, MOT, OTR, CSRS
Center Coordinator of Clinical Education
Rehabilitation Services
Eskenazi Health
Indianapolis, Indiana

—Theresa Rexroat MS, OTR, NTMTC
Occupational Therapy—NICU
Eskenazi Health
Indianapolis, Indiana

Having OTD capstone students at the Cancer Support Community has been invaluable. Not only are students able to meet one on one with survivors, they are able to develop broad educational programs. For instance, survivors and caregivers learned methods to manage their cancer-related fatigue in one program. Students were able to follow up with survivors as they progressed through the educational programs. This is a resource most of our survivor population would never be able to afford, or even know existed, if it were not for our capstone students. One capstone student wrote for a grant to fund a part-time occupational therapist at our community site, and it was awarded, allowing for sustainability of the programs.

—Lora Hayes, LMFT, RPT
Executive Vice President
Cancer Support Community Central Indiana
Indianapolis, Indiana

Description of Goals and Objectives and How They Relate to the Capstone

It is important that the student is able to articulate the purpose and goals of the proposed capstone experience and project and relate how achieving these goals will facilitate advanced knowledge. The overall purpose of the capstone is the overarching needs statement. Why is the capstone project important, and how is it supported by the evidence from current research? How is the project going to improve the lives of others and influence occupational performance? The overall outcome is what the capstone student strives to achieve. The capstone student will be answering these questions through the literature review and needs assessment that are required to be completed before the start of the capstone experience (ACOTE, 2018). Refer back to Chapter 3 for specifics on determining the purpose of the capstone experience and project. The goals that are developed are specific to what the student wants to accomplish, and the objectives are a step-by-step plan of how the student plans to meet those goals. Development of goals and objectives for the DCE is very different from that for fieldwork.

Guiding the student through the goals and objectives process is initially facilitated by the capstone coordinator and the faculty mentor. The site mentor will become involved as the capstone process moves into the planning stage, and it all starts with the initial idea. What does the site mentor or the student want to accomplish as part of the capstone experience? Is it a product, an experience, something learned, or a service? Is the doctoral capstone project realistic? Can it be completed within the time frame and with the resources available? Knowing some of this information will help facilitate the process of writing initial goals and objectives. Goals could be broad ideas to explore and then operationalize into a measurable objective within a stated time frame. The objectives are measurable steppingstones to reach that overarching goal. These small achievements can keep the process on track to ensure that the doctoral capstone project comes to fruition or may be reevaluated during the course of the experience. Chapter 6 goes into further detail on development of individualized student goals for the capstone.

Importance of Exploring State Licensure Implications

When direct individual client care is a part of the DCE and aligned with the student's goals and objectives, it is necessary for the doctoral capstone coordinator and the capstone student to investigate the impact of regulatory bodies. For instance, state licensure boards or third-party payers may dictate supervision requirements, and it is the ethical responsibility of the student and the site to comply with these. As mentioned previously, the site mentor or individual completing on-site supervision of the capstone student may or may not be an occupational therapy practitioner; however, is required that such individuals be experts in their field relative to the capstone focus.

If the site mentor is an occupational therapist, then there should be a discussion of the impact of occupational therapy licensure within the state in which the DCE is taking place. What language is used in the regulations and requirements for the occupational therapy practitioner or assistant? Does the state practice act include language specific to the student, fieldwork, or other language that suggests a supervisory process? If so, those requirements will influence the DCE with regard to selection of the site mentor, supervision guidelines, and implementation of the DCE objectives.

For instance, if the objectives of the DCE is to further the student's skills in an area of practice that is beyond entry level occupational therapy clinical practice, the site mentor will likely be an occupational therapy practitioner. If the state practice act for that occupational therapy site mentor states that there must be a certain level of student supervision by an occupational therapist, then those guidelines need to be followed and documented in the DCE memorandum of understanding. Some state practice acts and guidelines do not address students. For instance, in Indiana, "an individual who is practicing occupational therapy as part of a supervised course of study in an educational program" is exempt from the licensing requirement (IC 25-23.5-0.52). The onus, however, is on the supervising occupational therapy practitioner and how he or she is regulated by the state practice guidelines. Students will be using the processes of occupational therapy evaluation, programming planning, intervention, and discontinuation with input from occupational therapy faculty mentors as well as the site mentors.

Chapter Summary

This chapter has provided recommendations to inspire best practices and work systems that occur between the academic fieldwork coordinator and doctoral capstone coordinator and preparing the capstone student. It is clear that education and communication are essential key steps to the capstone site development. Assisting the capstone student and prospective sites to understand the differences between fieldwork and the capstone experience is a critical first step in site development. Once education is initiated, the process of procuring sites will evolve. As this relationship builds, the student will begin to work with the site to develop goals and objectives. Relationship development among the program, student, and site is essential to build a solid foundation for the DCE and project.

Learning Activities

1. Locate and review your occupational therapy program outcomes. These program outcomes have been established to measure student learning in your program and are based on the curricular design of the program. As you review your program outcomes, think about how your capstone purpose will link to program outcomes. Which program outcomes do you feel will relate to your capstone purpose? Write one potential capstone outcome you wish to achieve based on one of your program outcomes.

2. Determine the state in which you will complete your DCE and locate and review the occupational therapy licensure laws in that state. What items in the occupational therapy licensure law pertain to your doctoral capstone, and what is important to know or understand?

3. How do you define an expert? How will you determine that your site mentor is an expert?

4. Think about a time you had to deal with ambiguity and the results of experiencing this. Now determine how you will deal with the ambiguity of working through the process of locating a site for your capstone.

References

Accreditation Council for Occupational Therapy Education. (2018). *Standards and interpretive guide.* Retrieved from https://www.aota.org/~/media/Corporate/Files/EducationCareers/Accredit/StandardsReview/2018-ACOTE-Standards-Interpretive-Guide.pdf

American Occupational Therapy Association. (2009). Fieldwork education: value purpose. *American Journal of Occupational Therapy, 63*(6), 821-822. doi:10.5014/ajot.63.6.821

American Occupational Therapy Association. (2017). AOTA Fieldwork Data Form. Retrieved from https://www.aota.org/Education-Careers/Fieldwork/Supervisor.aspx

DeIuliis, E. D. (2017). Professionalism and fieldwork education. In E. DeIuliis (Ed.), *Professionalism across occupational therapy* (pp. 201-222). Thorofare, NJ: SLACK Incorporated.

Dickerson, A. E. (2006). Role competencies for a fieldwork educator. *American Journal of Occupational Therapy, 60,* 650-651. doi:10.5014/ajot.60.6.650.

Evenson, M. E., & Connor L.T. (2015). Perspectives on the doctoral experiential component. *OT Practice, 20,* 17-19.

Hanson, D. (2012, November 12). Benefits for fieldwork educators in working with students. *OT Practice, 18.*

Hanson, D., & DeIuliis, E. (2015). The collaborative model to fieldwork education: A blueprint for group supervision of students. Occupational Therapy in Health Care: *Occupational Educational Practices, 29,* 223-239.

Jirikowic, T., Pitonyak, J.S., Rollinger, B., Fogelberg, D., Mros, T.M. & Powell, J.M. (2015). Capstone projects as scholarship of application in entry-level occupational therapy education. *Occupational Therapy in Healthcare, 29*(2), 214-222. https://doi.org/10.3109/07380577.2015.1017788

Molitor, W. L., & Nissen, R. (2018). Clinician, educator and student perceptions of entry-level academic degree requirements in occupational therapy education. *Journal of Occupational Therapy Education, 2,* 1-23.

National Board for Certification in Occupational Therapy (NBCOT®). (2017, September 6). *NBCOT® Certification Renewal Activities Chart.* Retrieved from https://www.nbcot.org/-/media/NBCOT/PDFs/Renewal_Activity_Chart.ashx?la=en

Stutz-Tanenbaum, P., Greene, D., Hanson, D. J., & Koski, J. (2017). Professional reward in the academic fieldwork coordinator role. *American Journal of Occupational Therapy, 17,* 2-7. doi:10.5014/ajot/2017/022046

Appendix 4-A

EXAMPLES OF EMAIL COMMUNICATIONS

Student Contacting a Potential New Site

Hello,

My name is XXXX and I am an occupational therapy doctoral (OTD) student in the School of Occupational Therapy at the XXXX. As an OTD student, I am required to complete a Doctoral Capstone Experience (DCE) and project prior to graduation. This is a 14-week (40 hr/week) placement at a site working with a site mentor, who does not have to be an OT. My DCE will start in XXXX. At the point I start my DCE, I will have completed all Fieldwork requirements and coursework.

The DCE will allow me to gain advanced knowledge. It is an in-depth experience that will focus on one or more of the following: clinical practice skills, research skills, administration, leadership, program and policy development, advocacy, education or theory development. My area of focus is XXXX (program and policy development). I would like to partner with XXXX in order to develop an evidence-based healthy living program for seniors residing in your community.

I have enclosed my resume detailing my academic achievements and experience level. I hope to have an opportunity to speak with you further about my doctoral capstone. I look forward to hearing back from you soon. Thank you for your time.

Sincerely,

XXXX
Occupational Therapy Doctorate Student

Doctoral Capstone Coordinator Sending Mail to a Fieldwork Coordinator at a Current Fieldwork Site

Hello XXXX,

I have an occupational therapy doctoral (OTD) student, XXXX, who is very interested in completing her Doctoral Capstone Experience (DCE) with XXXX Health Network in the area of Home Health. I thought it might be best to first give you a brief description of the DCE here at XXXX since the Capstone is new to our profession. Our OTD students are required to complete a DCE and Project prior to graduation. This is a 14-week (40 hr/week) placement at a site working with a site mentor who does not have to be an OT depending on the site and project. The DCEs for our students start in XXXX. At the point the student starts the DCE they have completed all Fieldwork requirements and coursework.

The DCE is different than a Level I or Level II experience. It is an in-depth experience that allows the student to gain advanced knowledge. The student will focus on one or more of the following focus areas outlined by ACOTE: clinical practice skills, research skills, administration, leadership, program and policy development, advocacy, education or theory development. This is a very student self-directed learning experience. Students collaborate with a site mentor prior to the start of the experience to ensure goals and objectives for the experience and project are appropriate and meaningful to both the student and the site.

XXXX is interested in completing her DCE in the area of Home Health. She is interested in gaining advanced clinical skills in the area of home health and home modifications. She would like to work also on program development especially in the area of your home modification programming if there is a need.

I wanted to contact you to get your thoughts on the possibility of taking an OTD student for her DCE and project. I am attaching a brief description of the experience/roles and responsibilities and the mid-term and final evaluations.

Thanks so much and I hope to hear from you soon!

XXXX

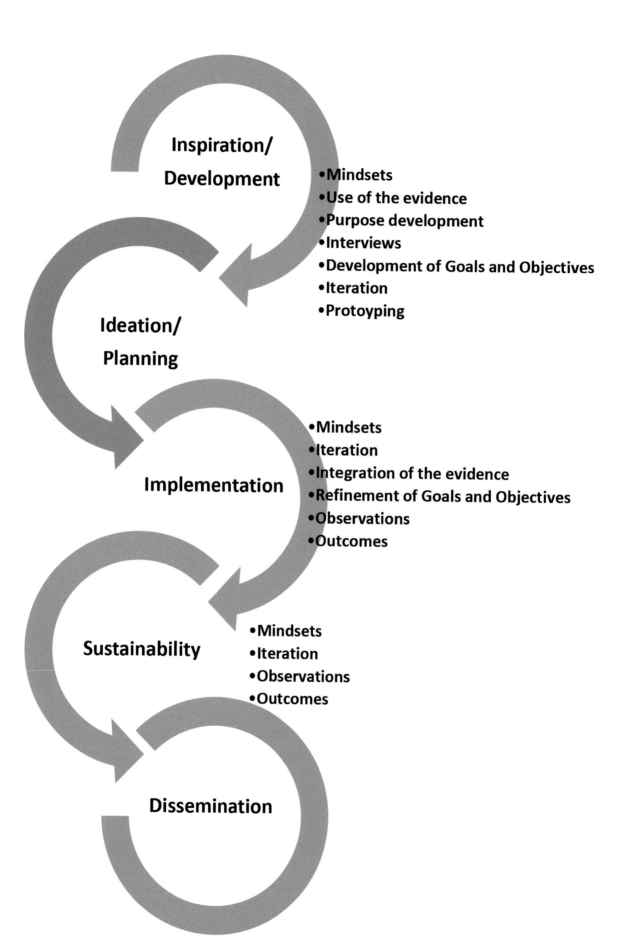

Inspiration/
Development

•Mindsets
•Use of the evidence
•Purpose development
•Interviews
•Development of Goals and Objectives
•Iteration
•Protoyping

Ideation/
Planning

•Mindsets
•Iteration
•Integration of the evidence
•Refinement of Goals and Objectives
•Observations
•Outcomes

Implementation

•Mindsets
•Iteration
•Observations
•Outcomes

Sustainability

Dissemination

Part II. Planning

The second step in the capstone process is **planning** the capstone experience and project, which aligns with the **ideation** process of human-centered design. This phase involves taking the information gathered that allowed the student to *develop* the problem and purpose and now begin problem-solving and generating ideas to solve a client, group, or population problem. During the ideation phase, the student is identifying opportunities and locating a site for the capstone. The student will begin the needs assessment process and begin testing and refining possible solutions. Working with people who share the capstone purpose to find real-life solutions is key to this planning phase. Goals and objectives are finalized to allow for iteration and prototyping to ensure a client-centered approach to the experience.

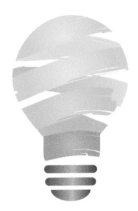

CHAPTER 5

Practice-Ready Skills for the Capstone

Amy M. Mattila, PhD, OTR/L

Human-Centered Design Mindsets for the Doctoral Students

The human-centered design mindsets of learning from failure and having optimism are important to reflect on as the capstone student begins to develop self-efficacy and emotional intelligence.

Learning From Failure: Don't get down on yourself if something you planned or developed does not work out in the first iteration—this is normal and expected. It is how you react to the failure that can affect change and growth. What is important is that you learn from something that failed because when you do you then are failing forward. You are reflecting on what went wrong and then making necessary adjustments, this is moving forward! As painful as it may seem, you grow from failures when you stop and reflect and don't take failures personally.

Optimism: Here's that word again—it must be important! Keep an optimistic mindset, and the entire experience will be much more productive and enjoyable. Find a way to keep your stress under control, which will help you remain optimistic and stay healthy throughout the process.

INTRODUCTION

The descriptor "practice-ready" has become a buzzword among higher education professional degree programs in depicting the desired outcomes of their graduates. For example, in law schools across the country, clinical legal education is moving toward providing the training required to graduate "practice-ready" lawyers, ready to take on the workforce. Barry (2012) defines the practice-ready law student

as, "equipped with a basic array of substantive knowledge, able to learn what they need to practice through apprenticeship in their first job" (p. 249). In addition to business and law, health care programs are defining what it means to be a practice-ready student. Pharmacy and nursing have explored key areas in which their graduates need to develop to be "work-ready" in each of their fields, such as critical thinking, problem-solving, and confidence in autonomous work (Missen, McKenna, Beauchamp, & Larkins, 2016; Murphy,

Deluliis ED, Bednarski JA.
*The Entry Level Occupational Therapy Doctorate Capstone:
A Framework for The Experience and Project* (pp 79-91).

2015). Skill sets of these professionals, and specifically occupational therapy, are often described as either hard skills or soft skills (Deepa & Seth, 2013). In many ways the term *practice-ready* is replacing the commonly used term *soft skills*. Occupational therapy educational programs have been historically focused on the hard skills, or competency and technical-based areas of practice, although concepts such as attitudes and behaviors (soft skills) are positively correlated with students' success in all levels of fieldwork learning (Campbell et al., 2015). In occupational therapy, practice-ready skills refers to graduates that are competent, safe, team-oriented, collaborative, professional, and efficient—not just in today's productive-driven environment but for future health care paradigm shifts as well.

As health care continues to move to outcome-based and performance-based reimbursement models, and, more specifically, the occupational therapy profession continues to embrace role emerging experiential learning and practice, it is crucial for occupational therapy education programs to foster, develop, and nurture practice-ready skills of occupational therapy students. In short, the end result for occupational therapy educational programs is for their graduates to be practice-ready at graduation. Rather than being a knowledge-generating research effort, the capstone is practice-focused, which requires the doctoral candidate to carry out a practice application-oriented experience and project. The entry level doctoral degree and advanced curricular standards create a shift in what practice-ready skills are now needed of occupational therapy doctoral students. Because of the dynamic health care system and ever-changing societal demands, occupational therapy consumers need practitioners who are confident and skilled in communication, clinical reasoning, problem-solving, and interprofessional teamwork. This chapter reflects on practice-ready skills that are necessary for the success of the capstone experience and provides recommendations for occupational therapy education programs to facilitate learning environments or tasks that foster growth in this area.

Capstone Student Reflective Questions

During the preparation phase of the doctoral capstone, the occupational therapy student may find it helpful to reflect on the following questions:

1. What challenges or barriers do you anticipate facing during your capstone experience?
2. What type of skills or abilities do you think would be essential to have to overcome these challenges or barriers?
3. What action steps can you commit to taking to becoming "practice-ready" for your capstone?

Chapter Objectives

By the end of reading this chapter and completing the learning activities, the reader should be able to:

1. Examine current and potential future challenges and barriers of the capstone experience.
2. Compare and contrast qualities of a successful fieldwork student vs the expectations of the capstone student.
3. Identify practice-ready skills that are instrumental to the successful completion of the capstone experience.

A PARADIGM SHIFT IN HEALTH CARE AND EDUCATION

With increasing complexity in the U.S. health care system at all levels, and more involved health issues facing society, it is imperative that occupational therapy practitioners be able to meet the needs of their clients, effectively and efficiently, by being prepared to provide advanced-level care immediately upon graduation. Health care administrators are increasingly challenged to reduce health care expenditures, leading to diminished opportunities to develop advanced skill competencies after entering the field. Student practitioners will need to obtain the additional training in practice-ready skills, leadership, and advocacy during their academic preparation before entering the field.

The preparation for occupational therapy students to understand themselves in terms of sociocultural diversity is also of great importance in the current health care system. Across the world, services are being provided to individuals and populations who historically have not been recipients of occupational therapy interventions (Talero, Kern, & Tupe, 2015). This shift in care requires a shift in occupational therapy curriculum, as well as opportunities for more diverse interactions while students are still in the educational setting. Taff and Blash (2017) suggested that a more systematized, comprehensive approach must be considered to address the need for a diversely trained and culturally competent workforce in our current health system. Currently, this is an issue because the workforce of practicing clinicians remains at 86% Caucasian and is practicing in mostly traditional settings (American Occupational Therapy Association [AOTA], 2015). To meet the needs of the focus areas and diversity in populations, capstone experiences may be frequently occurring in emerging areas of practice, such as health and wellness programs, veterans health, or aging in place, to name only a few of the available unique opportunities.

Accreditation Council for Occupational Therapy Education (ACOTE) standards specific to the entry level doctoral degree identify various advanced skills a student must demonstrate. Standard B.5.2 states that entry level doctoral students are to "identify, analyze, and advocate for existing and future service delivery models and policies, and their potential effect on the practice of occupational therapy and opportunities to address societal needs" (AOTA, 2018, p. 34). Standard B.7.4 states that the doctoral student will be able to "identify and develop strategies for ongoing professional development to ensure that practice is consistent with current and accepted standards" (ACOTE, 2018, p. 37). Both of these

Table 5-1. Greatest Reported Gaps in Employer Versus Student Perception of Proficiency in Career Readiness

COMPETENCY	% OF EMPLOYERS RATING GRADS PROFICIENT	% OF STUDENTS RATING THEMSELVES PROFICIENT
Professionalism/Work Ethic	42.5	89.4
Oral/Written Communication	41.6	79.4
Critical Thinking/Problem-Solving	55.8	79.9
Teamwork/Collaboration	77.0	85.1
Leadership	33.0	70.5
Career Management	17.3	40.9
Global/Intercultural Fluency	20.7	34.9

Adatped from National Association of Colleges and Employers. (2017). *Job outlook: Fall recruiting for the Class of 2018*. Retrieved from https://www.naceweb.org/job-market/trends-and-predictions/job-outlook-fall-recruiting-for-the-class-of-2018/.

standards require that the student possess practice-ready skills, such as a strong personal and professional identity.

MOVING FROM ACADEMIC READINESS TOWARD CAREER READINESS

Career readiness has been a continual focal point of professional degree programs. Although fieldwork education has historically prepared students for generalist, entry-level practice, there is still a gap between what students vs employers' feel are career ready skills and qualities (National Association of Colleges and Employers [NACE], 2017). In the NACE Class of 2018 surveys, there were large disparities in key areas of employment between students overreporting competency in skills required to be successful and effective in the workplace. Table 5-1 demonstrates there is now a greater demand than ever for occupational therapy educational programs to develop communication skills, critical thinking, collaboration, and creativity in all students, which aims to improve long-term employee productivity.

One way to begin to bridge this gap is through advancing the requirements and challenges of the experiential learning component within all programs. Experiential learning, as described by Kolb (1984), is commonly cited in professional programs in higher education and has relevance for designing the successful capstone placement. Kolb (1984) defined learning as a four-stage cycle in which students first encounter a "concrete experience," then take the time to reflect on the experience from new viewpoints through "reflective observation." Students then frame their ideas in a different light and assimilate these reflections and ideas into theories during "abstract conceptualization." In the final stage, they test their concepts and beliefs through "active experimentation" (Kolb, 1984). This cycle of learning is important during a capstone experience, in particular due to the increasing demands on the student and the more diverse practice settings

and clients they will encounter upon entering this type of placement. The student is challenged through this process at a greater level through the exploration of their learning (Jarvis, 2010; Kolb, 1984, 2014).

Jarvis (2010) suggested that when students begin the fieldwork phase of their occupational therapy education, they encounter a "primary experience of practice that presents them with an array of opportunities for new learning and development" (p. 78). This is equally true for the next phase of experiential learning through the doctoral capstone experience. Jarvis expands on Kolb's theory and defines the complexity of the adult learning process, adding the importance of drawing from past experiences and reflections. This is the area of knowledge that lies between an individual's awareness of an experience (based on the past encounter) and the authenticity of the current situation. When the two reflections begin to separate, questioning or dilemma occurs and learning begins. This is a critical moment for capstone students, as they begin to formulate their clinical questions and create a plan for a capstone experience. Figure 5-1 demonstrates the ongoing cycle that Kolb and Jarvis describe for successful experiential learning.

In addition to the social interaction that occurs in experiential learning, cultural interaction is an invaluable process to their learning experience. Similar to a health care context, where clients come from diverse backgrounds, experiential learning provides "a trusting and open learning atmosphere, where diverse ideas are shared, considered, tested, and modified" (Biedenweg & Monroe, 2013, p. 931). Of further importance to this interaction, researchers in the field find that the collaboration in these social and cultural contexts resulted in the acquisition of moral values through learning, something that often cannot be taught in the classroom setting (Talero et al., 2015).

As a result of this process, the student becomes transformed by their experience (Jarvis, 2010; Merriam, Caffarella,

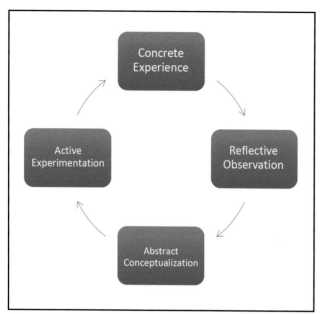

Figure 5-1. Kolb's experiential learning cycles.

& Baumgartner, 2007). Examples of these transformations from the literature include increased critical reflection, changed meaning of world views and beliefs, increased confidence, and increased connection to themselves and their community, all of which will help to bridge the gaps in employment as shared above (Bagatell, Lawrence, Schwartz, & Vuernick, 2013; Santalucia & Johnson, 2010).

TEXT BOX 5-1

The doctoral capstone experience process has been a transformative experience all around. Through my capstone experience at a veterans' hospital, I have improved my ability to critically reflect given the self-guided and self-directed nature of this process. As I lead a group of two to four veterans through sensory strategies in my program, I am faced with the challenge of constantly being aware of the atmosphere of the group, what dynamics I am working with, how to make the most beneficial adjustments or changes, providing examples that are relatable to each member, and many additional factors, all while ensuring the safety of the veterans and myself. 0 session and identify what went well, what could be changed, and maybe what could be taken out. This reflective process has allowed me to create a group that is both effective and efficient.

TEXT BOX 5-1 (continued)

This experience has increased my confidence tenfold. Before starting, I was worried that I would forget how to be an occupational therapist, traditionally speaking, during this experience. However, it has been quite the opposite. I have found my true passion within occupational therapy and have become confident in my ability to work with adults who have mental health disorders. Aside from the clinical aspect, I have also become more confident in my ability to lead interprofessional collaborations and train other professionals on the evaluation process and about sensory-based treatments. I have an increased confidence in my ability to document sessions and evaluations. This experience has increased my confidence in ways that I never could during fieldwork—it has made me feel more like an equal with the staff, rather than just another student.

As I spoke to earlier, this experience has helped me find my true passion within occupational therapy. Not only have I found that I love working with the mental health population, I have also discovered that I love program development, leadership, and educational roles within occupational therapy. I have been able to find my voice as an advocate and have a better understanding of identifying needs. Before this experience, I was not quite sure where I fit as an occupational therapist. I liked working with the veterans but was not as big a fan of the physical disability rehabilitation aspect. I enjoyed pediatrics but felt that it was not the right place for me. The doctoral capstone experience process has allowed me to find the missing pieces of the puzzle that make up my future as an occupational therapist.

—Nikki Yeckel, OTD
Class of 2018
Duquesne University
Pittsburgh, Pennsylvania

A REVIEW OF ATTRIBUTES OF THE SUCCESSFUL FIELDWORK STUDENT

Traditional fieldwork within occupational therapy has used the apprenticeship model of supervision in which students are supervised directly on-site by an occupational therapy practitioner (Hanson & DeIuliis, 2015; Mattila & Dolhi, 2016). Successful placements are often described by having detailed and clear expectations, quality feedback, and a structured learning environment (Rodger, Fitzgerald, Davila, Millar, & Allison, 2011). Students at this level of experiential learning are expected to embody the skills and traits of an entry-level practitioner at the culmination of the Level II fieldwork experiences. DeIuliis (2017) provided an overview of the traits of a successful fieldwork student, as summarized in Table 5-2.

Table 5-2. Highlights of Traits of Successful Fieldwork Students

A successful fieldwork student:

- Seeks and responds well to feedback
- Is inquisitive
- Demonstrates high emotional intelligence and maturity
- Is self-directed
- Builds positive therapeutic relationships
- Demonstrates strong communication and organization skills
- Takes risks
- Knows when to ask for help
- Collaborates effectively
- Exhibits a commitment to the profession
- Balances productivity, leisure, and rest

Adapted from Deluliis, E. (2017). *Professionalism across occupational therapy practice.* Thorofare, NJ: SLACK Incorporated.

Although these traits will still be essential to fieldwork education and occupational therapy curricula, additional opportunities and challenges for more autonomy and role development may help students to identify as a generalist practitioner whom now demonstrates in-depth knowledge of delivery models, policies, and systems. In addition, due to changes in health care service delivery, reimbursement demands, and the exponential growth of occupational therapy educational programs across the United States, greater and more diverse opportunities exist for the capstone experience to challenge this traditional model. Attributes that are unique to the successful capstone student are discussed in the next section.

ATTRIBUTES OF A PRACTICE-READY CAPSTONE STUDENT

To meet both the demands of the doctoral capstone experience and current health system needs, a variety of attributes are central to the success of a practice-ready capstone student. These suggested skills include *confidence* and *perceived self-efficacy*, *high emotional intelligence* and *maturity*, and an *openness to self-directed* and *self-regulated learning*. Academic programs will need to prepare students to expand the reach and impact of services, prepare to be practice-ready, and advance the quality of recognition of the profession, all with the confidence and maturity of a doctoral graduate. Each of these attributes is explored further in this section of the chapter through a social cognitive approach to learning.

A Social Cognitive Approach to the Capstone Experience

There is value to the social cognitive approach to learning practice-ready skills in clinical education. This theory assumes that adults have an intrinsic motivation to learn when the activity is meaningful, directly related to their current life roles, or they perceive a need for new knowledge and understanding (Bandura, 1977). Self-efficacy is an individual's belief in his or her capacity to perform the behaviors necessary to produce specific goals or task attainments (Bandura, 1977). The focus of learning from this approach is more about the student's self-development, such as self-efficacy (soft skills) rather than clinical competencies (hard skills). Eventually, through active involvement, changes in their learning capacity take place, meanings are created, a sense of belonging is developed, and identities are constructed (Dall'Alba, 2009; Lave & Wenger, 2003). This transformation not only potentially forms the experiences of the learner, but also the social context, as practice change can occur as a result of the contributions the learner makes, which is one of the key components of adding a capstone experience for occupational therapy doctorate programs (Lave & Wegner, 2003).

Social cognitive theory states four key factors can help create students' self-efficacy: (1) enactive mastery experiences, (2) vicarious (observational) experiences, (3) social persuasions, and (4) physiological and psychological states (Bandura, 1997). Enactive mastery experiences are authentic in nature and allow the student to deal with a situation in a successful manner. This type of mastery experience is considered the most influential in creating strong self-efficacy (Bandura, 1997). Mastery experiences can generally be attributed to one's own effort and skill. For example, a capstone student can increase his or her self-efficacy by successfully using therapeutic use of self (an internal skill) to build rapport with clients at their capstone site (Mattila, 2017). Students are able to interpret their results and outcomes, then use those interpretations to develop beliefs about their ability to repeat the task successfully. In these situations, strong self-efficacy is not created with easy success but requires persistence and drive in overcoming challenges.

TEXT BOX 5-2

Read the previous sentence again, specifically: "requires persistence and drive in overcoming challenges." This is an important revelation within the framework of human-centered design—learning from mistakes and failing forward is a part of the process. It is from failure that innovation (or reiterations and prototyping) occurs.

The next source to create self-efficacy is through vicarious learning, or having observational experiences provided by a "model" (Bandura, 1997). Ideally, capstone students will have had successful modeling in both their faculty and fieldwork educators before the capstone experience. A strategy students can use during the doctoral capstone experience is to perform their own self-assessment and comparison of capabilities based on the observation of others, such as through a role-play experience. In this example, having the opportunity to role-play or observe their site mentor, instructors, or peers in situations such as responding to the reactions of others or facing inaccurate assumptions can affect the student's assessment of self-efficacy.

TEXT BOX 5-3

This process of gathering feedback from various perspectives is often referred to as a **360 review** and is discussed in more detail in Chapter 9, which covers evaluation of the capstone.

Following this up with a structured journal prompt or written reflection can help capstone student explore how he or she responded, differences or similarities with the actors, and how the capstone student would change his or her response in the future if faced with that similar event. Thomas, Beyer, and Sealey (2018) found that through various "soft skills curriculum" role-playing vignettes in which occupational therapy students had the opportunity to watch and reflect, students reported increased awareness of the importance of soft skills and confidence in strategies to navigate difficult clinical situations. Although this source does not provide as strong a sense of self-efficacy, it can be helpful for students who are struggling with self-awareness (van Dinther, Dochy, & Segers, 2011).

TEACHING TIP 1: NAVIGATING DIFFICULT SITUATIONS Simulating situations in which difficult conversations or disagreements may arise in the clinical setting can provide an opportunity for students to practice soft skills. Here is one way to role-play challenging conversations, in which students can increase their confidence when faced with these situations in the capstone experience:

- Ask students to reflect on a time when they either had a difficult conversation or avoided a topic altogether. Prompt them that it was likely with someone important to them, such as a friend, family member, or classmate. Ask them to think about the perception they had on how the conversation would go (poorly, contentious, etc.).
- Once they have the situation in mind, teach them the SPIKES method and have them replay the conversation with a classmate. The SPIKES method trains them in the following communication techniques:
  - **S**etup: Ensure surroundings are appropriate for this conversation.
  - **P**erception: Ask open-minded questions to ascertain how the individual perceives the situation.
  - **I**nvitation: Find out how much information the individual is comfortable receiving or discussing at this time.
  - **K**nowledge: Stick to facts when possible, check for understanding as needed.
  - **E**mpathy: Respond to individual in a way that acknowledges his or her emotions and reassures that these responses are normal and expected.
  - **S**ummary: Determine whether the conversation should continue or find appropriate closure.

Adapted from Baile, W. F., Lenzi, R., Glober, G., Beale, E. A., & Kudelka, A. P. (2010). SPIKES-A six-step protocol for delivering bad news: Application to the patient with cancer. *The Oncologist, 5*, 302-311.

Social persuasion, the third source, states that students often receive information or feedback that affirms their ability to complete a task (Schunk, 1989). During difficult situations, capstone students can overcome obstacles if they have a significant other who can boost or instill confidence through communication and evaluative feedback. The importance of evaluation and recommendations to structure informal and formal evaluation of the doctoral student, site mentor, and doctoral capstone experience are discussed in Chapter 9.

Finally, Bandura (1997) states that people draw a sense of self-efficacy from their physiological, emotional, and mood states. Feelings such as anxiety, stress, or tension can allow for interpretation of failure, whereas positive feelings can strengthen overall self-efficacy.

TEXT BOX 5-4

Did you know that professionals outside of academia use Bandura's research and theory? Personal trainers and certified physical conditioning specialists use self-efficacy theory to develop physical fitness.

"A person with high self-efficacy within exercise will feel that he or she has the ability to be successful in exercise-related activities. Fitness professionals will help clients to be more successful if they can guide clients to higher levels of self-efficacy" (Jackson, 2010, p. 67).

Occupational therapy educators can benefit from using Bandura's self-efficacy theory to further enhance the preparation of occupational therapy students for the capstone.

Stress reactions can manifest in various ways, including physiological changes such as increased heart rate, sweating, hyperventilation, and can produce feelings of anxiety and fear that may negatively affect performance. Educators can observe some of these stress reactions in the classroom among students who suffer from test (performance) anxiety.

The impact of psychosocial stressors on well-being and quality of life is well known to the discipline of occupational therapy. Specific to higher education, occupational therapy literature has documented students' perceived stressors among their education (Clarke & Foxe, 2017; Pfeifer, Kranz, & Scoogin, 2008; Everly, Poff, Lamport, Hamant, & Alvey, 1994) and specifically linked to expectations of fieldwork education (Mitchell & Kampfe, 1990, 1993). Generation Y (also referred to as millennials) is the current student cohort entering the workforce and has the ability to have a positive impact on professional practice in occupational therapy (Hills, Ryan, Smith, & Warren-Forward, 2012) yet aligned with other generational stereotypes, are perceived as having positive and negative characteristics within education and workplace environments. Although Generation Y has documented strengths including being technology savvy, having a civic-minded attitude, demonstrating interest in team-based collaboration, and having an appreciation for work-life balance, there are also documented growth areas specific to concerns of how they respond to authority, having a sense of entitlement, and exhibiting underwhelming interpersonal skills (DeIuliis, 2017). More specific to the impact of one's psychological and physiological state, recent studies also have shown that millennials suffer from anxiety at a much higher rate than the generations that preceded them. A survey by the American Psychological Association (2018) found that millennials continued to be the most anxious generation overall.

This is important to recognize and respond to in advance because anxiety is currently the most common health diagnosis affecting all levels of occupational therapy students (Soja, Sanders, & Haughey, 2016). Depression and stress rank second and third as the most common psychosocial problems in college-age students. Due to the interrelationship of mood and self-efficacy, occupational therapy educators and students should proactively incorporate stress management techniques (such as deep breathing, imagery, and positive self-talk) from the start of the program, offer opportunities for regular reflection, and explore the concept of resilience, gratitude, and the growth mindset. There are strong suggestions that mindful and gratitude-based teachings result in positive outcomes for students. Dr. Robert Emmons has made large contributions to the ever-growing research on the positive impacts of gratitude. In one of his many studies, he found that individuals who kept gratitude journals on a weekly basis were more content with their lives as a whole and were more optimistic about the future than individuals who focused on negative or neutral occurrences of the week (Emmons & McCullough, 2003). Studies such as this suggest that there are ways for individuals to cope with stress in a healthy manner and lead more positive and productive lives. By all accounts, millennials are unlike preceding generations. They view the world differently and have redefined the meaning of success, both personally and professionally. A growing movement among occupational therapy educators is needed to create successful, ethical, well-rounded, and practice-ready students in terms of both their content knowledge and their mental well-being.

The work of Bandura (1997) is valuable for occupational therapy educators to prepare capstone students from these younger generations. Effective functioning for the capstone requires skills and efficacy beliefs. Because self-efficacy is influenced by mastery experience, vicarious experience, social persuasion, and physiological state, it is essential for occupational therapy educators to develop capstone preparation curricula aimed at increasing self-efficacy through each of these factors. This understanding of the majority makeup of the capstone student body provides a solid connection between perceived self-efficacy and the emotional intelligence (EI) of a student.

Confidence and Perceived Self-Efficacy

The level of perceived self-efficacy is defined as the degree to which people believe they can succeed at any given aspect of an activity; varying from total certainty to total uncertainty. The stronger the sense of self-efficacy, the greater the perseverance toward a successful experience. Traits of self-efficacy that align with practice-ready skills include confidence, willingness to take risks, adaptability, innovation, and overall professional competence.

Health science students who reported higher levels of perceived self-efficacy were found to have performed better in clinical rotations, had increased documentation and evaluation skills, and demonstrated increased clinical decision-making skills (Artino, 2012; Derdall, Olsen, Janzen, & Warren, 2002).

TEXT BOX 5-5

The capstone experience of my occupational therapy doctoral education has fostered my personal and professional growth. This experience has helped me achieve confidence in my clinical abilities, as well as my leadership skills and personal attributes. I was able to foster change at my doctoral capstone experience site by inspiring others to challenge their day-to-day processes. This connected me to other community members, furthering my inspiration to make a lasting impact throughout my site and within my small community.

This experience provided me with the opportunity to take leadership in my own doctoral capstone experience while also inspiring others to become followers. I was able to create lasting change in my community, increasing my overall confidence in my skills and abilities. I believe that I would be a typical entry-level clinical without this experience. The occupational therapy doctoral capstone experience, however, has inspired me to challenge the process and create change in my future. It has led me to have the confidence to meet with organizational leaders to create a potential job opportunity upon graduation. I now have the confidence to be a leader, rather than a follower, in my professional career.

—Cayla Leichtenberger, OTD
Class of 2018
Duquesne University
Pittsburgh, Pennsylvania

In relationship to experiential learning, perceived self-efficacy can serve as an indicator of the success or failure of a student in a stressful new clinical context, such as a capstone experience (Baird, Raina, Rogers, O'Donnell, Terhorst, & Holm, 2015). Students with higher perceived self-efficacy are also more likely to transfer knowledge on a single activity to other similar or different activities. In occupational therapy curriculum, we often refer to this as a core component of clinical reasoning. For example, Baird et al. (2015) evaluated the effects of transfer training in a simulated environment on occupational therapy students' perceived self-efficacy. The authors found that students who were completely confident in the training would have a higher level of perceived self-efficacy than those who were unsure of their skills for transferring patients. This is extremely valuable for the capstone, as doctoral students will continue to practice skills one way in the classroom but need to be able to translate those skills to varying populations and settings, often in a more advanced context during the capstone experience. Increasing self-efficacy can help the capstone student preserve and fail forward when faced with adversity during the capstone.

TEACHING TIP 2: MEASURING SELF-EFFICACY

An evidence-based tool you can incorporate into your work with capstone students to help them to self-assess areas of self-efficacy is the Student Confidence Questionnaire (SCQ). The SCQ, originally developed by Derdall, Olsen, Janzen, and Warren in 2002, allows students to evaluate their overall confidence in a variety of practice-ready areas. The SCQ is a 40-item Likert scale that assesses the student in the domains of professional competence, communication, adaptability, innovation, risk-taking, supervision, and clinical practice.

Adapted from Derdall, M., Olson, P., Janzen, W., & Warren, S. (2002). Development of a questionnaire to examine confidence of occupational therapy students during fieldwork experiences. *Canadian Journal of Occupational Therapy, 69,* 49-56.

Emotional Intelligence

EI describes how people, such as capstone students, may monitor and manage emotional responses to better communicate with and relate to others (Carmeli & Josman, 2006; Mayer, Salovey, & Caruso, 2008). Both EI theory and the principles of occupational therapy address the importance of relationship building skills that support the connection between self and others. In contrast to therapeutic use of self, EI is situated within the individual and indirectly influences relationships with others. The focus of the EI theory's process of how emotions influence thinking supports the interactive reasoning process commonly discussed in occupational therapy (McKenna & Mellson, 2013). Collaborative reasoning relies heavily on self-awareness and perception, which inform clinical reasoning, relationship-building, and decision-making—all important practice-ready skills for the capstone student (Cronin & Graebe, 2018). Previous studies have also found that fieldwork students with higher EI have demonstrated increased scores in competencies related to patient outcomes, teamwork skills, dealing with stress, and overall patient satisfaction (Andonian, 2013; Gribble, Ladyshewsky, & Parsons, 2017). In the capstone process, EI is situated within the capstone student and directly impacts other stakeholders in the capstone process, as shown in Figure 5-2.

Self-Directed and Regulated Learner

Students' ability to be a self-directed and self-regulated learners will lend to their success in the capstone experience and project. In terms of these practice-ready concepts, Gage and Berliner (1991) describe key objectives for self-regulated learning in relationship to educational psychology: (a) to promote positive self-direction and independence, (b) to develop the ability to take responsibility for learning, (c) to develop creativity, and (d) to promote curiosity. One could argue the inherent nature of the capstone experience addresses each of these objectives by design. These authors also emphasize that knowing how to learn is more important than purely gaining extensive knowledge, and the phases of self-regulated learning in Table 5-3 can help capstone students to better reflect and enhance their metacognition on the subject of learning. Students are required to be self-directed in their learning and therefore increase their clinical reasoning, critical thinking, and team-based communication skills (Sadlo, 1994; Scaffa & Wooster, 2004).

STRATEGIES TO DEVELOP PRACTICE-READY SKILLS

Although various strategies have been discussed throughout this chapter, there are other, more concrete ways that occupational therapy educators may be able to develop practice-ready skills in capstone students. Through exposure to more diverse learning environments and settings, critical reflection, and an emphasis on interpersonal and advocacy skills, educators and students can facilitate environments or tasks that foster growth.

First, educators and doctoral capstone coordinators can create unique learning experiences that encourage students to select nontraditional, community-based, or role-emerging settings. These types of settings that often provide services to communities or underserved populations where there is no current occupational therapy in practice can provide students with unique opportunities to refine the practice-ready skills discussed in this chapter. Role-emerging experiences offer an experiential learning approach that can better prepare students to be qualified practitioners and enhance a distinctive set of skills that differ from those learned in more traditional placements (Atler & Gavin, 2010; Scaffa & Retiz, 2013). There is also indication that students who participated in role-emerging or community-based fieldwork have positive gains in reflection, knowledge, and overall confidence in areas such as problem-solving, initiative, and creativity in practice (Hoppes, Bender, & DeGrace, 2005; Mattila, DeIuliis, & Cook, 2018). In addition, a different set of skills are often gained in these settings compared with a traditional fieldwork setting, including cultural awareness, therapeutic use of self, and self-efficacy (Atler & Gavin, 2010; Haro, Knight, Cameron, Nixon, Ahluwalia, & Hicks, 2014).

Another way to develop practice-ready skills is through the use of critical reflection during the capstone process. Critical reflection is an evidence-based teaching method that can foster personal growth and professional transformation in capstone students. According to Henderson (2010), critical reflection, communication, and support are the key components in fostering students' movement toward transformative learning. When students begin the doctoral capstone process, they are often challenged to question and rethink previously held thoughts and beliefs. Educators can facilitate

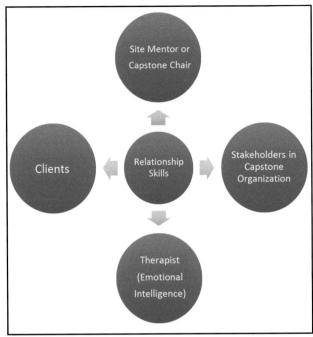

Figure 5-2. EI, situated with the capstone student, informs all relationships in the capstone process.

the student to consider options through exploratory prompts and critical reflection (Matthew-Maich et al., 2010; Mezirow, 2000). Promoting learning and achievement through critical reflection and self-assessment are integral components of developing self-efficacy and EI.

TEACHING TIP 3: FACILITATING SELF-REGULATION AND EMOTIONAL INTELLIGENCE
Keeping in mind that self-regulated learning and EI are explicit, practiced, and implemented over time, how will you help your students get there?

Think of a strategy you can incorporate with capstone students to foster self-regulation of learning and EI. Some evidence-based examples include the following (Zimmerman, 2002):

- Clarifying and modeling what good performance looks like (goals, criteria, expected standards, etc.)
- Facilitating the development of self-assessment and reflection
- Encouraging instructor and peer dialogue about the activity of learning
- Encouraging positive motivational beliefs and self-esteem
- Providing opportunities to close the gap between current and desired performance

For effective self-regulated learning to take place, students must develop the capability of monitoring what they

Table 5-3. Phases of Self-Regulated Learning During the Doctorate Capstone Experience and Project

SELF-REGULATION PHASE	CAPSTONE PROCESS PHASE	DESCRIPTION	QUESTIONS STUDENTS MIGHT POSE WHILE ENACTING THIS PHASE OF THE CAPSTONE EXPERIENCE
Forethought	Developing and planning phase	Processes and beliefs that occur before efforts to learn	• What is the task? What does the capstone assignment tell me to do? • Is it similar to something I have done before? • What information do I need to gather to accomplish this step of my capstone? • How, when, and where should I proceed? • What do I want to gain by completing this capstone project? Why? • Which factors of the project can I control? • Which factors are out of my control? How will I cope? • Where will I go when I need help?
Performance/Action	Implementation phase	Processes that occur during learning and/or activity	• What can I do to stay on track throughout the project? • Am I accomplishing what I set out to accomplish? • Am I being distracted? • Do I actually understand what I am implementing and why? Should I continue working, or is the task complete? • Is it time to seek help? • Do I need/deserve a break or incentive?
Self-Reflection	Evaluation phase	Processes that occur after each learning effort	• What is my reaction to the completed project? • What are others' reactions? • Have I taken all the important stakeholders' opinions into consideration? • What are the consequences of these reactions and the outcomes of my work? • Why did I perform well? What did I do poorly? • Did I choose the right steps? What can I do to improve?
Contributing factor throughout all phases	Motivation/Beliefs		• Am I capable of completing this capstone experience and project? • Why am I interested, curious, or frustrated? • Can I control my level of success? • Do I care more about the grade or the growth in my learning?

Adapted from Zimmerman, B. J. (2002). Becoming a self-regulated learner: An overview. *Theory Into Practice, 41*(2), 64-70.

do, and then modifying the skill or strategy appropriately (Boud, 2013). Students also need to have a realistic assessment of their own performance, of what they know, what they still need to know, and the path they will take to bridge theory into practice. In the capstone experience, students are required to be increasingly reliant on their own thinking. The ability to self-assess will allow the capstone student to be a more independent, critical thinker in realistic situations (Boud, 2013; Wald, Anthony, Hutchinson, Liben, Smilovitch, & Donato, 2015). Using this teaching and learning practice, students can explore greater meaning in the content, and through critical reflection and investigation, they may encounter a fundamental change in their beliefs, feelings, attitudes, perspectives, and assumptions (Costa, 2009; Santalucia & Johnson, 2010).

Finally, placing an emphasis on developing intrapersonal, interpersonal, and advocacy skills can assist in moving capstone students from a self-centric model of understanding the profession to "other-centered," where leading and serving others is at the core of their practice. This movement is critical, particularly when there are consistent findings that the U.S. health care system does not offer dependable, high-quality care to all people, due in part to the poor organization of the health care delivery system (Institute of Medicine, 2011). These changes in thoughts and behaviors can produce transformational and servant leaders as our capstone students graduate and enter the profession, which has been found to be a useful and practical pedagogical approach in occupational therapy education (King, Barclay, Ripat, Dubouloz, & Schwartz, 2015; Mattila & Dolhi, 2016). Fostering the practice-ready skills to graduate emerging health care leaders from our occupational therapy doctorate programs will be essential in addressing these systematic issues.

Chapter Summary

The doctoral capstone experience enhances occupational therapy students' abilities to interact, advocate, and collaborate with other health care professionals in more diverse settings. This process will allow programs to graduate into the health care system not only generalist, practice-ready practitioners but also transformational leaders. There needs to be a clear emphasis on practice-ready skills development that will allow capstone students to positively and confidently work through the human-centered design phases of inspire/ideate and promote more autonomous decision-making. Through precursory learning activities and purposeful selection of capstone settings that facilitate growth in self-regulated learning, leadership, and self-efficacy, capstone students will boldly enter the health care field as practice-ready professionals.

Learning Activities for the Student and Educator

1. Imagery activity: Picture yourself going through the capstone process. What do you know now that you didn't before you embarked on this advanced practitioner phase of your curriculum?

    a. Take a moment to reflect and write down some skills you have developed before, during, and after fieldwork to take inventory of what you need for the capstone.

    b. What are your strengths? What are your areas that need developed? How can you create SMART goals around these skills to help you to be successful?

2. Think of a task related to your capstone. It could be developing evidence-based questions, embarking on a literature review, or pragmatically preparing for the capstone experience itself. Use Table 5-2 and think through the phases of self-regulated learning.

    a. What questions and answers might you have in each phase of your learning?

    b. Reflect on your motivation and beliefs. How will these characteristics influence each of these phases?

3. Create a capstone experience planning journal. The intent of this journal is to help you set goals for each step of the capstone process. Successful students are known to set goals, monitor their progress, and make plans for how they are going to achieve those goals. In your initial post, think about the following questions:

    a. What are your specific, measurable learning objectives you hope to accomplish during your capstone experience?

    b. What are you going to do to meet these objectives? What do you expect of your faculty and/or capstone supervisor(s) to help facilitate your learning?

    c. How are you going to monitor your progress?

References

Accreditation Council for Occupational Therapy Education. (2018). *Standards and interpretive guide*. Retrieved from https://www.aota.org/~/media/Corporate/Files/EducationCareers/Accredit/StandardsReview/2018-ACOTE-Standards-Interpretive-Guide.pdf

American Occupational Therapy Association. (2015). Surveying the profession: The 2015 AOTA salary & workforce survey. *OT Practice, 20*(11), 7-11.

American Psychological Association. (2018). *Stress in America: Uncertainty about health care*. Retrieved from http://www.apa.org/news/press/releases/stress/2017/uncertainty-health-care.pdf

Andonian, L. (2013). Emotional intelligence, self-efficacy, and occupational therapy students' fieldwork performance. *Occupational Therapy in Health Care, 27,* 201-215.

Artino, A. R. (2012). Academic self-efficacy: From educational theory to instructional practice. *Perspectives on Medical Education, 1,* 76-85.

Atler, K., & Gavin, W. J. (2010). Service-learning-based instruction enhances students' perceptions of their abilities to engage in evidence-based practice. *Occupational Therapy in Health Care, 24,* 23-38.

Bagatell, N., Lawrence, J., Schwartz, M., & Vuernick, W. (2013). Occupational therapy student experiences and transformations during fieldwork in mental health settings. *Occupational Therapy in Mental Health, 29,* 181-196.

Baile, W. F., Lenzi, R., Glober, G., Beale, E. A., & Kudelka, A. P. (2010). SPIKES—A six-step protocol for delivering bad news: Application to the patient with cancer. *The Oncologist, 5,* 302-311.

Baird, J. M., Raina, K. D., Rogers, J. C., O'Donnell, J., Terhorst, L., & Holm, M. B. (2015). Simulation strategies to teach patient transfers: Self-efficacy by strategy. *American Journal of Occupational Therapy, 69*(Suppl. 2), 6912185030p1-6912185030p7.

Bandura, A. (1977). Self-efficacy: Toward a unifying theory of behavioral change. *Psychological Review, 84,* 191-215.

Bandura, A. (1997). *Self-efficacy: The exercise of control.* New York, NY: W.H. Freeman.

Barry, M. (2012). Practice ready: Are we there yet? *Boston College Journal of Law & Social Justice, 32,* 247-277.

Biedenweg, K. A., & Monroe, M. (2013). Cognitive methods and a case study for assessing shared perspectives as a result of social learning. *Society & Natural Resources, 26,* 931-944.

Boud, D. (2013). *Enhancing learning through self-assessment.* New York, NY: Routledge.

Campbell, M. K., Corpus, K., Wussow, T. M., Plummer, T., Gibbs, D., & Hix, S. (2015). Fieldwork educators perspectives: Professional behavior attributes of Level II fieldwork students. *Open Journal of Occupational Therapy, 3*(4), Article 7.

Carmeli, A., & Josman, Z. E. (2006). The relationship among emotional intelligence, task performance, and organizational citizenship behaviors. *Human Performance, 19,* 403-419. doi:10.1207/s15327043hup1904_5

Clarke, J., & Foxe, J. (2017). The impact of social anxiety on occupational participation in college life. *Occupational Therapy in Mental Health, 33,* 31-46.

Costa, D. M. (2009). Transformative learning in fieldwork. *OT Practice, 14*(1), 19-20.

Cronin, A., & Graebe, G. (2018). *Clinical reasoning in occupational therapy.* Bethesda, MD: AOTA Press.

Dall'Alba, G. (2009). Learning professional ways of being: Ambiguities of becoming. *Educational Philosophy and Theory, 41,* 34-45.

Deepa, S., & Seth, M. (2013). Do soft skills matter? Implications for educators based on recruiters' perspective. *IUP Journal of Soft Skills, 7*(1), 7-20.

DeIuliis, E. (2017). *Professionalism across occupational therapy practice.* Thorofare, NJ: SLACK Incorporated.

Derdall, M., Olson, P., Janzen, W., & Warren, S. (2002). Development of a questionnaire to examine confidence of occupational therapy students during fieldwork experiences. *Canadian Journal of Occupational Therapy, 69,* 49-56.

Emmons, R. A., & McCullough, M. E. (2003). Counting blessings versus burdens: An experimental investigation of gratitude and subjective well-being in daily life. *Journal of Personality and Social Psychology, 84,* 377-389.

Everly, J. S., Poff, D. W., Lamport, N., Hamant, C. & Alvey, G. (1994). Perceived stressor and coping strategies of occupational therapy students. *American Journal of Occupational Therapy, 48*(11), 1022-1028. doi:10.5014/ajot.48.11.1022

Gage, N., & Berliner, D. (1991). *Educational Psychology* (5th ed.). Boston, MA: Houghton Mifflin Harcourt.

Gribble, N., Ladyshewsky, R. K., & Parsons, R. (2017). Fluctuations in the emotional intelligence of therapy students during clinical placements: Implication for educators, supervisors, and students. *Journal of Interprofessional Care, 31,* 8-17.

Hanson, D. J., & DeIuliis, E. D. (2015). The collaborative model of fieldwork education: A blueprint for group supervision of students. *Occupational Therapy in Health Care, 29,* 223-239.

Haro, A. V., Knight, B. P., Cameron, D. L., Nixon, S. A., Ahluwalia, P. A., & Hicks, E. L. (2014). Becoming an occupational therapist: Perceived influence of international fieldwork placements on clinical practice. *Canadian Journal of Occupational Therapy, 81,* 173-182.

Henderson, J. (2010). Transformative learning: Four activities that set the stage. *Online Education.* Retrieved from http://www.uwex.edu/disted/conference/Resource_library/proceedings/28439_10.pdf

Hills, C., Smith, R. S., & Warren-Forward, H. (2012). The impact of "generation Y" occupational therapy students on practice education. *Australian Occupational Therapy Journal, 59,* 156-163.

Hoppes, S., Bender, D., & DeGrace, B. W. (2005). A service learning is a perfect fit for occupational and physical therapy education. *Journal of Allied Health, 34,* 47.

Institute of Medicine. (2011). *Crossing the quality chasm: A new health system for the 21st century. Report by the Committee on Quality of Health Care in America.* Washington, DC: National Academies Press.

Jackson, D. (2010). How personal trainers can use self-efficacy theory to enhance exercise behavior in beginning exercisers. *Strength and Conditioning Journal, 32,* 7-71.

Jarvis, P. (2010). *Adult education and lifelong learning, theory and practice* (4th ed.). Oxon, England: Routledge.

King, J., Barclay, R., Ripat, J., Dubouloz, C. J., & Schwartz, C. (2015). Response shift and transformative learning—do physical therapists and occupational therapists use concepts of change in their clinical practice? *Physiotherapy, 101,* e757-e758.

Kolb, D. A. (1984). *Experiential learning: Experience as the source of learning and development.* Englewood Cliffs, NJ: Prentice Hall.

Lave, J., & Wenger, E. (2003). *Situated learning: Legitimate peripheral participation.* Cambridge, England: Cambridge University Press.

Matthew-Maich, N., Ploeg, J., Jack, S., & Dobbins, M. (2010). Transformative learning and research utilization in nursing practice: A missing link? *Worldviews on Evidence-Based Nursing, 1,* 25-35.

Mattila, A. (2017). *Perceptions of occupational therapy students participating in role emerging fieldwork at community agencies: An explanatory case study.* Moon, PA: Robert Morris University.

Mattila, A., DeIuliis, E. D., & Cook, A. B. (2018). Increasing self-efficacy through role emerging placements: Implications for occupational therapy experiential learning. *Journal of Occupational Therapy Education, 2*(3). Retrieved from https://encompass.eku.edu/jote/vol2/iss3/3

Mattila, A. M., & Dolhi, C. (2016). Transformative experience of master of occupational therapy students in a non-traditional fieldwork setting. *Occupational Therapy in Mental Health, 32,* 16-31.

Mayer, J. D., Salovey, P., & Caruso, D. (2008). Emotional intelligence: New ability or eclectic traits? *American Psychologist, 63,* 503-517. doi:10.1037/0003-066x.63.6.503

McKenna, J., & Mellson, J. (2013). Emotional intelligence and the occupational therapist. *British Journal of Occupational Therapy, 76,* 427-430.

Merriam, S. B., Caffarella, R. S., & Baumgartner, L. M. (2007). *Learning in adulthood: A comprehensive guide.* San Francisco, CA: Jossey-Bass.

Mezirow, J. (2000). Learning to think like an adult: Core concepts of transformation theory. In J. Mezirow & Associates, (Eds.), *Learning as transformation: Critical perspectives on a theory in progress* (pp. 3-34). San Francisco, CA: Jossey-Bass.

Missen, K., McKenna, L., Beauchamp, A., & Larkins, J.A. (2016). Qualified nurses rate new nursing graduates as lacking skills in key clinical areas. *Journal of Clinical Nursing, 25,* 2134-2143.

Mitchell, M. M., & Kampfe C. M. (1990). Coping strategies used by occupational therapy students during fieldwork: An exploratory study. *American Journal of Occupational Therapy, 44,* 543-550.

Mitchell, M. M., &, Kampfe, C. M. (1993). Student coping strategies and perceptions of fieldwork. *American Journal of Occupational Therapy, 47,* 535-540.

Murphy, J. E. (2015). Practice-readiness of US pharmacy graduates to provide direct patient care. *Pharmacotherapy, 35,* 1091-1095.

National Association of Colleges and Employers. (2017). *Job out-look: Fall recruiting for the Class of 2018.* Retrieved from https://www.naceweb.org/job-market/trends-and-predictions/job-outlook-fall-recruiting-for-the-class-of-2018/

Pfeifer, T. A., Kranz, P. L., & Scoogin, A. E. Perceived stress in occupational therapy students. *Occupational Therapy International, 15,* 221-231.

Rodger, S., Fitzgerald, C., Davila, W., Millar, F., & Allison, H. (2011). What makes a quality occupational therapy practice placement? Students' and practice educators' perspectives. *Australian Occupational Therapy Journal, 58,* 195-202.

Sadlo, G. (1994). Problem-based learning in the development of an occupational therapy curriculum, Part 2: The BSc at the London School of Occupational Therapy. *British Journal of Occupational Therapy, 57,* 79-84.

Santalucia, S., & Johnson, C. R. (2010). Transformative learning: Facilitating growth and change through fieldwork. *OT Practice, 15,* CE1-CE7.

Scaffa, M. E., & Reitz, S. M. (2013). *Occupational therapy community-based practice settings.* Philadelphia, PA: F.A. Davis.

Scaffa, M. E., & Wooster, D. M. (2004). Effects of problem-based learning on clinical reasoning in occupational therapy. *American Journal of Occupational Therapy, 58,* 333-336.

Schunk, D. H. (1989). Self-efficacy and achievement behaviors. *Educational Psychology Review, 1,* 173-208.

Soja, J., Sanders, M., & Haughey, K. (2016). Perceived stressors and coping in junior, senior, and graduate occupational therapy students. *American Journal of Occupational Therapy, 70*(4, Supp. 1), 7011505178p1.

Taff, S. D., & Blash, D. (2017). Diversity and inclusion in occupational therapy: Where we are, where we must go. *Occupational Therapy in Health Care, 31*(1), 72-83.

Talero, P., Kern, S. B., & Tupé, D. A. (2015). Culturally responsive care in occupational therapy: An entry-level educational model embedded in service-learning. *Scandinavian Journal of Occupational Therapy, 22,* 95-102.

Thomas, J., Beyer, J., & Sealy, L. (2018). Emotional intelligence: Developing soft skills to Increase student success during fieldwork experience as practicing clinicians. *SIS Quarterly Practice Connections, 3*(2), 8-10.

Tomasello, M., Kruger, A. C., & Ratner, H. H. (1993). *Cultural learning. Behavioral and Brain Sciences, 16,* 495-511.

van Dinther, M., Dochy, F., & Segers, M. (2011). Factors affecting students' self-efficacy in higher education. *Educational Research Review, 6,* 95-108.

Wald, H. S., Anthony, D., Hutchinson, T. A., Liben, S., Smilovitch, M., & Donato, A. A. (2015). Professional identity formation in medical education for humanistic, resilient physicians: Pedagogic strategies for bridging theory to practice. *Academic Medicine, 90,* 753-760.

Zimmerman, B. J. (2002). Becoming a self-regulated learner: An overview. *Theory Into Practice, 41*(2), 64-70.

RESOURCES

Textbooks

Dann, J., & Dann, D. *The emotional intelligence workbook.* London, England: Hodder Education.

Kolb, D. A. (2014). *Experiential learning: Experience as the source of learning and development.* Englewood Cliffs, NJ: Pearson Education.

Nilson, L. B. (2013). *Creating self-regulated learners: Strategies to strengthen students' self-awareness and learning skills.* Sterling, VA: Stylus.

Shadiow, L. K. (2013). *What our stories teach us: A guide to critical reflection for college faculty.* San Francisco, CA: Wiley.

Websites

For a source addressing a variety of topics, see a special issue of *New Directions for Teaching and Learning,* Summer 2011, Issue 126, a Self-Regulated Learning Special Issue on engagement, goal orientation, help-seeking, the role of Web 2.0, computer-based learning, and more. Available online via Wiley Online Library: http://onlinelibrary.wiley.com/doi/10.1002/tl.v2011.126/issuetoc

The Highly Effective Teacher: www.thehighlyeffective-teacher.com

- Developing Self-Regulation
- Use of Mindfulness Exercises in the Classroom
- Incorporating Self-Assessment

Emotional Intelligence Consortium: www.eiconsortium.org

- References for Higher Education

Stanford Teaching Commons: www.teachingcommons.stanford.edu

- Student Self-Assessment

CHAPTER 6

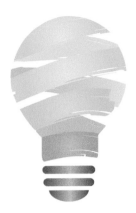

Finalizing the Planning Phase With the Capstone Team

Julie A. Bednarski, OTD, MHS, OTR
Elizabeth D. DeIuliis, OTD, MOT, OTR/L, CLA

Human-Centered Design Mindsets for the Doctoral Students

The human-centered design mindsets of optimism and empathy will be important for capstone students to embrace as they enter this final planning phase. Keeping optimistic and practicing empathy will allow the capstone student to delve deeper into the needs of the site, ensuring a client-centered approach and providing a meaningful project outcome.

Empathy: This is the time for you, as a capstone student, to "step into the shoes of your site" and begin to understand its needs to problem-solve solutions. This problem-solving will lead to more individualized goals and objectives and will create a meaningful experience for both you and your site. Spend time building the occupational profile with your site mentor. For your project to be successful and have sustainability, you need to listen to your clients and understand their problems and needs.

Optimism: Keep optimistic! By having a mindset of optimism, you will continue to try as hard as possible to find solutions to problems and develop goals that will be meaningful. Keep that attitude of optimism as you complete the final planning phase.

INTRODUCTION

This chapter provides recommendations to guide the final "planning" stage of the doctoral capstone experience (DCE) and project. Proactive and ongoing planning, communication, and collaboration among the capstone team (the student, doctoral capstone coordinator, the faculty mentor or chair, and site mentor) are important to ensure success. In this final planning stage, the capstone team is collaboratively

(a) securing the site, (b) developing the initial goals and objectives, (c) finalizing the capstone proposal, and (d) creating a memorandum of understanding (Accreditation Council for Occupational Therapy Education [ACOTE], 2018). This chapter guides the reader through these four steps to assist the capstone student in finalizing the project plan and timeline.

DeIuliis ED, Bednarski JA.
The Entry Level Occupational Therapy Doctorate Capstone:
A Framework for The Experience and Project (pp 93-118).
© 2020 Taylor & Francis Group.

Capstone Student Reflective Questions

When finalizing the planning of the doctoral capstone, capstone students may find it helpful to reflect on the following questions:

1. Where are you in the process of securing a site for your capstone experience and project?

2. How have you begun to plan for your project? Are you comfortable articulating your plan and purpose to others? Describe to a friend or family member your plan and purpose. Does it make sense to this person?

3. Express some of your thoughts and feelings toward the memorandum of understanding (MOU) process.

4. Reflect on your established goals; visualize the steps you will need to take to achieve your goals.

Chapter Objectives

By the end of reading this chapter and completing the learning activities, the reader should be able to:

1. Finalize a site for completion of the DCE and project.

2. Develop a project plan for the doctoral capstone project.

3. Develop initial goals and objectives collaboratively with the site mentor.

4. Determine the doctoral capstone timeline.

5. Understand the purpose of the MOU and develop the MOU.

FINALIZING THE CAPSTONE SITE

The first step in the final planning process is to ensure the capstone student has secured a site for the doctoral experience and project. In Chapter 4, the reader explored sites, how to communicate with potential sites, and site development. This chapter moves the capstone team to the finalization phase of collaboratively securing the site. As the capstone student begins to finalize the site for the DCE and project, it is required that the student has completed a literature review and needs assessment (ACOTE Standard D.1.3; ACOTE, 2018). Writing a literature review was discussed in Chapter 3 and the needs assessment is examined in Chapter 7.

Capstone Purpose

Through completion of the literature review, the capstone student has established a clear purpose for the DCE and project that is supported by evidence from the literature. It is important when finalizing the placement of a student to a capstone site that the problem the student wants to address is a problem the site wants to address so it can be a win-win for both the capstone student and the site. To ensure this is the case, the capstone student needs to be confident in articulating the capstone purpose to the site mentor to allow for the site mentor to make the final commitment. In this final planning stage, before the start of the capstone experience and project, the capstone student is finalizing the overall purpose of the capstone that will lead to the collaborative development of the goals and objectives for the experience and project. Establishing a final site for the DCE and project is a fluid process and often one that may have many iterations. Both the capstone coordinator and the student should keep a sense of optimism that a site and mentor will be located. It does take time, but, the capstone student working collaboratively with the capstone coordinator, will lead to a site placement that will allow students to develop in-depth knowledge in their focus area.

TEACHING TIP 1: *When I was the doctoral capstone coordinator at the University of Indianapolis, I set up specific office hours to meet individually with students in the semester between their capstone development course and capstone planning course to finalize placements. By doing this is, it allows the student more time to work with the site on goal development and establishing an MOU during their capstone planning course. By the end of the capstone planning course the student will then have a finalized proposal including a literature review, needs assessment, goals and objectives, evaluation plan, and a MOU in place in order to be prepared to begin the capstone experience and project after completion of all fieldwork.*

—Julie A. Bednarski, OTD, MHS, OTR
Clinical Associate Professor
Associate Program Director
School of Health & Human Sciences
Department of Occupational Therapy
Indiana University
Indianapolis, Indiana

TEXT BOX 6-1

The following are insights from an occupational therapy doctoral (OTD) student on how her DCE experience and project came to fruition based on a need found in the literature:

"Farmers and ranchers who undergo rehabilitation after injury are dissatisfied with the rehabilitation outcomes because the physical rehabilitative process does not necessarily assist them to return to farm life and agriculture work" (Jorge, 2006, p. 61). While planning the DCE, it was personally important to develop a project where I was interested, passionate, and could address current limitations in knowledge or care. Initial planning of the DCE included refinement of a practice area.

This was done by making a list of interested practice settings, followed by initial research, to gain a better understanding of the limitations currently being faced by the setting. During research, the above quote struck me. What was being done to address this issue, and how could I make an impact?

Based on personal experience within agriculture and limited research on the relationship between health professionals and the agriculture community, it was apparent that not enough efforts were being made to address the issue. Following additional research on this and related topics, the project idea was solidified. Through research on the project idea came the solidification of the DCE placement site.

—Danyele Clingan, OTD, OTR
Class of 2018
School of Occupational Therapy
University of Indianapolis
Indianapolis, Indiana

Determining Final Fit

Another component of finalizing the capstone student to a site is linking the capstone student's values to the site values to determine the fit. This is important because the DCE is a 14-week commitment (ACOTE, 2018) and is self-directed by the capstone student. Therefore, it is important that students develop an experience and project that aligns with their goals and values. One way to do this is to have capstone students examine their beliefs and values and create a personal mission statement.

Developing a Personal Mission Statement

A personal mission statement helps to identify a person's core values and beliefs and allows you to prioritize your life. Covey (2004) stated, "a personal mission statement describes what matters most to you, including your vision and values" (pp. 158-159). Components of a mission statement include stating a major goal in life, using positive language, creating positive energy, writing in the present tense, and keeping the statement concise. Creating a personal mission statement will guide students as they finalize their capstone site and throughout the capstone experience and project. After students have clearly defined a personal mission statement, they can link their mission to the mission of a site, and this may assist with determining a final fit for the student.

Here as some examples of mission statements that were developed by OTD students at the University of Indianapolis.

My personal mission is to provide a holistic and restorative service to individuals with physical and cognitive limitations. I am committed to creating a loving, compassionate, and respectful therapeutic environment for those who desire to improve their physical and cognitive functioning through client-centered intervention strategies and techniques.

My greatest desire is to help individuals integrate their body-mind-spirit aspects into their daily life activities so that they can lead healthy and fulfilling lives.

—Pamela Hess, OTD Student
Class of 2020
School of Occupational Therapy
University of Indianapolis
Indianapolis, Indiana

My life's mission statement is to always appreciate the little things and never take for granted what I have. I believe life should be about living and taking advantage of every moment and opportunity to learn and do something new. I believe that laughter and love should be at the core of all things. In my life, I strive to help others find their path that will lead them to a fulfilling life of love, laughter, and light.

—Tamzyn Mather, OTD Student
Class of 2020
School of Occupational Therapy
University of Indianapolis
Indianapolis, Indiana

To create relationships and partnerships to empower those who feel as if they are incapable in their abilities in themselves to engage in their occupations. To serve, motivate, and provide them the skills and confidence to conquer and problem solve whatever stands in their way.

—Amy Ragle, OTD Student
Class of 2020
School of Occupational Therapy
University of Indianapolis
Indianapolis, Indiana

My personal mission statement is to continually grow and better myself every day. To treasure the opportunities that come my way and make the best use of them. To focus on academics and build a reputation of being dedicated to each goal personally and professionally. To positively impact and make a difference in those surrounding me. To inspire, encourage, and use my education and experiences to motivate others to live respectable lives and reach their fullest potential.

—Kandyse Kaizer, OTD Student
Class of 2020
School of Occupational Therapy
University of Indianapolis
Indianapolis, Indiana

The steps to successfully (and efficiently) match a site with a capstone student can take time, and often a first idea for a capstone site may not be the right fit and the process will need to continue until the final site is found. Most often, the final acceptance is determined after all education, discussions, communications, and/or interviews have been completed. As a doctoral capstone coordinator, it will be important to have a written statement that the site agrees to take the student for the 14-week experience and provide the student a mentor that has expertise in the area of focus being addressed. When the capstone student is matched to a to site and site mentor, the process of finalizing; the goals and objectives, the doctoral capstone proposal, and the MOU will occur to prepare for the implementation phase.

DEVELOPING THE CAPSTONE PROJECT GOAL AND OBJECTIVES

As the site is finalized for the DCE, a collaborative effort needs to occur to develop the goals and objectives for the capstone project. The process of determining goals and objectives requires communication with the capstone team and should be directed by the capstone student. The following gives a narrative of how the process of goal development may require multiple iterations to ensure that the initial goals that student developed meet the needs of the site.

TEXT BOX 6-3

I found Island Dolphin Care (in Florida) and immediately got in contact with the internship coordinator. Originally, my primary focus area was clinical practice skills in this nontraditional practice setting. The area of secondary focus was program development in an area that was previously identified as a need by the therapy staff at Island Dolphin Care.

Through a review of the literature and communication with my site and faculty mentors, my topic was solidified to explore the role of occupational therapy in a nontraditional practice setting and create a home program to increase carryover of skills following a dolphin-assisted therapy program for children with special needs. We agreed that I would participate in all aspects of the therapeutic process, including evaluation of the client, intervention planning, and implementing a home program after the dolphin-assisted therapy program was complete.

—Taylor Millar, OTD, OTR
Class of 2018
School of Occupational Therapy
University of Indianapolis
Indianapolis, Indiana

Often, initial goals and objectives will be developed to have a starting point when talking with a site but will then be reworked and refined based on collaborative, ongoing communication. As a doctoral student, it can be helpful to conceptualize the overarching goals for your DCE as a long-term goal (LTG) and your individualized student objectives as short term goals (STG), that is, the steps that you need to take to accomplish your LTG. Goals and objectives should be measurable so that you can tell when your goals have been met (Bonner & Smith, 2018). Developmentally, the capstone student will have already had didactic curricula focused on establishing goals and objectives for clients through the occupational therapy process. A commonly used framework to create goals is the acronym SMART (Sames, 2014). When creating goals using the SMART framework, the capstone student is writing goals for the project that are Specific, Measurable, Action oriented, Realistic, and Timely. As SMART goals are developed, then objectives for each goal can be written to give the capstone student action steps to meet the goals. By creating specific goals and objectives as action steps, the capstone student is developing the plan for the DCE and project. Here are some examples of goals and objectives that capstone students have written within their final doctoral capstone proposal.

TEXT BOX 6-4

In this first example the capstone student collaborated with an older adult community partner and based her programming on the living legends program (Chippendale & Boltz, 2015).

GOAL 1: *The student will develop life review programming within the long-term care facility and assisted living facility by end of week 2.*

Objective 1: Complete needs assessment with key stakeholders in both settings by end of week 1.

Objective 2: Design 8-week life review writing/sharing/ discovery workshops and review with faculty mentor and site mentor by end of week 3.

Objective 3: Meet with administrators at the elementary school next door to the facility by end of week 2 to arrange for intergenerational exchanges between elementary students and older adults.

GOAL 2: *The student will implement life review programming in both settings by end of week 10.*

Objective 1: Instruct the older adults within both settings on how to develop, write, and share their stories.

Objective 2: Facilitate intergenerational exchange with the elementary school students by working with administrators to identify appropriate students for participation and educate students on communicating with older adults.

Objective 3: Determine sustainability plan by incorporating activities personnel in the program and providing education and training on the program.

GOAL 3: *The student will demonstrate efficacy of life review programming through program evaluation.*

Objective 1: Utilize pre/post testing measures with older adults participating in the program.

Objective 2: Complete post-program interviews with staff at each site including the school.

Objective 3: Create programming guide and train appropriate personnel on the program to facilitate continued implementation.

—Alexis LeCount, OTD, OTR
Class of 2019
School of Occupational Therapy
University of Indianapolis
Indianapolis, Indiana

TEXT BOX 6-4 (continued)

The second is an example of one goal and objectives for a DCE with the purpose to explore and define the role of occupational therapy in the prevention and treatment of Post Intensive Care Syndrome (PICS).

GOAL 1: *The student will implement an intensive care unit (ICU) Diary program serving at least five patients in the ICU by week 7 of the DCE.*

Objective 1: *Observation in the ICU with multiple disciplines during weeks 1 and 2.*

Objective 2: *Brief interviews with members of interdisciplinary team to discuss feasibility by end of week 2.*

Objective 3: *Trials with patient identified through site mentor and/or ICU team beginning week 3.*

Objective 4: *Assessment of trials and development of a plan to implement by week 7.*

—Claire Kittridge, OTD, OTR
Class of 2019
School of Occupational Therapy
University of Indianapolis
Indianapolis, Indiana

These goals and objectives will continue to be revised as the experience and project begins during the implementation phase. The goals and objectives are an essential part of the capstone proposal and will help to define a plan for what knowledge the student will gain by the conclusion of the experience. Appendix 6-A gives the reader an example of an overall capstone plan and how achievement of in-depth knowledge will occur. In this plan, the capstone student (a) defines goals and objectives, (b) creates an action plan to meet the objectives, (c) creates a proposed timeline, and (d) proposes evidence of meeting the objectives. The design of the capstone needs to be consistent with the program's design (ACOTE Standard D.1.2; ACOTE, 2018), and one way for the student to link to the design is to review the curriculum design and program outcomes. These documents are usually found in the occupational therapy education program's student handbook or are stated on course syllabi. The examples shown in Text Box 6-5 show how two OTD students related their DCE project to the curriculum design and outcomes of their occupational therapy program.

TEXT BOX 6-5

A Program outcome to ensure students are able to demonstrate client-centered practice is reflected in the following student capstone objective:
- The protocols designed will focus on the needs of the residents and education to caregivers and facility staff will promote sustainability of the project.

—Megan Shuret, OTD, OTR
Class of 2019
School of Occupational Therapy
University of Indianapolis
Indianapolis, Indiana

TEXT BOX 6-5 (continued)

A Program outcome in which students gain knowledge in evidence-based practice is reflected in the following student capstone objective:
- The DCE student will apply evidence-based practice of non-pharmacological management of delirium in the ICU and cognitive interventions for individuals with PICS.

—Claire Kittridge, OTD, OTR
Class of 2019
School of Occupational Therapy
University of Indianapolis
Indianapolis, Indiana

THE DOCTORAL CAPSTONE PROPOSAL

ACOTE (2018) Standard D.1.3 states to "ensure that preparation for the capstone project includes a literature review, needs assessment, goals/objectives, and an evaluation plan" (p. 44). In preparing for the implementation of the DCE and project, OTD programs may require the capstone student to create and disseminate to the capstone team a formal capstone proposal. See Appendix 6-B for an example of a "Doctoral Capstone Proposal" used by the School of Occupational Therapy at University of Indianapolis. When reviewing the capstone proposal example, you notice that the proposal is designed to meet ACOTE (2018) Standard D.1.3. Therefore, recommended components of a capstone proposal include the literature review (discussed in Chapter 3), an initial needs assessment (discussed in Chapters 7 and 10), goals and objectives (reviewed in this chapter), and a determination of how you will evaluate your capstone project—in other words, what is the evaluation plan? How to plan for and determine the outcomes of your project is discussed in Chapter 8. Another important aspect of the capstone proposal is determining the theory that will guide you in the development and implementation of your capstone project. The ACOTE (2018) definition of a capstone project is "a project that is completed by a doctoral-level student that demonstrates the student's ability to relate theory to practice and to synthesize in-depth knowledge in a practice area that relates to the capstone experience" (p. 46). Chapter 10 will assist the capstone student in determining how to link theory to the experience and project. An essential aspect of the preparation phase and the capstone proposal is alignment with the program's curriculum design. While the initiation of the proposal needs to occur before the start of the DCE, some items (such as the goals, objectives, and aspects of the needs assessment) may still evolve as the capstone experience begins.

INSTITUTIONAL REVIEW BOARD

A determination will need to be made as to whether the capstone project is considered "research" and if it will need to be submitted to the institutional review board (IRB) at the capstone student's institution or capstone site. The U.S. Department of Health and Human Services (2018) definition of research is "a systematic investigation, including research development, testing and evaluation, designed to develop or contribute to generalizable knowledge" (U.S. Department of Health and Human Services, 2017). An IRB is in place to protect human participants who take part in research, and each institution will have policies on what constitutes the need for approval. Some capstone projects may not be considered research or do not meet the research criteria. "Projects that are limited to program evaluation, quality improvement or quality assurance activities designed specifically to assess or improve performance within the department, hospital or classroom setting" may be determined by an IRB not to be research (University of Indianapolis, Human Subjects Research Determination Form, 2018). The IRB may consider a capstone project not to be research if, when students disseminate the information, they disseminate what they did in their capstone and the outcomes of their particular capstone and do not make suggestions on replication of the methodology and are not suggesting generalizing the results. In both of these instances, it is the IRB that determines whether the project is research, not the student. If the student is interested in publishing the results of the capstone project, it will be important to go through the IRB to obtain a letter stating an IRB review has taken place.

An IRB that considers a capstone project to be research may deem it to be exempt or expedited based on minimal risk to research participants. Minimal risk is,

> where the probability and magnitude of harm or discomfort anticipated in the research are not greater in and of themselves than those ordinarily encountered in daily life or during the performance of routine physical or psychological examinations or tests. (Federal Policy for the Protection of Human Subjects, 2017)

This, however, is determined by each IRB at the various institutions and not the researcher (Bonnel & Smith, 2018).

The capstone coordinator may first want to meet with the IRB chair when developing the capstone experience and project protocols. The IRB committee at the academic institution will want to be aware if there will be an increase of proposals submitted. This will enable the IRB committee to determine the best way to handle a large number of students submitting applications. Appendix 6-C gives an example of what is being utilized by the Department of Occupational Therapy at Duquesne University to expedite the process.

DEVELOPMENT OF THE MEMORANDUM OF UNDERSTANDING

An MOU is required per ACOTE (2018) Standard D.1.4: "Ensure that there is a valid MOU for the DCE, that, at a minimum, includes individualized specific objectives, plans for supervision or mentoring, and responsibilities of all parties" (p. 44). The MOU must be signed by both parties (ACOTE, 2018, p. 44). In fieldwork, the MOU is the contract or affiliation agreement between the site and the university. However, in the doctoral capstone, the MOU serves as a contract between the site mentor, the capstone student, and the capstone team. Other areas that the student may want to address in the MOU include a statement of authorship, credentials and qualifications of the site mentor, qualifications of the faculty mentor, relationship of DCE objectives to the curriculum design and professional outcomes of the program, and a statement of ownership of materials created as part of the capstone. See Appendix 6-D for an example of the MOU that the School of Occupational Therapy at the University of Indianapolis is using. The capstone student is responsible for the finalizing the MOU, but to create the MOU, the capstone student collaborates with the capstone team. The following will give direction to the capstone student and doctoral capstone coordinator as to what to include in the MOU.

Identification of the Capstone Team

The MOU is a document that outlines the members of the capstone team, which includes the site mentor, doctoral capstone coordinator, capstone student, and possibly a faculty member, who will serve as an additional mentor or chair for the capstone project. Depending on the number of capstone students, most often the doctoral capstone coordinator will work with the program director or department chair to identify faculty mentors (or capstone chairs) for the doctoral students and to serve as a capstone team member. ACOTE does not directly state that a faculty or capstone chair is required; however, ACOTE Standard D.1.2 does state the following: "Ensure that the doctoral capstone is designed through collaboration of the faculty and student, and provided in setting(s) consistent with the program's curriculum design, including individualized specific objectives and plans for supervision" (ACOTE, 2018, p. 44). Once the capstone team is in place, the student can begin working with the faculty mentor and will describe on the MOU how the qualifications of the faculty mentor will relate to the DCE. By having a faculty mentor as an added team mentor, capstone students are gaining a greater perspective in their specific area of focus. The site mentor will also be identified on the MOU and qualifications documented. ACOTE (2018) Standard D.1.6 states: "Document and verify that the student is mentored by an individual with expertise consistent with the student's area of focus prior to the onset of the DCE. The mentor does not have to be an occupational therapist" (p. 45). To verify expertise, a professional resume of the site mentor should be obtained, reviewed, and verified to ensure expertise consistent with the student's area of focus. Documents such as the resume to substantiate expertise should be attached to the MOU including any certifications or licensure verification.

Purpose

A clear purpose for the capstone experience needs to be stated along with support from the literature to assist in providing significance and need. It should be clear what the gap is in the literature and how the capstone project will address the gap. Refer back to Chapter 3 for more specifics on determining purpose.

Individualized Specific Objectives

The individualized student objectives are the tasks and actions that the capstone student will complete to achieve the in-depth knowledge and experience in the chosen focus area(s). These will be established collaboratively as described earlier in this chapter. It is important to have these goals and objectives on the MOU because all capstone team members are signing the MOU, and this will be verification that all parties agree. Refer to Appendix 6-E for a student example of individualized specific objectives written collaboratively with the capstone team.

Plans for Supervision or Mentoring

Having a plan for supervision is an ACOTE requirement and by having a plan the student and site mentor are setting up an environment for success. The conversation regarding expectations is important and by writing out these expectations all capstone team members will understand the plan. Referring to the MOU in Appendix 6-D gives the capstone student examples of documentation of responsibilities for each the student and the site mentor and to this, supervision guidelines can be added. Table 6-1 gives suggestions for questions for the capstone student and site mentor to consider as the supervision plan is developed.

Relationship of the Doctoral Capstone Experience Objectives to the Programs Curriculum Design and Professional Outcomes

The capstone experience needs to align with the curriculum design of the program (ACOTE, 2018). This allows the student to ensure that the plan for the experience and project aligns with the curriculum of the program. It is essential that capstone students review and understand their program's curriculum design and program outcomes during the initial development phase of the DCE. How does the capstone experience and project plan match the program's outcomes? Review the examples given in Text Box 6-5. As the capstone student is in the final phase of planning, it is now time to collaborate with the doctoral capstone coordinator and faculty mentor to document this link between the curriculum design and the capstone site to ensure compliance to Standard D.1.2 (ACOTE, 2018).

Statement of Authorship

Because dissemination is a required part of the doctoral capstone, an initial discussion about authorship needs to occur. Authorship should be given to those that make considerable contributions to the project, and acknowledgment is given to those who offer a lesser contribution (American Psychological Association [APA], 2010, pp. 18-19). Therefore, it may be that the site mentor and faculty mentor have authorship along with the capstone student on any dissemination presentations or publications. Depending on the level of involvement of the capstone coordinator, he or she may be given an acknowledgment or have authorship. Principal authorship is given to the person who is most involved (APA, 2010), and this most likely will be the capstone student. Initiating this discussion and making this determination at the start of the DCE will ensure that publication credit will be accurate and misconceptions will be avoided.

Statement of Ownership of Materials

If the doctoral student is planning on developing materials for the site (such as new handouts or training modules that follow best health literacy principles), there needs to be an understanding of ownership. What is created for the site most likely will be owned by the site and proper citations and permission for future use of materials will need to be followed. By having an ownership statement in the MOU, all parties agree and thus reducing any misunderstandings as to ownership of materials at the capstone completion.

COMMUNICATION WITH THE CAPSTONE TEAM

During this final planning stage, frequent and ongoing communication is critical among the capstone team to

Table 6-1. Items to Consider When Developing a Supervision Plan
• Roles and responsibilities for initial orientation?
• How often will we have formal face-to-face meetings?
• What is the best method of communication throughout the week?
• What is the students learning style?
• What is the site mentors leadership and/or mentorship style?
• How will conflict be resolved?
• A midterm and final evaluation is required—will there be other forms of evaluation?

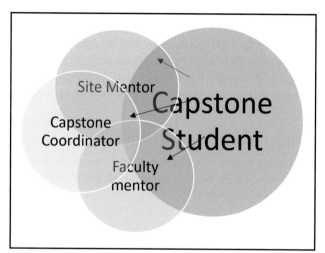

Figure 6-1. Communication with the capstone team.

ensure success of the capstone experience and project. Figure 6-1 gives the reader a visual of the communication taking place between the capstone team as the capstone experience and project become finalized. The capstone student at this point in time is the major communicator and is taking the initiative to remain in close contact with the site mentor, doctoral capstone coordinator and a faculty mentor (or capstone chair). Figure 6-1 illustrates the fluid communication that is occurring between members of the capstone team.

As stated in Chapter 1, assigning faculty mentors to capstone students is a process that will be different for each program, and some programs may choose to have a faculty member as the capstone chair for the student. This will be dependent on the number of students and program philosophy. If a faculty mentor (or capstone chair) is assigned, it is appropriate to ensure the faculty mentor has expertise in the capstone student's area of focus to best assist with goal development and final preparations. When there is faculty mentor involvement, it is important to begin the involvement early in the planning stage so he or she can be an active participant in goal development and assessment of site needs. The capstone student should be expected to establish meetings with both the faculty mentor and site mentor to (a) review the capstone proposal, (b) review and obtain signatures for the MOU, and (c) develop individualized goals and objectives.

Developing a solid foundation for communication with the capstone team will lead the capstone student into a successful start to the implementation phase.

CHAPTER SUMMARY

This chapter described the final planning stage of the capstone experience and project before moving into implementation. In this final planning stage, the capstone student writes the final capstone proposal, and the capstone team works together to complete the final individualized goals and objectives along with completion of the MOU. The DCE and project is drawing closer and ensuring all components are in place before the commencement of going on-site requires the capstone team working in congruence. This is an exciting time, as the next step in the process is the actual implementation.

Learning Activities

1. Review the mission statement of your proposed capstone site. Create a personal mission statement. Creating your own personal mission will help align your values and passion to a potential DCE project. How does your mission statement link to the potential site for your DCE? What is the connection of the two missions? How does your DCE project link to your personal mission?

2. Draw a tree on a large piece of paper. Make sure you draw roots, a large trunk, branches, leaves, and fruit. Once the outline of your tree is drawn complete the tree as follows:

   • The Roots: Your Values
   • The Trunk: Your Mission Statement
   • The Branches: Your DCE Purpose
   • The Leaves: Your Goals and Objectives
   • The Fruit: The proposed outcome/results

   Once you have completed your picture, share with another peer and discuss the meaning of your tree.

3. Think about your DCE and write one potential goal with two objectives. Share with a partner, and provide feedback to each other:

    •   Is the goal measurable?

    •   Does it sound doable?

    •   Is it clearly written?

    •   Does it have the components of a SMART goal?

    •   Discuss recommendations.

REFERENCES

Accreditation Council for Occupational Therapy Education. (2018). *Standards and interpretive guide*. Retrieved from https://www.aota.org/~/media/Corporate/Files/EducationCareers/Accredit/StandardsReview/2018-ACOTE-Standards-Interpretive-Guide.pdf

American Psychological Association. (2009). *Publication manual of the American Psychological Association* (6th ed.). Washington, DC: American Psychological Association.

Bonnel, W., & Smith, K.V. (2018). *Proposal writing for clinical nursing and DNP projects* (2nd ed.). New York, NY: Springer.

Chippendale, T., & Boltz, M. (2015). Living legends: Effectiveness of a program to enhance sense of purpose and meaning among community-dwelling adults. *American Journal of Occupational Therapy, 69*(4), 1-11.

Covey, S. R. (2004). *The 8th habit from effectiveness to greatness.* New York, NY: Free Press.

Jorge, M (2006). AgrAbility: Doctor of physical therapy (DPT) students learning to advocate for farmers and ranchers with disabilities. *Journal of Physical Therapy Education, 20*(3), 61.

U.S. Department of Health and Human Services. (2017, January 19). *Code of Federal Regulations*. Retrieved from https://www.gpo.gov/fdsys/pkg/CFR-2016-title45-vol1/pdf/CFR-2016-title45-vol1-part46.pdf

U.S. Department of Health and Human Services. (2018, revised). F*ederal policy for the protection of human subjects.* Revised Common Rule. Retrieved from https://www.hhs.gov/ohrp/regulations-and-policy/regulations/finalized-revisions-common-rule/index.html

Sames, K. M. (2014). *Documenting occupational therapy practice* (3rd ed.). Upper Saddle River, NJ: Pearson Education.

Appendix 6-A

ACTION PLAN

Doctoral Experiential Component Action Plan to Achieve In Depth Skills

Outline how you will achieve your self-authored goals (designed in collaboration with your site mentor) below by indicating your learning objectives, activities to achieve your objectives, and proposed evidence of achievement of your learning objectives (add rows to the table as needed)

Individualized Learning Objective	Activities, Strategies and/or Actions to Achieve Objective	Proposed Timeline for Each Objective	Proposed Evidence of Achievement of Learning Objective	Misc.
Increase program implementation skills with a spinal cord injury population	• Follow up with each patient to discuss ways to improve the program • Informally follow up with at least 2 patients per week to ensure they still understand concepts	• Follow up with each patient within a week of their post-test • Follow up with at least 2 patients per week, especially those with lower post-test scores	• Journaling feedback from meetings and patient satisfaction surveys • Journal which participants were met with and which topics were most difficult to understand	
Obtain advanced clinical knowledge of the spinal cord injury population	• Observe wound care, bowel/bladder care, respiratory therapy, and SLP to increase specialized clinical knowledge regarding SCI patients • Interview past SCI patients (at least 1 per week if on the unit) regarding additional topics that would have been beneficial to know prior to their initial discharge-can be done at outpatient	• Observe at least one discipline every other week • Interview at least one patient per week (if there is an old SCI patient on the unit)	• Journal the dates of the observations • Journal the date of interview and the important takeaways	
Enhance leadership skills pertaining to program implementation	• Recruit at least 2 patients per week to participate in the program (if applicable) • Discuss any other preventative techniques that should be added to the presentation with at least 3 other disciplines (PT, Speech, Nursing)	• Recruit at least 2 patient by the end of the week • Have a discussion with another profession at least every other week	• Log the number of patients the program was implemented with each week • Journal the techniques mentioned by each professional	

Signatures below signify acceptance of the above proposal and approval to move forward with implementation. It is the student's responsibility to access resources, carry out these and/or other strategies to increase their knowledge and skill, aligned with their chosen focus area.

Student Signature _____ *Justin McTish, Duquesne University, OTD Class of 2018* ___ Date: _____

Site Mentor Signature _____   Date: _____

Doctoral Experiential Component Action Plan to Achieve In Depth Skills

Outline how you will achieve your self-authored goals (designed in collaboration with your site mentor) below by indicating your learning objectives, activities to achieve your objectives, and proposed evidence of achievement of your learning objectives (add rows to the table as needed)

Signatures below signify acceptance of the above proposal and approval to move forward with implementation. It is the student's responsibility to access resources, carry out these and/or other strategies to increase their knowledge and skill, aligned with their chosen focus area.

Student Signature _____ *Justin McFish, Duquesne University, OTD Class of 2018* _____ Date: _____

Site Mentor Signature _____ Date: _____

Appendix 6-B

FINAL CAPSTONE PROPOSAL

UNIVERSITY of
INDIANAPOLIS

School of Occupational Therapy

Doctoral Capstone Experience and Project Proposal- Final Draft

CAPSTONE STUDENT NAME:

Name of DCE Site and Address	
Site Mentor Name and Contact Information	
Purpose of DCE (*must have literature to support purpose*)	

Please note the primary and secondary focus of your proposed AP by putting 1 and 2 in the appropriate boxes.

AP Focus	
Clinical Practice Skills	
Research Skills	
Administration	
Leadership	
Program/Policy Development	
Advocacy	
Education	
Theory Development	

UNIVERSITY *of* **INDIANAPOLIS**

School of Occupational Therapy

Literature Review	*Attach literature review to end of this document and reference list
Summary of Needs Assessment	

UNIVERSITY *of* **INDIANAPOLIS**

School of Occupational Therapy

Goals With Objectives	
Brief synopsis of model/theory and frame of reference to guide your DCE *(You must support with literature)*	

UNIVERSITY *of*
INDIANAPOLIS.

School of Occupational Therapy

Plan for evaluation *(How will you determine project outcomes—what outcome measures will you use and why? Use support from the literature)*	

Appendix 6-C

ADAPTED INSTITUTIONAL REVIEW BOARD SUMMARY FORM

> **DUQUESNE UNIVERSITY**
> **Rangos School of Health Sciences**
> **Department of Occupational Therapy**

Sample Abbreviated IRB Protocol

Instructions:

The Protocol Summary is limited to 3-6 single spaced pages using a 12-point font. Appendices may include but are not limited to items such as a consent form, data collection tools or recruitment flyers and these are not included in the page limits. Each appendix must be submitted to in a separate file and named accordingly (e.g. Recruitment Flyer.docx). Similarly, instruments for data collection may be submitted in WORD or PDF and included as an appendix. The page limitation does not include appendices or attachments. You are provided the specific content guidelines below. Once reviewed and approved by your capstone coordinator and/or faculty (or capstone chair), you will be asked to submit this protocol summary to the IRB Board.

SPECIFIC CONTENT: The following sections with headings MUST be addressed. Each of these components are evaluated by the Institutional Review Board. If you do not use these specific headings, your protocol summary may be rejected

1) **Statement of the research question:** You must use this heading, but you may not have a specific research question. It is appropriate to make this section only a sentence or two and to qualify your content by identifying the focus of your capstone, i.e.program development, program evaluation, quality improvement or staff training nature of your capstone project. When your capstone has multiple parts, you are encouraged to focus on any one of these. That is, even though your project may have many parts choose one component. In particular, choose a part of the project that may most lend itself to preparing for formal dissemination, such as presentation or publication.

2) **Purpose and significance of the study:** Use language like, "the purpose and significance of this program evaluation or this staff training project or this quality improvement project is ...". In this section you should draw directly from the earlier capstone drafts you have created. You are not providing and the IRB board does not want to see a full-blown literature review. A synopsis and summation will suffice. Bear in mind that you are not trying to convince the reader of your knowledge of all the relevant background literature. Your purpose in this section is to provide a context for the program or training that you are describing in the protocol. You are encouraged to judiciously choose statements from your needs assessment that helps you make strong arguments, e.g., a preliminary needs assessment revealed that the staff at this community facility had a strong interest in improving programming for adults with IDD and in improving their own skill sets for increasing participation with individual consumers - OR - a preliminary needs assessment revealed that parents and teachers alike identified several areas where communication in IEP meetings might be improved.

3) **Research design and procedures:** Use language like, "this project is designed as a program evaluation or this project is designed as a staff training project or this project is designed as a quality improvement project to ...". The work you have already completed to describe project

implementation can inform this section. Again, remember in a project that may have many component parts choose one or a few related parts that go hand in hand most effectively and which can be described efficiently.

4) **Instruments:** Be matter of fact. If the tool is a published tool, then your descriptions in your earlier capstone propsoal will suffice. If you created the tool, describe the tool BRIEFLY. You will need to upload each tool that your use and describe in your appendices section. Remember, don't load tools for components of your project that you are not including in this protocol summary submission.

5) **Sample selection and size:** Be matter of fact. Most of you are working with convenience samples. You are encouraged to not identify protected populations as your sample as this invited the highest level of scrutiny by the IRB. For example, many of you are working in programs that directly impact children while others are looking at adults with cognitive limitations such as IDD or dementia. These are protected populations for human subjects research. However, you all are also including the parents, caregivers, teachers or staff working with these protected populations and you want to emphasize that group as your sample.

6) **Recruitment of subjects:** Be matter of fact. How will you identify and recruit? If you use a flyer or some other mechanism like this, include a copy in your Appendices and write a short, succinct but clear description of your procedures.

7) **Informed consent procedures:** Be straightforward and define the process. Include the who, what, when and how. You will need to include a copy of the consent form in your appendices.

8) **Collection of data and method of data analysis:** Be specific and state what data will be collected and by what means. Again, only discuss the tools you will use that correspond to the parts of your project that you are describing in this protocol. Any tools you describe need to be loaded as appendices. You do not have to go into critical details of your data analysis plan but do provide a description of what you will do.

9) **Emphasize issues relating to interactions with subjects and subjects' rights:** The critically key element in your descriptions is DE-IDENTIFICATION. Only collect information that you absolutely need should be collected and human subjects concerns are all about confidentiality. I've included I've included an example of "template language" that has worked in previous proposals. You should feel free to delete what does not apply and to change titles of tools to consistently and accurately reflect what you will do.

Appendix 6-D

MEMORANDUM OF UNDERSTANDING

UNIVERSITY *of*

INDIANAPOLIS.

School of Occupational Therapy

Doctoral Capstone

Memorandum of Understanding

Title of the Doctoral Capstone Experience: _____

Area of Primary Focus: Please bold

Clinical Practice Skills	Program & Policy Development
Research Skills	Advocacy
Administration	Education
Leadership	Theory Development

Area of Secondary Focus: Please bold

Clinical Practice Skills	Program & Policy Development
Research Skills	Advocacy
Administration	Education
Leadership	Theory Development

Doctoral Capstone Experience Team

OTD Student:
Doctoral Capstone Coordinator:
Faculty Mentor:
Qualifications of the Faculty mentor relative to DCE focus:
Name of Site:
Primary Site Mentor: Name and Title:
Qualifications of Site Mentor (also attach resume and provide certifications):

Doctoral Capstone Experience and Project Purpose (evidence from the literature is required):

Doctoral Capstone Experience and Project Individualized Goals and Objectives:

Relationship of Doctoral Capstone Experience (DCE) Objectives to SOT Curriculum Design and Professional Outcomes:

Doctoral Capstone Experience Responsibilities & Supervision Plan:	
Student will demonstrate at a minimum: (not limited to the following): • Commitment to self-directed learning and fulfillment of all DCE and OTD 690 expectations • Adherence to the requirements for attendance and appropriate number of hours, including on site hours. • Consistent communication with DCE team and other appropriate entities/people • Adherence to Supervision Responsibilities & Guidelines • Demonstration of professional roles and responsibilities for both the site and school guidelines. **Additional responsibilities:**	**Site Mentor will demonstrate at a minimum: (not limited to the following):** • Adherence to the mentoring guidelines relative to the area of focus for this DCE • Provision of appropriate resources for the UINDY DCE student • Will serve as a professional role model for the UNIDY DCE student. **Additional responsibilities:**
Statement of planned dissemination of the final culminating project:	
Authorship agreement between the Student, Site Mentor, and Faculty Mentor (note; materials developed for the site (ie handouts, program protocols…) by the student are the property of the site unless otherwise noted):	

Signatures noting understanding and agreement to the above statement of responsibilities:

Student: Datc:

Site Mentor: Date:

Faculty Mentor: Date:

Doctoral Capstone Coordinator: Date:

Appendix 6-E

INDIVIDUALIZED STUDENT OBJECTIVES

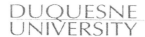
DUQUESNE
UNIVERSITY

JOHN G. RANGOS, SR, SCHOOL OF HEALTH SCIENCES
DEPARTMENT OF OCCUPATIONAL THERAPY
227 HEALTH SCIENCES BUILDING

600 FORBES AVENUE
PITTSBURGH, PA 15282
TEL 412.396.5945
FAX 412.396.4343
www.duq.edu

Occupational Therapy Doctoral Experiential Component Behavioral Objectives

Dear Doctoral Experiential Component Site Supervisor:

All occupational therapy academic programs are required by ACOTE (2011) to assure a documented plan for collaboration between the academic institution and the site and verify that all aspects of the fieldwork program are consistent with the academic institution's curriculum design. (Standard C.2.0 & C.2.1)

The objectives for the 16-week Doctoral Experiential Component for OTD students in Duquesne University's Occupational Therapy Program are listed below. In addition, you will see that there is space provided for the OTD Student and you, the Site Supervisor, to mutually decide upon 3 student-specific objectives that would be achievable within the 16-week experience.

Please collaborate with the OTD Student in setting student-specific learning objectives. **Please sign and date this form, (verifying that these objectives can be met at your site) make a copy for your files, and return the original to us by email (_____@duq.edu) or fax** _____. As always, thank you for the invaluable learning experience and support you provide to our students!

The OTD student will:
1. Demonstrate effective communication skills and work interprofessionally with those who receive and provide care/services
2. Display positive interpersonal skills and insight into one's professional behaviors to accurately appraise one's professional disposition strengths and areas for improvement.
3. Exhibit the ability to practice educative roles for consumers, peers, students, interprofessionals and others
4. Develop essential knowledge and skills to contribute to the advancement of occupational therapy through scholarly activities.
5. Apply a critical foundation of evidence based professional knowledge, skills, and attitudes.
6. Apply principles and constructs of ethics to individual, institutional and societal issues, and articulate justifiable resolutions to these issues and act in an ethical manner.
7. Perform tasks in a safe and ethical manner and adheres to the site's policies and procedures, including those related to human subject research when relevant
8. Demonstrate competence in following program methods, quality improvement and/or research procedures utilized at the site.
9. Learn, practice, and apply knowledge from the classroom and practice settings at a higher level than prior fieldwork experiences with simultaneous guidance from Site Supervisor and DU OT Faculty.

Education for the Mind, Heart, and Spirit

DUQUESNE
UNIVERSITY

John G. Rangos, Sr, School of Health Sciences
Department of Occupational Therapy
227 Health Sciences Building

600 Forbes Avenue
Pittsburgh, PA 15282
tel 412.396.5945
fax 412.396.4343
www.duq.edu

10. Relate theory to practice and demonstrate synthesis f advanced knowledge in a specialized practice area through completion of a doctoral field experience and scholarly project.

11. Acquire in-depth experience in one or more of the following areas: clinical practice skills, research skills, administration, leadership, program and policy development, advocacy, education, and theory development

12. (Student identified objective)

13. (Student identified objective)   *See attached.*

14. (Student identified objective)

I agree with the above stated objectives and feel that all learning objectives are obtainable within the established timeframe and encompass all aspects of the OTD student role at this site.

Goodwill YouthWorks   _Whitney Mills_   _5/19/17_
Name of Site   Signature of Site Supervisor   Date

Mail to:
       OTD, OTR/L Duquesne University
#216 Health Science Building
      Forbes Ave
Pittsburgh, PA 15282
Or fax to:

Education for the Mind, Heart, and Spirit

DEC SITE: Goodwill YouthWorks; Re-Entry through Industry-Specific Education (RISE) Program

CANDIDATE:

ANTICIPATED PROJECT TITLE & DESCRIPTION:
Preliminary Title –
At-Risk Youth and Re-Entry Through Vocation: An Occupational Therapy Application
An occupational therapy perspective has much to offer to the workings of a community re-entry program for at-risk and adjudicated youth. Through application of occupation-based group intervention framed by the Model of Human Occupation, Primary Occupations for Work and Employment Readiness (POWER) aims to facilitate functional integration of acquired knowledge to bolster vocational and educational outcomes.

SITE-SPECIFIC LEARNING OBJECTIVE 1: Over the course of the 16-week DEC, I will meet with individuals representing at least three external resources (organizations, programs, etc.) appropriate for the at-risk youth population and verbalize understanding of the process of referral to these resources.

LEARNING ACTIVITIES: To ensure successful completion of this objective, I will 1) engage in discussion with the three case managers of RISE, 2) research organizations in the Pittsburgh area with programs that may serve at-risk youth, 3) research public or social services available to this population and the process of referral to these services, and 4) have a list of potential individuals to meet outlined by July 1st, 2017.

RATIONALE FOR OBJECTIVE 1: This learning objective is appropriate for my engagement with RISE, as the program there addresses the vocational and educational aspects of community re-entry—however, it does not directly address other issues pertinent to the at-risk youth population such as housing, obtaining food, and management of mental health needs. By gaining an understanding of available external resources that can meet these needs, the process of referring a client to these resources, and building relationships with their providers—I will be better equipped to ensure that clients I encounter now and in the future will receive all services that they require and qualify for.

PLAN TO MONITOR/ASSESS OUTCOMES: I will monitor my progress towards this objective by setting specific timelines for completion; for example, by July 1st, I will have identified a list of potential meetings, by July 8th, I will have arranged the meetings, and by August 1st, I will have completed at least one meeting. I will assess my outcomes by documenting the information that I gain, and seek review of it by the case managers of RISE and my Site Mentor.

SITE SPECIFIC LEARNING OBJECTIVE 2: After the 16-week DEC, I will have completed a detailed activity analysis of the 9 trade fields that RISE trains its students to perform, with application to vocational exploration and work capacity determination.

LEARNING ACTIVITIES: To ensure successful completion of this objective, I will 1) complete 1-2 activity analyses per 2-week period over the 16-weeks of the DEC, 2) consult the occupational therapy literature, beginning with the Dictionary of Occupational Titles, to develop a specific structure to guide these analyses, and 3) research pre-existing occupational therapy literature regarding performance of tasks involved in the 9 trade fields.

RATIONALE FOR OBJECTIVE 2: Activity analysis is a practice at the base of occupational therapy intervention. By understanding, in-depth, the demands and process of tasks required for employment in the 9 trade fields incorporated into the RISE program, I will be better equipped to make adaptations and provide strategies for engagement in these work roles. Additionally, it will allow me to knowledgably guide my students through a work exploration and work capacity determination process. This will enhance my practice not only within the context of YouthWorks, but also in the future if I again encounter clients who are employed or are seeking employment in these fields.

PLAN TO MONITOR/ASSESS OUTCOMES: I will monitor my progress towards this objective by documenting my adherence to the schedule of my identified learning activities; if I complete 3 activity analyses per 2-week period of the DEC, I will be able to analyze all 9 trade fields over the 6-week period that will come before I begin my program implementation. This will allow me to be better prepared to guide my students through vocational exploration when program implementation begins. I will assess my outcomes with continual reflection on the products of these activity analyses to ensure the quality and thoroughness of process. I will also share the 9 trade field activity analyses with my Faculty Mentor/Capstone Chair, who is the only occupational therapist on my Capstone Advisory Committee.

SITE SPECIFIC LEARNING OBJECTIVE 3: At the end of the 16-week DEC, I will clearly and completely articulate the process, requirements, and strategies for a client to prepare for, be engaged in the process of, and attain their educational goals.

LEARNING ACTIVITIES: To ensure successful completion of this objective, I will 1) observe students as they engage in the GED process, 2) gather information about other educational goals that the students may have 3) discuss the educational processes implemented at YouthWorks with the teachers and case managers of RISE, 4) research and understand state/national requirements for GED completion and pursuit of continued education, and 5) familiarize myself with occupational therapy intervention pertaining to educational goals and outcomes..

RATIONALE FOR OBJECTIVE 3: The second component of RISE is educational, preparing and enabling the students to take the GED exams. Education is a process and outcome area that I am not deeply familiar with, but is nonetheless extremely important in the world of vocational rehabilitation-- since the GED alone is becoming an increasingly common minimum requirement for trade jobs, and continued education a requirement for advancement. In the future, clients I encounter in the future may have educational goals; therefore, by developing my understanding of the process and the outcome areas as a whole, I will be better equipped to assist clients in the future.

PLAN TO MONITOR/ASSESS OUTCOMES: I will monitor my progress towards this objective by setting and adhering to specific dates to complete my identified learning activities. I will assess the quality and thoroughness of my outcomes in this area by seeking review and feedback on my understanding from the case managers of RISE and my Site Mentor.

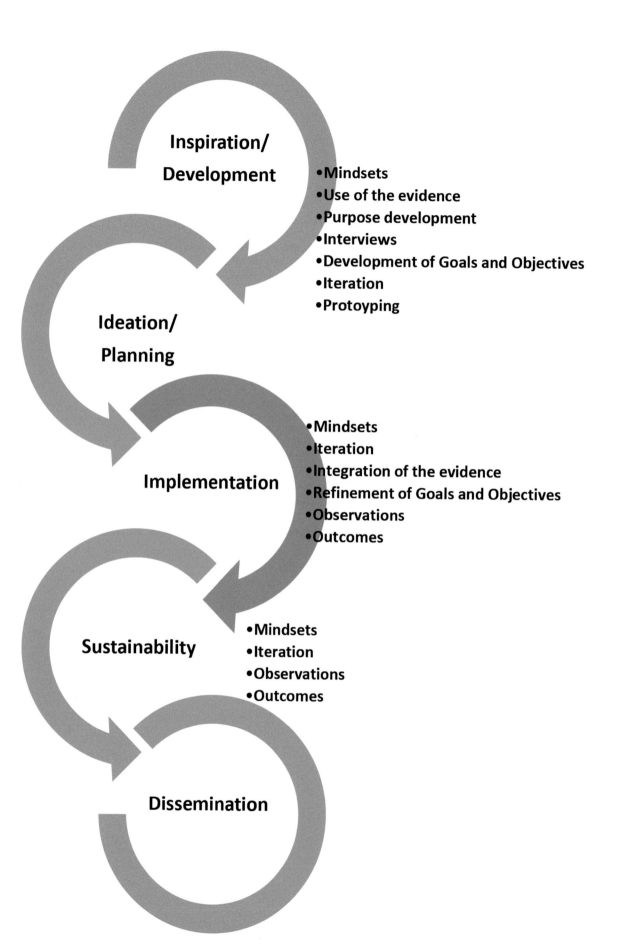

Inspiration/
Development

- Mindsets
- Use of the evidence
- Purpose development
- Interviews
- Development of Goals and Objectives
- Iteration
- Protoyping

Ideation/

Planning

Implementation

- Mindsets
- Iteration
- Integration of the evidence
- Refinement of Goals and Objectives
- Observations
- Outcomes

Sustainability

- Mindsets
- Iteration
- Observations
- Outcomes

Dissemination

PART III.
IMPLEMENTATION

The third step in the capstone process is **implementation and sustainability** of the doctoral capstone experience and project and aligns with the **implementation** process of human-centered design. This phase allows students to bring all their ideas and planning to life. Capstone students will continually be making adjustments during the implementation phase as they work with their specified population. Assessing and adjusting the planned solutions is important throughout the implementation. To be a human-centered designer means you are client-centered. Interacting and communicating with the client for feedback and adjusting goals and objectives as needed is important in this stage of the capstone. During the implementation phase, students are determining how their doctoral capstone project affects their identified client, group, or population and how the project will be sustained.

CHAPTER 7

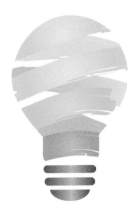

Capstone Project Management

Julie A. Bednarski, OTD, MHS, OTR
Elizabeth D. DeIuliis, OTD, MOT, OTR/L, CLA

Human-Centered Design Mindsets for the Doctoral Students

The human-centered design mindset concept of learning from failure is important for doctoral students to embrace as they begin the implementation phase of the doctoral capstone experience (DCE) and project. Students will continually refine their experience and learn from failures. Live prototyping will take place as students implement their projects at their sites, understand the feasibility of their ideas, and make needed adjustments. Iteration will continue to be important to ensure outcomes are meaningful to the client. Capstone students will continually monitor their experiences and make adjustments based on self-reflection and feedback from the clients. Adopting an iterative approach will assist the student to understanding how problem-solving with the site can lead to better outcomes.

Learning From Failure: Just remember to fail forward. This is a new project and as you initiate your DCE on-site, changes are being made daily to your initial goals and objectives. Each time you tweak and make adjustments, you are doing so to meet the needs of the client, which is positive. Keep initiating, communicating, and making needed adjustments because this is the way you will be successful with your capstone experience and project. The idea you came in with may not be where you are headed later, but you are still headed in the direction to solve the problem and meet the project purpose. You are going through the process of live prototyping, and often this means that the first iteration of an idea needs to be reworked. The first prototype, or idea, may have failed, but you learn from this and move forward.

Iterate, Iterate, Iterate: Remember to keep the focus on your client for this experience and project. You will be continually refining your plan, goals, and objectives to best meet the client's needs. Do not expect that your initial goals and objectives will be the same goals and objectives that you end up with. Through your ability to iterate, you are adjusting and adapting your project to meet the needs of the client.

DeIuliis ED, Bednarski JA.
The Entry Level Occupational Therapy Doctorate Capstone:
A Framework for The Experience and Project (pp 123-136).
© 2020 Taylor & Francis Group.

INTRODUCTION

The previous chapters focused on critical steps to prepare the occupational therapy student for the doctoral capstone experience (DCE) and project. This chapter further explores the initiation of the DCE and project as the student moves on-site and begins the in-depth experience. Management of the DCE and project can be overwhelming and establishing a clear timeline will set the capstone student (and capstone team) up for success. This chapter presents recommendations to structure a timeline, which divides the implementation stage of the DCE and project into five phases: (1) orientation, (2) screening and evaluation, (3) implementation, (4) discontinuation and sustainability, and (5) dissemination. Students will learn how to develop and implement an orientation plan, refine and polish the individualized goals and objectives based on the finalized needs assessment, develop a timeline for the experience and project, and finally create the individualized plan for the doctoral experience and project. Throughout the intervention phase of the doctoral capstone, evidence from the literature will continue to be integrated to ensure the most up-to-date evidence is used to support the project. This chapter also provides some examples of doctoral capstone projects and testimonials from real occupational therapy doctoral students.

STUDENT REFLECTIVE QUESTIONS

During the implementation phase of the doctoral capstone, the capstone student may find it helpful to reflect on the following questions:

1. How do I deal with change? As you begin the implementation phase, changes to your original goals and individual objectives are inevitable, and you need to be prepared to adapt accordingly.

2. What does it mean to you to fail forward? How will failing forward strengthen your capstone experience and project?

3. Are you feeling prepared (and optimistic) to act as a change agent with your site and population?

Chapter Objectives

By the end of reading this chapter and completing the learning activities, the reader should be able to:

1. Determine an orientation plan to guide the DCE.

2. Understand the steps to complete a needs assessment and apply results making necessary changes to project goals and objectives.

3. Develop a timeline for the implementation of DCE and project.

4. Create an implementation plan for the doctoral capstone project through development of goals and objectives.

IMPLEMENTATION PHASE

By the time the implementation phase begins, on average, 18 months of planning and developing the doctoral capstone have been completed. Table 7-1 gives an example of the preparation sequence the capstone student has completed prior to the start of the experience. Based on the occupational therapy program's curricular design, specifics of the development and planning will be different, however, Accreditation Council for Occupational Therapy Education (ACOTE) standards will guide this process.

After extensive development and planning, it is now time to implement. Figure 7-1 provides a visual for the implementation phase of the process of the capstone experience and project. This visual is intended to be a helpful reference knowing that each individual project may have a different timeline and weeks may be adjusted. Orientation is the first phase in implementation and most often takes place during week 1 of the DCE.

Orientation Phase of the Implementation

Orientation is important to allow the doctoral student to acclimate to the capstone site. As recommended for the fieldwork student (American Occupational Therapy Association [AOTA], 2009), ensuring a formalized orientation can contribute to the early success of the capstone student. First, the student must understand how the site defines orientation. Orientation can occur in varying ways based on the type of site. A traditional health care facility, such as a hospital, may have a formal orientation process and clear procedures for all students and new employees. This formalized process could range in length from 1 day to 1 week. Other sites will have less formal orientation procedures, and role-emerging sites such as a community nonprofit organization may have no formal, established orientation plans. Identifying the orientation process at the site is critical as the student begins implementation. The doctoral student will need to take the lead to ensure that there is a plan for orientation.

Creating an Orientation Plan

Once the procedures of the site orientation are known, this will lead to development of a plan for student orientation. The following are important areas to incorporate into an orientation plan and should be understood before the start of the capstone experience: (a) policy and procedures at the site and departmental level, (b) site environment, (c) site population, (d) key site employees and stakeholders, and (e) student supervision plan. Figure 7-2 provides a visual for the initial implementation phase of the capstone experience and project.

Policy and Procedures

Before the start of the DCE, it will be important for the student to understand all requirements related to health

TABLE 7-1. EXAMPLE OF THE STUDENT DEVELOPMENT AND PLANNING PRIOR TO IMPLEMENTATION

CAPSTONE DEVELOPMENT	Focus on: • Understanding the doctoral capstone process and capstone areas of focus (ACOTE Standard D.1.0) • Identifying an area of interest for the capstone (ACOTE Standard D.1.1) • Investigating potential communities and populations • Searching the literature for evidence in order to support an initial problem statement and purpose • Determine a "fit" with a capstone site that is consistent with the occupational therapy program's curriculum design (ACOTE Standard D.1.2)
CAPSTONE PLANNING	Focus on: • Developing individualized learning objectives and plans for supervision for the overall capstone (ACOTE Standard D.1.2) • Completing a literature review to provide support for the capstone project/experience (ACOTE Standard D.1.3) • Confirming site mentor and ensuring the mentor is an expert in the area of focus (ACOTE Standard D.1.6) • Completing and analyzing a site needs assessment (ACOTE Standard D.1.3) • Developing individualized learning objectives and planning for supervision for the overall capstone (ACOTE Standard D.1.2) • Creating goals and objectives for the capstone project (ACOTE Standard D.1.3) • Determining a plan for evaluation of the capstone project (ACOTE Standard D.1.3) • Creating the memorandum of understanding and obtaining necessary signatures (ACOTE Standard D.1.4)

history (such as immunizations), security and background checks, drug screenings, required trainings such as cardiopulmonary resuscitation (CPR) and first aid, and other professional documents or credentials. Some sites may also require electronic orientation modules to be completed before the start of the experience (such as training on the Health Insurance Portability and Accountability Act [HIPAA] or on the culture of care at the site). A determination of responsibility of obtaining requirements and follow through will be required. Will the student be responsible for communicating with the site mentor on these requirements or will the doctoral capstone coordinator be responsible?

TEACHING TIP 1: No need to reinvent the wheel—following the procedures that the academic fieldwork coordinator has established and has in place for immunizations, background checks, drug testing, CPR, and other document site requirements is recommended. Some programs use data management systems such as Castle Branch to track student compliance and can be easily accessed by a student when on-site.

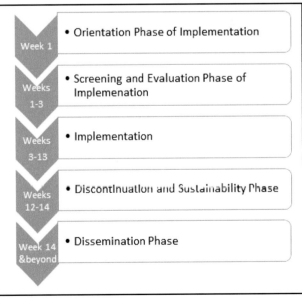

Figure 7-1. Timeline for the doctorate capstone experience implementation phase.

Next, understanding the formal policy and procedures at the site is important. Will the student need to attend a formal

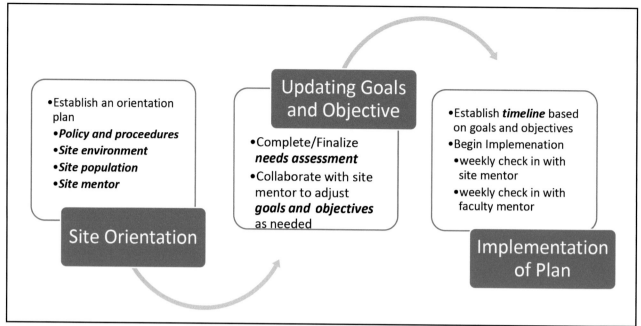

Figure 7-2. Implementing the DCE and project plan.

facility orientation? What are the formal policies and procedures, and how does the capstone student orient to these policies? Students will need to be responsible for understanding their sites orientation and participate in the orientation, whether that be in a formal workshop, informal reading of a manual, or completion of an online portal. Therefore, communication is vital, and capstone students must communicate with their site mentors to determine the orientation policy for the site.

Site Environment and Culture

As occupational therapists, we are trained to assess the environment to enable our clients to perform at their highest occupational level. This same philosophy is true for the capstone student. Capstone students need to take intentional efforts to understand the environment and context of their capstone site to ascertain how to adapt and thus perform at their highest level during the capstone experience. It is important to tour the site to gain a better understanding of the physical space where work will take place. Capstone students should have a workspace and knowledge of what will be provided in this space. For example, at nonprofit community sites, capstone students may be required to work using their own personal electronic devices. Capstone students working within a health care system will be expected to become competent with the organization's electronic documentation system; however, they will most likely use their personal computer to work on components of the capstone manuscript. Determining other areas of the site to tour will

also be important. Students need to begin to understand the physical space of their immediate surroundings and, it is also essential that they gain understanding of the "big picture," which may include interacting with space, individuals, and contexts outside of their particular capstone site. Looking through the lens of the Person Environment Occupation Model, it is the capstone student who determines his or her unique roles at the site, and this is a dynamic process. The environment is the site for the DCE, and once the capstone student understands the context, it is important to modify or adapt to achieve the just-right fit (Law et al., 1996).

Understanding the culture of the site is also important. For instance, the site's dress code should be ascertained before the start date. Will medical scrubs, business dress, business casual, or casual dress be required? Nametags are usually required. Some sites will require students to wear their nametag provided by the school, whereas others will require facility name badges. Whatever the requirement, it is important to make sure this is fully understood. Work hours are also important to understand. What is the expectation of days and hours worked? ACOTE Standard D.1.5 requires a minimum of 14 weeks, 560 hours, with no more than 20% of time working being off-site (ACOTE, 2018). How will on-site and off-site hours be documented? The capstone student needs to take responsibility of documentation of hours, and doctoral capstone coordinators should have a plan in place to ensure that hours are met so the doctoral experience will be successfully completed. Some schools may use an electronic data management system such as CORE-ELMS to document hours, while other schools may provide the students with a time log that must be turned in to the school on a scheduled basis (see Appendix 1-C in Chapter 1 for a template of a time log to track capstone student hours). Whichever method the program uses for documentation of hours, the policy needs to be fully explained to capstone students so that they are aware of the expectations and process to document on-site and off-site hours.

Site Population

Understanding the culture includes knowing the population the site serves. What term is given to the population the site serves? In a medical model site, the term is most often patient, whereas in a community-based site, the term may be *participants, clients, students, residents, members,* or other terms. Understanding and establishing terminology like this is crucial during the first days of the capstone experience, if not ascertained beforehand. Another crucial detail to think about and devise a plan for is how the capstone student will be introduced to the site and relevant stakeholders. This can occur formally or informally and most likely will depend on the culture of the site. The introduction may be informal, and the capstone student may simply mingle with the participants, or it may be more formal with the site mentor introducing the capstone student via a group meeting at the site. As discussed in Chapter 5, initiative, self-confidence, and self-directedness are important practice-ready skills for the capstone student to consistently exercise throughout the DCE and especially during these initial introductions.

Key Site Employees and Stakeholders

Identify the key site personnel and stakeholders and make a plan for introductions. Before the capstone student is introduced, make sure to have a clear and concise explanation of the capstone purpose and how the project will be an asset to the organization. The capstone student may want to have an "elevator speech" practiced and prepared. Learning Activity 1 at the end of the chapter provides students an opportunity to develop an elevator speech and think about how to explain the difference between Level II fieldwork and the DCE and capstone project. Students will be making a first impression, so they need to make it a good one!

Review of Supervision Plan

The plan for supervision (or mentorship) should already be established in the memorandum of understanding (MOU) that was collaboratively agreed on before the start of the DCE. Now is the time to review the plan and develop a schedule that meets the goals set. If the capstone student and site mentor plan to meet once a week for a formal meeting, then make sure the days and times are scheduled and on the calendar. Initially, the capstone student and site mentor

may plan more informal interactions within the first several weeks. Make sure both parties are clear with the expectations for supervision and this is documented. The MOU (as discussed in Chapter 6) is one place the formal determination of the supervision plan can be documented.

Screening and Evaluation Phase of Implementation

Weeks 1 through 3 of the DCE should be a time for the capstone student to complete the screening and evaluation portion of the implementation. This is a time for the capstone student to finalize the needs assessment of the client, organization, or population to develop and implement a client-centered project. The process can look very different to each capstone student depending on the nature of the project. A needs assessment is an important part of the screening and evaluation phase of implementation; however, ACOTE (2018) Standard D.1.3 requires a needs assessment be completed before commencement of the DCE. A needs assessment will need to be completed with the site mentor along with a thorough review of the literature before the start of the experience; however, it is important to update the needs assessment during the initial 1 to 2 weeks at the start of the experience based on experience and knowledge gained.

Needs Assessment

A needs assessment will assist the student in evaluating the context of the experience and discover new data to clarify problems and gaps in practices enabling refinement of the capstone project. Needs assessment approaches can include the following:

- Literature search
- Interviews or focus groups with site employees, stakeholders, and/or clients served by the site
- SWOT (strengths, weaknesses, opportunities, threats) analysis (Bonnel & Smith, 2018)

Once on site, finalizing the needs assessment is important so that the student can gather more information on what is important to the site, and any barriers, gaps, or opportunities. The capstone student may only have had access to the site mentor before the start of the capstone experience; therefore, the initial days and weeks of the experience are a good time to continue to develop the needs assessment. A needs assessment at the site level is often the first way a student can gather more information to refine the capstone project and ensure that the site needs are met and sustainability is addressed. Sustainability of the doctoral capstone project is discussed in detail in Chapter 8.

Table 7-2. Needs Assessment Questions Based on the Occupational Profile

1. Please describe why a majority of your clients are seeking services through your organization.

2. In your opinion, what do you feel are supports to engagement in meaningful activities, and what are barriers to engagement?

3. Can you describe any typical roles, routines, and habits your clients may have?

4. What types of life experiences do your clients have?

5. What priorities and desired targeted outcomes do you have for the clients?

Adapted from American Occupational Therapy Association. (2017). *Occupational profile template.* Retrieved from https://www.aota.org/~/media/Corporate/Files/Practice/Manage/Documentation/AOTA-Occupational-Profile-Template.pdf.

Conducting Needs Assessments

The first steps of a needs assessment should be a literature review that has been completed before the start of the experience (ACOTE, 2018), which was discussed in detail in Chapter 3. The literature review is important to identify gaps in services for a population, evidence-based content, and support for the project. The capstone student has completed the literature review before the start of the on-site experience; however, the process of obtaining literature should continue and the literature review should be updated as additional evidence and literature is found that support the project or provide new gaps or ideas.

A second step in the needs assessment and what is typically defined as a needs assessment is interviewing the site mentor, population served, site employees, and other stakeholders. This is to determine needs, goals, and understand the client, population served, and the environment. It will be important to develop targeted questions to each of these entities. Thinking in terms of an *Occupational Profile* for the site is a great way for a capstone student to frame the needs assessment interview to the site mentor. Table 7-2 gives some initial questions that may be used for a needs assessment.

Another way to determine site needs is conducting a SWOT analysis with the site. A SWOT analysis allows the capstone student to understand strengths (S) and weakness (W) of the organization, as well as opportunities (O) and threats (T) that are driven by forces outside the organization, such as new governmental determined health care policies (Bonnel & Smith, 2018). Text Box 7-1 provides an example of a SWOT analysis completed by an occupational therapy doctoral student from the School of Occupational Therapy at the University of Indianapolis while at a hospital and working on a pediatric program initiative.

TEXT BOX 7-1

For this project, a SWOT analysis was completed via two means. Initially, I took notes from interviews with stakeholders and community members and categorized each item into the relevant SWOT category. I then posted a large chart in the staff office with definitions and examples of strengths, weaknesses, opportunities, and threats. I educated staff on the purpose of this analysis and engaged in conversation regarding correct placement of items. This chart remained in the office for 1 week, with five service providers contributing to the chart.

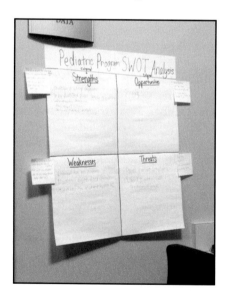

Questions:

Strengths: What do we do better than others?

Weaknesses: What is holding us back? What resources are we lacking? What could we improve? What do our competitors do better than we do?

Opportunities: What are opportunities to serve our community? Where is there an unmet need?

Threats: What do you see at threats to our program from outside our facility?

Results were compiled and reported as follows:

Strengths
- Knowledge of sensory integration
- Individualized plans, focused on the child and the family
- Interdisciplinary model and communication
- Holistic approach—nutrition and dietetics, environmental
  Adequate Environment—two rooms dedicated to pediatric clients
- Location
- Communication with outside stakeholders (schools)

Weaknesses
- Limited marketing opportunities due to decreased time
- Time frame for insurance approvals
- Limited pediatric specializations
- No standard documentation (electronic medical record and intake forms)
- Limited assessment resources
- Incontinent children do not have access to aquatic therapy
- Tracking certifications and recertifications with insurance (not letting kids fall through the cracks)

Opportunities
- Screening Day
- Parent support
- Family events/respite
- Need expressed by parents, teachers, and therapists in varying settings
- Use of social media to advertise
- Use of students to market services and complete projects
- Need for behavior modification/feeding services

Threats
- Low socioeconomic status community
- Home contexts/environments—drug epidemic
- Transportation difficulties
- Parent and client compliance
- Low referrals from area physicians
- School therapists restricted from offering referrals to outside services
- Limited knowledge of pediatric scope of practice for occupational therapy in the community
- Low reimbursement rates
- Limited visits approved by insurance

I created a list of possible "action items" that arose from the needs assessment and SWOT analysis. This list comprised 10 items, which a team of service providers from the site ranked into three tiers of importance. The items marked in the top two tiers became the basis for my Goal Attainment Scale (GAS). The goals were approved by my supervisor to ensure realistic expectations.

—Michaela Wadsworth, OTD, OTR
Class of 2018
School of Occupational Therapy
University of Indianapolis
Indianapolis, Indiana

The SWOT analysis led to refinement of the initial goals and objectives for the doctoral experience and project and the use of the GAS for the evaluation plan. This example demonstrates the many iterations initial capstone goals and objectives go through once on site. Relating back to human-centered design, taking on a mindset of empathy allows you to understand the client more fully and change the prototype as needed based on the client's needs and feedback (IDEO. org, 2015.) Having this open systems process may identify additional site needs that the capstone student will address, as part of the capstone experience however, might not be necessarily a part of the capstone project.

Once the needs assessment is fully completed and results assessed, capstone students will need to review and update goals and objectives. By doing this, students will be able to more easily complete their implementation phase. Goals and objectives that are clearly developed give the capstone student a *structure and timeline* for their doctoral project and experience. The goals and objectives by the start of implementation have usually been through many iterations and developed as the collaborative relationship with the site evolves.

Implementation

To ensure adequate time, it is suggested that by week 3, implementation of the capstone project begins. This, however, will be dependent on each capstone student's individualized plan and individual course objectives of the education program. An example of being ready to begin the actual implementation is a capstone student whose area of focus is on policy and program development working in the community with older adults at an adult day center. The capstone student is working toward addressing community-based programming, which is defined as working with clients in the community targeting a certain population that has identified a specific need (Scaffa, Reitz, & Pizzi, 2010). As noted, the student completes a literature review and a needs assessment with the site mentor before the start of the experience.

Fazio (2001) describes this as phase I of the needs assessment. The capstone student is determining the needs of the targeted population, adult day-center participants. Through this, the needs assessment of a falls prevention program is determined. Once on-site, it is important to continue with phase II of the needs assessment (Fazio, 2001) in which the capstone student assesses the perceived needs of participants at an adult day center and discovers whether falls prevention is an important issue for this specific population. The student discovers that the clients at the adult day center do indeed feel a falls prevention program is valued, and thus the capstone student moves forward with the proposed program. In this example, the capstone student is ready by week 3 to implement the evidenced-based falls prevention program at the site.

To assist the capstone student to stay on track, it may be helpful to participate in an online course from the occupational therapy program that parallels the capstone experience. An online "capstone course" may occur as a course in the capstone doctoral curriculum and can serve as a process of project management for the doctoral student. Within the online course, the use of asynchronous weekly discussion forums can allow the faculty mentor (if the student has been assigned a faculty mentor), student, doctoral capstone coordinator, and a small group of peers to keep focused and in contact. Think back to Chapter 5 and the discussion of the Kolb (1984) four-stage learning cycle. The forum discussion allows for self-reflection each week, and providing and receiving peer feedback can promote the development of new learning and self-efficacy (Kolb, 1984). The online forum will also allow for peer-to-peer reviews, which provide valuable feedback to the student and promote the practice-ready skills discussed in Chapter 5.

TEACHING TIP 2: The following are examples of weekly forum questions posted to the learning management system.

1. Discuss where you are in the process of your doctoral capstone project—are you at the implementation phase? If you are entering the implementation phase, give a brief synopsis of what you are doing and if you are meeting the goals and objectives you have set. If you are not yet to the implementation phase, give a brief synopsis of where you are and how you are progressing toward your goals and objectives.

TEACHING TIP 2 (continued):

2. Please read the following article before responding this this question. Hammell, K. R. (2016). Empowerment and occupation: A new perspective. *Canadian Journal of Occupational Therapy, 83,* 281-287. doi:10.1177/000841741665291. In reflecting on the clients served at your DCE site, discuss issues of occupational injustices and how those injustices may be negatively influencing the well-being of clients served. Describe how you are facilitating occupational engagement with clients served and how this engagement may be facilitating occupational well-being. Be thoughtful in your answers and give specifics. Please reference your post, especially when describing definitions of occupational engagement, occupational justice, and occupational injustices.

Example Question 1 allows the faculty mentor and doctoral capstone coordinator to understand where each student is in the process and ensure that the student is moving forward at a pace that will allow the project to be completed in 14 weeks.

Example Question 2 may help capstone students bridge the gap between what they are doing for their capstone and the philosophy of the program, allowing the doctoral capstone coordinator to ensure ACOTE (2018) Standard D.1.2 is being met.

As capstone students move through the implementation phase, they are focused on following the timeline for the established capstone project goals and objectives. Week 7 will mark the midpoint of the capstone project and experience. This is an excellent time to more formally assess progress toward goals and objectives through a midterm evaluation and make adjustments as needed. Opportunities may be presented and added to the capstone experience, enabling the student to provide more value to the site or gain more in-depth knowledge. If this occurs, make the needed adjustments to the goals and objectives. It is recommended that the midterm evaluation be completed between the student and site mentor. (See Chapter 9 for more recommendations about evaluation of the DCE.) A plan for moving forward should be discussed. Is the student on track to meet the goals and objectives? Are adjustments needing to be made? What other issues might the capstone student need to address before the completion of the experience and project? As the academic fieldwork coordinator does with fieldwork midterm evaluations, it is recommended that the doctoral capstone coordinator review each midterm to ensure that all students are on track and no problems are identified. If issues do arise on the midterm evaluation, it is important for the capstone coordinator to initiate contact with the student directly to begin the process for planning a remediation. This will vary based on the issue. Evaluation of the capstone student is discussed further in Chapter 9. Throughout the intervention, the capstone student will continue to work toward completion of the set goals and objectives. As the student works toward the end of implementation, a decision about discontinuation and sustainability needs to be addressed.

Discontinuation and Sustainability Phase of Implementation

As capstone students enters weeks 12 through 14 of the DCE, they will be thinking about discontinuation of the project and what that entails. A reassessment of progress toward goals and objectives is key at the midway point, and adjustments have already been made to update the goals and objectives. During the discontinuation phase, it is important for students to determine outcomes of the doctoral capstone project. Whatever outcome measure the student used will form the summative assessment of the capstone project. For program development, the student may be determining outcomes based on the GAS. The GAS is a mathematical way to quantify the achievement of goals and the achievement of goals can be measured on a 5-point scale (Turner-Stokes, 2009). Using the GAS for an outcome measure will also provide the capstone student with well-defined goals and a plan for implementation. Table 7-3 gives an example of a GAS used by a doctoral student in the School of Occupational Therapy at the University of Indianapolis in response to the completed SWOT analysis and needs assessment with the site (the goals in **bold** were achieved).

Determining an outcome measure before the start of the capstone is essential to able to report overall capstone project outcomes and is discussed in detail in Chapter 8. The program outcomes will be assessed during the final phase of the implementation. Depending on the capstone project, sustainability of the program will need to also be addressed. A student determining the role of occupational therapy in dolphin-assisted therapy created a full-time position of employment for herself at the site and was hired as a staff occupational therapist after graduation with her occupational therapy doctoral degree. In this role-emerging community setting, the capstone student, now an occupational therapist, will be able to further explore the benefits of dolphin-assisted therapy with children, adults, and veterans. This is truly the best outcome for sustainability of a capstone project.

TEXT BOX 7-2

The experience has been great, and I have learned so much about myself personally and professionally. Through a literature review and personal experience, the therapy team and I collaboratively determined the home program should address five domains: fine motor skills, gross motor skills, sensory integration, self-regulation, and speech/language skills. The home program was well received by the families and met the need of the facility. Both families who participated in the home program reported that the activities helped increase carryover after completion of the dolphin-assisted therapy program and that they would continue to complete the activities despite completion of the student project. The facility determined having an occupational therapist on staff would provide a unique approach to the interdisciplinary therapy team at Island Dolphin Care. Once graduation festivities are complete, I will be going back to Island Dolphin Care to begin my experience as a therapy staff member.

—Taylor Millar, OTD, OTR
Class of 2018
School of Occupational Therapy
University of Indianapolis
Indianapolis, Indiana

Dissemination Phase

As week 14 approaches, the capstone student will have a plan in place for dissemination. Dissemination of the doctoral capstone project is fully explored in Chapter 11. It is, however, important to ensure students disseminate the results of their capstones at the site level. This will demonstrate to the site the benefit of the student being on-site for 14 weeks and also assist with acceptance of future capstone students. Dissemination with the site may also lead to further needs the site may have and in turn lead to future capstone students working at the site. Often, program outcomes may not be able to be evaluated until a later date because of the nature of the project. Therefore, a dissemination meeting is important so that the site understands what the needs may be for program evaluation as the program continues forward.

TEACHING TIP 3: One way to keep capstone students on track and assist with project management is having them write a final written report (or a formal manuscript) that documents this implementation phase as students are moving through implementation. What is important to note here is that you are not asking for one document at the end of the 14-week capstone to sum up the learning that occurred; instead, students write the paper as they are learning and moving through the capstone process.

Table 7-3. Goal Attainment Scale

LEVEL OF EXPECTED OUTCOME	GOAL 1	GOAL 2	GOAL 3	GOAL 4	GOAL 5
+2	**I will request eight to 10 resources that would benefit the growth of the occupational therapy program from XXX Center administration including assessment tools, treatment tools, or continuing education.**	A team from the XXX Center will visit five or more pediatrics offices to educate staff about pediatric services offered at the XXX Center and request referrals.	**Eight to 10 families will attend an event hosted by the XXX Center for families in the community to provide parent support and promote the XXX Center.**	**I will create promotional handouts that educate caregivers about pediatric services and providers at the XXX Center and deliver them to 11 or 12 schools/day cares in the area.**	**The XXX Center will track an increase in pediatric caseload >80% from January 8, 2018, to April 27, 2018.**
+1	I will request six or seven resources that would benefit the growth of the occupational therapy program from XXX Center administration including assessment tools, treatment tools, or continuing education.	**A team from the XXX Center will visit four pediatrician's offices to educate staff about pediatric services offered at the XXX Center and request referrals.**	Six or seven families will attend an event hosted by the XXX Center for families in the community to provide parent support and promote the XXX Center.	I will create promotional handouts that educate caregivers about pediatric services/ providers at the XXX Center and deliver them to nine or 10 schools/day cares in the area.	The XXX Center will track a 60% to 80% increase in pediatric caseload from January 8, 2018, to April 27, 2018.
0	I will request at least five resources that would benefit the growth of the occupational therapy program from XXX Center administration including assessment tools, treatment tools, or continuing education.	A team from the XXX Center will visit three pediatrician's offices to educate staff about pediatric services offered at the XXX Center and request referrals.	Five families will attend an event hosted by the XXX Center for families in the community in order to provide parent support and promote the XXX Center.	I will create promotional handouts that educate caregivers about pediatric services/ providers at the XXX Center and deliver them to eight schools/day cares in the area.	The XXX Center will track a 40% to 60% increase in pediatric caseload from January 8, 2018, to April 27, 2018.

continued

Table 7-3. Goal Attainment Scale (continued)

LEVEL OF EXPECTED OUTCOME	GOAL 1	GOAL 2	GOAL 3	GOAL 4	GOAL 5
–1	I will request three or four resources that would benefit the growth of the occupational therapy program from XXX Center administration including assessment tools, treatment tools, or continuing education.	A team from the XXX Center will visit two pediatrician's offices to educate staff about pediatric services offered at the XXX Center and request referrals.	Three or four families will attend an event hosted by the XXX Center for families in the community to provide parent support and promote the XXX Center.	I will create promotional handouts that educate caregivers about pediatric services/ providers at the XXX Center and deliver them to six or seven schools/day cares in the area.	The XXX Center will track a 20% to 40% increase in pediatric caseload from January 8, 2018, to April 27, 2018.
–2	I will request one or two resources that would benefit the growth of the occupational therapy program from XXX Center administration including assessment tools, treatment tools, or continuing education.	A team from the XXX Center will visit one pediatrician's office to educate staff about pediatric services offered at the XXX Center and request referrals.	One or two families will attend an event hosted by the XXX Center for families in the community to provide parent support and promote the XXX Center.	I will create promotional handouts that educate caregivers about pediatric services/ providers at the XXX Center and deliver them to four or five schools/day cares in the area.	The XXX Center will track <20% increase in pediatric caseload from January 8, 2018, to April 27, 2018.

This GAS indicated the level of expected outcome expected and achieved within this DCE. Levels are determined as follows: +2 = much more than expected; +1 = somewhat more than expected; 0 = Patient achieves the expected level; –1 = somewhat less than expected; –2 = much less than expected. The levels achieved are shown in boldface.

—Michaela Wadsworth, OTD, OTR
Class of 2018
School of Occupational Therapy
University of Indianapolis
Indianapolis, Indiana

Table 7-4. The Capstone Deliverable Timeline

PHASE OF WRITTEN CAPSTONE FINAL REPORT	DUE DATE
Literature review/background information (Even though this was completed before the start of the experience, it is important to update the literature and the needs assessment.)	End of week 3
Screening and evaluation	End of week 4
Implementation	End of week 13
Discontinuation, program outcome, sustainability	End of week 14
Dissemination plan	End of week 14

TEACHING TIP 3 (continued): Feedback can be given for each section as the capstone student is writing so edits can be made. Therefore, at the end of the 14-week experience, the student will have a well-developed manuscript that describes what was completed and will have demonstrated advanced learning (ACOTE, 2018). Chapters 10 and 11 go into much more detail on types of capstone deliverables.

Depending on the project, the timeline for the capstone and the deliverable may be different for each student. To keep on track as students move through the capstone experience, establishing a timeline for the deliverable is important. The finalized capstone project can provide a summative assessment of the capstone student's integration of knowledge. Table 7-4 gives an example of a timeline for the capstone deliverable.

Communication throughout the 14-week DCE is key to a successful experience. Communication between the faculty mentor (or chair) and/or doctoral capstone coordinator and capstone student can be more formal through weekly online forums. Communication between the site mentor and capstone coordinator is also important. Site visits can be an important form of communication for the capstone team. Refer to Appendix 9-A in Chapter 9 for an example of a site visit form used by the Department of Occupational Therapy at Duquesne University.

TEACHING TIP 4: As the faculty mentor (or capstone chair), you can help the doctoral student keep on track by following and participating in the learning management system online forums, scheduling check-in meetings in person or on the phone, grading/reviewing papers in a timely fashion so that edits can be made and updated before the next section of the paper is due, and finally ensuring that capstone students are keeping you up to date on their movement through the capstone timeline.

CHAPTER SUMMARY

Organization is crucial to the success of capstone students as they enter the implementation phase of the doctoral experience and project. Months of preparation and planning have gone into the development of the capstone experience and project, and now is the time to show the fruits of the labor. A well-developed plan for orientation and project implementation is important to set the student up for initial success. This chapter has presented the doctoral student with a plan for project management and described the five stages of the capstone experience and project. Following the five stages and documenting the in-depth learning that has taken place are essential to a successful experience.

Learning Activities

1. Think, Pair, Share (Ridgway, Sachs, & Stephenson, 2015). Think: Create an elevator speech. How will you describe to someone the purpose of your capstone experience and project in the time you may spend with a person in a hotel elevator? Pair: Pair up with another student. Share: As partners, practice your elevator speeches and give feedback.

2. Create an overall timeline based on your goals and objectives for your capstone experience and project. See Appendix 7-A.

3. Determine questions for your needs assessment. What questions will you ask of what people? Write three to five questions each for site employees, the population served, and other stakeholders.

REFERENCES

Accreditation Council for Occupational Therapy Education. (2018). *Standards and interpretive guide, effective July 31, 2020.* Retrieved from https://www.aota.org/~/media/Corporate/Files/EducationCareers/Accredit/StandardsReview/2018-ACOTE-Standards-Interpretive-Guide.pdf

American Occupational Therapy Association. (2017). *Occupational profile template.* Retrieved from https://www.aota.org/~/media/Corporate/Files/Practice/Manage/Documentation/AOTA-Occupational-Profile-Template.pdf

American Occupational Therapy Association. (2009). *Self-assessment tool for fieldwork educator competency.* Retrieved from https://www.aota.org/~/media/Corporate/Files/EducationCareers/Educators/Fieldwork/Supervisor/Forms/Self-Assessment%20Tool%20FW%20Ed%20Competency%20(2009).pdf

Bonnel, W., & Smith, K. V. (2018). *Proposal writing for clinical nursing and DNP projects, Second edition.* New York, NY: Springer.

Fazio, L. (2001). *Developing occupation-centered programs for the community: A workbook for students and professionals.* Englewood Cliffs, NJ: Prentice Hall.

IDEO.org. (2015). *The field guide to human-centered design.* Retrieved from http://www.designkit.org/resources/1

Law, M., Cooper, B., Strong, S., Steward, D., Rigby, P., & Letts, L. (1996). The person-environment occupational therapy model: A transactive approach to occupational performance. *Canadian Journal of Occupational Therapy, 63,* 9-23.

Ridgway, A., Sachs, D., & Stephenson, D. (2015). *14,641 lesson plans: A flipbook for designing engaging lessons.* Terre Haute, IN: Speaker Fulfillment Services.

Scaffa, M. E., Reitz, S. M., & Pizzi, M. A. (2010). *Occupational therapy in the promotion of health and wellness.* Philadelphia, PA: F.A. Davis.

Turner-Stokes, L. (2009). Goal attainment scaling (GAS) in rehabilitation: A practical guide. *Clinical Rehabilitation, 23,* 362-370. doi:10.117/0269215508101742

Appendix 7-A

Doctoral Capstone Experience and Project Weekly Planning Guide					
WEEK	DCE STAGE (Orientation, Screening/ Evaluation, Implementation, Discontinuation/ Sustainability, Dissemination)	WEEKLY GOAL	OBJECTIVES	TASKS	DATE COMPLETE
1					
2					
3					
4					
5					
6					
7					
8					
9					
10					
11					
12					
13					
14					

CHAPTER 8

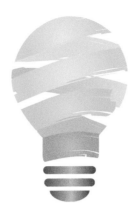

Supporting Sustainability of the Capstone Project Through Program Evaluation

Amy M. Mattila, PhD, OTR/L; Elena V. Donoso Brown, PhD, OTR/L;
Meghan Blaskowitz, DrPH, MOT, OTR/L

Human-Centered Design Mindsets for the Doctoral Students

Human-centered design mindset concepts of optimism and creative confidence are important for doctoral students to embrace as they begin to problem-solve sustainability of their project.

Optimism: As you think through how your project can be sustained, keep a positive focus. Be optimistic that your project can continue. Determine how you can overcome barriers and limit constraints that might be preventing your project from being carried on after you are no longer at the site.

Creative Confidence: You gained confidence in your ability to find solutions and create a meaningful project at your site now keep up that creative confidence as you think about how your project sustainability. Trust yourself; trust that you will find a solution.

INTRODUCTION

The concept of sustainability is gaining importance in all aspects of health care, from project design and management to service delivery. Sustainability can also often refer to the health of the clients that are served—for example, how programs designed around prevention or evidence-based practice ultimately lead to sustained independence and quality of life. To ensure sustainability in a doctoral capstone project that is delivered in this current system, students need to be well-versed in the feasibility of the project, the desirability

from all stakeholders, and in the end, the viability of the program long term. For successful implementation of a doctoral capstone project, students need to be knowledgeable in not only these design-centered concepts but the evaluation processes that should occur in each phase of planning, implementation, and finalization of the doctoral capstone experience (DCE). This chapter begins with the overarching theme of sustainability and uses this as a frame to explore evaluation of process and outcomes and the development of a data analysis plan.

- 137 -

Deluliis ED, Bednarski JA.
The Entry Level Occupational Therapy Doctorate Capstone:
A Framework for The Experience and Project (pp 137-154).
© 2020 Taylor & Francis Group.

Capstone Student Reflective Questions

During the implementation phase of the doctoral capstone, the capstone student may find it helpful to reflect on the following questions:

1. How can you consider sustainability, feasibility, and desirability in each stage of your capstone project?
2. How does program evaluation used during the DCE support evidence-based practice?
3. Using the tables available in this chapter, what study design and statistical analysis would be most useful to you in establishing whether you have achieved statistically or clinically significant DCE program outcomes?

Chapter Objectives

By the end of reading this chapter and completing the learning activities, the reader should be able to:

1. Describe processes that will support the sustainability of the doctoral capstone project.
2. Identify three ways that sustainability is supported through program evaluation.
3. Define the purpose of a logic or conceptual model in the program evaluation process.
4. Compare and contrast outcome and process evaluations and their corresponding research methods.
5. Describe methods for planning, implementing, and analyzing data from a program evaluation.
6. Identify characteristics that will support success in managing unexpected challenges in the program evaluation process.

SUSTAINABILITY

The sustainability of a DCE and capstone project should be a key outcome of the overall student experience. *Sustainability*, a term often used in project and health care management, can be defined as "how organizations manage financial, social, and environmental risks to ensure their organization can continue to operate, regardless of obstacles" (Project Management Institute, 2018). In project management (PM), sustainability also often refers to continuity planning and stakeholder engagement, two concepts that are particularly important in the DCE, where the capstone student is often the "outsider" in the organization. The understanding of sustainability from a PM perspective will be further explored in this section of the chapter.

The World Health Organization (WHO; 2018) defines health care project sustainability as "the ability of a project to continue to function effectively … with high treatment coverage, integrated into available (community resources), with strong community ownership using resources mobilized by the community and local government." In many cases for the DCE, community engagement and buy-in is an extremely important part of whether the program remains stable, particularly for students placed at a role-emerging or community-based practice setting.

Having the goal of sustainability in mind throughout the planning, implementation, and finalization of the DCE process will help to ensure that successful programs are supported not only at the occupational therapy level but for the organization and even community as a whole. Fostering a mindset of sustainability and understanding the concept of capacity building can help the student increase the organization's ability to respond to the changes put in place with innovative solutions created by the DCE and capstone project.

Capacity-building is the idea that organizations can use a range of activities to expand or change directions that add to the functioning or "health" of the organization. The United Nations was one of the first organizations to develop the term and defines capacity as "the ability of individuals, institutions, and societies to perform functions, solve problems, and set and achieve objectives in a sustainable manner" (United Nations, 2006, p. 7). The two concepts can go hand-in-hand to allow the capstone student to infuse sustainability and capacity building practice into their DCE and capstone project.

Frameworks of Sustainability

As mentioned earlier, sustainability and capacity-building are used in many practices, from business and PM, to health care systems, and even in environmental design and development. Three key frameworks of sustainability are discussed in this chapter: PM models, the Substance Use and Mental Health Services Administration (SAMHSA) model, and the Occupational Therapy Intervention Process Model (OTIPM). Each of these models can provide a blueprint for a capstone student to continually plan, reflect, and respond to sustainable project practices.

PM is gaining interest with many health care managers, including occupational therapists. With ever-increasing costs, waste, and diversity in the health care system, a growing number of practitioners are taking courses in PM, such as Lean Six Sigma, the Project Management Academy, or even the number of PM programs rising in the country (Lavoie-Tremblay et al., 2017). There is also a rising number of stakeholders in the health care environment. It is no longer a simple "therapist-client relationship" but often the provider, client, insurance, organization, or even the government who dictate how, why, and when the care can occur. For example, for occupational therapy practitioners to be successful in their clinical reasoning of an individual post-stroke, they need to understand the complex relationship between the client, the authorized length of stay, the continuum of care, and the interdisciplinary plans, to name just a few of the important factors at hand. As capstone students learn the greater impact of their potential project, it is more apparent than ever that they need to have the skills to identify and work, from conception to completion, with all parties involved.

In addition to the stakeholders, PM provides a framework for understanding the social, economic, and environmental consequences associated with the design and execution of projects, such as the capstone (Thomson, El-Haram, & Emmanuel, 2011). The consideration of each of these concepts in the early stages of the DCE can allow for capstone students to obtain the necessary models, metrics, and tools that will ultimately allow for sustainable outcomes, which are further described later in this chapter. Figure 8-1 provides an overview of some of the key PM-based dimensions of sustainability that should be reflected on throughout the capstone experience.

The idea of sustainability and capacity building is also heavily present in health care prevention and community services, such as the WHO and SAMHSA. These concepts have a great fit in these organizations because their primary roles are to respond to the needs and resources of communities and populations as a whole. According to SAMHSA's Strategic Prevention Framework (SPF), the organization uses capacity-building to "understand various types and levels of resources available to establish and maintain a community prevention system that can identify and respond to community needs" (SAMHSA, 2017, para. 1). Capstone students can utilize the logic model set forth by this organization as a step-by-step guide to developing relationships, including stakeholders, and becoming champions for their projects and roles. (Logic models will be defined and discussed in detail later in this chapter.)

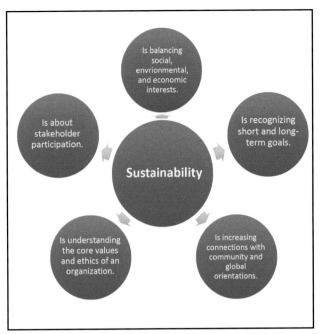

Figure 8-1. Dimensions of sustainability. (Adapted from Silvius, A. J. G., & Schipper, R. [2012]. *Sustainability in the business case.* Proceedings of the 26th IPMA World Congress, Crete, Greece, pp. 1062-1069.)

students could potentially use for ensuring the sustainability of their project. The model includes the following stages:

1. Assess Needs: What is the problem within the organization or population? How can I learn more and dig deeper into this issue?

2. Build Capacity: What are the resources available that I have to work with? Are there ways I can acquire further resources to help my mission and vision?

3. Plan: What is it that I actually hope to accomplish? How should I carry this out and ensure I have included the appropriate stakeholders?

4. Implement: How can I put this plan into action?

5. Evaluate: What data-driven tools have I gathered to ensure sustainability? Can I define whether my project is succeeding, as well as meeting the original needs of the organization or population?

One of the distinctive features of this model is that it encourages assessment as more than just a starting point. As capstone students use this framework, they will return to assessment repeatedly throughout their project because it allows them to recognize that as the needs of their organization changes, their capacity to meet those needs or create programming will also evolve. The additional benefit of this model is that it goes beyond simply identifying stakeholders but also encourages a team-based approach, consistent with most health care environments where capstone students will work beyond graduation. Additional resources, online courses, and tools are available through the SAMHSA Center for the Application of Prevention Technologies and are listed in the Resource section of this chapter.

TEACHING TIP 1: HELPING STUDENTS BUILD CAPACITY AND RAISE COMMUNITY AWARENESS
The following ideas may help capstone students better understand their role and increase readiness for their capstone projects to occur:

- Meet one-on-one with public opinion or community organization leaders.
- Submit articles to local newspapers, club newsletters, and other resources to spread the word on ideas and services.
- Convene focus groups to get input on capstone project ideas and plans.
- Go to the stakeholders in their own environments to share information on wants and needs. As a capstone student, think holistically about this process. If the capstone project is in a community or large organization, the capstone student should seek feedback from other providers, local government, neighborhood and cultural organizations, law enforcement, or even local university or research institutions that could ultimately form a sustainable partnership.

SAMHSA's (2017) SPF has suggested a five-step process using a data-driven, change-based model that capstone

The final framework explored in this chapter is unique to occupational therapy: the OTIPM. This model, originally introduced in 2002 by Anne G. Fisher and Kristin Bray Jones (Fisher & Jones, 2009), has been practiced more recently as a framework for long-term improvement projects by Sirkka, Zingmark, and Larsson-Lund (2014). The authors of this study aimed to understand how the OTIPM could drive long-term improvement work on an occupational therapy unit and found it to be a meaningful process to support sustainable improvements in practice. Capstone students could potentially use a similar framework as they evolve their project and ensure sustainability and long-term improvement outcomes are met in all phases of design. Table 8-1 provides an example of how aligning the components of the OTIPM with factors to consider in a sustainable capstone project could potentially benefit an organization.

The use of this occupational therapy model of practice can guide capstone students in an improvement process that ensures sustainability is infused throughout each phase of the DCE and capstone project.

Regardless of what framework is chosen to guide sustainability and capacity-building, having the tools to make a lasting impact at the DCE site will be an invaluable skill for the entry-level doctoral student. Sustainability practice requires constant planning, reflection, and reevaluation. The plan needs to be practical and feasible to ensure not only student success but also buy-in and implementation on the part of the capstone site.

EVALUATION OF PROCESS AND OUTCOMES

Overview of Evaluation Methods

For a doctoral capstone project to sustain itself over time, it is imperative, as noted in several of the models described here, that the project provide data to support how it was implemented as well as the benefit of its implementation. In this section, an overview of the types of program evaluation that can be done with corresponding examples is provided. Health program evaluation has been referred to as a "three-act play" of creating appropriate evaluation questions, answering the questions through well-designed and implemented evaluations, and using the answers to make decisions (Grembowski, 2016, p.19). Therefore, the following sections present the process of program evaluation from the initial planning stages, through implementation, and ending with data analysis, interpretation, and program modifications (Figure 8-2).

Before walking through the three stages of program evaluation, understanding the two general categories of evaluation is critical. There are two types of program evaluations typically presented in health care and public health literature. The first is known as an *outcome, impact* or *summative evaluation*. The purpose of this evaluation is to determine whether a particular program has met its objectives and intended outcomes (Braveman, Suarez-Balcazar, Kielhofner, & Taylor, 2017; Grembowski, 2016). This type of evaluation typically uses experimental or quasi-experimental research designs to determine whether the program has had an effect on target outcome areas (Braveman et al., 2017; Grembowski, 2016). The second type of program evaluation that can be highly relevant during the DCE experience is known as *process or implementation evaluation*. This type of evaluation can focus on a variety of topics including reach, attendance, use of materials or resources, as well as areas such as experience of the program and participant satisfaction (Baranowski & Stables, 2000). This type of evaluation can assist in a myriad of ways, such as ensuring that the program can be implemented as designed and identifying key areas that contribute to program success or failure (Braveman et al., 2017; Grembowski, 2016). Implementation evaluations can therefore use quantitative or qualitative methods to answer these evaluation questions.

Doctoral Capstone Experience Program Evaluation Planning

In many of the models described here, the concept of evaluation is presented as the last step, but the process of how the capstone student will evaluate the doctoral capstone project should be planned in concert with the project itself.

TEXT BOX 8-1

Accreditation Council for Occupational Therapy Education (2018) Standard D.1.3 indicates that the **evaluation plan is a required preparatory activity PRIOR TO** engaging in the DCE.

This begins with an understanding of how you think your program works (Grembowski, 2016). This is often represented in the form of a logic model or conceptual model. This concept is common throughout program development and is a key element of not only planning your program but also planning the evaluation (Grembowski, 2016). Logic models contain information on resources, activities, outputs, and outcomes at the short-term, midterm, and long-term time points. For example, Figure 8-3 is an example of a logic model for a doctoral capstone project at as skilled nursing facility that was designed to address the issue of agitation for residents with dementia through the use of technology with both residents and their families. The logic model outlines both outputs and outcomes. Outputs are direct results of the program that will indicate the feasibility of a program, such as the number of family members who use the iPad to access materials. Outputs are often measured as part of a process evaluation. Outcomes are the areas in which change is anticipated given the selected interventions, such as agitation. This example illustrates that a solid understanding of how the doctoral capstone project is expected to work can support an understanding of what to measure in a program evaluation. Conceptual models outline similar areas, but have a stronger

Table 8-1. Phases of the Occupational Therapy Intervention Process Model With Capstone Student Examples

PHASES	STEPS WITHIN THE PHASE*	POTENTIAL QUESTIONS AND CONSIDERATIONS FOR THE CAPSTONE STUDENT
Evaluation and goal-setting phase	Establish the client-centered performance context.	• What are the organization's values, mission, interest, and goals? • What roles are important to the organization? What does the organizational leadership look like? What is the expertise of the staff? • Does the organization have connections and relationships with others in the community or other health care context? • What are the daily routines of the organization? • What are the economic factors (funding) that influence the organization? • What are the rules, regulations, and policies that impact the organization? • What other conceptual models within occupational therapy will allow me to better understand the organization's perspective?
	Identify the organizations reported and prioritized strengths and problems with occupational performance.	• Conduct a SWOT analysis (as described in Chapter 7). • On the basis of the needs, what occupation-focused tools can be used to gather to prepare for the next step in this process?
	Observe organizational performance.	• Engage in observation, interviews, focus groups, surveys, or other data-collection methods to gain a holistic picture of the organization and its needs. • Ensure these assessments are occurring within the natural context of the organization and allow for multiple vantage points.
	Define and describe task actions the organization does and does not perform effectively.	• Using collected data, create a list of all task actions within the organization that are effective and another list of those that are ineffective. • Select no more than 10 task actions from each list, that best "capture" the performance of the site.
	Establish, redefine, or finalize goals of the organization.	• In this final step of the evaluation process, consider what might be the reasons for the gaps in services, decreased performance, or other organizational issues. • In direct collaboration with the organization, sustainable program development should be considered only from what is on this list.

continued

Table 8-1. Phases of the Occupational Therapy Intervention Process Model With Capstone Student Examples (continued)

PHASES	STEPS WITHIN THE PHASE*	POTENTIAL QUESTIONS AND CONSIDERATIONS FOR THE CAPSTONE STUDENT
Intervention phase	Select the goals to plan and implement a capstone project that either addresses educational programs, collaborative consultation, development of occupational skills, or acquisition/restoration of person factors and body functions.	• In terms of sustainability and feasibility, the capstone student should consider the following factors for capstone project implementation: ◦ Effective marketing ◦ Price or funding for services ◦ Length of project/timeline ◦ Available resources (staff, equipment, time, etc.)
Reevaluation phase	Reevaluate for enhanced and satisfying performance of the organization.	• What was the effectiveness of my project/program? • What is my lasting relationship with the organization or community? • How will funding affect the sustainability of this project? • Do the staff have the expertise to continue, or should an occupational therapy practitioner be part of the organization? • What are opportunities for additional program integration?

SWOT = strengths, weaknesses, opportunities, threats.
*In this example, the client is the organization.

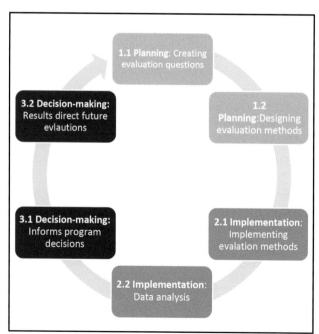

Figure 8-2. Planning, implementation and decision-making cycle. (Adapted from Grembowski, D. [2016]. *The practice of health program evaluation* [2nd ed.] Thousand Oaks, CA: Sage.)

focus on the processes used to produce outcomes. See an example of a conceptual model in Figure 8-4. Once you have used either of these processes to gain an understanding of how the program should work, the next step is developing a program evaluation plan.

Program Evaluation Plan

Once a logic model/conceptual model has been developed, the capstone student can begin to identify which questions are of greatest importance to the site. Depending on the project, this may be an outcome-focused question, such as, "Do the comprehensive therapy services provided through interaction with and caring for animals in a farm context result in changes to social participation skills for children with autism spectrum disorder?" In this case, the program is already established, and the capstone student's focus may be more on supporting rigorous outcome measurement to use in future grant applications for the program. At the other end of the spectrum, a capstone student may be working with a site that has noted challenges with transition services and wishes for the doctoral student to complete a process evaluation that would answer the question "What are the barriers to addressing transition services?" and possibly "How do their clients, staff and stakeholders want to address these challenges?" It is also possible for a capstone student to

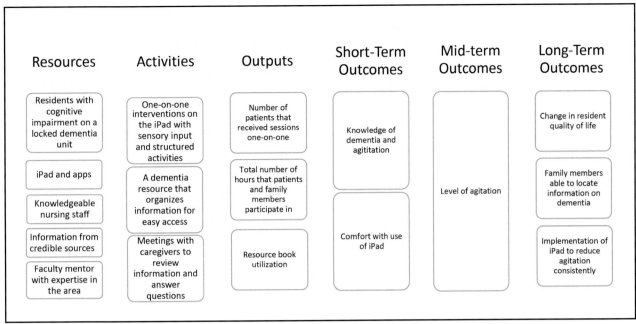

Figure 8-3. Sample DCE logic model of the interpersonal approach to dementia program. (Reprinted with permission from Anna Olexsovich, OTD, 2016, Duquesne University.)

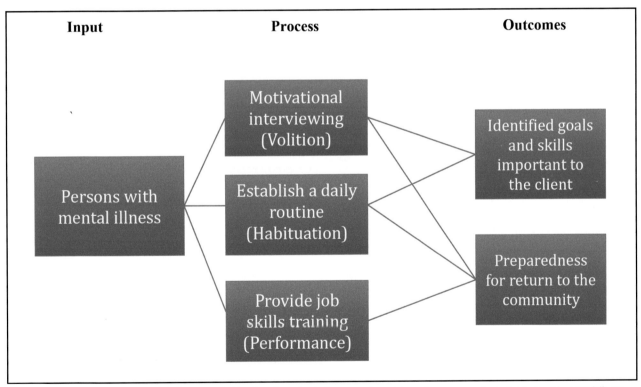

Figure 8-4. Simple conceptual model of cause and effect for a hypothetical community re-integration program for individuals with mental illness, guided by components of the model of human occupation.

complete both types of evaluation simultaneously, answering questions about the effectiveness, experience, and feasibility of the program that was implemented. Using both designs may allow for the most robust picture of the program, which could support future sustainability. Once program evaluation questions have been determined, an appropriate design to answer these questions should be selected.

Outcome Evaluation

As noted previously, outcome evaluations are typically quantitative in nature and are intended to measure whether a program made changes in the anticipated outcome areas (Braveman et al., 2017; Grembowski, 2016). As capstone students may recall from prerequisite didactic courses in evidence-based practice and research methods, one of the strongest types of research designs is a randomized controlled trial (Nelson, Kielhofner, & Taylor, 2017).

> **TEACHING TIP 2:** Per language provided by the Accreditation Council for Occupational Therapy Education (2018), academic programs cannot use fieldwork or the DCE to meet learning objectives in the B standards.

In this design, participants are prospectively assigned at random to either the control group or the experimental group. This design is strong because it reduces threats to internal validity, such as selection bias, through the process of randomization (Nelson, Kielhofner, & Taylor, 2017). It also increases the ability of a researcher to determine whether any observed change is due to the program. Despite the strengths of this type of design, it is generally impractical for implementation during a DCE and project, due to time and resources needed to complete this design well. Given that the capstone student has limited time and resources to complete an outcome evaluation, it is strongly suggested that one of the following designs be considered in the DCE and capstone project: (a) pretest/posttest, (b) pretest/posttest with comparison group, (c) repeated measures design, or (d) single-subject design. Strengths and weakness of each design, as well as examples of use in DCE projects, are outlined in Table 8-2. These types of designs, although limited in their ability to demonstrate whether a change in outcome is due directly to the program, are feasible to complete within the time frame and resources most capstone students will have available to them for their projects.

Process Evaluation

As process evaluations answer different kinds of questions, designs for these types of evaluations span both quantitative and qualitative methods. For quantitative investigations, designs are generally descriptive in nature and may use direct observation or survey methods to obtain the desired information. Qualitative methods can also be useful in gathering process evaluation data as interviews and focus groups allow participants and other stakeholders involved in the program to provide feedback on experiences and perceived strengths and barriers to the program. See Table 8-3 for process evaluation examples.

SELECTING MEASUREMENT TOOLS AND METHODS

After program evaluation questions have been finalized and an appropriate design to shape your evaluation has been selected, it is time to identify the outcomes and process areas that will be measured. Again, this is where reference to the logic model is helpful because it was through that process that the capstone student identified short-term, midterm, and long-term outcomes. Given that the capstone project that is implemented over a short period of time (14 weeks), when thinking of outcome areas, it is important to focus on short-term outcomes that are closest to the intervention. For example, imagine a capstone student has implemented a patient education program for individuals with spinal cord injury in an acute inpatient rehabilitation hospital. The short-term outcome identified was change in knowledge and the long-term outcome identified was quality of life. It would likely be most appropriate to focus measurement on the change in knowledge because it may take a longer duration of program implementation and follow-up to see changes in quality of life. This example illustrates the challenging nature of selecting outcome measures for the capstone project; however, this process in many ways parallels the selection of assessment tools for the evaluation of clients because many of the same key pieces of information are considered. To select appropriate outcome measures, it will be beneficial for the capstone student to answer the following questions:

1. Who is being evaluated?
2. What type of measurement tool would be best to capture this outcome or process area?
3. What tools can be implemented in this setting?
4. Can these measures provide a consistent and accurate picture of the desired area?

Who Is Being Evaluated?

For the capstone student, this may be a challenging question to answer precisely because, until the student moves on-site and begins the implementation phase of the DCE, the exact mix of people in their program may fluctuate. For example, students may know that the clients at their site all have a diagnosis of an eating disorder, but the specific disorder may vary, as does the age, gender, and comorbidities of each client. However, regardless of the specifics of the population, selecting an outcome measure can be supported by knowing their DCE population's general diagnostic category

Table 8-2. Doctoral Capstone Experience Outcome Evaluation

DESIGN	STRENGTHS	CHALLENGES	EXAMPLE
Pretest/posttest: Single group receives the intervention. Data collection occurs at two times points, before and after intervention.	• Ease of implementation. • Can measure a change over time (Braveman et al., 2017; Grembowski, 2016).	Changes observed could be due to several other factors, including time passing, an outside external event, the measurement tools used, or retesting (Braveman et al., 2017; Grembowski, 2016).	*Patient education after spinal cord injury uses a knowledge test before and after participation in program to determine whether there is a change in knowledge.* —Justin McTish, OTD Class of 2018 Duquesne University Pittsburgh, Pennsylvania
Pretest/posttest with comparison group: Two groups. One receives the intervention one does not. Data collection occurs at two times points, before and after intervention.	• Increased rigor of design means more confidence in results potentially being attributed to your program. • Provides a reference group to compare results of program (Braveman et al., 2017; Grembowski, 2016).	• Selection bias main threat to internal validity as groups are not randomized. • Need to locate a reasonable nonequivalent comparison group. • Increased demand for data collection (Braveman et al., 2017; Grembowski, 2016).	*A staff training program on the importance of visual perception to participation in daily activities and newly implemented screening procedures, in addition to a pretest/posttest for those in attendance, the tests could also have been given to others at a facility who did not receive the training, creating a naturally occurring nonequivalent group.* —Abbey Moonis, OTD Class of 2017 Duquesne University Pittsburgh, Pennsylvania
Repeated measures: Single group with measurements at multiple times (i.e., three or more).	• Can establish a baseline level of performance for participants before intervention, which can reduce threats due to maturation. • Evaluates simple behaviors well (Braveman et al., 2017; Grembowski, 2016).	• Requires establishment of a baseline, which, given the 14-week timeline, will require advanced planning. • Vulnerable to threats related to instrumentation if new instruments are added at the same time as the intervention. • Also requires increased time for assessment as data collection points are greater (Braveman et al., 2017; Grembowski, 2016).	*A program to address agitation in adults with dementia measured level of agitation with an observation of behavior scale at two time points before implementing the use of mobile applications to decrease agitation and two times after.* —Anna Olexsovich, OTD Class of 2016 Duquesne University Pittsburgh, Pennsylvania
Single-subject: Experimental design with one or more cases completed across time. Several designs could be applied, including reversal (A-B-A-B) and alternating treatment (A-B-C) (Deitz, 2017).	• Decreases threats to internal validity such as change due to the passing of time or occurrence of outside events. • Good for populations with high variability (Braveman et al., 2017).	• Depending on the number and diversity of cases, limited generalizability. • Requires measurement of observable behavior (Braveman et al., 2017).	In an outpatient hand therapy clinic, an alternating treatment design could be used to compare the effectiveness of different modalities to decrease pain and increase duration of participation in functional activities in a client with complex regional pain syndrome.

Table 8-3. Doctoral Capstone Experience Process Evaluation

DESIGN	STRENGTHS	CHALLENGES	EXAMPLE
Observation	• Can provide quantitative data that informs understanding of how program was implemented and/or how program resources were used. • Feasible implementation in the timeline provided. • Ecologically valid as it will occur in the context the DCE is delivered (Taylor & Kielhofner, 2017).	• Vulnerable to other variables impacting observation. • Dependent on the rigor and neutrality of the observer. • Behavior could be different if individuals know they are being observed (Taylor & Kielhofner, 2017).	Implementation of a program to address falls on the orthopedic unit, tracking the use of fall safety measures after two in-service sessions.
Survey	• Provides descriptive information that can help identify areas of need or measure patient satisfaction. • Can be administered via questionnaire or interview. • Allows for correlational analysis if characteristics of respondents are collected. • Can feasibly be implemented in the time frame of the DCE (Forsyth & Kviz, 2017).	• Requires consideration of the sample and how they are gathered. • Individuals who may respond are different from those who do not or, if administered in person, participants may not feel comfortable being honest. • Individuals may interpret questions differently, not recall information, or may not have a choice that represents their opinion (Forsyth & Kviz, 2017).	Capstone student in a state political action committee uses a cross-sectional survey to gain information from state association members about areas of concern related to policy. Could also use a survey to gain insight into participant satisfaction with the program or use of program materials after the conclusion of the program.
Interview	• Can provide narrative data that clearly describes participants experience (Braveman et al., 2017).	• Time-consuming to complete with a large number of individuals. • Response bias, especially if interviewer is the student who completed the project (Braveman et al., 2017; Forsyth & Kviz, 2017).	In a higher education setting after implementing a mentoring program, one-on-one interviews are completed to understand the benefits and key elements to the program as perceived by the students.
Focus Group	• Allows for social component in responding to questions. • Provides narrative understanding of experience from more people in a single setting (Finlayson, 2017).	• Requires competent moderator to facilitate. • Fewer questions can be asked, as time to respond from the group increases (Finlayson, 2017).	After the completion of a 6-week social participation program for families with children with intellectual development disorder, a focus group could be held with parents to support a better understanding of their experience of the program and what were perceived supports and barriers to program participation.

because it is generally good practice to first look at tools that have been validated with your population of interest.

The additional details about the individuals who actually attend the program should be collected through the completion of a demographics form. This form should contain information that would help describe to others key characteristics about your sample that could influence how they understand and apply the findings of your program evaluation.

What Type of Measurement Tool Would Best Capture This Outcome or Process Area?

As occupational therapists, we are trained to have a unique skill set to assess a wide variety of areas, and numerous strategies and methods to evaluate them. We will look at selecting outcome areas and process areas separately, although there can be overlap between the two. When selecting an outcome measure, it is critical that you consider the best way to capture information on this outcome. For example, if you want to understand a program participant's perceived performance and satisfaction on personal goal areas, use of the Canadian Occupational Performance Measure or Goal Attainment Scale (GAS) may be a good option as both of these tools are patient report measures that look at goal areas identified by the client (Doig, Fleming, Kuipers, & Cornwell, 2010). However, if you are creating a community-based activity program that is intended to improve motor function of the impaired upper extremity for persons poststroke, you may want to use a tool that evaluates performance through observation such as the Fugl-Meyer Upper Extremity Subtest or Chedoke Arm and Hand Activity Inventory (Barreca, Stratford, Masters, Lambert, & Griffiths, 2006; Lin et al., 2009). In some cases, standardized assessment tools may not be available for an outcome area. For example, in staff or patient education programs, standardized knowledge tests are not often readily available for all areas of content. Therefore, capstone students may need to develop their own tools or adapt tools found in the literature. With creation or adaptation of a measurement tool, it is important for the capstone student to recognize the limitations that come from its lack of previous use. These limitations include limited reliability and unknown validity (Grembowski, 2016). When considering methods to measure process areas, you will need to match the method with what you want to know and also consider logistical factors (Grembowski, 2016). For example, if you wish to evaluate use of a community resource book provided at a staff training, you have several measurement options, including observation of the number of times staff members are observed using the book to administering a survey that asks staff members for this information. Deciding how to measure any given area will involve several factors and collaboration with the capstone team, but once you have a set of possible measures and methods, you can begin to compare them.

What Tools Can Be Implemented in the Setting of the Doctoral Capstone Experience?

Once possible assessments and methods have been identified for implementation within the program evaluation, capstone students will need to refer back to their knowledge of the site and the expertise of their capstone team to determine which of the identify measurement tools are most feasible for implementation. This is known as *utility* and considers the time to complete the assessment or method, the materials and space needed, as well as any potential staff training that might need to occur to use that measurement tool (Brown & Bourke-Taylor, 2014). This is important to consider because although an assessment or data collection method may look at your desired area in your population, if it is not practical to complete in the setting, a capstone student may become discouraged at the time of implementation.

Can These Measures or Methods Provide a Consistent and Accurate Picture of the Desired Area?

After feasibility is ensured, it is important to consider which of the remaining choices has the strongest profile related to consistent and accurate measurement. For standardized assessments, this would include a review and consideration of psychometric properties, including test-retest reliability, responsiveness, standard error of measure, content validity, and criterion validity or construct validity (Grembowski, 2016; Portney & Watkins, 2009).

Again, it is noted that assessment tools in some areas of practice may have limited psychometrics data available. This does not mean that such assessments cannot be used for a capstone project; however, it does mean that the limitations and negative impact on the strength of the evaluation need to be reflected in the data analysis and interpretation phase of the project. For example, if an outcome measure has not been evaluated for test-retest reliability, it needs to be noted that any change observed in a pretest/posttest design could be due to measurement error from the assessment and not change due to the intervention (Grembowski, 2016).

For process evaluations, to generate a consistent and accurate data set, considerations of bias and influence are often in the forefront. For instance, when evaluating participant satisfaction, one can consider either an interview or an anonymous survey. A capstone student would need to reflect on whether data collected via an interview would be unduly influenced if the capstone student who ran the program was also completing the interview (Braveman et al., 2017; Forsyth & Kviz, 2017). Therefore, students will want to identify the method for collection that will be least vulnerable to these types of influences. Another method that can increase the trustworthiness of the qualitative findings is the use of triangulation. Triangulation "refers to the use of two or more strategies to collect and/or interpret or analyze information" (Lysack, Luborsky, & Dillaway, 2017, p. 208) and, by doing so, the confidence in findings increases (Portney & Watkins, 2009). For example, if a staff education program on how to prevent falls on an orthopedic unit instructs staff to use a resource book, both observation of the number of times the book is used and interviews of staff on the use of the book can be triangulated to determine the value of this piece of the program. Triangulation can also occur by analysis and will be described later in the chapter.

Selecting measurement methods for use in outcome and process evaluations is an important step in the planning process. This activity builds on knowledge of assessments and methods gained throughout the earlier phases of occupational therapy training and often applies it to a larger programmatic perspective. Again, conversation with the capstone team, and especially the site mentor, will support the selection of measures that will be sustainable after the DCE and capstone project is completed to allow for continued program evaluation.

PROGRAM EVALUATION PLANNING LOGISTICS

After selection of program evaluation design and measurement tools, the capstone student can begin to define logistics around data collection. This begins with a continued discussion of who will be included in the DCE project. For instance, will the doctoral capstone project be something that all persons who are admitted to a facility go through, or will participants need to be gathered from the community? Depending on the mode of recruitment, different levels of marketing will be required. It is best to go into this with an agreed-on plan to ensure that the doctoral capstone project is successful in gaining participants.

In addition to planning how participants will be recruited, creating a timeline and processes for implementation of assessment measures will support implementation. When developing a timeline, it is important to recognize that this is a guide and that it may need to change as unexpected circumstances arise during the DCE and adjustments may need to be made. As discussed in Chapter 7, having a timeline for implementation of the program evaluation will support communication between the capstone student and site mentor, thus increasing the likelihood for seamless implementation.

Developing a Data Analysis Plan

In preparation for the start of the DCE, the capstone student should revisit the overarching program evaluation

questions and components of their project, as outlined in the logic model. It is imperative to the success of the project that the student create alignment between their program evaluation questions, program components, data collection, and analysis. It is highly recommended that a student develops not only a data collection plan, but also a data analysis plan before DCE implementation in an effort to guide organization of outcome measures, data entry, summarization of data, and testing of program evaluation hypotheses through data analysis and to minimize unexpected changes during DCE project implementation.

A data analysis plan typically consists of (a) identification of key dependent (a.k.a. outcome) and independent (a.k.a. predictor) variables to be measured during the DCE, (b) definition of the levels of measurement of each variable measured, (c) consideration of the number of participants needed to detect a clinically significant change or reach saturation of themes with program evaluation quantitative and qualitative data (discussed later in this chapter), and (d) the quantitative and qualitative analyses and software the student intends to use to make sense of data collected and test program evaluation hypotheses (Centers for Disease Control and Prevention, 2013). Variables are "characteristics of people, activities, situations, or environments that are identified or measured in a study" (Brown, 2017, p. 52). Independent variables are those that are manipulated in a doctoral capstone project and typically represent the "intervention" or "comparison" (no-intervention) in a program evaluation project, whereas dependent variables are the outcomes or observed results of a project, which potentially occur in response to the manipulation of one or more independent variables. Drawing on foundational research knowledge, variables can be classified generally as categorical (i.e., nominal or ordinal variables) or continuous (i.e., interval or ratio variables). When creating their own measurement tools (e.g., demographic surveys, satisfaction surveys), capstone students should make every effort to gather variables from participants at the highest level of measurement possible (continuous data).

For example, a capstone student implementing a social skills program for school-age children with autism spectrum disorder may seek to evaluate the program participants' social skills pre- and postprogram implementation using the Social Profile (Donohue, 2013). The capstone student may also want to create a survey to gather valuable process evaluation data on the number of children who participated in her program and their demographic characteristics. In this example, the social skills program or intervention is considered the independent variable, as well as the personal, social and environmental characteristics of each child, their parents, and their home/school life. The dependent variable is the change in social skills observed in the children and measured over a given period of time. In gathering demographic characteristics for each child, rather than asking parents to place their children in a given age bracket (which would represent categorical data), gathering their actual age (a continuous variable), would provide more meaningful information about each child and allow for more advanced statistical analyses to be conducted using this demographic information.

Organization and Implementation of the Doctoral Capstone Experience Program Evaluation

The strength of a doctoral capstone project's program evaluation is only as good as the quality and completeness of the data collected from its participants. Each capstone project is individualized to the capstone student and site. Therefore, program evaluation data will vary; however, to maximize the quality of data collected, initial steps should be undertaken to ensure organization of the data collection and data entry process and to avoid missing data and errors on the back end.

Capstone students are encouraged to first locate and obtain the assessment tools and outcome measures they intend to use to collect data on participant and program outcomes as part of their doctoral capstone project. Because capstone students may not have funds available to purchase new assessment tools and outcome measures, there are a variety of other sources where tools can be sought including the occupational therapy doctoral program's assessment library, academic institution's library, or online through open-access channels or free digital resources. For example, two frequently used occupational therapy assessment tools that are located online and have copyrights that allow permission for clinical use include the Montreal Cognitive Assessment (MoCa; Nasreddine et al., 2005) and Modified Interest Checklist (Kielhofner & Neville, 1983).

Capstone students who choose to create their own outcome and process evaluation measures, such as knowledge tests, demographic surveys, or program satisfaction surveys, are encouraged to pilot test these measures before the start of their DCE, with special consideration given to the health literacy and readability of these tools. Health literacy refers to a person's ability to obtain, process, and understand health information so that he or she can make informed decisions about his or her care (Berkman et al., 2011). The highest prevalence of low health literacy is observed in men, the elderly, racial and ethnic minorities, and individuals with low socioeconomic status (Ayotte, Allaire, & Bosworth, 2009; Rikard, Thompson, McKinney, & Beauchamp, 2016). When creating patient education materials or new outcome measures, capstone students should consider principles for improving health literacy—for example, create materials at or below a sixth-grade reading level, avoid medical terminology and abbreviations, include ample white space on the page, use pictures, and check readability statistics using Word processing systems (e.g., Microsoft Word's Flesch-Kincaid Readability tool).

Once all assessments and outcome measures have been obtained or created, a schedule of administration of these measures should be developed in concert with the faculty mentor (or capstone chair) and site mentor. This assessment schedule should strike a balance between ensuring that enough data is collected to answer program evaluation questions and adequately test hypotheses but that the capstone student can still manage DCE time effectively and that program participants are not subject to overassessment or assessment fatigue.

A critical step in collecting and organizing high-quality program evaluation data is setting up database(s) for data entry, confidential security, and storage of records. A data spreadsheet can be created in software, such as Microsoft Excel, as soon as assessment tools and outcome measures have been identified for use in the DCE project, and independent and dependent variables defined. A common method used in establishing a data spreadsheet involves organizing independent and dependent variables as column headers and entering one program participant's assessment data per row. It is recommended that a capstone student create a data spreadsheet, document and enter data on a regular basis throughout the DCE project because it is easy to fall behind in data entry and management. Human error is also common in data entry and management. Therefore, capstone students should take the lead in managing the data spreadsheet, providing limited access to others involved in the DCE project. High attention to detail is necessary when entering program data to minimize the amount of missing data gathered for independent and dependent program evaluation variables. For example, when entering pairwise data for program participants, preassessment data should be entered and matched to the same participant's postassessment data.

To protect the confidentiality of doctoral capstone project program participants, all data collected while on the DCE should be de-identified, coded numerically, and recorded in a password-protected data spreadsheet (Jacobsen, 2017). One solution to increasing security of participant data is the upkeep of a separate password-protected code sheet, in which numeric identifiers are assigned to each program participant and their demographic characteristics. These numeric identifiers are the only link between individual-level demographic information and assessment data for the program participants. It is also recommended that capstone students and their site mentors have sole access privileges to these files and to any locked filing cabinets where hard copies of assessment data are stored.

Subsequently, identification of statistical analysis software that interfaces well with a student's data spreadsheet is equally as important. See Table 8-4 for a list of statistical analysis software systems that may be available to capstone students, with a special focus on health and social sciences

Table 8-4. Review of Quantitative Statistical Analysis Software Systems

STATISTICAL SOFTWARE PACKAGE	BASIC FEATURES	STRENGTHS	WEAKNESSES
Excel (Microsoft, n.d.)	• Point-and-click software • Can be used for descriptive statistics (median, mean, standard deviation, frequencies, and percentages), correlations, *t* tests, ANOVA, regression	• Inexpensive • Easily accessible • Widely used in many workplaces as part of Microsoft Office • Can easily create databases for data entry	• Decreased ease of use (e.g., Excel formulas are not intuitive and require macro downloads) • Creating tables and figures and exporting them is challenging
R (The R Foundation, n.d.)	• Code-based software • Can be used for descriptive statistics, correlations, bivariate analyses (chi-square test), *t* tests, ANOVA, regression	• Free software • R can be used to analyze large data sets • Creates high-quality tables and figures	• Learning code/syntax for R requires increased time (this can be ameliorated by R Studio) • Limited/no customer support; can seek help only via online forums
Statistical Analysis Software (SAS) 9.4 (SAS Institute, n.d.)	• Code-based software • Can be used for descriptive statistics, correlations, bivariate analyses (chi-square test), *t* tests, ANOVA, regression	• SAS can easily analyze large data sets • Used by state and federal government/health agencies • Strong customer support	• Expensive • Writing code/syntax is not always intuitive for health care professionals and other social scientists
Statistical Package for the Social Sciences (SPSS) 25.0 (IBM, n.d.)	• Point-and-click software with a coding option • Can be used for descriptive statistics, correlations, bivariate analyses (chi-square test), *t* tests, ANOVA, regression	• User can choose to use point-and-click and/or write syntax • Increased ease of use for health care professionals and other social scientists • Tables and figures can be easily created, modified, and exported from SPSS	• SPSS license is more expensive than other statistical software • Few workplaces purchase SPSS license(s) • Memory intensive, thus difficult to manage large data sets and run other programs
Stata 15 (StataCorp, n.d.)	• Code-based software with a point-and-click option • Can be used for descriptive statistics, correlations, bivariate analyses (chi-square test), *t* tests, ANOVA, regression	• Inexpensive • Highly intuitive coding system • Many available customer support resources (e.g., online guides, manuals, textbooks)	• Decreased ease of data entry compared with Excel and SPSS • Stata is not designed to manage analysis of large data sets

ANOVA = analysis of variance.

data analysis. It is important to consider factors such as the type of data collected (quantitative vs qualitative), usability (point-and-click vs code-based programming), cost, level of customer support available, interface with other programs and operating systems, amount of memory needed to run the program, types of statistical analyses that can be conducted using the software, and quality of tables and graphs produced to choose the best statistical processing system for the doctoral capstone project and data analysis. Statistical analysis software systems and factors for consideration are highlighted in greater detail in Table 8-4.

Program Evaluation Data Analysis

Analysis of data collected over the course of a doctoral capstone project is one of the most important steps of the capstone process, as it allows the student to generate answers to their program evaluation questions and test hypotheses set at the beginning of the DCE planning process.

Whether the capstone student collects quantitative, qualitative, or mixed data, descriptive statistics should be used to summarize and describe the main features and patterns that emerge from participants included in the program evaluation (Brown, 2017; Simpson, 2015). See Table 8-5 for a sample descriptive statistics table used to present demographic data gathered from participants with intellectual and developmental disabilities (IDD).

TEACHING TIP 3: Occupational therapy educators and students can refer to other prominent resources regarding research methodology by referring to the following texts that are rated as most frequently used, according to the National Board for Certification in Occupational Therapy's *OTR Curriculum Textbook and Peer-Reviewed Journal Report*. Retrieved from http://www.nbcot.org.

- DePoy, E., & Gitlin, L. N. (2016). *Introduction to research: Understanding and applying multiple strategies* (5th ed.). St. Louis, MO: Mosby Elsevier.
- Kielhofner, G. (2006). *Research in occupational therapy: Methods of inquiry for enhancing practice*. Philadelphia, PA: F.A. Davis.
- Law, M., & MacDermid, J. (Eds.). (2014). *Evidence-based rehabilitation: A guide to practice* (3rd ed.). Thorofare, NJ: SLACK Incorporated.
- Portney, L. G., & Watkins, M. P. (2015). *Foundations of clinical research: Applications to practice* (3rd ed.). Philadelphia, PA: F.A. Davis.

Quantitative Data Analysis

In determining the statistical tests that can be used to analyze quantitative data collected in the DCE project, capstone students must, first and foremost, understand whether the data they have collected meets the assumptions of normality.

A normal distribution represents a symmetrical distribution of scores on either side of the mean, or a "bell curve," in which the majority of scores fall in the middle of a scale and fewer scores fall at the extremes of a scale (Portney & Watkins, 2009). Parametric tests assume that a sample is drawn from a population with a distribution that approximates a normal distribution; therefore, to use a parametric statistical test, such as a t test or analysis of variance (ANOVA), the sample data must meet the assumptions of normality. To assess for normality, capstone student can use statistical analysis software to create a histogram, or bar graph that displays all assessment scores for a given sample of program participants, and then visually inspect the graph for a normal distribution curve. A more precise method for assessing normality would be to run a Shapiro-Wilk test using statistical analysis software, recommended as one of the best tests for assessing normality in small samples (Ghasemi & Zahediasl, 2012). If a data set meets normality assumptions, *parametric tests*, such as independent samples t tests, paired samples t tests, between-subjects ANOVA, mixed ANOVA, and repeated-measures ANOVA, can be used in analyzing DCE participant data. However, if this normality assumption is not met, then equivalent nonparametric tests, such as a chi-square test, Mann-Whitney U test, Wilcoxon signed rank test, or Krukal-Wallis, will need to be used instead.

Determining the Significance of Program Evaluation Findings

At the end of the DCE, capstone students ultimately want to be able to use the data they have collected to answer questions such as "Did this program work?" or "Did this program have an impact on the clients served over the course of the DCE and doctoral capstone project?" Determining the significance of the findings will be dependent on the capstone focus and type of doctoral capstone project.

TEACHING TIP 4: A DCE and project with a focus on research may use quantitative data to measure program outcomes and statistical significance as an indicator of success.

Statistical significance is a measure that expresses the likelihood that program outcomes or findings are due to chance (Brown, 2017). A significance level of .05 is used by most researchers and program evaluators to indicate a statistically significant effect.

Drawing on foundational statistics knowledge, a p value, or probability value, is typically used to decide whether the result obtained reflects true differences between groups of participants (Jacobsen, 2017). If the p value derived from a statistical test is less than the established level of significance (.05), there is sufficient evidence that the findings are not due to chance.

Table 8-5. Sample Demographics

INDIVIDUAL-LEVEL CHARACTERISTICS TOTAL SAMPLE (n=597)

Age, mean (SD), years
    Youth: 18 to 24, n (%)
    Young adult: 25 to 44
    Midlife: 45 to 64
    Late life: 65 and older

Gender, n (%)
    Female
    Male
    Transgender
    Other

Type of developmental disability, n (%)
    Autism spectrum disorder
    Cerebral palsy
    Down syndrome
    Neurological disorder
    Other

Level of intellectual disability, n (%)
    None/unspecified
    Mild
    Moderate
    Severe
    Profound

Self-identified race/ethnicity, n (%)
    American Indian or Alaska Native
    Asian
    Black or African American
    Hispanic/Latinx
    Native Hawaiian or other Pacific Islander
    White
    Other

Living arrangement, n (%)
    Institution
    Group home
    Family home
    Supported apartment

Determining the clinical significance of program evaluation findings can also be accomplished by analyzing changes in occupational performance that are deemed meaningful to a client or treating clinician. A minimally clinically important difference (MCID) is the "the amount of change on a particular measure that is deemed clinically important to the client" (Brown, 2017, p. 140). At the heart of measuring the MCID for an outcome, capstone students must use their professional and clinical judgment to estimate how much meaningful change they would expect to see in an assessment of occupational performance to make it "clinically significant." For example, a capstone student who is working with adolescents with psychiatric disabilities who are "at risk" may choose to use GAS to measure achievement of vocational outcomes before and after implementation of a 14-week vocational training program. The student might identify a change from "somewhat less than expected" (–1) to "expected level of outcome" (0) on the GAS pre- to post-training program to be a MCID for her adolescent client.

Although there may be certain doctoral capstone projects that implement qualitative methodologies, such as phenomenology or ethnography, which require complex analysis, most capstone projects are likely to use qualitative analysis for responses to open-ended questions on a survey or as a part of process evaluation interviews or focus groups. In this case, a content analysis approach that aims to summarize the information into categories and possibly implement counts (Morgan, 1993) is often sufficient to determine the perspectives of the participants related to program processes or key ingredients. While the goal in most qualitative research is to reach data saturation or the point at which no new information is being gathered (Lysack, Luborsky, & Dillaway, 2017), reaching this point may not be feasible given the short timeline of the DCE unless the sole focus of the project is to complete a qualitative investigation. Therefore, it is important for the capstone student to consider other ways to increase the trustworthiness and rigor of their findings. One way to do this is for the capstone student to consider ways to triangulate the data through use of multiple analysts who analyze the data separately at first and then join and compare coding structures to decrease the influence of bias (Dillaway, Lysack, & Luborsky, 2017). Another way to increase the trustworthiness of the qualitative findings is to complete member checking, in which the initial interpretation of the findings is sent to those who participated to determine if it represents their perspectives (Lysack, Luborsky, & Dillaway, 2017). Use of these strategies can support the validity of the qualitative findings but does require advanced planning and additional resources.

Managing the Unexpected

Although the PM principles outlined here, as well as the use of a logic model and development of data collection and data analysis plans, are meant to minimize the myriad problems that can occur during program implementation and evaluation, a variety of unexpected changes can still occur. For example, DCEs and projects conducted in community-based mental health settings can be affected by low funding streams and thus decrease participant recruitment to the program. A low census on an acute care unit in the hospital can have an impact on a capstone student's sample size and change his or her data analysis plan. Changes to the initial program evaluation and data analysis plans are inevitable.

To minimize unexpected modifications to the DCE and problem solve through unexpected changes, capstone students must maintain open lines of communication with their faculty and site mentors, drawing on the resources within the capstone team. The capstone team should be engaged in every step of the planning process and DCE program implementation and evaluation to support appropriate selection of methods that will work effectively with the DCE site's current organizational processes. Capstone students who remain flexible and communicate regularly with their faculty mentor (or capstone chair) to actively solve problems will produce successful DCE results, despite unexpected changes.

DRAWING CONCLUSIONS AND DISSEMINATING PROGRAM EVALUATION FINDINGS

Findings from the doctoral capstone project can and should be disseminated to a broader audience to contribute evidence-based practice knowledge to the field of occupational therapy and to the DCE site so that they can receive valuable information on the impact of the services provided at their organization. Program evaluation findings can be used to advocate for much-needed policy change, procure additional funding for occupational therapy services, or to inform future iterations of the program, making any necessary changes to the logic model should the capstone student choose to continue to implement the program moving forward. Chapter 11 reviews best practices and recommendations on how and where to disseminate capstone findings.

CHAPTER SUMMARY

The DCE is an optimal opportunity for occupational therapy students to create sustainable, meaningful projects in diverse settings. To achieve this goal, it is imperative that capstone students have a solid understanding of program evaluation and appropriate data analysis throughout each stage of the experience. Having a well-thought-out process in place will allow students not only to experience a successful placement but also potentially have a direct impact on populations in the health care system. If doctoral programs can place an emphasis on skills such as sustainable design, assessment, measurement, and evaluation, capstone students can confidently work through human-centered design phases of feasible and desirable projects.

Learning Activities for the Student

1. Think about a program you consider to be "sustainable." Reflect on why you think the program has outlasted others. What resources do they have? What does their leadership and staffing look like? What makes this program important to its community or organization? What lessons can you learn from the program's mission, vision, funding structure, staffing, or other factors that have led to its sustainability?

2. Think of a program. This could be one that currently exists at your DCE site or one you are hoping to create.

Use a logic model to identify the resources, activities, outputs, and short-term outcomes from this program.

REFERENCES

Accreditation Council for Occupational Therapy Education. (2018). *Standards and interpretive guide, effective July 31, 2020*. Retrieved from https://www.aota.org/~/media/Corporate/Files/EducationCareers/Accredit/StandardsReview/2018-ACOTE-Standards-Interpretive-Guide.pdf

Ayotte, B. J., Allaire, J. C., Bosworth, H. (2009). The associations of patient demographic characteristics and health information recall: the mediating role of health literacy. *Neuropsychology, development, and cognition. Section B, Aging, neuropsychology and cognition, 16*(4), 419-432.

Baranowski, T., & Stables, G. (2000). Process evaluations of the 5-a-day projects. *Health Education and Behavior, 27*, 157-166. doi: 10.1177/109019810002700202

Barreca, S. R., Stratford, P. W., Masters, L. M., Lambert, C. L., & Griffiths, J. (2006). Comparing 2 versions of the Chedoke Arm and Hand Activity Inventory with the Action Research Arm Test. *Physical Therapy, 86*, 245-253.

Berkman, N. D., Sheridan, S. L., Donahue, K. E., Halpern, D. J., Vierra, A., Holland, A., … Viswanathan, M. (2011). Health literacy interventions and outcomes: An updated systematic review. *Evidence Report Technology Assessment, 199*, 1-8.

Braveman, B., Saurez-Balcazar, Y., Kielhofner, G., & Taylor, R. R. (2017). Program evaluation research. In R. R. Taylor (Ed.), *Kielhofner's research in occupational therapy: Methods of inquiry for enhancing practice* (pp. 410-423). Philadelphia, PA: F.A. Davis.

Brown, C. (2017). *The evidence-based practitioner: Applying research to meet client needs*. Philadelphia, PA: F.A. Davis.

Brown, T., & Bourke-Taylor, H. (2014). Accommodating diversity issues in assessment and evaluation. In J. Hinojosa & P. Kramer (Eds.), *Evaluation: Obtaining and interpreting data* (4th ed.). Bethesda, MD: American Occupational Therapy Association.

Centers for Disease Control and Prevention. (2013). *Creating an analysis plan*. Atlanta, GA: Author. Retrieved from https://www.cdc.gov/globalhealth/healthprotection/fetp/training_modules/9/creating-analysis-plan_pw_final_09242013.pdf

Deitz, J. C. (2017). Single-subject research. In R. R. Taylor (Ed.), *Kielhofner's research in occupational therapy: Methods of inquiry for enhancing practice* (pp. 360-374). Philadelphia, PA: F.A. Davis.

Dillaway, H., Lysack, C., & Luborsky, M.R. (2017). Qualitative approaches to interpretation and reporting data. In R. R. Taylor (Ed.), *Kielhofner's research in occupational therapy: Methods of inquiry for enhancing practice* (pp. 228-243). Philadelphia, PA: F.A. Davis.

Doig, E., Fleming, J., Kuipers, P., & Cornwell, P. L. (2010). Clinical utility of the combined use of the Canadian Occupational Performance Measure and Goal Attainment Scaling. *American Journal of Occupational Therapy, 64*, 904-914.

Donohue, M. V. (2013). *Social Profile: Assessment of social participation in children, adolescents, and adults*. Bethesda, MD: American Occupational Therapy Association.

Finlayson, M. (2017). Needs assessment research. In R. R. Taylor (Ed.), *Kielhofner's research in occupational therapy: Methods of inquiry for enhancing practice* (pp. 395-409). Philadelphia, PA: F.A. Davis.

Fisher, A. G., & Jones, K. B. (2009). Occupational therapy intervention process model. In J. Hinojosa, P. Kramer, & C. Brasic Royeen (Eds.), *Perspectives on human occupation: Theories underlying practice* (pp. 237-286). Philadelphia, PA: F.A. Davis.

Forsyth, K., & Kviz, F. J. (2017). Survey research. In R. R. Taylor (Ed.), *Kielhofner's research in occupational therapy: Methods of inquiry for enhancing practice* (pp. 375-394). Philadelphia, PA: F.A. Davis.

Ghasemi, A., & Zahediasl, S. (2012). Normality tests for statistical analysis: A guide for non-statisticians. *International Journal of Endocrinology and Metabolism, 10,* 486-489. doi:10.5812/ijem.3505

Grembowski, D. (2016). *The practice of health program evaluation* (2nd ed.) Thousand Oaks, CA: Sage.

IBM. (n.d.). IBM SPSS Statistics [software]. Retrieved from https://www.ibm.com/products/spss-statistics

Jacobsen, K. (2017). *Health research methods: A practical guide* (2nd ed.). Burlington, MA: Jones & Bartlett.

Kielhofner, G., & Neville, A. (1983). *The modified interest checklist.* Model of Human Occupation Clearinghouse, Department of Occupational Therapy, University of Illinois Chicago. Retrieved from https://www.moho.uic.edu/products.aspx?type=free

Lavoie-Tremblay, M., Aubry, M., Cyr, G., Richer, M. C., Fortin-Verreault, J. F., Fortin, C., & Marchionni, C. (2017). Innovation in health service management: Adoption of project management offices to support major health care transformation. *Journal of Nursing Management, 25,* 657-665.

Lysack, C., Luborsky, M. R., & Dillaway, H. (2017). Collecting qualitative data. In R. R. Taylor (Ed.), *Kielhofner's research in occupational therapy: Methods of inquiry for enhancing practice* (pp. 196-213). Philadelphia, PA: F.A. Davis.

Lin, J. H., Hsu, M. J., Sheu, C. F., Wu, T. S., Lin, R. T., Chen, C. H., & Hsieh, C. L. (2009). Psychometric comparisons of 4 measures for assessing upper-extremity function in people with stroke. *Physical Therapy, 89,* 840-850. doi:10.2522/ptj.20080285

Microsoft. (n.d.). Microsoft Excel [software]. Retrieved from https://products.office.com/en-us/excel

Morgan, D. L. (1993). Qualitative content analysis: A guide to the path not taken. *Qualitative Health Research, 3,* 112-121.

Nasreddine, Z. S., Phillips, N. A., Bédirian, V., Charbonneau, S., Whitehead, V., Collin, I., Cummings, J. L., & Chertkow, H. (2005). The Montreal Cognitive Assessment (MoCA): A brief screening tool for mild cognitive impairment. *Journal of the American Geriatric Society, 53,* 695-699.

Nelson, D. L., Kielhofner, G., & Taylor, R.R. (2017). Quantitative research designs: Defining variables and their relationships with one another. In R. R. Taylor (Ed.), *Kielhofner's research in occupational therapy: Methods of inquiry for enhancing practice* (pp. 244-273). Philadelphia, PA: F.A. Davis.

Portney, L. G., & Watkins, M. P. (2015). *Foundations of clinical research: Applications to practice.* Upper Saddle River, NJ: Pearson/Prentice Hall.

Project Management Institute. (2018, August 1). *Sustainability.* Retrieved from http://www.pmi.org

The R Foundation. (n.d.). The R project for statistical computing [software]. Retrieved from https://www.r-project.org/

Rikard, R. V., Thompson, M. S., McKinney, J., & Beauchamp, A. (2016). Examining health literacy disparities in the United States: A third look at the National Assessment of Adult Literacy (NAAL). *BMC Public Health, 16*(975), 1-11.

SAS Institute, Inc. (n.d.). SAS Products, Technology & Solutions A to Z. Retrieved from https://www.sas.com/en_us/software/all-products.html

Silvius, A. J. G., & Schipper, R. (2012). *Sustainability in the business case.* Proceedings of the 26th IPMA World Congress, Crete, Greece, pp. 1062-1069.

Simpson, S. H. (2015). Creating a data analysis plan: What to consider when choosing statistics for a study. *Canadian Journal of Hospital Pharmacy, 68,* 311-317.

Sirkka, M., Zingmark, K., & Larsson-Lund, M. (2014). A process for developing sustainable evidence-based occupational therapy practice. *Scandinavian Journal of Occupational Therapy, 21,* 429-437.

StataCorp LLC. (n.d.). Stata Release 15. Retrieved from https://www.stata.com/products/

Substance Abuse and Mental Health Services Administration. (2017, August 25). *What is the SPF? An introduction to SAMHSA's Strategic Prevention Framework.* Retrieved from https://www.samhsa.gov/capt/tools-learning-resources/what-is-spf

Taylor, R. R., & Kielhofner, G. (2017). Collecting quantitative data. In R. R. Taylor (Ed.), *Kielhofner's research in occupational therapy: Methods of inquiry for enhancing practice* (pp. 296-312). Philadelphia, PA: F.A. Davis.

Thomson, C. S., El-Haram, M. A., & Emmanuel, R. (2011). Mapping sustainability assessment with the project life cycle. *Proceedings of the ICE—Engineering Sustainability, 164*<2>, 143-157.

United Nations. (2006). *Definition of basic concepts and terminologies in governance and public administration* (UN Publication E/C.16/2006/4). New York, NY: United Nations Economic and Social Council.

World Health Organization. (2018, October 3). *What is meant by sustainability?* Retrieved from http://www.who.int/apoc/sustainability/definition/en/

RESOURCES

Textbooks

Asher, I. E. (2014). *Annotated index of occupational therapy evaluation tools* (4th ed.). Bethesda, MD: American Occupational Therapy Association.

Brown, C. (2017). *The evidence-based practitioner: Applying research to meet client needs.* Philadelphia, PA: F.A. Davis.

Jacobsen, K. (2017). *Health research methods: A practical guide* (2nd ed.). Burlington, MA: Jones & Bartlett.

Kielhofner, G. (2017). *Research in occupational therapy: Methods of inquiry for enhancing practice.* Philadelphia, PA: F.A. Davis.

Law, M., Baum, C., & Dunn, W. (2017). *Measuring occupational performance: Supporting best practice in occupational therapy* (3rd ed.). Thorofare, NJ: SLACK Incorporated.

Portney, L. G., & Watkins, M. P. (2009). *Foundations of clinical research: Applications to practice.* Upper Saddle River, NJ: Pearson/Prentice Hall.

Websites

SAMHSA Center for Application of Prevention Technologies (CAPT): https://www.samhsa.gov/capt/

Offers tools, resources, funding, and online courses related to projects that focus on practicing innovate and effective prevention.

CHAPTER 9

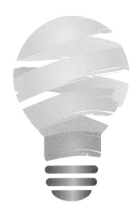

Evaluation of the Capstone Experience

Elizabeth D. Deluliis, OTD, MOT, OTR/L, CLA
Julie A. Bednarski, OTD, MHS, OTR

Human-Centered Design Mindsets for the Doctoral Students

Human-centered design mindsets of learning from failure and iteration are important for the doctoral capstone student to continue to embrace as they finalize implementation of the doctoral capstone experience and project. Evaluating the overall experience, the student, and mentors is important to reflect and make adjustments for the future. As an instructional designer, occupational therapy faculty and the capstone coordinator should create student learning activities and assessment measures that make a difference to your learners' lives. We want to create courses, learning activities, and evaluations that inspire them, change mindsets, and drive performance during the capstone and future practice.

Iterate, Iterate, Iterate: You have been iterating throughout the implementation stage and this is the final iteration period. Final changes are made based on outcomes and decisions are made for future ideas based on outcomes. Evaluating your iterations and understanding how you came to the final product are important and important to be able to communicate. Be able to communicate how your iterations have led to the final product.

Learn From Failure: Throughout the implementation phase, you have been learning from your failures, learning from things that did not go just right. Evaluating your experience and project in this final stage of implementation allows you to make further changes and recommendations for the future. "When human-centered designers get it right, it's because they got it wrong first" (IDEO.org, 2015, p. 21).

INTRODUCTION

Not unlike the occupational therapy process, assessment (or evaluation) is an essential step in the teaching-learning process. The interrelationship between adult learning theory (andragogy) and assessment is well documented by major educational theorists such as Bandura (1971), Cross (1981), Knowles (1970), Kolb (1984), Lave (e.g., Lave & Wenger, 1991), Revans (1980), and Rogers (1969). Although there is no single theory of adult learning that can be applied to all adults, the models represented by the aforementioned pioneers of education provide useful frameworks to conceptualize the evaluation mechanisms for experiential learning such as the capstone. Experiential learning has influenced adult

Deluliis ED, Bednarski JA.
The Entry Level Occupational Therapy Doctorate Capstone:
A Framework for The Experience and Project (pp 155-190).
© 2020 Taylor & Francis Group.

education by making educators responsible for creating, facilitating access to, and organizing experiences to facilitate higher order learning. Experiential learning coincides closely with one of the fundamental pieces of the philosophy of occupation—learning by doing (Lewis & Williams, 1994). Evaluation of learning is a meaningful process for the learner and the instructor. Assessments are critical elements of instruction; they determine accomplishment of learning objectives and can provide feedback to instructors on their effectiveness. Are capstone students learning what we want them to learn throughout their capstone experience and project? Is the site mentor (and/or site) providing a substantive impact on the performance of the capstone student? Did learning and growth occur within the student's chosen focus area(s)? Occupational therapy educators, specifically doctoral capstone coordinators, should be empowered to design these assessments to be more than an evaluation of what has been learned. The evaluation mechanism for the doctoral capstone can be designed to be a part of the learning process itself and a process to get data to support program evaluation measures, required by the Accreditation Council for Occupational Therapy Education (ACOTE). This chapter provides an overview of student assessment for experiential education and recommendations to guide the evaluation process during the doctoral capstone experience (DCE).

Capstone Student Reflective Questions

As the implementation phase of the capstone experience nears completion, the occupational therapy student may find it helpful to reflect on the following questions:

1. How will your learning and performance be assessed during the DCE?

2. What role you will play in evaluating and providing feedback to your site mentor (and other stakeholders involved in your capstone experience)?

3. What is your understanding how your expectations and goals on the DCE differ from Level II fieldwork?

4. What are your education program's policy and expectations regarding formal assessment and overall grading procedures for the doctoral capstone?

Chapter Objectives

By the end of reading this chapter and completing the learning activities, the reader should be able to:

1. Discuss theoretical approaches used to evaluate experiential learning.

2. Compare and contrast evaluation mechanisms of Level I and Level II fieldwork and the DCE.

3. Understand different strategies to design evaluation mechanisms for the DCE.

BRIEF OVERVIEW OF ADULT LEARNING THEORY

Awareness of adult learning theories is needed to develop and select evaluation systems and instruments that can measure the expected competencies and outcomes. What (to measure), how, when, and by whom are important key questions, and their answers are not always easy. Assessment should be tied to specific learning outcomes, and learners should be given whatever feedback will help them develop or consolidate their knowledge, skills or attitudes. One principle of adult learning theory is to allow learners to determine their own learning goals. In most instructional settings, specific learning objectives must be met and are traditionally established, reinforced, and monitored by the educator. The accreditation standards surrounding the capstone require a shift in this paradigm and requires that capstone student play an integral role in structuring how they show evidence of skill proficiency within their chosen focus area(s). ACOTE (2018) Standard D.1.4 enforces this adult learning principle to be instituted by the creation of student-directed learning objectives as part of the memorandum of understanding (MOU; discussed in Chapters 1 and 6). Knowles (1984, 1992) has contended that adults differ from younger learners in the following ways.

TEXT BOX 9-1

What are the basic principles of adult learning?
- They derive from adults' experiences and needs.
- Adults need to be involved in planning their instruction and evaluating their results. (This is encompassed in the co-creation of the individualized student learning objectives in the MOU.)
- Adults are often self-directed, and their motivation to learn is internal.
- Adults also learn well in situations where they can experience using their new knowledge.
- Adult learning should center on solving problems and not on absorbing content.
- Adults prefer experiential learning.

Not unlike the various lenses that practitioners use to view the occupational therapy process, assessment strategies can be developed using theoretical frameworks. For instance, Alexander Astin, a clinical and counseling psychologist, proposed the Input-Environment-Output (I-E-O) model to develop assessment and evaluation activities in higher education. The premise of this model is that educational assessments are not complete unless the evaluation includes information on three essential elements: student inputs (I), the educational environment (E), and student outcomes (O) (Astin, 1993). Figure 9-1 shows the interrelationship among the three components of the I-E-O model.

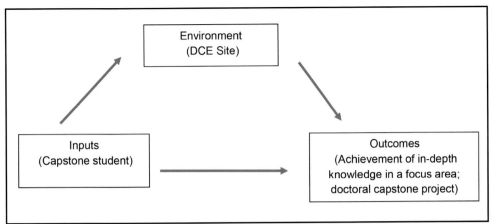

Figure 9-1. Schematic of Astin's I-E-O model.

Astin's model contends that outcomes in terms of student development are determined by both inputs (I) and learning environments (E); at the same time, inputs also influence outcomes (O). Astin's theory can be useful to occupational therapy educators as we further explore strategies to evaluate the doctoral capstone (Table 9-1).

The holistic perspective of the I-E-O Model and the significance of the interaction (interdependence) among the three postulates parallels many signature occupational therapy theories and models of practice such as Person-Environment-Occupation Performance (PEOP) Model (Christiansen, Baum, & Bass, 2005), Person-Environment-Occupation (PEO) model (Law et al., 1996), and the Canadian Model of Occupational Performance (CMOP; Polatajko, Townsend, & Craik, 2007). Capstone students' learning and performance are a function of the students themselves, their context, and their experience. Application of the I-E-O model results in more accurate assessment of the effects of the learning environment. Use of this model in student assessment "forces" educators to address not only outcomes but also inputs and environmental variables when evaluating student performance. Again, like the occupational therapy process, evaluation measures should be an ongoing process of establishing clear, measurable expected outcomes of student learning, ensuring that students have sufficient learning opportunities to achieve those outcomes. Assessment should include a systematic process of gathering, analyzing, and interpreting the evidence to determine how well the learner matched the stated expectations (Allen, 2004; Banta, 2002; Banta, Jones, & Black, 2009; Maurrasse, 2002; Suskie, 2009; see Figure 9-2). Although outcomes are important to measure, they reflect the end product of assessment, not a "complete assessment cycle" (Qualters, 2010, p. 56). It is therefore necessary to devise unique assessment methods to measure success in both the process and the product (Moon, 2004).

Assessment strategies, consistent with Knowles's philosophy, might include case studies, role-play, simulations, and self-evaluation that enable adults to learn the process as much as the content itself. Many of these assessments are commonly used in occupational therapy education, yet do they provide a mechanism that offers holistic and ongoing feedback on the doctoral capstone student's performance?

ASSESSMENT IN OCCUPATIONAL THERAPY EXPERIENTIAL EDUCATION

ACOTE (2018) provides an excellent structure for diversifying evaluation of student learning. Via the standards and the accreditation process, each occupational therapy program is required to provide evidence of student learning in the B, C, and D standards. ACOTE offers several measures for student learning assessment via their accreditation process and related documents. These include assignment, lab test, objective test, essay test, project, presentation, and demonstration. There is also an "other" selection that can be used to describe pedagogical approaches that may not be encompassed in the previous seven assessment measures. Experiential learning can be simply described as "hands-on" learning, yet it can occur via several approaches. Formal, regulated, and accredited experiential learning in occupational therapy includes fieldwork education and the doctoral capstone. Other pedagogical methods to foster "hands-on" learning can occur via community engaged learning (Greene, 1997; Hoppes, Bender, & DeGrace, 2005) and simulation (Bethea, Castillio, & Harvison, 2014), which are often cited in occupational therapy literature yet not required by ACOTE. In Chapter 1 of this book, you learned that the primary objective of Level I fieldwork is to "introduce students to fieldwork, to apply knowledge to practice, and to develop understanding of the needs of clients" (ACOTE, 2018, p. 40). Newly adopted standards provide additional oversight needed by the academic fieldwork coordinator in regard to having clearly documented student learning competencies expected of the Level I fieldwork experience. ACOTE Standards indicate that there needs to be mechanisms for formal evaluation of student performance for Level I fieldwork. More recently, the American Occupational Therapy Association (AOTA) endorsed a new tool "Level I Fieldwork Competency Evaluation for OT and OTA Students" (AOTA, 2017). This tool was designed to complement the AOTA Fieldwork Performance Evaluation

Table 9-1. Astin's Model

INPUT	Assess capstone students' knowledge, skills, and attitudes before a learning experience	Capstone students are required to demonstrate
ENVIRONMENT	Assess capstone students' actual experience during the capstone	Impact of site mentor and site
OUTPUT	Assess the success (or talents) that we are trying to develop	In-depth skills/knowledge developed aligned with the focus area

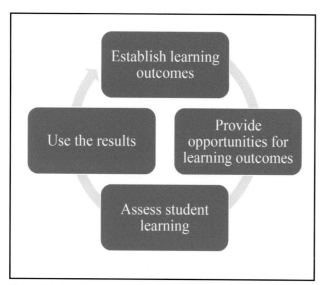

Figure 9-2. Iterative process of the evaluation of student learning.

(FWPE) for the occupational therapy and occupational therapy assistant students and uses similar categories for the indicators:

- Fundamentals of Practice
- Foundations of Occupational Therapy
- Professional Behaviors
- Screening and Evaluation
- Intervention

More important, this evaluation is used to assess performance skills that build a foundation for successful completion of Level II fieldwork.

TEACHING TIP 1: The Level I Fieldwork Competency Evaluation tool for occupational therapy and occupational therapy assistant students can be found at http://www.aota.org under "Resources for Fieldwork Education."

Chapter 1 also discussed that the goal of Level II fieldwork is to develop competent, entry-level, generalist occupational therapy practitioners (ACOTE, 2018). Standard C.1.2 and C.1.5 requires that the occupational therapy education

program documents mechanisms for evaluating the effectiveness of supervision (e.g., student evaluation of fieldwork) and formal evaluation of student performance on Level II fieldwork. Evaluation of the student performance can be completed via the AOTA FWPE or an equivalent evaluation mechanism.

TEXT BOX 9-2

Other evaluation mechanisms for fieldwork education include the **FEAT** and **SAFECOM** tools.

The **Self-Assessment Tool for Fieldwork Educator Competency** (SAFECOM) is a tool to facilitate student self-reflection and self-assessment throughout the fieldwork process. The SAFECOM can be used formally via the midterm and final evaluation time periods, or informally to guide conversation between the student and fieldwork educator and guide the student's growth based on site-specific learning objectives and to promote continued professional development (AOTA, 2018).

The **Fieldwork Experience Assessment Tool** (FEAT) provides a structure for the fieldwork student and the fieldwork educator to have a meaningful discussion aimed to identify strategies to facilitate the just-right challenge. This tool is meant to be used collaboratively and help within the fieldwork educator and the fieldwork student understand the unique and dynamic interaction among the environment, the fieldwork educator and the student (Atler et al., 2001).

There are clear resources provided to occupational therapy faculty, academic fieldwork coordinators, fieldwork educators and students provided by the AOTA regarding fieldwork education.

ACOTE D standards outline the minimum educational requirements for the capstone (ACOTE, 2018). In previous chapters, keys aspects of the doctoral capstone were discussed, such as the differentiation of the capstone project vs experience (Chapter 1), correlation with an in-depth focus areas (Chapter 2), congruence with the program's curriculum design (Chapter 4), and necessary collaboration among faculty, site mentor, and student (Chapter 6). Specific to the assessment process, Standard D.1.7 requires that occupational therapy doctoral (OTD) programs "document a formal evaluation mechanism for objective assessment of the student's performance during and at the completion of the DCE" (ACOTE, 2018, p. 45). Although there is not a formally endorsed tool provided by AOTA or ACOTE to use for evaluation of the capstone experience, the AOTA Commission on Education has posted on its website approved documents from current accredited OTD programs, which include an example of an evaluation form for the doctoral capstone. This chapter is intended to provide additional recommendations and resources for the evaluation of the capstone student during and at completion of the capstone experiences, as well as evaluation of the mentorship provided by the site mentor.

Evaluation of the Capstone Student's Performance During the Experience

The capstone student's performance and progress during the DCE should be closely monitored by the student, site mentor, and capstone coordinator, and perhaps even by the faculty mentor (or capstone chair). Evaluation can occur informally and formally. Informal evaluation of the capstone student can occur during feedback sessions with various members of the capstone team and during phone calls or site visits supported by the capstone coordinator. Sample forms to guide feedback sessions or for phone check-ins or site visits can be found in Appendix 9-A at the end of this chapter. These informal methods of evaluating the student's performance and providing feedback for growth can be used to satisfy evaluation mechanisms "during the capstone experience" aspect of the D.1.7 standard (ACOTE, 2018). Other strategies to evaluate student feedback during the capstone experience can be through the use of required student reflections. The capstone coordinator can use the academic institutions learning management system (such as Blackboard, Canvas, Design2Learn, Moodle, etc.) as means to connect, collaborate, and evaluate student performance during the capstone experience. Self-reflections and student discussion board postings can be required elements of the course listed on the syllabus and provide useful information to the capstone coordinator to the overall grading outcome of the experience. Engaging the capstone student in reflection is crucial to organize, interpret, and bring meaning and coherence to their learning experience. Similar to Level II fieldwork, although the site mentor or faculty mentor (or capstone chair) can provide valuable feedback on the capstone student's performance via the evaluation forms and established feedback mechanisms, as the primary faculty member responsible for the capstone, it is the doctoral capstone coordinator's responsibility to assign the overall grade for the experience. Reflections or postings can be used creatively by the doctoral capstone coordinator to exemplify congruence to curricular threads or curriculum philosophy, acknowledge the in-depth knowledge within the chosen focus area(s), and gain feedback on the capstone student's overall growth and development at specific intervals of the 14-week experience (see Text Box 9-3). Strategies to approach the grading of the capstone are discussed later in this chapter.

TEXT BOX 9-3

Week 1
Can you believe it is the XYZ semester of your doctoral program? CONGRATULATIONS on passing your proposal defense! Now it is time to put all of your hard work into practice and make it a reality! Throughout the capstone journey, I would like each of you to respond to questions and also respond to your peers. I will also offer my own thoughts and suggestions. For this week, please respond to the following questions:

1. How did your site mentor respond to the final draft of your project proposal? Did they provide feedback? Share some details.
2. What updates have been made to your individual student objectives through collaboration with your site mentor?
3. How are things going in general? Any questions or concerns? Any questions from you or your site supervisor regarding the paperwork?

Week 4
Identify effective mentorship strategies that work for you why this type of supervision works for you. Do you feel that you are receiving the type and amount of mentorship/feedback that you need for successful completion of your DCE? How has your site supervisor/external mentor provided you with feedback and how has this supported your capstone project and DCE experience thus far? Does anything need to change, and if so, how could you ask for this type of feedback?

Week 8
You are halfway through your capstone! How is the journey thus far?
For this week's post, please describe one aspect of interprofessional collaboration that you participated in. Who were the different professionals involved, and what role did they play? How did you participate? Why is interprofessional collaboration important at your site?

Week 12
Share with your peers how you have incorporated evidence-based practice into your role as an occupational therapist (student) at your site. Do other professionals at your site use evidence to guide their decision-making, and if so, how do they demonstrate this practice?

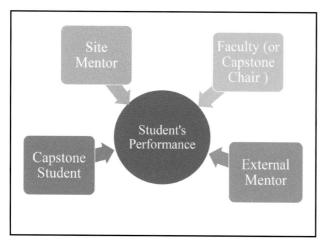

Figure 9-3. Using the 360-degree evaluation approach with the capstone team.

Week 14

You are nearing the end of the DCE! I hope that you enjoyed the journey and grew as you experienced curves and bumps in the road along the way.

The goal of the capstone is to develop occupational therapists with in-depth knowledge. Share with your peers about an in-depth experience with the following: clinical practice skills, research skills, administration, leadership, program development, policy development, advocacy, education, and/or therapy development. Provide an example of two advanced skills, using the terms above, that you have had a chance to develop during the DCE.

360-Degree Evalutation Approach

In addition to these informal strategies to provide feedback and evaluate capstone student performance, the use of a more formal evaluation mechanism (tool) is recommended for consideration. Similar to Level II fieldwork, which uses a tool to evaluate student performance at midterm and at completion of the 12-week experience, an evaluation report can be created by the occupational therapy program to be used by the site mentor, doctoral capstone coordinator, or faculty mentor (or capstone chair). This approach to evaluation is often described as a *360-degree approach* (Braken, 2009; Cormack, Jensen, Durham, Smith, & Dumas, 2018) and can be used to help maximize the functions of feedback to enhance the capstone student's learning and improve curriculum outcomes. This multisource feedback approach is a useful method to ensure that the evaluation process is holistic and interactive among the capstone team. The goal is to encourage reflection among the capstone team and collect feedback that will help capstone students grow and develop in their focus area. By including the site mentor, faculty

member (or capstone chair), capstone student, and perhaps an external mentor in the evaluation process, the student has an opportunity to get balanced feedback and encouragement for increased self-awareness (Figure 9-3). This allows students to gain a clearer picture of their progress and desired goal. It may also be beneficial to have a mechanism for the consumers (clients) who interact with the capstone student to provide feedback, if appropriate, based on the type of DCE and focus area (Figure 9-3).

Evidence indicates that the 360-degree evaluation approach can create behavior change (Goldsmith & Morgan, 2004; Goldsmith & Underhill, 2001; Smither, London, & Reilly, 2005), yet it is recommended that four critical design factors are taken into consideration: (1) relevant content, (2) credible data, (3) accountability, and (4) consensus (Bracken & Rose, 2011). See Table 9-2.

In addition to the evaluation of the capstone student being a holistic appraisal, this tool can be designed to measure progress and provide feedback at specific intervals of the DCE, such as midterm (week 7) and at completion (week 14).

TEACHING TIP 2: Specific resources that capstone coordinators and OTD faculty may find useful when creating evaluation measures for the capstone can be found in the following resources:

- Fitzpatrick, J. L., Sanders, J. R., & Worthen, B. R. (2010). Program evaluation: *Alternative approaches and practical guidelines* (4th ed.). Boston, MA: Pearson.
- Presser, S., Couper, M. P., Lessler, J. T., Martin, E., Martin, J., Rothgeb, J. M., & Singer, E. (2004). *Methods for testing and evaluating survey questions.* Hoboken, NJ: Wiley.
- Saris, W. E., & Gallhofer, I. N. (2014). *Design, evaluation, and analysis of questionnaires for survey research.* Hoboken, NJ: Wiley.

General Recommendations for Designing an Evaluation Tool

- Be concise.
- Have clear instructions for use and purpose of tool.
- Focus on measurable, objectives (American Association for Public Opinion Research, 2018).
- Have a clear and understandable rating scale.

Table 9-2. Recommended Design Features for Evaluation Tools

DESIGN FEATURE	IMPLICATIONS FOR DEVELOPMENT OF A TOOL FOR THE DOCTORAL CAPSTONE
Relevant content	Constructs being measured (hard or practice-ready skills) Accessibility of tool
Credible data	Response scale Training of raters Frequent of rating
Accountability	Reviewing results among the capstone team Awareness and acceptance of feedback
Consensus	Having all members of the capstone team participate to "maximize message" (Braken & Rose, 2011, p. 6)

Adapted from Bracken, D. W., & Rose, D. S. (2011). When does 360-degree feedback create behavior change? And how would we know it when it does? *Journal of Business and Psychology, 26*(2), 183-192. doi:10.1007/s10869-011-9218-5.

TEXT BOX 9-5 (continued)

- Keep the questions relevant.
- Arrange the questions using topic areas, in a organized manner (for example you can purposefully group all of the practice-ready [soft skills] together) (American Statistical Association [ASA], 1997).
- Be aware of possible limitations and biases (ASA, 2018).
- Keep the interest of the client as focus.

Designing an evaluation tool is much like writing a research paper: Before you write about your findings, you need to ask questions about and clarify your research goal and your process and break down your topic into manageable parts. Questions to ask yourself can include the following:

- "What is the purpose of this evaluation?"
- "What do I hope to learn?"
- "How will the data I collect influence my decisions?"
- "What is my target population?"

By target population, we mean the people who you want to take your survey.

Another critical consideration when developing assessments has to do with the variability of experiential activities during the capstone experience. Because capstone students are working on different projects and in different focus area(s), they cannot all be expected to learn the exact same things, and each student may take away something different from the experience. Beyond the variability of activities, there is also variability among the students. Additional focus points to consider when creating a formal evaluation mechanism to measure the student's performance on the capstone can include rooting evaluation components in the individualized learning objectives, established in the MOU. See Appendices 9-B and 9-C for sample evaluation forms. Several of these sample evaluations in the appendices offer blank space for the capstone student to specify (i.e., write in)

their individualized learning objectives. Evaluation components can include a combination of technical skills (related to their chosen focus area) and practice-ready skills (elaborated on in Chapter 5). Capstone coordinators can also use Bloom's domains of learning (often referred to as KSA—Knowledge, Skills, and Attitudes) as a guide to structure constructs of the capstone evaluation (Anderson & Krathwohl, 2001; Bloom, 1956; Table 9-3).

Within the 360-degree evaluation process, providing opportunities for self-reflection and self-assessment of the capstone student is crucial. Boud (2013) indicated how important self-assessment is in the learning process and the value of involving students in determining how success or achievement is defined. As part of the learning objectives for the capstone experience course, educators and doctoral capstone coordinators can specifically require that the capstone student complete and submit a self-assessment (using the same tool that their site mentor uses to evaluate their performance). Not only is this strategy an important component of adult learning that fosters self-reflection, it can also be used to facilitate discussion among the capstone team. The use of self-assessment could occur at midterm and at completion of the DCE.

Recommendations for Rating Scales

A Likert scale is typically a 5- or 7-point scale used to allow individuals to express how much they agree or disagree with a particular statement (McLeod, 2008). The rating scale offers a range of answer options—from one extreme to another—and includes a moderate or neutral point. In survey design, Likert scales are commonly used to measure attitudes and opinions with a greater degree of nuance than a simple "yes-no" question. The AOTA FWPE tool uses a Likert scale for the fieldwork educator to evaluate the performance of a Level II fieldwork student (Table 9-4).

There are various types of response scales that can be used in a 360-degree evaluation approach:

- Effectiveness scale
- Observed frequency scale (4 point)

Table 9-3. Overview of Bloom's Domain of Learning and the Capstone

DOMAIN OF LEARNING	DESCRIPTOR	RELATIONSHIP TO THE DCE
Cognitive domain	Mental skills (knowledge)	• Adhering to the procedures of the capstone site • Problem-solving, troubleshooting an unanticipated scenario • Metacognition
Affective domain	Growth in feelings or emotional areas (attitude or self)	• Listens with respect • Culturally aware • Participation and initiation • Motivation • Self-efficacy
Psychomotor domain	Manual or physical skills (i.e., doing)	These may pertain more specifically to the focus area chosen and the type of capstone project.

Adapted from Bloom, B. S. (1956). *Taxonomy of educational objectives: The classification of educational goals.* New York, NY: Longmans, Green.

Table 9-4. Rating Scale of the AOTA Fieldwork Performance Evaluation

4 = EXCEEDS STANDARDS	Performance is highly skilled and self-initiated. This rating is rarely given and would represent the top 5% of all the students you have supervised.
3 = MEETS STANDARDS	Performance is consistent with entry-level practice. This rating is infrequently given at midterm and is a strong rating at final.
2 = NEEDS IMPROVEMENT	Performance is progressing but still needs improvement for entry-level practice. This is a realistic rating of performance at midterm and some ratings of 2 may be reasonable at the final.
1 = UNSATISFACTORY	Performance is below standards and requires development for entry-level practice. This rating is given when there is concern about performance.

Reprinted with permission from American Occupational Therapy Association. (2002). *Fieldwork performance evaluation for the occupational therapy student.* Retrieved from https://www.miota.org/docs/AOTA.FWPE.SAMPLE.pdf.

- Anchored observed frequency scale (typically a recommended approach where 360 is being used for behavioral development)
- Developmental rating scale

Examples of each of these types of response scales are presented in the following subsections.

Effectiveness Scale

To counter a skew of ratings when using a 5-point scale, this type of scale should be designed to have three positive response options and two negative response options (Expert Training Systems [ETS], 2018; Table 9-5).

Observed Frequency Scale (4 Point)

This scale asks raters about the frequency with which an individual displays certain behaviors (ETS, 2018). It also has an "unable to comment" response, which accounts for the fact that some of those providing feedback may not feel they have had the opportunity to observe a particular behavior. For example, if the faculty mentor (or capstone chair) is using the same tool as the site mentor, there may be certain components of the evaluation that they would not be able to formally rate if they did not observe (Table 9-6).

Anchored Observed Frequency Scale

This scale uses percentage bandings to guide raters and ensure greater consistency in ratings (ETS, 2018). This method can reduce the likely discrepancies in ratings based on individuals' different interpretation of frequencies. This scale can help bring more objectivity to the process by providing guidance on how often is "often" to enable more distinction between ratings (Table 9-7).

Table 9-5. Effectiveness Scale

RESPONSE OPTION CODE	DESCRIPTION
NE	Not effective (–)
SE	Somewhat effective (–)
E	Effective (+)
VE	Very effective (+)
EE	Extremely effective (+)

Table 9-6. Observed Frequency Scale

VALUE	DESCRIPTION
4	Always does this
3	Does this more often than not
2	Sometimes does this and sometimes does not
1	Rarely or never does this
N/A	Unable to comment (not observed)

Developmental Rating Scale

This type of rating scale is focused on rating a person's capabilities on a particular behavior (ETS, 2018). This scale has a greater number of positive descriptors to enable a more spread of ratings and reduce a positive skew. Naturally, it is often chosen where 360-degree feedback is being used to directly inform personal or professional development plans. A developmental scale is focused on helping raters reinforce their strengths and take action to improve their development needs. It should only be used for developmental purposes and is not suitable for performance management. The "no opportunity to observe" option can be helpful for feedback providers if they are newly interacting with the capstone student or do not work closely with the individual in certain capacities and so have not seen a particular behavior or skill being demonstrate (Table 9-8).

Some examples of terminology to consider when building a tool to evaluate the doctoral capstone can be seen in Text Box 9-6 and 9-7.

TEXT BOX 9-6

1 = needs attention
2 = not making progress
3 = making progress
4 = met
5 = exceeding

TEXT BOX 9-7

NE = no evidence
S = somewhat (incomplete/needs improvement)
A = approaching (acceptable yet developing)
G = grasped (present)

It also be beneficial to use qualifying words to help the evaluator further understand the rating, seen in Text Box 9-8 and 9-9.

TEXT BOX 9-8

Consistently exceeds
Often exceeds expectations
Meets expectations
Some improvement needed
Major improvement needed

TEXT BOX 9-9

Strongly disagree
Disagree
Neutral/neither agree nor disagree
Agree
Strongly agree

An open or blank space for qualitative comments should also be provided. It should be encouraged that any scores that are rated as extremely low or high on a Likert scale should include a qualitative comment from the evaluator to help substantiate the score. An example of comments to satisfy a rating of 5 out of 5, or above expectations/exceptional, can be seen in Text Box 9-10.

TEXT BOX 9-10

"Capstone student established interprofessional team rounds with rehabilitation staff on daily basis and created a virtual communication log that led to increased care coordination."
"Capstone student completed systematic review of literature regarding rehabilitation care of the patient with traumatic brain injury and developed evidence-based protocol to be implemented on the brain injury unit."

Examples of comments to satisfy a 1 out of 5 rating, which may indicate performance that is significantly below expectations or at risk can be seen in Text Box 9-11.

Table 9-7. Rating Scale of the AOTA Fieldwork Performance Evaluation

LABEL	PERCENTAGE	VALUE
Always	95% or more	6
Nearly always	75% to 94%	5
Often	50% to 74%	4
Sometimes	25% to 49%	3
Rarely	6% to 24%	2
Hardly ever	5% or less	1
No opportunity to observe	—	N/A

Table 9-8. Developmental Rating Scale

Significant development need	Slight development need	Competent	Slight strength	Definite strength	Exemplary—a role model	No opportunity to observe

TEXT BOX 9-11

"Capstone student has difficulty initiating conversation with site mentor as well as the interprofessional team members, including other occupational therapy staff, rehabilitation aides, and nurses. Interprofessional input to the capstone project has been limited due to poor communication."

"Capstone student has demonstrated poor use of evidence, citing Wikipedia and Google as primary sources used to inform the capstone project."

An important aspect of the DCE is that capstone students ultimately demonstrates in-depth skills within their focus area, through the experience and the project. One strategy to specify that the individualized learning objectives were met by the capstone student is to include a statement or attestation on the evaluation tool, such as Text Box 9-12.

TEXT BOX 9-12

Please check one:

___ All the learning objectives have been accomplished and I recommend that the student pass the DCE.

___ The Student has NOT fulfilled the objectives for the DCE and is NOT recommended to pass.

The preceding information is meant to inform and inspire doctoral programs that are seeking to develop or enhance the evaluation mechanisms regarding the capstone. Regardless of the evaluation mechanisms created and chosen, the capstone coordinator should educate all members of the capstone team on the evaluation tool, and related procedures and processes. One strategy to educate the capstone team, specifically the site mentor, is to develop a webinar-like training that can be used to onboard all site mentors and compare and contrast fieldwork education and the capstone.

Recommendations for Grading Schemes for the Doctoral Capstone Experience

In addition to establishing the evaluation mechanism, educational programs will need to determine the grading practice to be used in the capstone experience course. Programs could synthesize formative and summative evaluation feedback from the capstone team to assign a letter grade (using a traditional A through F letter grade scale) or have more of a benchmark measure, which may determine a final rating such as

- Pass with honors (H—to recognize exemplary performance of the capstone student)
- Pass (P)
- Not pass (NP)

Policies and procedures related to the doctoral capstone should include clear expectations of performance, grading process, and remediation plan. Similar to what occurs with Level II fieldwork, the site mentor is able to provide input and feedback on the capstone student's performance during the experience, yet it is ultimately the responsibility of the doctoral capstone coordinator to assign the final grade or rating for the capstone student.

Requirements for successful completion of the DCE can include the following components:

- Satisfactory completion of the 14-week (560-hour) full-time experience
- Satisfactory completion and submission of all learning objectives, learning activities, and evidence via completion of the evaluation form
- Satisfactory completion of all required assignments (e.g., reflection postings and submission of other required forms)
- Completion of the "Student Evaluation of Capstone Experience" form

The doctoral capstone coordinator can synthesize information obtained from the evaluation tools as well as the capstone student's effectiveness in completing required paperwork, according to the established policy and syllabus. An example of how to use the Pass-Fail-Honor grading system for the DCE is provided in Table 9-9.

The literature on pass-fail grading schemes in medical and health science education provides several advantages that should be considered by doctoral capstone coordinators and occupational therapy faculty. Pass-fail grading allows for assessment of the learner by assessing competency of an outcome rather than earning a grade. There is evidence to suggest that a significant reduction in perceived stress and potential for improvement in positive attitude is associated with pass-fail grading (Rohe et al., 2006). Dyrbye et al. (2005) stated that letter grading systems promote a competitive environment that promotes maladaptive psychosocial well-being (e.g., stress and anxiety) and increases peer competition rather than cooperative learning. A pass-fail system for experiential education has the potential to promote intrinsically self-directed learners motivated through personal growth and development (Spring, Robillard, Gehlbach, Moore, & Simas, 2011). The inclusion of "honors" or a "high pass" grade (as noted in Table 9-9) can be a nice way to recognize students that are above average and consistently go above and beyond expectations set by the academic program and the site.

Suggestions for Remediation for the Capstone Student

Remediation of student deficiency is another essential element of the teaching-learning process, and integral to adult learning andragogy. The word *remediation* can be described a correction of maladaptive or defective performance. However, an important aspect of remediation as a teaching intervention is that it does not always have to be punitive in nature. The result of remediation can include modification of teaching strategies, giving clear, corrective feedback, and positive reinforcement for the learner. The use of feedback and formal remediation plans (such as a learning contract or performance improvement plan) can be used to proactively identify at risk attitudes or behavior to improve the success of the student.

A learning contract is a long-standing remedial intervention also used in fieldwork (Gutman, McCreedy, & Heisler, 1998; Hanson & DeIuliis, 2015) and can certainly also be a useful strategy to help support the development of capstone students.

TEXT BOX 9-13

A learning contract is a written document developed collaboratively among the capstone team members. And should:

- Identify clear, smart individualized performance goals.
- Include a time frame in which the goals should be completed.
- List action steps, resources, or strategies that the learner commit to using to be successful.
- Have responsibilities of both parties included (the site mentor should play an active role in supporting the student's success).
- Serve as formal agreement and include signatures of all parties involved.
- Outline consequences if performance does not meet the identified goals (which could include additional counseling and advisement, extension of the capstone experience, failure of the experience, etc.).

Learning contracts can be used to improve success with hard or practice-ready skills (see Appendix 9-D for a sample learning contract). Occupational therapy educational programs should have clear policies and procedures outlining expectations regarding remediation and specifically handling a capstone student who is not successful during the DCE. Specific aspects that should be considered in the development of remediation policies related to the doctoral capstone can include the following:

- What if the student has a history of a previous failed experiential (or fieldwork) experience?
- What if the student is on academic probation?
- Are there any ethical or legal implications?

TEACHING TIP 3: Similar to fieldwork, site mentors need to be encouraged to initiate contact with the academic program via the doctoral capstone coordinator with any signs of concern about the capstone student. Also, document, document, document! Having a paper trail that consists of things such as when concerns developed, meetings and communications that occurred, and student response to feedback and the learning contract is important data that may come in handy with a student who is not successful on the doctoral capstone.

Table 9-9. Examples of a Pass-Fail-Honor Grading System for Doctoral Capstone Experience

GRADE	DESCRIPTOR	DATA
Honors or High Pass	• Beyond Exceeded Score for 80% of DCE Evaluation of the OTD Student • Exceptional comments on DCE • Evaluation of the OTD Student	90% to 100% on assignments (including reflections and other required tasks)
Pass	• Beyond Exceeded and met for 70% of DCE Evaluation of the OTD Student • Above average comments on DCE • Evaluation of the OTD Student	80% to 89% on assignments
Fail/Not Pass	• Did not receive a passing score on DCE • Evaluation of the OTD Student	Did not turn in assignments or missed assignment deadlines

Educational programs should have policies that outline whether students who do not earn a passing grade on the DCE are offered a second opportunity after a plan of remediation has been successfully completed or at discretion of the doctoral capstone coordinator. If deemed eligible to continue, the capstone student would need to repeat the DCE course (experience), which may include registering again for the same course (and payment for additional credits). The capstone student should also be made aware that the dates and location of the new DCE site are dependent on the availability of placement sites, potential site mentors, and match to student's needs. Occupational therapy programs should also have polices that clearly communicate to the capstone student that he or she may be allowed to repeat only one failed DCE placement.

TEACHING TIP 4: Doctoral capstone coordinators and occupational therapy faculty should investigate their academic institution policies of how a "fail" or "not pass" grade may affect a student's standing in the program, based on academic requirements.

EVALUATION OF THE CAPSTONE MENTOR, SITE, AND EXPERIENCE

Evaluation of the doctoral capstone should be a mutual experience among members of the capstone team. The capstone student plays a central role in the capstone process and should have the opportunity to have their voice heard. According to Knowles (1970; 1990), a pioneer in adult learning theory, optimal learning occurs when adults are self-directed and actively engaged in the learning process. Feedback from the student can have multifaceted purposes. It can be used to measure the student's perception of the overall experience, collaboration with the mentor, and whether the site was welcoming to the student. Feedback from the student can also be used from a program evaluation method to determine the need to develop, refine, or eliminate fieldwork and capstone sites and curriculum enhancement. Depending on the capstone focus, type of setting, or individual mentoring the capstone student, there can be great diversity among the end product of the doctoral capstone. It is important to develop assessments that measure success in both the process and the product—each area may require separate learning outcomes and criteria. One example to evaluate student performance and progress during the capstone is for the occupational therapy education program to use structured reflection prompts, which was discussed earlier in this chapter (refer back to Text Box 9-3). Obtaining feedback from capstone students about their experience at the site and their mentorship from the site mentor is also important. This tool can include a combination of open- and closed-ended questions and might have a similar Likert scale that is used on the student evaluation. Other important elements of the evaluation that capstone students should complete will gauge their perception on meeting the MOU objectives and achieving competence in their focus area and their perception of the supervision and mentorship received from their mentor.

Sample indicators on an evaluation tool that capstone students would use to evaluate their experience and the role of the site mentor may include their perception of the:

• Orientation process at the DCE site
• Communication and feedback system with their mentor or other stakeholders at their site
• Availability of supervision from site mentor
• Site mentor as a role model
• Meeting the MOU objectives

- Achieving in-depth knowledge or competence in the chosen focus area(s)
- Site mentor's contribution and impact on project

See Appendix 9-E for an example.

Students can also be prompted to consider how their new skills (in their focus area), knowledge, and experiences are transferable to other situations or environments, including those outside of a formal academic course. The evaluation tool to measure the experience from capstone students' perspective and their feedback on the mentorship received from the mentor can be gleaned in a combination of open- and closed-ended questions and the use of a Likert scale, as noted previously. Results of the evaluation completed by the capstone student can be used to develop, refine, or eliminate capstone sites.

Use of an Exit Survey

In addition to getting subjective feedback from the capstone team using developed evaluation tools, the doctoral capstone coordinator may be interested in developing and deploying an exit survey at the completion for the entire capstone course sequence. The exit survey could also include open- and closed-ended questions and be set up to be completed anonymously by students. Exit surveys should be designed with the notion that students provide valuable insight and can help enhance curriculum and department processes and procedures. Questions can be designed to capture key data required by the academic institution or accreditors such as ACOTE, including job placement rate and amount of student debt. (See Appendix 9-F for sample exit survey.)

TEACHING TIP 5: To get feedback for their own professional development and growth, doctoral capstone coordinators can create and deploy student evaluation surveys specific to their role as capstone coordinator. Check with your academic institution to see if there are already surveys developed specifically for clinical, teaching, and coordinator roles that could be applicable to the DCE. See Appendix 9-G for an example of a doctoral capstone coordinator effectiveness survey.

CHAPTER SUMMARY

This chapter has provided recommendations of how to envision and develop a holistic evaluation system, including all members of the capstone team. In addition to their own mission, vision, and curriculum philosophies at their respective academic institutions, seminal teaching and learning pillars including Bloom's taxonomy and domains of learning can be useful resources for doctoral capstone coordinators to use to become inspired and develop evaluation mechanisms

for the capstone. Educating members of the capstone team on the evaluation tools themselves as well as the importance of their specific vantage point are important responsibilities of the doctoral capstone coordinator. Creating and maintaining clear policies (including those within a policy handbook, included on syllabi, or posted on a website) are critical aspects to ensure fair, equitable, and consistent grading practices. This chapter specifically focused on the DCE; subsequent chapters provide recommendations and strategies to design and evaluate the capstone project and final written capstone document.

Learning Activities

1. Review the AOTA Level II FWPE. For each of the 42 items, brainstorm how the skill or competency could be enhanced to measure a higher level of learning according to Bloom's taxonomy.
2. Review the evaluation process at your academic institution used to get student feedback on the Level II fieldwork experience. Brainstorm ideas of how it could be adapted to use on the capstone.
3. Envision one of your Level II fieldwork placements. Pick an ACOTE focus area. Using the sample learning contract in Appendix 9-D, outline several action steps you could take to develop in-depth knowledge that coincides with the focus area.

REFERENCES

Allen, M. J. (2004). *Assessing academic programs in higher education.* Bolton, MA: Anker.

Accreditation Council for Occupational Therapy Education. (2018). *Standards and interpretive guide.* Retrieved from https://www.aota.org/~/media/Corporate/Files/EducationCareers/Accredit/StandardsReview/2018-ACOTE-Standards-Interpretive-Guide.pdf

American Association for Public Opinion Research. (2018). *Best practices for survey research.* Retrieved from https://www.aapor.org/Standards-Ethics/Best-Practices.aspx

American Occupational Therapy Association. (2002). *Fieldwork performance evaluation for the occupational therapy student.* Retrieved from https://www.miota.org/docs/AOTA.FWPE.SAMPLE.pdf

American Occupational Therapy Association. (2017). Level I fieldwork Competency evaluation for OT and OTA Students. Retrieved from https://www.aota.org/~/media/Corporate/Files/EducationCareers/Educators/Fieldwork/LevelI/Level-I-Fieldwork-Competency-Evaluation-for-ot-and-ota-students.pdf

American Occupational Therapy Association. (2018). *Self-assessment tool for fieldwork educator competency.* Retrieved from https://www.aota.org/~/media/Corporate/Files/EducationCareers/Educators/Fieldwork/Supervisor/Forms/Self-Assessment%20Tool%20FW%20Ed%20Competency%20(2009).pdf

American Statistical Association. (1997). What is a Survey? Retrieved from http://ludwig.missouri.edu/405/SurveyData.pdf

American Statistical Association. (2018). *Ethical guideline for statistical practice.* Retrieved from http://www.amstat.org/asa/files/pdfs/EthicalGuidelines.pdf

Anderson, L. W., & Krathwohl, D. R. (2001). *A taxonomy for learning, teaching, and assessing: A revision of Bloom's taxonomy of educational objectives.* New York, NY: Longman.

Astin, A. W. (1993). *What matters in college: four critical years revisited*. San Francisco, CA: Jossey-Bass.

Atler, K., Brown, K., Griswold, L. A., Krupnick, W., Melendez, L. M., & Stutz-Tanenbaum, P. (2001). *Fieldwork experience assessment tool (FEAT)*. Retrieved from https://www.aota.org/-/media/Corporate/Files/EducationCareers/Accredit/FEATCHARTMidterm.pdf

Bandura, A. (1971). *Social learning theory*. New York, NY: General Learning Press.

Banta, T. W. (2002). *Building a scholarship of assessment*. San Francisco, CA: Jossey-Bass.

Banta, T. W., Jones, E. A., & Black, K. E. (2009). *Designing effective assessment: Principles and profiles of good practice*. San Francisco, CA: Jossey-Bass.

Bethea, D. P., Castillo, D. C., & Harvison, N. (2014). Use of simulation in occupational therapy education: Way of the future? *American Journal of Occupational Therapy, 68*(Suppl. 2), S32-S39. doi:10.5014/ajot.2014.012716

Bloom, B. S. (1956). *Taxonomy of educational objectives: The classification of educational goals*. New York, NY: Longmans, Green.

Boud, D. (2013). *Enhancing learning through self-assessment*. New York, NY: Routledge Falmer.

Bracken, D. W. (2009). The art and science of 360 degree feedback (2nd ed.) [book review]. *Personnel Psychology, 62*, 652-655.

Bracken, D. W., & Rose, D. S. (2011). When does 360-degree feedback create behavior change? And how would we know it when it does? *Journal of Business and Psychology, 26*(2), 183-192. doi:10.1007/s10869-011-9218-5

Chi-Kwan, S. (2015). High-fidelity simulation: A tool for occupational therapy education. *The Open Journal of Occupational Therapy, 3*(4). https://doi.org/10.15453/2168-6408.1155.

Christiansen, C. H., Baum, C. M., & Bass, J., 2005. *Occupational therapy: Performance, participation and well-being* (3rd ed.). Thorofare, NJ: SLACK Incorporated.

Cormack, C. L., Jensen, E., Durham, C. O., Smith, G., & Dumas, B. (2018). The 360-degree evaluation model: A method for assessing competency in graduate nursing students. A pilot research study. *Nurse Education Today, 64*, 132-137. doi:https://doi.org/10.1016/j.nedt.2018.01.027

Cross, K. P. (1981). *Adults as learners: Increasing participation and facilitating learning*. San Francisco, CA: Wiley.

Dyrbye, L. N., Thomas, M. R., & Shanafelt, T. D. (2005). Medical student distress: Causes, consequences, and proposed solutions. *Mayo Clinic Proceedings, 80*, 1613-1622. doi:10.4065/80.12.1613

Expert Training Systems. (2018). *360 degree feedback rating scales: What's best practice?* Retrieved from https://www.etsplc.com/360-degree-feedback-rating-scales-whats-best-practice/

Goldsmith, M., & Morgan, H. (2004). Leadership is a contact sport: The "follow-up" factor in management development. *Strategy + Business, 36*, 71-79.

Goldsmith, M., & Underhill, B. O. (2001). Multisource feedback for executive development. In D. W. Bracken, C. W. Timmreck, & A. H. Church (Eds.), *The handbook of multisource feedback: The comprehensive resource for designing and implementing MSF processes* (pp. 275-288). San Francisco, CA: Jossey-Bass.

Gutman, S.A., McCreedy, P., & Heisler, P. (1995). Student level II fieldwork failure: strategies for intervention. *American Journal of Occupational Therapy, 52*(2), 143-149. doi:10.5014/ajot.52.2.143

Greene, D. (1997). The use of service learning in client environments to enhance ethical reasoning in students. *American Journal of Occupational Therapy, 51*, 844-852.

Hall, D. L., & Taft, T. B. (1976). Pass/fail versus AF grading: A comparative study. *Journal of Dental Education, 40*(5), 301-303.

Hansen, A. M. W., Muñoz, J., Crist, P. A., Gupta, J., Ideishi, R. I., Primeau, L. A., & Tupé, D. (2007). Service learning: Meaningful, community-centered professional skill development for occupational therapy students. *Occupational Therapy in Health Care, 21*(1-2), 25-49. doi:10.1080/J003v21n01_03

Hanson, D. & DeIuliis, E. (2015). The Collaborative Model to Fieldwork Education: A blueprint for group supervision of students. *Occupational Therapy in Health Care, 29*(2), 223-239. doi:10.3109/07380577.2015.1011297

Hoppes, S., Bender, D., & DeGrace, B. W. (2005). Service learning is a perfect fit for occupational and physical therapy education. *Journal of Allied Health, 34*, 47-50.

IDEO. (2015). *The field guide to human-centered design*. San Francisco, CA: Ideo.org.

Knowles, M. S. (1970). *The modern practice of adult education: Androgogy versus pedagogy*. New York, NY: Association Press.

Knowles, M. S. (1984). *The adult learner: A neglected species* (3rd ed.). Houston, TX: Gulf.

Knowles, M. S. (1990). *The adult Learner: A neglected species* (4th ed.). Houston, TX: Gulf.

Knowles, M. S. (1992). Applying principles of adult learning in conference presentations. *Adult Learning, 4*(1), 11-14. doi:10.1177/104515959200400105

Kolb, D. (1984). *Experiential learning: Experience as the source of learning and development*. Englewood Cliffs, NJ: Prentice Hall.

Lave, J., & Wenger, E. (1991). *Situated learning: Legitimate peripheral participation*. New York, NY: Cambridge University Press.

Law, M., Cooper, B,. Strong, S., Stewart, D., Rigby, P., & Letts, L. 1996. The Person-Environment-Occupation Model: A transactive approach to occupational performance. *Canadian Journal of Occupational Therapy, 63*, 9-23.

Lewis, L. H., & Williams, C. J. (1994). In L. Jackson & R. S. Caffarella (Eds.), *Experiential learning: A new approach* (pp. 5-16). San Francisco, CA: Jossey-Bass.

Maurrasse, D. J. (2002). Higher education-community partnerships: Assessing progress in the field. *Nonprofit and Voluntary Sector Quarterly, 31*, 131-139.

McLeod, S. (2008). *Likert scale*. Retrieved from https://www.simplypsychology.org/likert-scale.html

Moon, J. A. (2004). *A handbook of reflective and experiential learning: Theory and practice*. New York, NY: Routledge Falmer.

Polatajko, H. J., Townsend, E. A., & Craik, J. (2007). Canadian Model of Occupational Performance and Engagement (CMOP-E). In E. A. Townsend & H. J. Polatajko (Eds.), *Enabling occupation II: Advancing an occupational therapy vision of health, well-being, & justice through occupation* (pp. 22-36). Ottawa, Canada: CAOT.

Qualters, D. M. (2010). Bringing the outside in: Assessing experiential education. *New Directions for Teaching and Learning, 124*, 55-62. Retrieved from http://ezproxy.lib.ryerson.ca/login?url=http://search.ebscohost.com/login.aspx?direct=true&db=eric&A N=EJ912853&site=ehost-live

Revans, R. W. (1980). *Action learning: New techniques for management*. London, England: Blond & Briggs.

Robins, L. S., Fantone, J. C., Oh, M. S., Alexander, G. L., Shlafer, M., & Davis, W. K. (1995). The effect of pass/fail grading and weekly quizzes on first-year students' performances and satisfaction. *Academic Medicine, 70*, 327-329.

Rogers, C. R. (1969). *Freedom to learn*. Columbus, OH: Merrill.

Rohe, D. E., Barrier, P. A., Clark, M. M., Cook, D. A., Vickers, K. S., & Decker, P. A. (2006). The benefits of pass-fail grading on stress, mood, and group cohesion in medical students. *Mayo Clinic Proceedings, 81*, 1443-1448. doi:10.4065/81.11.1443

Smither, J. W., London, M. & Reilly, R. R. (2005). Does performance improve following multisource feedback? A theoretical model, meta-analysis, and review of empirical findings. *Personnel Psychology, 58*,33-66.

Smither, J. W., & Walker, A. G. (2004). Are the characteristics of narrative comments related to improvement in multirater feedback ratings over time? *Journal of Applied Psychology, 89*, 575-581.

Spring, L., Robillard, D., Gehlbach, L., & Moore Simas, T.A. (2011). Impact of pass/fail grading on medical students well-being and academic outcomes. *Medical Education, 45*, 867-877.

Suskie, L. (2009). *Assessing student learning: A common sense guide* (2nd ed.). San Francisco, CA: Jossey-Bass.

Appendix 9-A

DUQUESNE UNIVERSITY
Rangos School of Health Sciences
Department of Occupational Therapy

Appendix A Sample DCE Site Visit / Call Form

Capstone Student name: _____ Site:_____

Site Mentor: _____

Contact: ☐ Call ☐ Visit   Dates of DCE:_____   Phone #:_____

Today's Date:_____ Setting:_____

Population(s): _____

Focus Area: _____

Comments:

Discussion Items	Student	Site Mentor
DEC	**Orientation to site:** ☐ Yes ☐ No **Met staff:** **Discuss Specific Objectives:** **On track to meet?** ☐ Yes ☐ No **Comments:** **Workplace for student:** ☐ Yes ☐ No	**Orientation to site:** ☐ Yes ☐ No **Met staff:** **Discuss Specific Objectives:** **On track to meet?** ☐ Yes ☐ No **Comments:** **Workplace for student:** ☐ Yes ☐ No
Level of Supervision / Mentorship ☐ Discrepancy noted between site mentor and student	**Level of Supervision/Mentorship:** ☐ Type/level of supervision/mentorship **Supervision conducive to learning experience:** ☐ Yes ☐ No **Comments:**	**Level of Supervision/Mentorship:** ☐ Type/level of supervision/mentorship **Supervision conducive to learning experience:** ☐ Yes ☐ No **Comments:**

Communication Skills ☐ Discrepancy noted between site mentor and student	<u>**Methods of communication/feedback:**</u> ☐ Formal meeting times set If yes, how often:_____ ☐ Ongoing, informal communication ☐ Use of weekly communication sheets ☐ Other:_____ <u>**Who initiates the communication?**</u> ☐ Student ☐ Site Mentor ☐ Student or Site Mentor <u>**Site Mentor provides constructive feedback**</u> ☐ Always ☐ Most of the time ☐ Sometimes ☐ Never <u>**Communication / Collaboration with other professionals:**</u>	<u>**Methods of communication/feedback:**</u> ☐ Formal meeting times set If yes, how often: _____ ☐ Ongoing, informal communication ☐ Use of weekly communication sheets ☐ Other:_____ <u>**Who initiates the communication?**</u> ☐ Student ☐ Site Mentor ☐ Student or Site Mentor <u>**Student accepts constructive feedback**</u> ☐ Always ☐ Most of the time ☐ Sometimes ☐ Never <u>**Non-verbal communication:**</u> ☐ Appropriate ☐ Inappropriate <u>**Communication / Collaboration with other professionals:**</u>

Professional Behaviors ☐Discrepancy noted between site mentor and student	**Problem-solving skills require guidance:** ☐ Some of the time ☐ Most of the time ☐ All of the time **Integration of Site Supervisor's feedback:** ☐ Some of the time ☐ Most of the time ☐ All of the time **Time Management:** **Use of free time:** **Professional Dress:** ☐ Yes ☐No	**Problem-solving skills require guidance:** ☐ Some of the time ☐ Most of the time ☐ All of the time **Integration of Site Supervisor's feedback:** ☐ Some of the time ☐ Most of the time ☐ All of the time **Time Management:** **Use of free time:** **Professional Dress:** ☐ Yes ☐No
Project Planning / Implementation ☐Discrepancy noted between site mentor and student	**Evals/Asessments Used:** **Interventions:** **Does student incorporate EBP into practice:** ☐ Yes ☐ No **Utilization of EBP:** ☐ Texts ☐Web ☐Journals ☐ Professionals ☐Others	**Evals/Assessments Used:** **Interventions:** **Does student incorporate EBP into practice:** ☐ Yes ☐No **Utilization of EBP:** ☐ Texts ☐Web ☐ Journals ☐Professionals

Preparation for DEC	Was academic preparation appropriate: ☐ Yes ☐ No	Was academic preparation appropriate: ☐ Yes ☐ No
☐ Need to discuss points at faculty meeting	Comments:	Strengths of Program:
Strengths/ Weaknesses ☐ Discrepancy noted between site supervisor and student	Strengths: Areas for Development:	Strengths: Areas for Development:
Additional learning opportunities	Assignments / Projects:	Other activities: Any unique activity opportunities:

Signature acknowledges that Capstone coordinator performed on-site visit.

Student Signature: _____

Site Mentor Signature: _____

Capstone Coordinator Signature: _____

Date: _____

Site Call/Visit Form Continued

<u>**Site Mentor Description:**</u>

Is this your first doctoral student? ☐ Yes ☐ No

Have you been FwEd credentialed? ☐ Yes ☐ No

If no – would you like to be? ☐ Yes ☐ No

Would you like to be notified of any credentialing courses in the area?
☐ Yes ☐ No

Other site supervisor certifications:

Professional memberships:

Did the DEC placement process run smoothly   Yes ☐   No ☐

What could the Capstone Coordinator do to facilitate success and improve communication?

Have you attended a continuing education course this year? ☐ Yes ☐ No

Any course topics you are interested in? _____

How many years in current position? _____

What school did you attend?: _____

<u>**Midterm Evaluation Forms:**</u>

Midterm completed and discussed: ☐ Yes ☐ No

Goals & feed back discussed and agreed upon : ☐ Yes ☐ No

Goals:

<u>**Overall performance:**</u>

Above expected level of competence   ☐

At expected level of competence   ☐

Below expected level of competence   ☐

<u>**Comments:**</u>
☐ On track   ☐ Follow-up needed   ☐ Intervention Required

_____

_____

_____

<u>**If performing site visit:**</u>

First site visit at this site: ☐ Yes ☐ No

Size of site: _____

Staffing of site: _____

Additional opportunities: _____

If any discrepancies noted between site supervisor and student responses what action was performed?

☐ Clarification only was needed from   ☐ Site Mentor   ☐ Student   ☐ Both

☐ Follow-up was performed via phone

☐ Follow-up was performed during a visit

Appendix 9-B

| DUQUESNE UNIVERSITY |
| Rangos School of Health Sciences |
| Department of Occupational Therapy |

Appendix B Doctoral Capstone Experience: Evaluation of the OTD Student

Student Name: Site Mentor Name:

DCE Dates: Site/Setting:

Date of Midterm Review: Date of Final Review:

Select the focus of the DCE:
☐ Research   ☐ Administration   ☐ Teaching
☐ Adv Clinical Practice ☐ Leadership   ☐ Theory Development
☐ Adv Community Practice ☐ Advocacy   ☐ Other: please describe: _____

INSTRUCTIONS:
The Site Mentor will complete this Evaluation form at midterm (~7weeks), and final (14 weeks). The Site Mentor and the OTD Student will review the evaluation collectively and sign that they agree on the evaluation. The OTD Student is encouraged to complete a self-assessment to guide discussion and the learning process. Learning objectives 1–11 are derived from the Curriculum Philosophy of the OTD program and DCE Behavioral Objectives.

Note that there is space provided (potential objectives 12–14) for both the fieldwork student and the site supervisor to add 3 Student-specific objectives, mutually decided upon by the OTD Student and Site **Mentor** based on what the student wants/needs to know, and what skills the student needs to develop. All objectives must be: (1) Relevant to the **DCE** setting **and project**; (2) understandable to the Student, Site **Mentor**, and **Capstone Coordinator**; (3) measurable; (4) behavioral/observable; and (5) achievable within the specified time frame.

Please use this scale to rate the objectives below:
5= Exceeding, **4**= Met, **3**= Making Progress, **2**= Not Making Progress, **1**= Needs Attention
Provide comments to indicate evidence, as indicated.

OTD Objective #1: Student will demonstrate effective communication skills and work interprofessionally with those who receive and provide care.
Evidence of Accomplishment, to be completed by Student and Site Mentor
_____
_____

Midterm: ☐ 5 ☐ 4 ☐ 3 ☐ 2 ☐ 1
Comments: _____
_____

Final: ☐ 5 ☐ 4 ☐ 3 ☐ 2 ☐ 1
Comments: _____
_____

OTD Objective #2: Student will demonstrate positive interpersonal skills and insight into one's professional behaviors to accurately appraise one's professional disposition, strengths, and areas for improvement.
Evidence of Accomplishment, to be completed by Student and Site Mentor

_____

Midterm: ☐ 5 ☐ 4 ☐ 3 ☐ 2 ☐ 1
Comments: _____

Final: ☐ 5 ☐ 4 ☐ 3 ☐ 2 ☐ 1
Comments: _____

OTD Objective # 3: Student will demonstrate the ability to practice educative roles for clients, peers, students, interprofessionals, and others.
Evidence of Accomplishment, to be completed by Student and Site Mentor:

_____

Midterm: ☐ 5 ☐ 4 ☐ 3 ☐ 2 ☐ 1
Comments: _____

Final: ☐ 5 ☐ 4 ☐ 3 ☐ 2 ☐ 1
Comments: _____

OTD Objective # 4: Student will develop essential knowledge and skills to contribute to the advancement of occupational therapy through scholarly activities.
Evidence of Accomplishment, to be completed by Student and Site Mentor

_____

Midterm: ☐ 5 ☐ 4 ☐ 3 ☐ 2 ☐ 1
Comments: _____

Final: ☐ 5 ☐ 4 ☐ 3 ☐ 2 ☐ 1
Comments: _____

OTD Objective # 5: Student will apply a critical foundation of evidence-based professional knowledge, skills, and attitudes.
Evidence of Accomplishment, to be completed by student and site mentor:

_____

Midterm: ☐ 5 ☐ 4 ☐ 3 ☐ 2 ☐ 1
Comments: _____

Final: ☐ 5 ☐ 4 ☐ 3 ☐ 2 ☐ 1
Comments: _____

OTD Objective # 6: Student will apply principles and constructs of ethics to individual, institutional, and societal issues, and articulate justifiable resolutions to these issues and act in an ethical manner.
Evidenco of Accomplishment, to be completed by Student and Site Mentor:

_____

Midterm: ☐ 5 ☐ 4 ☐ 3 ☐ 2 ☐ 1
Comments: _____

Final: ☐ 5 ☐ 4 ☐ 3 ☐ 2 ☐ 1
Comments: _____

OTD Objective # 7: Student will perform tasks in a safe and ethical manner and adhere to the site's policies and procedures, including those related to human subject research, when relevant
Evidence of Accomplishment, to be completed by Student and Site Mentor:

_____

Midterm: ☐ 5 ☐ 4 ☐ 3 ☐ 2 ☐ 1
Comments: _____

Final: ☐ 5 ☐ 4 ☐ 3 ☐ 2 ☐ 1
Comments: _____

OTD Objective # 8: Student will demonstrate competence in following program methods, quality improvement, and/or research procedures utilized at the site.
Evidence of Accomplishment, to be completed by Student and Site Mentor:
_____

Midterm: ☐ 5 ☐ 4 ☐ 3 ☐ 2 ☐ 1
Comments: _____

Final: ☐ 5 ☐ 4 ☐ 3 ☐ 2 ☐ 1
Comments: _____

OTD Objective # 9: Student will learn, practice, and apply knowledge from the classroom and practice settings at a higher level than prior fieldwork experiences, with simultaneous guidance from Site Mentor and OTFaculty.
Evidence of Accomplishment, to be completed by Student and Site Mentor:
_____

Midterm: ☐ 5 ☐ 4 ☐ 3 ☐ 2 ☐ 1
Comments: _____

Final: ☐ 5 ☐ 4 ☐ 3 ☐ 2 ☐ 1
Comments: _____

OTD Objective # 10: Student will relate theory to practice and demonstrate synthesis of advanced knowledge in a specialized practice area through completion of the doctoral capstone experience and capstone project.
Evidence of Accomplishment, to be completed by Student and Site Mentor:
_____

Midterm: ☐ 5 ☐ 4 ☐ 3 ☐ 2 ☐ 1
Comments: _____

Final: ☐ 5 ☐ 4 ☐ 3 ☐ 2 ☐ 1
Comments: _____

OTD Objective # 11: Acquire in-depth experience in one or more of the following areas: clinical practice skills, research skills, administration, leadership, program and policy development, advocacy, education, and theory development.
Evidence of Accomplishment, to be completed by Student and Site Mentor:
_____

Midterm: ☐ 5 ☐ 4 ☐ 3 ☐ 2 ☐ 1
Comments: _____

Final: ☐ 5 ☐ 4 ☐ 3 ☐ 2 ☐ 1
Comments: _____

OTD *Student*-Selected Objective #1: _____

Evidence of Accomplishment, to be completed by Student and Sit eMentor:

_____
_____

Midterm: ☐ 5 ☐ 4 ☐ 3 ☐ 2 ☐ 1
Comments: _____
_____

Final: ☐ 5 ☐ 4 ☐ 3 ☐ 2 ☐ 1
Comments: _____
_____

OTD _Student_–Selected Objective #2: _____

Evidence of Accomplishment, to be completed by Student and Site Mentor:

_____
_____

Midterm: ☐ 5 ☐ 4 ☐ 3 ☐ 2 ☐ 1
Comments: _____
_____

Final: ☐ 5 ☐ 4 ☐ 3 ☐ 2 ☐ 1
Comments: _____
_____

OTD _Student_-Selected Objective #3: _____

Evidence of Accomplishment, to be completed by Student and Site Mentor:

_____
_____

Midterm: ☐ 5 ☐ 4 ☐ 3 ☐ 2 ☐ 1
Comments: _____
_____

Final: ☐ 5 ☐ 4 ☐ 3 ☐ 2 ☐ 1
Comments: _____
_____

We are interested in obtaining an accurate profile of the OTD Student's capacity for the profession. We would appreciate your additional comments regarding the areas in which you rated the student on the previous pages.

Overall Strengths:

Areas for Growth:

Please Check one:

___ All the learning objectives have been accomplished and I recommend that the student pass the Doctoral Capstone Experience.

___ The Student has NOT fulfilled the objectives for the Doctoral Capstone Experience and is NOT recommended to Pass

Student's Signature _____   Date _____

Site Mentor PRINT NAME: _____

Phone _____

Email Address _____

Site Mentor's Signature _____

Appendix 9-C

UNIVERSITY *of*

INDIANAPOLIS.

School of Occupational Therapy

Doctoral Capstone Experience Evaluation Form
Midterm and Final

Please respond to all items by placing checks in the satisfactory (S), needs improvement (NI), or unsatisfactory (U) columns. Designate N/A if the item is not applicable. Please add clarifying statements and /or examples in the comments column. (S) = 2 points, (NI) = 1 point, (U) = 0 points. There are a total of 54 points if there are no (NA) ratings. **For the Final Evaluation, students must achieve a total score 80% to pass with no more than 1 item rated as Unsatisfactory.**

Date: Midterm Score: Student Signature: Site Mentor Signature:	Please evaluate the effectiveness of the student's performance relative to the individualized goals & objectives. **Midterm Summary Statement:**
Date: Final Score: Student Signature: Site Mentor Signature:	**Final Summary Statement:**

	S	NI	U	NA		S	NI	U	NA	Comments/Suggestions
Planning		Midterm					Final			
Designs, selects, and conducts an appropriate needs assessment.										
Utilizes appropriate theory to guide the process.										
Interprets the data appropriately.										

	Midterm				Final			
Assessment reflects the DCE area of focus & individualized objectives.								
Utilizes appropriate outcome tool to quantify goals.								
Development	**Midterm**				**Final**			
Collaborates with site/organization & staff to determine goals/objectives.								
Identifies appropriate strategies for completion of goals and objectives.								
Uses appropriate resources, theory, and evidence.								
Designs programming that is relevant to the client needs.								
Implementation	**Midterm**				**Final**			
Articulates the rationale and use of theory.								
Intervention is appropriate for the goals and objectives.								
Professionally implements program in a manner appropriate to the area of focus, client needs, and setting.								
Quality Improvement	**Midterm**				**Final**			
Uses appropriate methods to measure effectiveness of the program goals and objectives.								
Communication	**Midterm**				**Final**			
Uses effective strategies to interact and collaborate with staff, clients, and other stake holders								
Completes written work accurately and professionally and in a timely manner.								

OTD 690 Evaluation Form

Keeps site mentor informed of schedule in a timely manner.									
Communicates problems or issues in an appropriate and timely manner to site mentor, faculty mentor and/or DCC.									
Professionalism			**Midterm**				**Final**		
Exhibits effective leadership skills.									
Exhibits good work habits and effective use of time.									
Participates appropriately in the supervision process.									
Effectively advocates for occupational therapy within this setting.									
Utilizes professional ethics.									
Exhibits professional demeanor.									
Adheres to all site policies and procedures.									
Exhibits ability to be self-directed.									
Keeps site mentor aware of schedule and completes required hours.									
Demonstrates ability to be on-time to all meetings and scheduled events.									

OTD 690 Evaluation Form

Appendix 9-D

DUQUESNE UNIVERSITY
Rangos School of Health Sciences
Department of Occupational Therapy

Appendix D Learning Contract/ Action Plan

Performance Issue/Concern (Be specific	Expected Performance Goal (Behavioral Goal- SMART)	Strategies, Actions & Resource(s) required to meet the goal	Plan for Follow- up / Timeline (establish date/time for performance to be re-evaluated)	Consequences if performance not improved

By providing signature, both parties are acknowledging the above performance issues and agree to participate in the performance improvement plan as outlined above. It is the student's responsibility to access resources, carry out these and/or other strategies to improve their performance and implement feedback in the identified problem areas. Failure to meet expected performance in established timeline may indicate disciplinary action and/or failed capstone experience.

Student signature:_____ Date:_____

Site Mentors signature(s):_____

Date:_____

Capstone Coordinator and/or Chair's Signature:_____

Date:_____

For use at follow-up meeting (cont)

Evidence to demonstrate change in performance /Outcome:

_____ Review met expectations   _____ Review did not meet expectations * Disciplinary action may be necessary.

Student signature:_____ Date:_____
Site Mentors signature(s):_____ Date:_____
Capstone Chair's Signature:_____
Date:_____

Appendix 9-E

Appendix E
(sample) Capstone Student Evaluation of the Doctoral Capstone Experience and Site Mentor

OTD Student:
Site Mentor
Doctoral Capstone Site:

INSTRUCTIONS: The OTD Student will complete this evaluation form at completion of the 14 week experience. The Site Mentor and OTD Student will review the evaluation collectively and sign that they have discussed. The Student will then submit the form to the Capstone Coordinator, according to the due dates in the course syllabus.

I. Briefly Describe the Doctoral Capstone Site/Setting:

II. Please use the scale below and rate the following:
1 = Strongly Disagree
2= Disagree
3 =Neither disagree / agree (neutral)
4 = Agree
5 = Strongly Agree

Objective	Rating					Comments
1. My Site Mentor was accessible and available.	1	2	3	4	5	
2. My Site Mentor communicated regularly with me.	1	2	3	4	5	
3. My Site Mentor's behavior and attitude are an example of professionalism.	1	2	3	4	5	
4. My Site Mentor made sure to provide ample time to ask questions and provide feedback.	1	2	3	4	5	
5. I was provided ongoing feedback in a timely manner.	1	2	3	4	5	
6. My Site Mentor reviewed written work in a timely manner.	1	2	3	4	5	

7. My Site Mentor made specific suggestions to improve my performance	1	2	3	4	5	
8. My Site Mentor provided clear performance expectations.	1	2	3	4	5	
9. My Site Mentor sequenced learning experiences to grade progression.	1	2	3	4	5	
10. My Site Mentor used a variety of instructional strategies. List those used:	1	2	3	4	5	
11. My Site Mentor identified resources to promote student development.	1	2	3	4	5	
12. My Site Mentor facilitated advanced clinical reasoning.	1	2	3	4	5	
13. I learned new things about myself and how they relate to future OT practice.	1	2	3	4	5	
14. Professional growth occurred for me during this DCE experience.	1	2	3	4	5	
15. Overall, this DCE met my expectations.	1	2	3	4	5	

III. ACADEMIC PREPARATION

Rate the relevance and adequacy of your academic coursework relative to the needs of your DCE, *circling* the appropriate number.

Sample List of OT Courses	Preparation					Comments
	Minimal			Excellent		
Foundations & Concepts of OT	1	2	3	4	5	
Human Development	1	2	3	4	5	
Human Anatomy	1	2	3	4	5	
Kinesiology	1	2	3	4	5	
Neuroscience	1	2	3	4	5	
OT Theory and Practice Models	1	2	3	4	5	

Activity Analysis	1	2	3	4	5	
Occupational Therapy Evaluation and Assessments	1	2	3	4	5	
Medical Conditions	1	2	3	4	5	
Clinical Reasoning	1	2	3	4	5	
Group Dynamics	1	2	3	4	5	
Psychosocial and Behavioral Health & OT	1	2	3	4	5	
Biomechanical Function	1	2	3	4	5	
Cultural Competence	1	2	3	4	5	
Pediatric OT Practice	1	2	3	4	5	
Quantitative Research	1	2	3	4	5	
Qualitative Research	1	2	3	4	5	
Physical Disabilities	1	2	3	4	5	
Evidence-Based Practice	1	2	3	4	5	
OT as a Manager	1	2	3	4	5	
Population Health	1	2	3	4	5	
Assistive Technologies	1	2	3	4	5	
Advanced EBP	1	2	3	4	5	
Program Development	1	2	3	4	5	
Leadership	1	2	3	4	5	
Instructional Learning Theory & Technology	1	2	3	4	5	

IV. Capstone Student Reflections

1. What courses or experiences contributed the MOST to your success on your DCE?

2. What changes would you recommend in your academic program relative to the needs of your DCE?

3. Before beginning a DCE at this site, a capstone student should study/read/prepare by:

4. The most rewarding part of this DCE experience was:

5. The most challenging part of this DCE experience was:

Site Mentor Signature: _____Date: _____

Student Signature: _____ Date: _____

Appendix 9-F

SAMPLE EXIT SURVEY

Select the PRIMARY focus area your DCE
- ❏ Clinical Practice
- ❏ Research
- ❏ Program Development
- ❏ Education
- ❏ Theory Development
- ❏ Advocacy
- ❏ Policy
- ❏ Leadership
      Administration

In general, how well did the OTD curriculum prepare you for the DCE?
- ❏ No Preparation
- ❏ Poor Preparation
- ❏ Moderate Preparation
- ❏ Good Preparation
- ❏ Excellent Preparation

Do you feel that your DCE experience aligned with your chosen focus area(s)?
Yes
No (please explain:)

Do you feel that your DCE site mentor aligned with your chosen focus area(s)?
Yes
No (please explain:)

What do you see as the strengths of the academic preparation for your DCE?

What do you see as the areas of improvement for the academic preparation for your DCE?

Please indicate the degree to which you were satisfied with your overall DCE experience;
- ❏ Not at all
- ❏ Somewhat
- ❏ Moderately
- ❏ Mostly
- ❏ Completely

Appendix 9-G

SAMPLE CAPSTONE COORDINATOR EFFECTIVENESS QUESTIONNAIRE

*this is an example of a tool that could be used to obtain feedback from doctoral students on the role and effectiveness of of the capstone coordinator.

The capstone coordinator ….	Likert Scale Strongly Disagree ←-----------> Strongly Agree
Provided an adequate orientation to the requirements of the doctoral capstone experience. .	1 2 3 4 5
selected an appropriate setting to meet the chosen focus area(s)	1 2 3 4 5
implemented procedures for experiential placements based on the department's policies	1 2 3 4 5
was available to me as a resource person/consultant as needed via email, phone, site visits, blackboard sit, and/or during office hours	1 2 3 4 5
actively solicited my input concerning my doctoral capstone experience at the site via an evaluation, questionnaire or survey post- rotation	1 2 3 4 5
felt comfortable contacting the capstone coordinator via email, phone or during office hours regarding this clinical experience	1 2 3 4 5
was responsive to my questions/concerns regarding my doctoral capstone experience.	1 2 3 4 5
provided feedback about my performance or requirements as needed	1 2 3 4 5
reinforced expectations for demonstrating professionalism during the capstone experience	1 2 3 4 5
	1 2 3 4 5

was an effective professional role model overall faculty member was an effective capstone coordinator	1	2	3	4	5
(optional open-ended question) What aspects of the capstone coordinator's teaching was _**most effective**_?					
(optional open-ended question) What aspects of the capstone coordinator's teaching was _**least effective**_?					

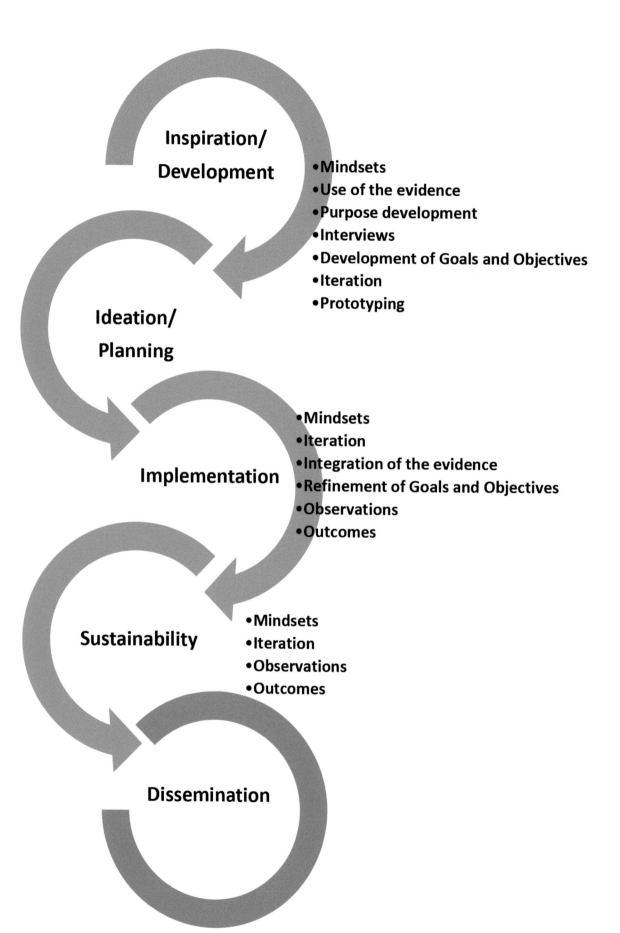

Inspiration/
Development

• Mindsets
• Use of the evidence
• Purpose development
• Interviews
• Development of Goals and Objectives
• Iteration
• Prototyping

Ideation/
Planning

Implementation

• Mindsets
• Iteration
• Integration of the evidence
• Refinement of Goals and Objectives
• Observations
• Outcomes

Sustainability

• Mindsets
• Iteration
• Observations
• Outcomes

Dissemination

PART IV. DISSEMINATION

The final step in the doctoral capstone process is addressing **dissemination** of results. This phase allows students to share the doctoral capstone experience and project with others, including the site; the client, group, or population involved; stakeholders; occupational therapists; and other health professionals. In this phase, capstone students communicate what was done, why it was important, and how the results have had an impact on the client. The dissemination allows capstone students to reflect on how taking on the mindset of a human-centered designer and the process phases of inspiration, ideation, and implementation lead them to have an impact in the world. Share this impact!

CHAPTER 10

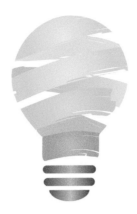

Suggested Components of the Final Capstone Report

Ann B. Cook, OTD, OTR/L

Human-Centered Design Mindsets for the Doctoral Students

The mindsets of iterate, iterate, iterate and creative confidence are important as capstone students are developing their final capstone report. These reports take on different characteristics depending on the student, the area of focus, and program requirements. Capstone students will be creating some type of summative report that meets set program requirements and Accreditation Council for Occupational Therapy Education Standards. By being able to express their creative confidence and how iterations led to a completed project, capstone students pave the way for other students and occupational therapists interested in taking on a human-centered designer mindset.

Iterate, Iterate, Iterate: This will be the time to express and document how iterations took shape and ultimately solved a problem and provided a solution. You will explain how by refining each iteration, learning occurred, and ideas advanced. Continuous iterations may be initially frustrating, but during the writing of the final capstone report, it allows you to reflect on the iterations that ultimately led to the success of the project.

Creative Confidence: You can better understand your client by being creative and documenting how this creativity led to a solution for the client. By this stage in the capstone experience and project, you will have built a creative confidence within yourself; now it is time to utilize this confidence to create a superior final capstone report.

INTRODUCTION

The capstone project is a high-stakes learning activity within occupational therapy doctoral education curricula. It is critical that both capstone students and faculty within occupational therapy doctoral programs understand the process of designing a capstone project, as well as strategies of how to structure the outcomes of the project. The end result

of the capstone project can take many forms. Most familiar to practice-related doctoral degrees is a written capstone report. However, it is important to identify that a doctoral capstone report is not the same as a doctoral dissertation. Depending on the setting of the doctoral capstone experience and chosen focus area, the end result can appear in various formats. This chapter provides an overview of suggestions of how to

Deluliis ED, Bednarski JA.
The Entry Level Occupational Therapy Doctorate Capstone:
A Framework for The Experience and Project (pp 195-214).
© 2020 Taylor & Francis Group.

format and write a solid capstone report with examples and suggestions for capstone students and faculty.

Capstone Student Reflective Questions

When planning the dissemination of the doctoral capstone project, the occupational therapy student may find it helpful to reflect on the following questions:

1. How do I measure my professional writing abilities and skills?
2. What resources are available to me through my academic institution and program to assist in my scholarly writing?
3. What are my program's requirements for a final written capstone report?
4. What literature in the occupational therapy profession can support scholarly writing (e.g., journal articles, position papers, evidence-based practice protocols), and how can I use them as inspirations to structure my own work?

Chapter Objectives

By the end of reading this chapter and completing the learning activities, the reader should be able to:

1. Compare and contrast a doctoral dissertation and a doctoral capstone project.
2. Understand the purpose and process of professional writing in the field of occupational therapy.
3. Explain recommendations for components of the written doctoral capstone report.
4. Identify additional formats for the completion of the capstone report.

COMPARING AND CONTRASTING A DOCTORAL DISSERTATION AND A DOCTORAL CAPSTONE PROJECT

There are several differences between a doctoral dissertation and a doctoral capstone project. Both require significant scholarly effort, but they differ in their process and outcomes. First, the focus of a doctoral dissertation differs from that of a capstone project. A dissertation applies action research methodology to specific situations to generate localized solutions to problems that must then be supported through a review of the literature (Herr & Anderson, 2015). A dissertation is the author's original contribution to the existing literature and theory in a particular field, and is intended to fill the gap in literature while addressing a research problem (Herr & Anderson, 2015). The individual completing a dissertation is expected to create new evidence by conducting formal and rigorous research.

The dissertation process typically involves several steps. First, a problem needs to be identified and lead the author to formulate a research question. Next, a review of the existing literature should be completed to determine whether an answer to the question already exists. If the review reveals a gap in the existing literature—that is, the research question cannot be answered by the existing literature—appropriate methodology should be determined to go about answering the question. From there, research should be conducted, including detailed analysis of data. Finally, the results should be disseminated, thus adding to the existing literature and filling the previous gap regarding the problem.

In contrast, a doctoral capstone project is meant to have a direct impact on a real-world, practice problem that may extend or apply existing research. A capstone project involves application of best evidence, as it exists in current literature, to occupational therapy practice.

The capstone project not only expands the capstone student's knowledge but also informs occupational therapy practice within the student's focus area through scholarly inquiry and critical analysis. The capstone project can be viewed as a culminating project where the capstone student demonstrates synthesis and application of knowledge gained during the focused area of study through the capstone experience (Accreditation Council for Occupational Therapy Education [ACOTE], 2018). Similar to a dissertation, there is a process to completing a capstone project. See Table 10-1 for the suggested steps of completing a capstone project.

HISTORY OF DOCTORAL CAPSTONE PROJECTS

Although relatively new to the occupational therapy education requirements, the idea of a capstone project is not new to health science education. Both nursing and audiology doctoral degree programs have used capstone projects to meet accreditation standards within their curricula and can provide useful information regarding the structure of such projects. In 2004, the American Association of Colleges of Nursing (AACN) voted to endorse a position statement that required the field of nursing to transition from a master's level of preparation to a doctoral level for advanced practice by 2015 (AACN, 2017). Due to changes in health care and to improve patient outcomes, advanced scientific knowledge and practice skills would be met through the academic curriculum for the practice doctorate in nursing (DNP).

The DNP degree requires a final DNP project, often referred to as a capstone project. Similar to the occupational therapy doctoral capstone project, it is not a dissertation but requires mastery of an advanced specialty area in nursing (AACN, 2006). It is not the creation of original research (such as with a dissertation) but requires the application of existing research and literature into practical application in clinical practice. Regarding accreditation standards, it provides evidence that the DNP program has more advanced outcomes than the master's level of preparation (Berkowitz, 2015). Like occupational therapy doctoral students, DNP

Table 10-1. Steps of Completing a Capstone Project

1. Identify a real-world practice problem to address through the capstone project process. This problem can be identified through the completion of a **needs assessment**.

2. Complete an in-depth review of the current **literature** regarding the problem and identifying solutions to the problem evidenced in the literature. Reviewing existing literature not only ensures that the solution is evidence based but that the solution has proved to be successful in practice.

   Occupational therapy capstone students may find that there exists a gap in the literature regarding the particular practice problem, and therefore, the capstone project may intend to fill that gap by finding solutions to the problem identified.

3. Apply evidence-based, practical strategies to find solutions to the specific problem encountered in practice and identified through the needs assessment. This is the "implementation phase" of the capstone project.

4. Contribute to individual, organizational, institutional, or societal change. The capstone project should be something that not only advances the capstone student's skills in a particular focus area (refer to Chapter 2 for more information on the focus areas); it should also benefit the site or community and participants. The benefits of the capstone project should not end when the project is finished.

   ACOTE (2018) Standard D.1.8 states that the dissemination of the capstone should demonstrate synthesis of knowledge in the focused area of study. In addition, the student should share any knowledge gained and pertinent information needed for the site or community to continue to carry out the project.

   The capstone project could be disseminated in various formats, such as a written report, a manuscript, an evidence-based practice protocol, or a hand book (see Table 10-5 for examples of various formats). In addition, products created as part of the capstone project should continue to be used at the site or in the community (e.g., patient or staff training materials, webinars, outcome measurements).

5. Communicate the outcomes of the capstone project with key stakeholders and staff at the site or community organization impacted by the project, including any accompanying artifacts or deliverables. Information related to the overall process and specifically the results of the capstone project should be shared for the site or organization to continue to benefit from the project after it is complete.

   This could be completed through a presentation at a regularly scheduled staff meeting or in-service, through small group meetings with key stakeholders involved in or affected by the student's capstone project, or even virtually through a live webinar. It is important that the outcomes of the project are clearly communicated and that those at the site or organization are able to ask questions to ensure the results of the project are understood.

   All necessary information for follow-through or continuation of the capstone project should be provided so that the site can continue to use the information after the capstone student has completed the project. (Strategies on sustainability of the capstone are discussed in Chapter 8.)

6. Disseminate the outcomes of the capstone project (Standard D.1.8). The capstone project process, including identification of the practice problem, the review of literature, the method of addressing the problem, data analysis, and impact are to be disseminated and appropriate for publication or scholarly presentation (ACOTE, 2018). The requirement for dissemination ensures contribution to the existing literature surrounding this practice area as well as the knowledge of the occupational therapy community of practice.

   Dissemination could be completed in the form of a professional poster or platform session at the local, national, or international level, a written publication for a scholarly journal, or both. Refer to Chapter 11 for more details on potential means for disseminating knowledge and information gleaned from the capstone.

students are required to disseminate the results of their capstone projects. The DNP project is to produce an academic product that results from the student being immersed in a practice experience. It is reviewed by a committee, which serves as an evaluation of their growth in knowledge and expertise (AACN, 2006).

The text *DNP Capstone Projects: Exemplars of Excellence in Practice* (Anderson, Knestrick, & Barroso, 2015) provides detailed examples of actual nursing capstone projects,

including the written capstone document. Table 10-2 provides topic areas for the capstone projects.

The DNP capstone projects in Table 10-2 highlight the importance of applying evidence to practice. Although each capstone project was very different in focus and structure, each identified an area of need and addressed it in practice. This differs from a dissertation, in which the expectation is to produce new evidence. Similar to the DNP capstone, application is key to the occupational therapy doctorate capstone.

Table 10-2. Examples of Practice Doctorate in Nursing Capstone Projects

Burnout as a Barrier to Practice Among Nurse-Midwives: Examining the Evidence
A replica of the 1986 national nurse-midwife study conducted by Beaver et al. (as cited in Barroso, 2015), this project reexamined the prevalence of burnout among members of the American College of Nurse-Midwives (ACNM) currently in clinical practice in Pennsylvania. Various factors associated with burnout were evaluated. This capstone project compared findings with the original study (Barroso, 2015, p. 47).

Changing the Paradigm: Diabetic Group Visits in a Primary Care Setting
The purpose was to assess the impact of introducing one component of the Chronic Care Model (CCM), group visits, on the delivery of health care to diabetic patients in a family medicine clinic and residency training program. The group visit is one strategy to attempt improvements in redesigning the delivery of health care delivery services. The scope of this project was to measure patient perceptions of their health care and changes in specific diabetes clinical indicators as a result of attendance at the group visits (Short, 2015, pp. 55-56).

Promoting Compassion Fatigue Resiliency Among Emergency Department Nurses
Emergency nurses work in an environment that is intellectually, emotionally, and physically demanding with repeated exposure to the stressors of the emergency department. Compassion fatigue may result. This capstone focused on prevention of compassion fatigue and promotion of resiliency among emergency department nurses (Flarity, Holcomb, & Gentry, 2015, pp. 67-68).

Many programs that offer the doctor of audiology (AuD) degree require a capstone project to meet accreditation standards set by the Accreditation Commission for Audiology Education (ACAE; 2016). Standard 25, which outlines student research and scholarly activity, states that students must demonstrate knowledge of research design, be critical consumers of professional literature, and evaluate research to apply this knowledge related to evidence-based practice (ACAE, 2016). The guidelines also suggest the completion of a "mentored experiment" to meet this standard. Many audiology programs opt to require a project that demonstrates students' abilities to evaluate research and apply evidence-based practice in the form of a clinical project.

While the capstone is required for the degrees just discussed, it is not necessarily required for all practice doctorates. The physical therapy profession made the transition to the entry-level doctorate of physical therapy degree (DPT) to meet the Commission on Accreditation in Physical Therapy Education (2017) time frame. During the time of the transition to the entry-level doctorate, the physical therapy profession envisioned a degree that would glean greater respect from health care professionals, the potential for autonomous practice with increased skills, and preparation for clinical scholarship (Plack & Wong, 2002; Rothstein, 1998; Woods, 2001). Although the transition to a doctoral degree meant that programs needed to change their curriculum, it did not require the completion of a capstone.

TEXT BOX 10-1

Current data indicate that 36% of accredited DPT programs offer a designated capstone (Barlow, Hanks, & Tate, 2018).

Similarly, the doctorate of pharmacy degree (PharmD) does not require a capstone project; however, some programs choose to include it as part of their curriculum (Accreditation Council for Pharmacy Education, 2015).

Although the doctoral capstone project is not a new concept in health science curricula, it is a relatively new requirement for entry level occupational therapy doctoral curricula. It is important for all key stakeholders (faculty, capstone students, occupational therapy practitioners, and site mentors) to understand the differences between a dissertation and a doctoral capstone project, as well as to understand the expectations of the occupational therapy capstone student throughout the completion of the capstone project and culminating capstone report.

MEETING THE ACOTE STANDARDS FOR THE CAPSTONE PROJECT

The capstone experience and project are significant pieces of the ACOTE requirements for the occupational therapy doctorate. It is important for faculty in entry-level doctoral programs to ensure that the standards are met within their curricula. Standard D.1.8, which refers specifically to the doctoral capstone project, states: "Ensure completion and dissemination of an individual doctoral capstone project that relates to the doctoral capstone experience and demonstrates synthesis of in-depth knowledge in the focused area of study" (ACOTE, 2018, p. 45).

To demonstrate synthesis of in-depth knowledge in the focused area of study, the program may meet this standard by requiring the capstone student to complete a written capstone report. This document may take various forms, and the style chosen should fit with the nature of the capstone project as well as the student's focus area. For example, one form is a written manuscript to be bound and made available through hard copy in the academic institution's library or electronically through the library's virtual databases. Another form of capstone report is a written practice guideline or evidence-based protocol. Examples of content to be included in forms of culminating documents are provided in Table 10-5 later in the chapter.

In addition, an oral presentation or "defense" of the doctoral capstone project may be required. Key stakeholders from the capstone site, faculty, students, and perhaps family and other supporters of the capstone student could be invited to the presentation. This provides an opportunity for capstone students to share the overall process and outcomes of their work while also informing key stakeholders and clarify any questions that may arise.

Depending on the focus area, doctoral capstone experience and project, occupational therapy students may also be required (or encouraged) to prepare a manuscript of sufficient quality to be submitted to a peer-reviewed publication or a professional trade periodical (such as the American Occupational Therapy Association's [AOTA] *OT Practice* publication) or to submit a proposal to present their capstone as a poster or oral presentation at a local, state, or national professional conference. The capstone student should seek advisement from the capstone team to determine the most appropriate audience for dissemination. Chapter 11 provides additional discussion on key scholarly deliverables from the capstone.

OVERVIEW OF PROFESSIONAL WRITING

Writing is an occupation that occupational therapy practitioners complete regularly. Regardless of practice setting, documentation or writing of some form must take place. The types of writing occupational therapy professionals complete include progress notes, evaluation reports, and other writing tasks such as annual performance appraisals, strategic plans, or a patient-education home program. As a writer, occupational therapy professionals need to be able to write for varying audiences and use an other-centered philosophy. Regardless of the writing task, the occupation of writing requires the development and implementation of key skills to effectively communicate. A written report of the capstone is one example. In the final capstone report, the student is required to communicate outcomes of the project in an organized, accurate, and concise manner with the readers in mind.

ACOTE Standard B.6.3 states that the occupational therapy doctorate student is required to be able to "create scholarly reports appropriate for presentation or for publication in a peer-reviewed journal that support skills of clinical practice. The reports must be made available to professional or public audiences" (ACOTE, 2018, p. 36). It is clear that writing is an important skill for capstone students to develop, especially given that they are required to disseminate the results of the capstone project.

TEACHING TIP 1: Because ACOTE Standard B.6.3 is a B standard, it must be met in the didactic occupational therapy curriculum and ultimately help prepare the capstone student to be able to compose written communication for various audiences. For instance, the student might create an evidence-based practice protocol for an audience consisting of the capstone site mentor and other practitioners at the site. The student might also prepare a written manuscript describing the process and outcomes of creating and implementing such a protocol for submission to a peer-reviewed, clinical practice journal. The style of writing will differ between the evidence-based practice protocol and the manuscript submission. As primary author, the capstone student needs to be able to skillfully shift writing styles to disseminate the information effectively.

Along with other behavioral and social sciences, the occupational therapy profession uses the style of writing and formatting published by the American Psychological Association (APA). The *Publication Manual of the American Psychological Association* (6th ed.) provides guidelines for concise scientific writing with information regarding the use of punctuation and abbreviations, the construction of tables, selection of headings, citation of references, and presentation of statistics (APA, 2010). It is recommended that capstone students use APA style and the available resources through the APA when creating any written scholarly product, whether it be a manuscript for a professional journal, a conference proposal submission, or a presentation to disseminate information.

Both capstone students and faculty should become familiar with the supports and resources offered at their academic institution (both on campus and online). Academic institutions may have a writing center that assists students regarding APA formatting and grammar. The APA (2010) manual is a helpful resource to purchase or use if available through the university library.

TEXT BOX 10-2

Online formatting resources such as Purdue Online Writing Lab (OWL; The Purdue OWL, 2018) and reference generators such as Endnote, Zotera, and Mendeley, can be resourceful to help with the literature search and organization of relevant literature, including managing bibliographies, citations, and references. Because some capstone students may be completing their capstone experience at a site that is not near their academic institution, students are encouraged to determine whether their academic institution provides online or virtual writing supports.

TIPS FOR SCHOLARLY WRITING

Scientific writing is a particular style of scholarly writing with which occupational therapy students and practitioners effectively communicate information regarding practice. It is the style of writing that is recommended when writing the doctoral capstone report, a proposal submission for presentation at a conference, or a manuscript for publication. According to DeIuliis (2017), the goal of scholarly writing is to communicate information clearly, concisely, and accurately. It is not typically used to share one's opinions or beliefs, but to convey facts and data. Following are tips for using scholarly scientific writing for the capstone report.

- *Consider the purpose of writing and the intended audience.* The purpose of the capstone report is to describe the capstone project, how it was conducted, and its results. The outcomes of the capstone project are meant to be disseminated and shared not only with the key stakeholders at the site where the project is completed but with the profession as a whole. The language used in the capstone report should reflect the language of the profession, but any occupational therapy jargon should be explained and abbreviations (e.g., ADL) should be expanded on first use.

TEACHING TIP 2: As a learning activity, doctoral capstone coordinators can divide capstone students into various groups and have each group read one section of an occupational therapy journal article (the introduction, methods, discussion, etc.). Ask each group to highlight any words, phrases, or abbreviations that are specific to occupational therapy. Have students reflect on the amount of occupational therapy-specific language that is used and whether someone outside the field would understand the article. Consider asking the groups to edit their assigned journal sections to be more descriptive for a non–occupational therapist audience.

- *Use proper grammar.* Scientific writing avoids use of the first person (e.g., "I," "we") and is more formal than conversational grammar (Hofman, 2017). Capstone students need to carefully choose vocabulary that reflects the specific message they wish to communicate. Avoid the use of slang. For example, "When the client struggled, I encouraged him to hang in there." The pronoun "I" should be replaced with a noun, and the phrase "hang in there" is informal grammar, or slang. Instead, consider "When the client struggled, the capstone student encouraged the client to do his or her best work."
- *Write in the past tense.* The capstone report is written after the capstone project has occurred; therefore, in most cases, past tense should be used throughout the report. Present tense is to be used for general rules and accepted facts (Hofman, 2017). For example, when writing the results section of the capstone report, the student might write, "Following the training program, staff knowledge increased by 70%." However, in the theory section or conceptual model section of the capstone report, the student might write, "The Model of Human Occupation seeks to explain how occupation is motivated, patterned, and performed."
- *Write with active verbs* (Hofman, 2017). Instead of using abstract nouns, use verbs to energize your writing. For example, "The client's home program was to be completed 3 days per week" uses abstract nouns. Instead, "the client was instructed to complete the home program 3 days per week" uses an active verb. The former is passive, whereas the latter captures the reader's attention.

TEACHING TIP 3: Doctoral capstone coordinators and/or occupational therapy faculty could have capstone students practice transforming passive sentences into active ones. This could be a simple in-class activity or an entire assignment. Consider writing a short article or paragraph with passive phrasing throughout and ask the capstone students to rewrite the article or paragraph to reflect the active voice.

- *Focus on novel ideas.* One possible outcome of the doctoral capstone is to contribute to the existing literature of the profession. Completing a thorough literature review will ensure that the capstone student's project is not replicating something that has already been done or is already answered in the literature. The outcomes of the doctoral project are intended to be useful for the site but also provide professional clinical utility. The literature should be cited and referenced as appropriate.
- *Be concise and objective.* Scientific writing avoids the subjective, and therefore, capstone students must avoid inserting their opinions and assumptions into the writing. Focusing on observations, facts, and data will help students to write objectively and avoid bias. Scientific writing also needs to be concise and to the point. The capstone student should avoid using too many adjectives and unnecessary descriptors. For example, instead of writing, "The capstone student implemented an exciting, new program at the summer camp, and the children seemed to loved it!" consider, "The capstone student implemented an evidence-based sensory integration program at the summer camp across a 6-week period. The children appeared to enjoy it based on their interaction level and facial expressions, and the data confirm that their quality of life improved." The latter provides a much clearer picture and includes objective data.

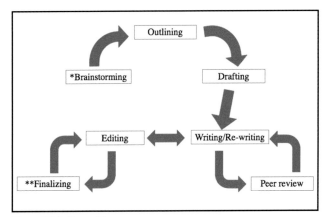

TEACHING TIP 4: Doctoral capstone coordinators and/or occupational therapy faculty could have capstone students watch a brief video clip of an occupational therapy session with a client and write only what they observed, avoiding inserting their own opinion or interpretation. Have them share their written observations in a group, allowing group members to edit for any subjective information and excessive adjectives or to add missed data.

- *Provide evidence to support claims.* Along with being objective, the capstone student needs to provide evidence regarding outcomes of the project. Outcomes data can be qualitative and/or quantitative in nature and clearly articulate the outcomes of the capstone project.
- *Give credit where credit is due.* It is important to give credit to any secondary authors and significant contributors to the scholarly work. The order of authorship is based on the contribution of that author (with the primary author listed first having done the majority of the work). Additionally, individuals who have made a significant contribution to the capstone project should be recognized. This may be done by including an "Acknowledgments" section toward the beginning of the written scholarly work (before the body).

According to the APA (2019):

An author is considered anyone involved with initial research design, data collection and analysis, manuscript drafting, and final approval ... The primary author assumes responsibility for the publication, making sure that the data are accurate, that all deserving authors have been credited, that all authors have given their approval to the final draft; and handles responses to inquiries after the manuscript is published. (n.p.)

TEACHING TIP 5: It is beneficial for the doctoral capstone coordinator to include a statement of authorship in the memorandum of understanding (MOU). The MOU should be signed by the capstone student's site mentor before the capstone experience, agreeing to be included as a contributor on the capstone report.

The Scholarly Writing Process

Scholarly writing is a process. Capstone students should not expect the process to be linear, in that they create the title page and continue writing until the document is finished. Writing a capstone report involves ongoing steps, such as editing, rewriting, and seeking peer review. Due to the dynamic nature of a capstone project, students will be continuing to search and incorporate literature throughout the capstone

Figure 10-1. The writing process.

report, reflecting on feedback received and noting changes made during implementation and critically evaluating their writing as a scholarly product.

As previously mentioned, using any reputable resources, such as the academic institution's writing center, can help the capstone student at any point in the writing process. It is better to receive consultative assistance early on and frequently throughout the writing process than toward the end as any substantial revisions may take time. Peer review is an important aspect of writing because it allows the author to receive feedback from various individuals with a specific skill set and viewpoint. For example, a student may have a peer reviewer who has expertise in his or her focus area to provide feedback on content. Another peer reviewer might have strong writing skills to provide feedback on scholarly writing. See Figure 10-1 for a schematic of the writing process.

TEACHING TIP 6: Doctoral capstone coordinators could have students peer review certain aspects of their peers' capstone reports, focusing on content and writing style.

RECOMMENDATIONS FOR THE FORMAT OF THE FINAL CAPSTONE REPORT

Although not every capstone report will fit neatly into the following headings, these are general suggestions for creating a well-defined, evidence-based, and feasible final written capstone report. To help the capstone student conceptualize how the components fit together, the headings of the capstone report can be viewed through a lens aligned with the occupational therapy process (AOTA, 2014). See Figure 10-2.

Title Page

The title of the capstone report gives the reader a clear idea of the subject matter and should be formatted according

Figure 10-2. A capstone report using the structure of the occupational therapy practice.

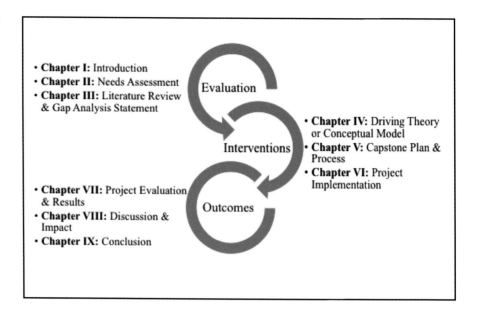

- **Chapter I:** Introduction
- **Chapter II:** Needs Assessment
- **Chapter III:** Literature Review & Gap Analysis Statement

Evaluation

Interventions

- **Chapter IV:** Driving Theory or Conceptual Model
- **Chapter V:** Capstone Plan & Process
- **Chapter VI:** Project Implementation

- **Chapter VII:** Project Evaluation & Results
- **Chapter VIII:** Discussion & Impact
- **Chapter IX:** Conclusion

Outcomes

to APA (2010) guidelines. Next, the capstone student's name is listed. Then list any contributing authors, such as the capstone site mentor and faculty capstone chair, along with their credentials and title (e.g., Ann B. Cook, OTD, OTR/L, Capstone Chair). Next, include the name of the academic institution. A running head and page number is included in the header and will be carried throughout the capstone document. Each institution may require different information on the title page, such as the address of the university; capstone students need to follow any guidelines provided by their institution. Refer to Appendix 10-A for an example.

Acknowledgments

The acknowledgments section is unrelated to the capstone content itself but is an important place to recognize individuals who made meaningful contributions to the capstone project. Capstone students may recognize members of the capstone team, including the site mentor and any faculty who played an important role in their capstone project, as well as other key stakeholders at the site who provided guidance or feedback on their project. It is also an area where the students may want to thank those who supported or inspired them throughout the doctoral program, such as family, friends, and significant others. A more formal dedication may also be included as a separate section, following the acknowledgments.

Table of Contents

The table of contents clearly outlines the contents of the capstone report with page numbers. The report may be organized by chapters, with headings and subheadings created as needed. The capstone student may also include the titles of any tables, figures, and appendices the table of contents as well. If the list is extensive, each may be listed as a separate section or heading.

Chapter I: Introduction

The introduction captures the reader's attention and provides a context for the capstone report. Information about the site itself is included. Details may include the practice setting, population served (common diagnoses, ages, or number of clients), programs offered, professionals employed, or other information that provides the reader with a mental picture of the site and its operations. The capstone student describes the chosen focus area(s) for the capstone experience and how the site provides a context for the focus area(s). The issue addressed by the capstone project is clearly defined and based in literature, addressing a larger problem of practice; therefore, rudimentary information related to the issue being addressed is used as a transition to lead into the needs assessment.

Chapter II: Needs Assessment

The purpose of the needs assessment section is to identify the issue or problem at the site. Following are examples of various purposes for completing a needs assessment:

- To document existence of an ongoing/exacerbating problem
- To prioritize the need for services in communities
- To determine whether interventions and other resources to address the identified needs exist in a community, including strengths and weaknesses
- To determine whether existing interventions are known to or are acceptable to potential clients
- To examine strengths and limitations of various service delivery models (e.g., medical, educational, community, social) on occupational therapy programing
- To determine major barriers (e.g., access, policies, reimbursement) preventing clients from accessing existing services

Table 10-3. Questions to Consider to Identify Issues

Who are the participants?
The capstone student will need to consider various possibilities including the clients themselves, family members or caregivers of clients, and the staff themselves.

What are the common wants and needs of the participants?
Informal discussions or interviews with the participants and key stakeholders (e.g., administration at the site) will provide insight into such needs. Asking open-ended questions regarding current needs will encourage participants to freely share their thoughts and opinions. Follow-up, probing questions can then be used to target more specifics about the need. It is important to gain input from more than one participant if possible to ensure that there is agreement that this is indeed something that is an issue that can and should be addressed.

What are the barriers for achieving these wants and needs?
Once the need has been identified, determining why the need has not been addressed will uncover barriers that the capstone student will need to overcome. Common barriers include lack of time to address the need, limited resources or staff availability, and/or lack of knowledge on how to best address the need. Discussions with participants and key stakeholders are key to determining barriers as well as why they have not been addressed.

Are there gaps in the service that you could fill to support these needs?
There may be several areas of need identified; however, it is important that the capstone student determine which area(s) can be realistically addressed as a capstone project. The student should consider the structure and operations of the site, potential supports and barriers, and their own knowledge and time frame. The capstone project should address an area that is within the profession's scope of practice as well as meet the objectives of the capstone itself.

- To determine whether there are enough clients with a particular problem to justify creating a new program
- To obtain information for tailoring a program to a specific target population

Table 10-3 contains questions that the capstone student should consider to identify issues or problems at the site.

It is important to include details regarding how the needs assessment was conducted in the capstone document. First, the capstone student shares where and when the needs assessment took place. It could have taken place across several days or weeks, and it may have been on-site or virtual. Documentation of meetings with the site mentor, administration, staff, and other key stakeholders is included. The student also includes the types of questions that were asked, themes that emerged during face-to-face or virtual discussion or interviews, and relevant observations made on-site. Finally, the capstone student includes the outcomes of the needs assessment. Although many needs may be identified, capstone students focus on the need or needs that directly influenced their capstone project and any supports or barriers presented. A problem statement is included to clearly identify the area of need to be addressed by the capstone project.

After completing the needs assessment, a written or verbal proposal should be presented to the site stakeholders for approval. Information regarding this proposal process should be included. See Table 10-4 for tips for writing a persuasive proposal. The capstone report will then include any feedback that was received from key stakeholders after the proposal presentation.

Chapter III: Literature Review and Gap Analysis Statement
Literature Review

As discussed in Chapter 3, when determining whether a particular need at a site should be addressed by a capstone project, the student needs to complete a thorough literature review. The review of literature may occur at various points before the actual capstone project, such as before visiting the capstone site, during the formal needs assessment on-site, and after the on-site needs assessment has occurred. In addition, it is important that the literature review continue during the doctoral capstone experience because capstone students should remain current with any new literature being published regarding their capstone topic. It is important to provide a comprehensive, current, and evidence-based review of what information is available regarding the topic and what related research has already been completed.

When reviewing the literature, the student considers quality sources of information such as peer-reviewed journal articles and texts. After exhausting all possibilities for information, the literature will then be appraised, and the student will select only the evidence that is relevant, recent (unless theoretical or foundational in nature), and of high quality (consider the level of evidence from Level I evidence being a randomized controlled trial to Level V evidence being expert opinion). Refer to Chapter 3 for more information regarding the literature search process and synthesis.

Within the literature review section, the capstone student includes methods used to search the literature, such as databases and search terms used, as well as how the articles were

Table 10-4. Tips for Writing a Persuasive Paper

MEET A NEED	When performing the needs assessment, the capstone student should keep in mind that the capstone project is other-centered in design and focus. The capstone proposal must meet a need identified by the site stakeholders. It is key that the student collaborate with stakeholders during the needs assessment to clearly identify what is needed at the site as well as the barriers to meeting that need. If the student presents a proposal for a project that is not needed, site stakeholders will likely reject the proposal. Even so, with any proposal, students should be prepared to alter the details of their proposal based on feedback from the stakeholders.
HAVE INTELLECTUAL MERIT	The capstone proposal needs to be written clearly and be intellectually sound. Robinson, Stroller, Costanza-Robinson, and Jones (2008) suggest that proposals meet the "Three C's" (p. 371): • Creativity—Use innovative ideas to solve the problem at hand. Consider what has already been attempted in the past to solve the problem and why it did not work. • Credibility—Proposals should be evidence based. Capstone students should cite literature throughout their proposal to support the proposed program components. • Competence—Capstone students also need to outline their competence and the role of occupational therapy in meeting the need. This is especially important for role-emerging sites.
HAVE A BROADER IMPACT ON SOCIETY	The capstone project should align with the AOTA's Vision 2025 which states that "As an inclusive profession, occupational therapy maximizes health, well-being, and quality of life for all people, populations, and communities through effective solutions that facilitate participation in everyday living" (AOTA, 2018).

selected. Search parameters such as publication date will also be included. This data may be presented in a table.

Next, the report will contain the actual literature review findings. The capstone students should state what was found in the literature in regard to the identified need. Presenting the literature in an organized manner is important for the reader to understand the project focus and the gap found in the literature. General information on the topic should be presented first, with specifics toward the end of the literature review section. Gaps in the literature relevant to the needs assessment will lead to the question or problem statement, also known as a gap analysis statement (what was not known or had not yet been researched).

Gap Analysis Statement

The question or problem statement will be used to write the gap analysis statement. Once the gap in the current literature has been identified, the student clearly identifies the lack of literature or evidence. To indicate to the reader what was missing from the literature, certain key phrases might be used. Robinson, Stoller, Costanza-Robinson, and Jones (2008, p. 205) provided numerous examples of gap statements:

• "Questions remain unanswered about…"

• "Much as been learned about X, Y remains poorly understood…"

• "The next step is to apply X to…"

• "Additional studies are needed…"

Following are examples of gap analysis statements:

• "Although the literature clearly indicates that occupational therapy plays an important role in the recovery of clients who are burn-injured, the role of occupational therapy in addressing self-image of burn survivors has not been studied."

• "Occupational therapists play a key role in addressing sensory deficits in children with autism spectrum disorder; however, it is important to address the carryover of sensory interventions in the home."

Next, the student explains how he or she intends to "fill the gap." This can be done by simply stating the purpose of the capstone in one to two sentences. Some phrases that writers might use to indicate how they intend to "fill the gap" are as follows:

• "The student will analyze…"

• "In this study, the student will investigate…"

• "Therefore, the purpose of this project is to…"

• "In this paper, the student reports…"

Students should keep in mind that when writing the capstone report, they will eventually need to write in the past tense because the project will be complete. Following are examples of purpose statements written in the past tense:

• "The student therefore analyzed the perceived role of occupational therapy practitioners in an inpatient acute care hospital in addressing self-image with burn-injured clients."

- "Therefore, the purpose of this project was to determine if and how occupational therapy practitioners are addressing carryover of sensory interventions in the home and to address any barriers identified through the capstone project."

After providing the gap analysis statement and before discussing the project plan, the capstone student will discuss the driving theory or conceptual model used to frame the capstone project.

Chapter IV: Driving Theory or Conceptual Model

The capstone student may choose to include a conceptual model or theory to support and frame the design of the capstone project. While the description and rationale for the theory may be written in a defined chapter of the capstone report, the theory itself will be woven throughout the report because it informs the entire process of designing and completing the doctoral capstone project.

Boniface and Seymour (2012) supported the use of theory and its role in informing evidence-based practice for occupational therapy practitioners. "Conceptual professional models not only enable therapists to connect with the theoretical foundation of their work, but they also articulate the nature of their profession" (Reagon, 2012, p. 160). Models and frameworks specific to occupational therapy often consider the person or client, environment or context, and the task or occupation. In other words, a model helps the capstone student to think conceptually about the potential participants, the identified problem or need, and any influencing factors (e.g., environmental, societal, cultural, institutional). In line with Vision 2025 (AOTA, 2018), a model helps the capstone student consider how to best address the problem through creative solutions. An occupation-based focus is key to ensuring the project is grounded in the domain of the profession (AOTA, 2014).

Chapter V: Capstone Plan and Process

Plan

In this section, the capstone student describes the goals that were identified through the literature review and needs assessment as well as the plan and process to achieve the goals. The capstone student needs to keep in mind that the occupational therapy profession is client-centered and that goals and objectives to reach the goals need to have been developed in collaboration with the site mentor to ensure that the project was meaningful to the site and benefitted key stakeholders. It is recommended that capstone students consider writing SMART goals (Specific, Measurable, Action oriented, Realistic, and Timely), just as they would when working with client during traditional fieldwork. Then, students should list short-term objectives or steps to meet the goals. The following is an example of a goal with short-term objectives:

- Goal: Within 4 weeks of program implementation, rehabilitation staff members will implement their knowledge of fall prevention measures as evidenced by an average weekly decrease of one fall incident per unit.
  - Objective: Within 1 week of program implementation, 90% of rehabilitation staff will attend one in-service on fall prevention measures.
  - Objective: Within 3 weeks of program implementation, 90% of rehabilitation staff will demonstrate two strategies for fall prevention during patient handling.

Process

The capstone student would be wise to provide an outline of the process for carrying out the project. The outline should also include a timeline to give the audience a sense of how the capstone student planned to spend 14 weeks accomplishing the project. The capstone student may want to consider including the following:

- Time spent orienting to the site, becoming familiar with processes and procedures, and meetings with key stakeholders
- Refinement of the project plan based on feedback from the site mentor, stakeholders, and faculty mentor
- Any meetings planned in accordance with administration, stakeholders, or site mentor for information regarding approvals, budgeting, recruitment, etc.
- Regular meetings with site mentor, faculty mentor, and/or doctoral capstone coordinator including student evaluation meetings (midterm and final)
- Time for updating the literature review or for any research needing to be done to set a foundation for the doctoral project
- Creation of any products or artifacts for the project (training materials, webinars, protocols, outcome measurements, etc.)
- Marketing/recruitment period for participants (staff, patients, clients, families, etc.)
- The implementation period
- Time for data analysis
- Planning of final presentation
- Final presentation date and time, in collaboration with site mentor, stakeholders, faculty mentor, and capstone coordinator
- Time for final paperwork required by the site or student's occupational therapy program

See Appendix 10-B for an example outline. Other important information to include in the plan is an overall budget for materials needed and any specific resources to which the student will need access to complete the doctoral project.

Chapter VI: Project Implementation

Following the plan and process, the capstone student will discuss how the doctoral project was actually implemented. Although the plan provides an overview of what was intended, it is not uncommon that changes are made to the plan throughout the implementation phase of the project.

Within this chapter of the final capstone report, first the student describes the participants. The demographics of the participants will vary based on the student's project focus area and the site. Participants may have been clients or patients, their families or caregivers, occupational therapy practitioners, other staff, volunteers, administration, students, or others. The capstone student may choose to provide specific inclusion and exclusion criteria for participants, dependent on the type of project implemented. For example, inclusion criteria for clients might include the diagnosis, age, comprehension level, and/or function level. Inclusion criteria for staff might include occupational therapy practitioners, years of practice, and practice setting.

Next, the process to recruit participants is described. If approval from the academic institution's or capstone site's institutional review board was needed and obtained, this information should be included in the capstone report. Documents such as templates for gaining informed consent, recruitment letters, or marketing flyers should be included in appendices. Any contact made with participants should be described, such holding an in-service for therapy staff or contacting a specific group of individuals via phone or email to ask for their participation.

The student notes any pertinent information regarding the participants; however, no identifying information should be included in the report. The capstone report discusses the actual number of participants and any retention issues that occurred. For example, if 10 participants were originally recruited but only eight fully participated, reasons for attrition should be mentioned.

Next, the student includes the project components and specific methods that were used to carry out each component of the plan. It is recommended that a timeline of events is included. Dependent on the project itself, implementation may take several consecutive weeks or a certain day(s) each week, across several weeks. Any resources used should be listed, as well as an updated budget for the project. This information may be included as appendices in the capstone report. The site may have offered the student use of its resources, or it may have been up to the capstone student to obtain resources. If grant funding was a source of funding, detailed information regarding the grant should be included.

Project components and methods may vary greatly from one capstone project to another and will be dependent on the student's area of focus. For example, a report discussing a program involving patient education on health and wellness should include information on the frequency and length of the education sessions, whether they were face-to-face or virtual, group vs individual sessions, and any actual material

discussed. A project that focused on advocacy might discuss how advocacy occurred, such as letters written to legislators, information on events attended to raise awareness, and how consumers were educated regarding the issue. It is important that any deliverables be included in the report. They may be added as appendices. Examples of deliverables that might be included for a variety of capstone reports are as follows:

- Evaluation tools or outcome measurements (e.g., standardized and nonstandardized, pre and post measures)
- Written treatment protocols
- Webinars or educational/learning modules
- Training materials (e.g., educational handouts)
- Curricular materials
- Community resources handbook
- Written letters
- Photos* of products (now owned by the site)

TEXT BOX 10-3

*Occupational therapy capstone students need to seek permission and comply with all policies from the academic institution and capstone site regarding the use of **any** photographs and/or video.

Deviations from the original plan will need to be noted, as well as the cause or reasoning for the change. Supports and barriers during the implementation phase should be clearly described.

Chapter VII: Project Evaluation and Results

Evaluation

An explanation of how the data were collected and analyzed as well as why such methods were used will need to be included. Capstone students will include any relevant literature to support their process of project evaluation. The evaluation will be objective in nature, including factual information and be free from author bias. Any individuals involved in the evaluation process, such as the capstone student or others such as the site mentor, need to be mentioned. If the evaluation was completed by anyone in addition to the capstone student, any collaborative processes are to be described to provide information regarding the consistency of results. The capstone report should include any training on the measures used, if applicable. Depending on the project focus area and methods used, this may include standardized or nonstandardized outcome measures (or both), pre-post implementation measures, and others. See Chapter 8 for more information regarding recommendations and strategies for outcome measurement of the doctoral capstone.

Results

The results section is written after the data have been gathered and analyzed. The results describe the findings in relation to the project evaluation. This may include quantitative data (e.g., statistics), qualitative data (e.g., descriptive themes), or a combination of the two. Refer to Chapter 8 for general recommendations of how to complete data analysis procedures properly. Tables, graphs, charts, or other visuals to help the reader understand the data should be included in the results. See Appendix 10-C for examples.

Chapter VIII: Discussion and Impact

Discussion

The discussion helps to summarize the results of the project through interpretation of the data in relation to the original problem or question. The capstone student should keep in mind the information discussed in the literature review, the gap analysis statement that was formed, and the goals and objectives set for the doctoral project. Addressing each of these areas in a concise manner based on the results of the project will make for a thorough discussion. The capstone student will also need to include any limitations of the doctoral project. Limitations could relate to barriers to participation (e.g., attrition), barriers to project implementation (e.g., restrictive site policies), a lack of resources or funding, to list a few.

Impact

The impact section discusses the project's impact on the site, the participants, and the occupational therapy profession. The doctoral capstone project is to be mutually beneficial, as the student gains in-depth knowledge and skills and the site has a project that will continue to make an impact long after the 14-week capstone experience has concluded. This section of the capstone report is more subjective in nature than the results section. The capstone student needs to include feedback received regarding the project. Feedback may have been from participants, the site mentor, or administration. If the project will continue after the student has left the site, information regarding any changes or refinement are to be shared. In addition, plans for carryover should be included. The capstone student may also choose to discuss the project's broader implications for society or the profession.

Chapter IX: Conclusion

The capstone student needs to provide a concise conclusion that leaves the reader with a "take-home message." This section should be to the point and may restate the purpose of the project and a concise summary of the outcomes. It is recommended that no new information be shared in the conclusion.

References

The reference section is intended to give credit to any sources of information the capstone student cited throughout the capstone document. If information is not considered "general knowledge," it should be cited in the body of the document. A good rule of thumb is, when in doubt, cite the source. Capstone students should use APA (2010) formatting to properly format their reference list.

Appendices

An appendix is information that is informative but not essential. By including appendices, the capstone student provides readers with information that they can easily locate and refer to without cluttering the body of the paper itself. Each appendix should be lettered, titled, and included in the table of contents.

Students may include various items in their appendices. Following is a list of items to consider for this purpose:

- Program marketing materials
- Letters of consent for participants
- Pre-post assessment measures
- Budgeting spreadsheets
- Flow charts or diagrams to illustrate data collection or analysis procedures
- Actual products or portions of products created for the project

The next section in this chapter provides examples of scholarly capstone products that relate to each of the focus areas and that may be included as appendices of the capstone report.

Examples of Scholarly Products Based on Focus Areas

Throughout the capstone experience, students may create scholarly products to meet the needs of their stakeholders. The type and scope of the product will vary based on site, population, and focus area. Within the written capstone report, the student may wish to include products such as the outcomes of an evidenced-based practice guideline or a critical pathway. Table 10-5 provides examples of scholarly products that can be derived from the capstone experience and included as appendices within the capstone report.

> **TEACHING TIP 7**: It is beneficial for doctoral capstone coordinators to understand each of the focus areas (clinical practice skills, research skills, administration, leadership, program and policy development, advocacy, education, and theory development) and to be able to provide examples of related capstone projects and products to both students and potential sites. Table 10-5 provides examples of doctoral capstone products in each of the ACOTE focus areas.

Table 10-5. Examples of Scholarly Products To Be Included as Appendices

FOCUS AREA	DESCRIPTION	EXAMPLE OF CULMINATING PRODUCT
Clinical practice skills	The capstone student is interested in advancing his or her clinical skills in an area of advanced practice, specifically, lymphedema management. The student advances her skills through clinical training and via direct supervision (mentorship) of a certified lymphedema therapist. The student engages in continued education and takes advanced certification courses to prepare to obtain her lymphedema certification after receiving licensure.	An evidence-based, comprehensive protocol for lymphedema management for the facility. The product could be a binder that included lymphedema wrapping instruction with visuals, precautions and contraindications, resources for wrapping materials, and handouts for patient education.
Research skills	The capstone student completes a needs assessment in an elementary school and determines that several students require occupational therapy in the kindergarten class to address decreased attention and sensory needs. A literature review reveals that two sensory integration techniques have proven to be effective in addressing these issues in the classroom. After obtaining approval from key stakeholders, parents, and the university's institutional review board, the capstone student uses a standardized assessment to evaluate each student for attention and sensory needs to obtain a baseline score. One intervention is provided to a group of students and the other intervention to a second group of students. This occurs over a period of 4 weeks with intervention occurring twice each week. Student attention and sensory needs are reevaluated to determine progress and identify whether one treatment technique is more effective than the other.	A sensory diet protocol to be used across the school district. The protocol is based on the intervention that was found to work more effectively for the students, with suggestions for individualizing the protocol based on various needs. The student provides a typed protocol, along with a link to a webinar training, teachers, classroom aides, and therapists district-wide.
Administration	The capstone student is interested in gaining advanced skills in administration and therefore uses an apprenticeship model under the owner of a pediatric outpatient clinic. The student assists in preparing for reaccreditation by the Commission on Accreditation of Rehabilitation Facilities (CARF), collecting data points and preparing staff for the on-site visit by CARF.	The survey application packet, which includes detailed information about leadership, the programs and services offered at the site, and quality improvement initiatives in process. All materials needed to provide evidence of quality service are included.
Leadership	The capstone student is interested in completing advanced leadership training to create a vision for inclusion and diversity in a community organization. He or she completes advanced leadership training through continued education courses, readings, and webinars. After training, the student creates a series of leadership in-services for staff regarding respect for cultural and social diversities and steps to take for including individuals with intellectual and physical disabilities in the organization. This includes contacting speakers with expertise in in these areas and creating pre-post assessments to measure change in staff knowledge and awareness.	A series of webinars based on the leadership in-services provided to staff, which can be used repeatedly as new staff are hired as a part of the orientation process. At the completion of the webinar, staff are required to pass online quizzes with lifelike scenarios regarding decision-making surrounding inclusion.

continued

Table 10-5. Examples of Scholarly Products To Be Included as Appendices (continued)

FOCUS AREA	DESCRIPTION	EXAMPLE OF CULMINATING PRODUCT
Program development	The capstone student is interested in social inclusion for children with disabilities. An elementary school offers summer camps, but they lack programs that are inclusive of children with disabilities. The capstone student creates a summer program for children with disabilities with a focus on socialization and age-appropriate play. Parents are included in parent training sessions on community resources for children with disabilities and social events for their children. Quality-of-life measurements are completed pre-post programming to determine parents' perceived change in their children's quality of life.	A training video for parents based on the summer camp program series with instruction and demonstrations regarding increasing social opportunities for their children. Included are links to community resources for children with disabilities as well as events for socialization.
Policy development	The capstone student is interested in policy development and becomes aware of recent issues in a community outreach program regarding staff knowledge of how to best meet the needs of clients among the lesbian, gay, bisexual, transgender, queer/questioning, intersex (LGBTQI) community. The student administers a self-assessment to staff members regarding their own preconceptions and bias regarding individuals who are LGBTQI. The student researches best practices in addressing and meeting the needs of clients who are LGBTQI. She obtains approval of the policies and procedures from administration and completes staff education on implementation of the policy.	A policies and procedures manual regarding best practices in addressing and meeting the needs of individuals who are LGBTQI. The manual includes a self-assessment to measure staff member's own pre-conceptions and bias, resources such as links to additional information for staff, as well as community supports that the staff can share with clients.
Advocacy	The capstone student organizes a campaign to increase community and policymaker awareness of health disparities affecting individuals in the local community. The student attends rallies, organizes petitions, writes letters, and attends meetings with various stakeholders to create change.	A website for consumer advocacy is created with information on health disparities, an online discussion forum, downloadable campaign materials including letter templates, and links to local rallies and advocacy events.
Education	The capstone student is interested in academia as a practice setting. The student attends continued education on teaching pedagogy, curricular development, educational technology, classroom management, and best practices in student assessment at an academic institution. He or she is mentored by an experienced faculty member. The student creates a series of lectures and hands-on learning activities to meet course objectives and ACOTE standards. The student delivers the lectures as a guest speaker in collaboration with the primary instructor.	A lecture series with PowerPoints, handouts, and learning activity instructions. Information related to course objectives and accreditation standards met by the lecture series is included.
Theory development	The capstone student wants to learn how motor control and overall function in children with cerebral palsy (CP) is influenced by the child's experience, the task at hand, and the environment. The capstone student applies the dynamic systems theory in structuring animal-assisted therapy interventions for children with CP to measure outcomes on motor control and overall function.	A written manuscript submitted to a peer-reviewed journal regarding use of theory to guide intervention with a particular population, environment, and task.

FINALIZING THE CAPSTONE REPORT

There are various ways in which capstone students may disseminate the outcomes of their capstone project. The academic institution may require that students submit the capstone report in hard copy or electronically as an assignment as well as provide evidence of completion of their capstone project. In addition, students may choose to disseminate the results to a larger audience, such as through a poster or platform presentation at a conference or through publication in a professional magazine or peer-reviewed journal. Regardless, the completion of the capstone project needs to be officiated through dissemination, sharing the knowledge gained in the area of focus (ACOTE [2018] Standard D.1.8).

Regardless of how the capstone is to be disseminated, before final submission, capstone students are wise to receive feedback on their report. Students may choose to have one or more peers in their cohort provide feedback, or they may ask for a faculty member such as the capstone chair or other professional to review the report. It is helpful if the reviewer is familiar with the subject matter, as well as APA formatting and scholarly writing. Many professional journals require a specific review process, and students should closely follow guidelines provided by the journal.

Regarding formal submission to the academic institution, the occupational therapy program may have guidelines or requirements that the capstone student should follow. If the program requires that the capstone report be bound, determining the specifications for the bound document is important. The program may recommend a specific binding company, color and material for the cover, or require the academic institution's crest to be displayed. The academic institution may require an electronic copy for the library database. In this case, the academic librarians may be contacted for details regarding that process. Chapter 11 goes into more detail on creating a dissemination plan.

> **TEACHING TIP 8**: Doctoral capstone coordinators should become familiar with their academic institution's library processes for submitting reports to the library's catalogue. The library may have specific guidelines and processes for doing so, and it is best to let students know before writing their capstone report. Provide the students with this information early in the writing process because reformatting the capstone report could be time-consuming if not done properly from the initial draft.

CHAPTER SUMMARY

This chapter has provided several recommendations and guidelines to consider structuring the written culmination of the doctoral capstone. A capstone project is completed by a doctoral student to demonstrate the synthesis and application of knowledge gained in an area of focus (ACOTE [2018] Standard D.1.0). It is a culminating project that must be disseminated (ACOTE [2018] Standard D.1.8). The capstone report may take on various forms, and it is essential that the capstone report clearly communicates the nature of the doctoral project and the greater impact that it had and will continue to have on the site, the profession, and society.

Learning Activities

1. "Think, Pair, Share." Write a gap analysis statement for your capstone. Pair with a peer in your cohort, share your analysis statement and provide feedback to each other.

2. Make an appointment with the writing center within your academic institution for review/discussion of at least one section of your written manuscript to gain feedback.

3. Access Purdue OWL (2018) website and bookmark it in your search browser or review your APA Manual and tab important/frequently utilized sections.

REFERENCES

Accreditation Commission for Audiology Education. (2016). *Accreditation standards for the doctor of audiology (Au.D.) Program*. Retrieved from https://acaeaccred.org/standards/

Accreditation Council for Occupational Therapy Education. (2018). *Standards and interpretive guide*. Retrieved from https://www.aota.org/~/media/Corporate/Files/EducationCareers/Accredit/StandardsReview/2018-ACOTE-Standards-Interpretive-Guide.pdf

Accreditation Council for Pharmacy Education. (2015). *Accreditation standards and key elements for the professional program in pharmacy leading to the doctor of pharmacy degree*. Retrieved from https://www.acpe-accredit.org/pdf/Standards2016FINAL.pdf

American Association of Colleges of Nursing. (2006). *The essentials of doctoral education for advanced nursing practice*. Retrieved from http://www.aacnnursing.org/DNP/DNP-Essentials

American Association of Colleges of Nursing. (2017). *DNP fact sheet*. Retrieved from http://www.aacnnursing.org/News-Information/Fact-Sheets/DNP-Fact-Sheet

American Occupational Therapy Association. (2014). Occupational therapy practice framework: Domain and process (3rd ed.). *American Journal of Occupational Therapy, 68*(Suppl. 1), S1-S48. http://dx.doi.org/10.5014/ajot.2014.682006

American Occupational Therapy Association. (2018). Vision 2025. Retrieved from https://www.aota.org/Publications-News/AOTANews/2018/AOTA-Board-Expands-Vision-2025.aspx

American Psychological Association. (2010). *Publication manual of the American Psychological Association* (6th ed.). Washington, DC: American Psychological Association.

American Psychological Association. (2019). Publication practices and responsible authorship. Retrieved from https://www.apa.org/research/responsible/publication/

Anderson, B. A., Knestrick, J. M., & Barroso, R. (Eds.). (2015). *DNP capstone projects: Exemplars of excellence in practice*. New York, NY: Springer.

Barlow, S. J., Hanks, J., & Tate, J. J. (2018). A study of capstone courses utilized in United States doctor of physical therapy program curricula. *Journal of Allied Health, 47*, 147-151.

Barroso, R. (2015). Burnout as a barrier to practice among nurse-midwives: Examining the evidence. In B. A. Anderson, J. M. Knestrick, & R. Barroso (Eds.), *DNP capstone projects: Exemplars of excellence in practice* (pp. 45-53). New York, NY: Springer.

Berkowitz, B. (2015). The emergence and impact of the DNP degree on clinical practice. In B. A. Anderson, J. M. Knestrick, & R. Barroso (Eds.), *DNP capstone projects: Exemplars of excellence in practice* (pp. 3-16). New York, NY: Springer.

Boniface, G., & Seymour, A. (Eds.). (2012). *Using occupational therapy theory in practice*. Ames, IA: Wiley.

Commission on Accreditation in Physical Therapy Education. (2017). *Standards and required elements for accreditation of physical therapist education programs*. Retrieved from http://www.calstate.edu/app/dpt/documents/CAPTE-criteria-2009.pdf

DeIuliis, E. D. (2017). *Professionalism across occupational therapy clinical practice*. Thorofare, NJ: SLACK Incorporated.

Flarity, K., Holcomb, E., & Gentry, J. E. (2015). Promoting compassion fatigue resiliency among emergency department nurses. In B. A. Anderson, J. M. Knestrick, & R. Barroso (Eds.), *DNP capstone projects: Exemplars of excellence in practice* (pp. 67-78). New York, NY: Springer.

Herr, K., & Anderson, G. L. (2015). *The action research dissertation: A guide for students and faculty* (2nd ed.). Thousand Oaks, CA: Sage.

Hofmann, A. H. (2017). *Scientific writing and communication: Papers, proposals, and presentations* (3rd. ed.). New York, NY: Oxford University Press.

Plack, M. M., & Wong, C. K. (2002). The evolution of the doctorate of physical therapy: Moving beyond the controversy. *Journal of Physical Therapy, 16*, 48-58.

The Purdue Online Writing Lab. (2018). Retrieved from https://owl.english.purdue.edu/owl/resource/551/01

Reagon, C. (2012). Using occupational therapy theory within evidence-based practice. In G. Boniface & A. Seymour (Eds.), *Using occupational therapy theory in practice* (pp. 155-164). Ames, IA: Wiley.

Robinson, M., Stroller, F., Costanza-Robinson, M., & Jones, J. K. (2008). *Write like a chemist: A guide and resource*. New York, NY: Oxford University Press.

Rothstein, J. (1998). Education at the crossroads: For today's practice, the DPT. *Physical Therapy, 78*, 358-360.

Short, P. (2015). Changing the paradigm: Diabetic group visits in a primary care setting. In B. A. Anderson, J. M. Knestrick, & R. Barroso (Eds.), *DNP capstone projects: Exemplars of excellence in practice* (pp. 55-65). New York, NY: Springer.

Woods, E. N. (2001). The DPT: What it means for the profession. *PT Magazine, 9*(5), 36-43.

Appendix 10-A

EXAMPLE TITLE PAGE

Title of Capstone Report

First M. Last

Contributing Author Name(s) and Credentials

Academic Institution Name

School/College/Division

Appendix 10-B

TITLE OF CAPSTONE PROJECT

Timeline of Program Development

Weeks 1-2
Finalizing & Orienting
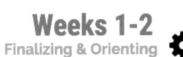

- Orient to site
- Meet with all key stakeholders
- Edit and finalize capstone project process
- Gather all materials for project

Weeks 3-4
Recruitment & Evaluation

- Recruit participants based on inclusion criteria
- Evaluate participants
- Collaborate with capstone team

Weeks 5-9
Program Implementation

- Implement program
- Continue recruitment
- Refinement of program
- Continue mentorship from site

Weeks 10-11
Outcome Measurement

- Complete outcome measurements with all participants
- On-going mentorship from site-mentor and collaboration with tea

Weeks 12-14
Data Analysis & Debriefing

- Complete data analysis
- Train staff on outcomes & steps for continued implementation
- Debrief with site mentor

Appendix 10-C

EXAMPLE OF RESULTS

Quantitative

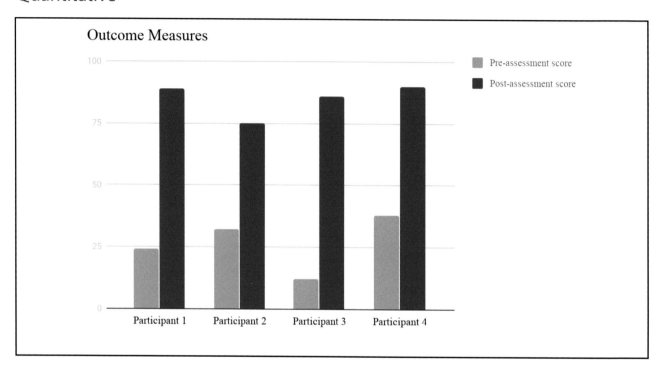

Qualitative

Participants were asked to describe their experience participating in the program. All participants noted positive experiences, and two shared that they hoped to continue to utilizing the information shared even after the program had concluded. Participant 1 stated, "I really enjoyed the social nature of group therapy. It was beneficial to hear from other patients who were going through something very similar to what I'm going through, and how they are adjusting."

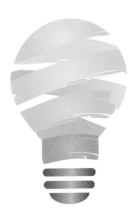

CHAPTER 11

Scholarly Deliverables and Impact of the Capstone

Sally Wasmuth, PhD, OTR
Katie M. Polo, DHS, OTR, CLT-LANA

Human-Centered Design Mindsets for the Doctoral Students

The doctoral capstone experience and project are ending and your choice to disseminate is an important one. How will you let other professionals, consumers, and stakeholders know what you have done and the outcomes of your work? You need to disseminate, and using the human-centered design mindset concepts of optimism and learning from failure will assist you in this endeavor.

Optimism: You have come so far. It is important to keep an open mind and an optimistic outlook as you think about dissemination. What is the best way to disseminate your work? Optimism will drive you forward as you think of all the potential possibilities. Keep an open mind, and understand that you will find the best way to disseminate your work.

Creative Confidence: Do not be limited by fear of failure as you think about how you will disseminate. Often, proposals for papers or presentations are not accepted on first attempts. Learn from feedback, and keep submitting until you are accepted. Do not give up!

INTRODUCTION

Occupational therapy doctoral capstone students may have widespread impact, with the potential to change the lives of the clients served within the capstone site, their family members and loved ones, the site's employees (including other occupational therapy practitioners and people from other disciplines), and the surrounding community. On a broader scale, some of the work of capstone students may have an impact on society (e.g., by reducing stigma held by society at large), health care policy decisions, and the profession of occupational therapy (e.g., by illustrating the need to mandate occupational therapy services for a specific population). The scholarly deliverables resulting from doctoral capstone experiences (DCEs) serve to deepen and extend the impact a capstone student can have in these areas. This

Deluliis ED, Bednarski JA.
The Entry Level Occupational Therapy Doctorate Capstone:
A Framework for The Experience and Project (pp 215-226).
© 2020 Taylor & Francis Group.

chapter outlines several potential means for disseminating knowledge and information gained through the DCE. It will examine factors to consider when deciding how to disseminate work as well as some potential challenges and will illuminate the impact doctoral capstone students can have through various forms of dissemination.

Capstone Student Reflective Questions

During the dissemination phase of the capstone, occupational therapy students may find it helpful to reflect on the following questions:

1. How does your doctoral capstone project link to the Vision of the American Occupational Therapy Association (AOTA)?
2. Think about dissemination. Why is it important? What is your plan?
3. What are the next steps after your doctoral capstone project is complete? How will you continue the work you have begun during this experience?

Chapter Objectives

By the end of reading this chapter and completing the learning activities, the reader should be able to:

1. Analyze the impact of his or her DCE and project.
2. Appraise how his or her doctoral capstone project links to the AOTA Vision 2025.
3. Compare and contrast dissemination of results possibilities.
4. Determine best method to disseminate the results of the DCE and project.
5. Design a plan for next steps.

LINKING THE DOCTORAL CAPSTONE PROJECT TO AOTA VISION 2025

Vision 2025 of AOTA (2018) states, "As an inclusive profession, occupational therapy maximizes health, well-being, and quality of life for all people, populations, and communities through effective solutions that facilitate participation in everyday living" (p. 1). Three critical elements can be gleaned from this vision as pertinent when considering the impact and scholarly deliverables of a DCE. First, the profession is focused on health, well-being, and quality of life. This basic tenet provides focus to the DCE. Regardless of the population served and whether the project focuses on individual clients, policy issues, therapists' clinical skills, or organizational staff and structure, the results of students' efforts should enhance health, well-being, and quality of life for those affected. Second, occupational therapy practitioners strive to provide services that reach all people, emphasizing occupational justice—the notion that all people should be afforded the right to engage in and benefit from personally meaningful

activities (Kronenberg, Pollard, & Sakellariou, 2011). Thus, occupational therapy practitioners especially focus their efforts toward people who are stigmatized, marginalized, or for other reasons are likely to lack opportunities for occupational participation or access to occupational therapy services. In addition to providing services to individuals, occupational therapy practitioners consider population health approaches and community-based practices (including service to organizations) as central to the profession. Third, the means by which occupational therapy practitioners promote health, well-being, and quality life is by facilitating participation in everyday living. This aspect of Vision 2025 emphasizes the centrality of occupation-based intervention and the belief within the profession that meaningful participation in life is critical to human health and can reverse disease processes, improve quality of life, and enhance well-being (AOTA, 2014). Taking Vision 2025 into consideration, the DCE should include an exploration of ways to use and emphasize the health-promoting power of meaningful participation in life, especially for those likely to be deprived of this universal human need.

Five guideposts define in more detail the tenets of AOTA's Vision 2025:

1. Accessible: Occupational therapy provides culturally responsive and customized services.
2. Collaborative: Occupational therapy excels in working with clients and within systems to produce effective outcomes.
3. Effective: Occupational therapy is evidence based, client centered, and cost-effective.
4. Leaders: Occupational therapy is influential in changing policies, environments, and complex systems.
5. Equity, Inclusion, and Diversity: We are intentionally inclusive and equitable and embrace diversity in all its forms (AOTA, 2018).

These guideposts can further focus a capstone project and provide structure for discussions between students and their site or faculty mentors. Table 11-1 lists some discussion questions rooted in theses guideposts. Conversations steered by these questions can help pinpoint opportunities for collaborative scholarship that capitalize on the strengths of all involved. Answers to these questions may illuminate potential avenues for scholarly deliverables.

TEACHING TIP 1: *Learning Activity 1* at the end of this chapter offers two case examples of students' answers to some of these questions and the ways in which those answers helped shape projects with unique scholarly deliverables.

Table 11-1. Discussion Questions to Determine Focus and Scholarly Deliverables

AOTA VISION 2025 GUIDEPOSTS	QUESTIONS TO CONSIDER WITH SITE AND FACULTY MENTORS
Accessible: *Occupational therapy provides culturally responsive and customized services*	• Who receives services at my site—what is the client population? • Is the primary population racially, ethnically, or otherwise diverse? • Are the majority of clients of a marginalized or stigmatized group? • Do the conditions of clients at the site entail stigma? • Is the population inherently diverse? • Are current assessments at the site able to capture nuanced differences between clients?
Collaborative: *Occupational therapy excels in working with clients and within systems to produce effective outcomes*	• What are considered effective outcomes at this site according to personnel? • What would clients consider to be effective outcomes of services? • What systemic factors impact client care within the site? • What type of outcomes need attention at the site?
Effective: *Occupational therapy is evidence based, client centered, and cost-effective*	• Does the site provide services supported by current evidence? • How does the site determine client needs and wants? • To what extent or in what way are client needs and wants addressed by current services? • Are occupational therapy services currently provided at the site? • Are other professionals providing services that fall in the scope of occupational therapy practice? • Would service changes related to occupational therapy impact cost at the site? How?
Leaders: *Occupational therapy is influential in changing policies, environments, and complex systems*	• In what ways can occupational therapy benefit clients within the capstone site? • What barriers currently prevent beneficial occupational therapy services within the site? • How does/can change occur within the site?
Equity, Inclusion, and Diversity: *We are intentionally inclusive and equitable and embrace diversity in all its forms*	• How do inequities and health disparities impact clients within the capstone site? • What steps could be taken within the site to promote equity, inclusion, and diversity? • Are all client forms and practices sufficiently updated to promote inclusive and equitable care to diverse groups?

Adapted from American Occupational Therapy Association. (2018). Vision 2025. Retrieved from https://www.aota.org/Publications-News/AOTANews/2018/AOTA-Board-Expands-Vision-2025.aspx.

IMPACT POTENTIAL OF THE DOCTORAL CAPSTONE PROJECT

DCE of occupational therapy students have enormous impact potential. The multilevel impact of a DCE on various stakeholders is discussed next.

Clients

As mentioned in the introduction, capstone student projects may change the lives of clients served within the capstone site as well as their family members and loved ones. Capstone students have created client-centered, occupation-based groups to address the needs of marginalized populations that would not otherwise receive occupational therapy, thereby promoting occupational justice and offering new opportunities for wellness. This has been especially true in mental health hospitals and addiction recovery centers where occupational therapy practitioners are not typically employed. Therapeutic groups have centered on client needs, especially in the areas of recovery engagement, social participation, and leisure and enjoyment opportunities. Brief surveys given to clients after a new group protocol can be helpful in analyzing the impact at the level of client satisfaction and wellness outcomes.

Families of Clients

Therapeutic groups have been developed that not only provide wellness opportunities for clients but that also benefit family members, either directly or indirectly.

TEXT BOX 11-1

We tried to create positive relationships, roles, and routines through social interaction at what we called "High Impact Parties," designed to be a time when families could join together and, rather than discussing addictions and all their related problems, enjoy a supportive environment where they could experience and create positive roles and routines through sharing games, food, and social interaction.

—Aubriana Adney, OTD, OTR
Class of 2018
School of Occupational Therapy
University of Indianapolis
Indianapolis, Indiana

Another example of a project that indirectly involved family members was a theater group that rehearsed and performed scenes that enacted family disputes. Clients performed these scenes and discussed varying perspectives about the experiences, thoughts, and attitudes of characters, and how these factors influenced the interactions between characters. Clients reported enhanced awareness of others' perceptions as a result of the group. One client reported being able to interact more effectively with his ex-wife the following week. This type of theater-based occupational therapy has been piloted in medical and community settings (Wasmuth & Pritchard, 2016) and provides a creative means for engaging clients and their families in nontraditional capstone experience settings. Qualitative feedback from clients, family members, and the community audiences of therapeutic theatre groups can serve as analyzable data to determine the extent of the impact that this sort of capstone project may have within social networks.

An occupational therapy student completing her capstone experience in an inpatient mental health hospital setting created another group protocol that exemplifies how a capstone student can directly affect family members of clients served at the capstone site. This student created occupation-based groups in which participants wrote letters to family members and loved ones, detailing their recovery journeys and goals as they related to family dynamics. For example, one client described the steps he was taking toward obtaining employment to pay child support fees and provided a plan to maintain accountability to his family member. Postsession surveys suggested that these experiences were powerful for individual clients and their family members.

Community

The impact of a DCE often extends beyond individual clients and their families. For example, a capstone student placed in a rural, faith-based addiction recovery organization discovered that both client workshops and large-scale community events would be needed to adequately address the harms brought on by drug addiction in a small Midwestern city. Based on findings from a needs assessment performed in the beginning weeks of the DCE, this student created client-centered, occupation-based workshops to address the needs of clients and their families. Recognizing, however, that the effects of addiction extend beyond individuals and their families (Alexander, 2015), the student decided to host a community event to reduce stigma, provide education and resources, and create an atmosphere of acceptance and compassion within the community.

TEXT BOX 11-2

A needs assessment showed that across the state, there was a lack of knowledge about addiction. To address this need, we organized and launched a community resource fair to provide all community members education, awareness, and resources offered through local organizations. The event also aimed to promote community involvement, decrease stigma, and increase community members' knowledge and understanding of addiction by having various speakers share their personal experience with addiction and/or working with the population. Information packets on local treatment centers, sober living homes, homeless shelters, and support meetings for individuals with addiction and family members were available at the event. Event outcomes were measured through attendance and satisfaction surveys.

—Mariah Haffner, OTD, OTR
Class of 2018
School of Occupational Therapy
University of Indianapolis
Indianapolis, Indiana

This student was also able to secure funding to sustain these efforts through successful application for a grant from a local charitable organization. The grant provided funds for additional community events and financial support to allow eight clients to receive detox and treatment services. Funds were also secured to cover the costs of hosting workshops and purchasing promotional products and food for events. Thus, this doctoral capstone project contributed to changing community perspectives while also connecting a large number of people to needed resources and information on how they can help address the rising opioid epidemic (Ostling et al., 2018) in American society.

Multilevel Impact(s)

Finally, doctoral capstone projects have the potential to have an impact on employees within a capstone site, such as other occupational therapy practitioners, practitioners from other disciplines, administrators, managers, and grant writers.

TEXT BOX 11-3

I was able to envision the role of occupational therapy in a preestablished team within an emerging area of practice. As organic conversations between the team and I arose, specifically regarding the needs of the clinic, it was imperative to collaborate and identify common goals. While the clinic had a variety of needs, these were not occupation-based in their entirety. I collaborated with the patient care coordinator on the topic of support groups, explaining that social participation is considered an occupation within the profession's scope of practice. Advocacy and evidence-based practice were inherently symbiotic in the early stages of the DCE. Before advocating for occupational therapy's role in an emerging area of practice, it was imperative to refamiliarize myself with the fundamental nature of occupational therapy, as well as the small body of literature supporting the profession's role in transgender care. It was through this deep level of understanding beyond a generalist's knowledge that I was able to educate about and advocate for the intricate relationship between occupation and gender. Although intentional, the retroactive awareness of my role indirectly aided in the clinic's receptiveness toward these ideas, thus creating a healthy atmosphere for subsequent staff development. Through advocacy and education, the clinic is now acutely aware of occupational therapy's role in a psychosocial setting.

—Annie DeRolf, OTD, OTR
Class of 2018
School of Occupational Therapy
University of Indianapolis
Indianapolis, Indiana

This section features detailed descriptions of the experiences of two students placed in a nontraditional settings and working with marginalized populations. The examples illustrate how projects can influence a wide variety of individuals within and outside of a site and truly illuminate how widespread the impact of a capstone student project might be. They also highlight several levels at which the impact of the capstone experience can be analyzed.

The impact of the first student's doctoral capstone project extended to the level of influencing the profession of occupational therapy as a whole. The student was placed among medical doctors and social workers in a clinic serving individuals who are transgender and/or gender non-conforming. It was quickly discovered through a needs assessment that clients within this setting had a variety of unmet occupational needs, including a lack of social participation, fear of or difficulty with "passing" as their preferred gender (which primarily involved dressing and self-care), general knowledge on how to perform self-care that is congruent with their

preferred gender, and numerous postsurgical needs. For instance, upper extremity exercises to maintain functional range of motion are needed for people undergoing double mastectomies when transitioning from female to male (Dell, 2001). The postsurgical needs of this population can be time-consuming and thus place occupational demands regarding time management on daily routines such as performing morning activities of daily living. Additional occupational needs pertinent to this population include medication management, learning to navigate one's own new identity, and dealing with discrimination at work. For example, urinary tract infections have been a significant concern as a result of individuals who are transgender, fearing public restroom use within their places of employment (James et al., 2016). The capstone student at the transgender clinic was able to educate the other professionals within the clinic on the many ways in which occupational therapy practitioners have a distinct role to assist clients in this population. The clinicians were unfamiliar with occupational therapy and therefore unaware of how many of their clients' struggles were essentially occupational in nature.

As part of the DCE, the student also created an occupational therapy screening tool to help clinicians determine whether a client within the clinic had a need for occupational therapy. In addition, the student collected information on the lives of clients within the clinic to write an occupation-based frame of reference to assist occupational therapy practitioners working with this population. Upon recognizing the immense value of having an occupational therapy doctoral capstone student, the clinic commenced grant-writing efforts to create a grant-funded occupational therapy position for this student upon graduation.

Finally, after the capstone experience, this student also guest lectured at a mental health course for occupational therapy students on the importance of understanding and incorporating appropriate "sexual orientation and gender identity" data when working with clients to communicate an openness and welcoming attitude toward all (but especially marginalized) clients (National LGBT Health Education Center, n.d.).

A second capstone student example that had multilevel impacts was that of a student placed at a nonprofit national cancer support center. The cancer community center had existing programming in the areas of support and wellness groups; however, it did not offer health promotion and wellness education to improve occupational performance of their cancer survivors. The main theme among the needs assessment included a desire of the survivors to improve their occupational performance and participation in daily activities. The student's main purpose was thus to bring health and wellness services to this cancer survivorship community setting to meet the needs of an underserved population by providing health promotion and wellness education in group and individual sessions.

Both group sessions and individual sessions were held to address overarching cancer-related topics supported through evidence-based practice, such as managing fatigue, compensation strategies for cognitive issues, improving sleep hygiene, and stress management and mindfulness. Participants were encouraged to attend individual follow-up appointments that involved more hands-on interventions or discuss education in further detail. Educational handouts were created in relation to evidence found in research with compensatory strategies, stress management, energy conservation to combat cancer-related fatigue, chemotherapy-induced peripheral neuropathy, fall prevention, sleep hygiene, and cognitive issues for this population. For program sustainability, it was indicated that grant funding would be beneficial to provide continued occupational therapy services at this community site. The capstone student searched and identified a community partnership grant that she applied for and was awarded in partnership with her faculty and site mentor to sustain provision of occupational therapy services at the site. After she graduated, she was able to fulfill this part-time job position, delivering occupational therapy services in this emerging practice area.

These case examples illustrate DCEs that impacted clients, families, occupational therapy practitioners, the discipline of occupational therapy as a whole, occupational therapy students, grant funders and policy (hiring), and other health care professionals. These examples provide a helpful reminder that the extent of the impact of doctoral capstone projects is vast.

> **TEACHING TIP 2**: *Learning Activity 2* at the end of this chapter provides some questions and a diagram to assist capstone students in identifying and articulating the impact(s) of their doctoral projects.

PURPOSE AND IMPORTANCE OF DISSEMINATION OF PROJECT

At the culmination of the DCE, students have performed a needs assessment, fine-tuned the focus for their capstone project, and documented the process and findings that resulted from their work. After completing the final papers and receiving a passing grade for the DCE and project, it may be tempting to avoid or indefinitely postpone dissemination of scholarly works. At this stage, it is important for students to recognize the expertise they have gained by undergoing a unique experience in the field of occupational therapy. DCEs result in students gaining unique insight into the workings of an organization, understanding the needs of a specific population of clients, and recognizing issues pertaining to occupational justice, evidence-based practice, and effective policy. Students identify gaps in health care that occupational therapy practitioners can address. Without dissemination of scholarly works, other clinicians cannot learn from this

expertise. Clients outside of an individual capstone site cannot benefit from the treatment planning and service models students have created. Organizations cannot acquire knowledge about the widespread roles of occupational therapy practitioners and the impact they can have. Upon completion of the capstone experience, students are equipped with insights and new knowledge that others can benefit from. It is an ideal time to disseminate scholarly work.

Dissemination Planning

The main goal of dissemination is to share with others the knowledge, information, or results that capstone students have gathered or produced with their project. It is important first to understand knowledge translation as a paradigm to close the gaps that exist between what the findings are from the capstone student's project and carrying them out to change practice. The World Health Organization (WHO; 2018) defines knowledge translation as "the synthesis, exchange, and application of knowledge by relevant stakeholders to accelerate the benefits of global and local innovation in strengthening health systems and improving people's health" (n.p.). There are many knowledge translation models or frameworks that one can adopt when initially preparing for a dissemination plan to ensure application of the project results into practice.

When developing a dissemination plan, it is important to be strategic with the overall approach to ensure that the capstone student's project results will be utilized. For the capstone project dissemination plan, the student will want to write several objectives outlining the following information:

- The information or message that will be disseminated
- The audience or to whom the message will be delivered
- The methods that will be used to disseminate the information
- The resources that will be used and who will deliver or disseminate the information
- Timing (timeline) of dissemination

When starting to develop a plan and writing objectives, it is helpful to consider overall steps in developing a dissemination strategy. See Table 11-2 for steps in developing a dissemination strategy.

Developing Project Dissemination Purpose

There are three steps that occur in developing the capstone student's project dissemination purpose. These include building the dissemination objectives, developing the message, and determining the audience(s).

Step 1: Devise Dissemination Objectives

When considering objectives, it is helpful to identify what the capstone student hopes to achieve by delivering the results of the doctoral capstone project. When writing objectives, consider why the capstone student wishes to communicate

Table 11-2. Steps in Developing a Dissemination Strategy

1. Devise dissemination objectives
2. Determine audience
3. Develop messages
4. Decide on dissemination approaches and methods
5. Review available resources
6. Consider timing and window of opportunities
7. Evaluate efforts

findings to particular stakeholders. Additionally, it is important to consider purpose. Is the purpose of dissemination to increase awareness, understanding, or action? Keep in mind that the capstone student's project will have multiple stakeholders that will require different ways for disseminating findings and results. *Dissemination for awareness* refers to delivering and receiving of a message and is often used for those target audiences that do not need detailed knowledge of the capstone student's work but it is still important for them to be aware of the outcomes of the project (Harmsworth, Turpin, & the TQEF National Coordination Team, 2000). *Dissemination for understanding* refers to engaging an individual into a process, or allowing for those target audiences to build a deeper understanding of the project and results (Harmsworth, Turpin, & the TQEF National Coordination Team, 2000). *Dissemination for action* is the transfer of a process or product, or changing of practice or process due to the results of the project (Harmsworth, Turpin, & the TQEF National Coordination Team, 2000). Dissemination for action targets audiences that are in a position to influence and bring about change.

Clear and easy-to-understand language should be used to articulate the objectives the capstone student is writing for dissemination. Objectives should identify the message(s) targeted for delivery, to what audience(s) they are intended, who will deliver the messages, and in what time frame.

Step 2: Determine Audience(s)

Understanding the various stakeholders of the project and more broadly the target audience(s) is pertinent in developing your projects dissemination strategy. A stakeholder is a group or an individual that is affected or who can affect the achievement of the capstone project, and a target audience is the different groups of stakeholders connected to the project (Harmsworth, Turpin, & the TQEF National Coordination Team, 2000). Therefore, the need to identify stakeholders as well as target audiences that the capstone student will need to report results or findings from the project is essential. Keep in mind the various target audiences will perhaps require a different message and delivery (dissemination approach).

Step 3: Develope the Message

In this step, capstone students identify what message(s) they want to disseminate that relate to the capstone findings and tie each to the previously identified targeted audiences. Messages should be clear with easy-to-understand language (avoid professional jargon) if any of the target audiences are beyond the occupational therapy profession. For example, if the doctoral capstone project used an assessment tool that is familiar to the occupational therapy profession to capture individual change, the capstone student will want to ensure that audiences beyond occupational therapy can understand the tool's purpose, as well as why it is appropriate to demonstrate change for the project. Therefore, messages should be written solely for one audience with an identification of a dissemination approach that caters to their needs.

Step 4: Decide on Dissemination Approaches and Methods

Many doctoral capstone projects have multiple stakeholders and target audiences involved within the process of collaboration, development, designing, and implementation. As such, the dissemination of project results and findings can and should be distributed to various communities, stakeholders, and appropriate wider audiences affected by the outcomes of the project. Although there is a plethora of dissemination methods or approaches, it is of utmost importance to select the correct one(s) to get the message to target audience(s) clearly and efficiently and achieve the capstone student's purpose. Therefore, thinking of the purpose of the dissemination will better assist with identification of appropriate methods. See Table 11-3 for examples of purpose and methods of dissemination.

Targeting methods of dissemination is essential because it will guide requirements, tools, and resources needed for dissemination; writing style; and inclusion of pertinent information for the designated stakeholder.

Step 5: Review Available Resources

It is important to consider what resources the capstone student has access to for dissemination either from the university level or from the capstone site and who might help assist

Table 11-3. Aligning Purpose With Method of Dissemination

PURPOSE OF DISSEMINATION	POTENTIAL METHODS
Create awareness about the project	Newsletters, flyers, press releases
Transmit information about the project	Written reports, journal articles, and websites
Promote the project and reported outcomes	Presentations and websites

Adapted from Agency for Healthcare Research & Quality. (2014). *Quick-start guide to dissemination for practice-based research networks.* Retrieved from https://pbrn.ahrq.gov/sites/default/files/AHRQ%20PBRN%20Dissemination%20QuickStart%20Guide_0.pdf.

with dissemination efforts. Resources can include copies of materials or handouts for newsletters, reports, workshops, conference presentations, and support for poster printing or publication fees for journal submission. Additionally, the capstone student will want to consider who will assist with dissemination efforts. The capstone team can include the site mentor, faculty mentor (or capstone chair), doctoral capstone coordinator, or any other content and site experts who assisted with supervision, mentorship, and feedback of the capstone experience and project. Often those who are on the team will have varied resources to pull together to assist with dissemination efforts, so knowing what each person brings to the table will be important in driving the method(s) of dissemination. When writing the dissemination objectives, the capstone student will want to include who will be a part of disseminating each objective. Often this entails discussion of authorship, inclusion and order for publications, and professional conference opportunities. Refer back to Chapter 6 for discussion of the importance of an initial authorship agreement determination when developing the memorandum of understanding (MOU).

Step 6: Consider Timing and Window of Opportunities

A timeline for disseminating the capstone project results to each of the specified targeted audiences should be included in the dissemination plan. Each objective should clearly state the anticipated due date of dissemination. Keep in mind that some dissemination efforts might happen after graduation. When writing the dissemination objectives, include who will assist with each objective and the timeline.

Step 7: Evaluate Efforts

An effective dissemination strategy embodies a constant developing process. Therefore, it will be critical to review project progress toward the dissemination objectives continuously to ensure success. Keep in mind that during implementation of the doctoral capstone project, adjustments may need to be made to the dissemination plan objectives.

IMPLEMENTING THE DISSEMINATION PLAN

While implementing the dissemination plan, the capstone student needs to keep in mind that each stakeholder or target audience might have various expectations that will guide method(s) of delivery. Some of the stakeholders that the capstone student will want to build within the dissemination plan are the university, the capstone site, the community, and the occupational therapy profession; expectations of each of these stakeholders should be understood and verified. Given each stakeholder's expectations or culture, preferred method of delivery for the capstone results could range from presentation(s), papers or journal articles, briefings, or engagement in community events, each of which require sound communication and professional preparation.

Communication Principles

Regardless of the method of delivery chosen, it is critical to ensure that your message is carefully designed to enhance the audience's understanding of the capstone results. Following are recommended principles from the Agency for Healthcare Research and Quality (2014) to enhance communication with various target audiences:

- *Have a clear and factual message.* The message should be clear, easy to understand, and use language suitable for the target population. For example, if capstone students are disseminating results to a community partner that does not have occupational therapy services, they would want to avoid using professional language that the stakeholder might not fully understand. Additionally, capstone students will want to ensure that the message is correct and realistic.
- *Tailor the message to the receiver.* The message should be targeted to each audience and should deliver what it *should know about the results of the doctoral capstone project.*
- *The message should invoke action and may be repeated.* The message should create an understanding of action among the audience members and how they can produce that action. For example, if a capstone student is disseminating results to a community site to which he or she brought occupational therapy services, stakeholders

at the site should understand how they can act with the presented results in the future. Additionally, the capstone student may repeat key messages to the audience to reinforce them.

Determining and Negotiating Authorship

Authorship is a primary means of recognizing the capstone student's contributions to the project process as well as the collaborators involved. Order of authorship should be discussed from the beginning with the site mentor and university faculty mentor, and the discussion should be ongoing throughout the course of the project if necessary, as dissemination can be a dynamic process. Once authorship order and responsibilities have been agreed on by all parties, a statement should be placed into the capstone MOU delineating the agreed-on terms. Beginning this process early on will ensure that all contributors' expectations are considered. It is important that everyone in the process understands that order of authorship can change throughout the project to best mirror all collaborators contributions. Often authorship order changes are situation dependent but should be decided on by taking into account all collaborators' perspectives and their contributions. Revisions to the MOU should be updated throughout the process to continuously reflect changes in authorship terms. Keep in mind that order of authorship might vary depending on which method of dissemination is chosen (presentation at a conference vs a peer reviewed-journal article). Some of the capstone student's mentors might have more guidance and expertise in a selected method of delivery; therefore, their contributions might increase and warrant authorship order changes. Ongoing and open communication while navigating the authorship process is key to ensuring the dissemination of the capstone project is professional, respectful, and, above all, successful.

Methods of Delivery

Presentations

Presentations can be a way to promote the capstone student's doctoral project and its outcomes to various stakeholders. Keep in mind that multiple presentations might be a possibility to ensure that outcomes have been disseminated to the proper stakeholders, such as the academic institution, community and site partners, state associations, and national associations. If the capstone student is considering preparing a presentation for a professional conference, whether state, national, or international, it is critical to align the writing of the proposal to the purpose of the conference. The capstone student will also want to carefully consider what type of presentation will effectively disseminate results, whether it be poster sessions, short courses, platform presentations, workshops, or another format. When responding to a call for submissions to a particular conference, it is important that the capstone student follows the designated criteria set forth from the organization, such as length requirements,

number of adequate references, objectives, and abstract materials. Allow for plenty of time before submission for the entire capstone team to review and proofread multiple times to provide feedback for change.

The audience of the capstone student's presentation(s) will vary, so changing the delivery of content and language depending on the knowledge base of the listener is important. For example, if the capstone student is disseminating results to a community board of directors at a collaborating community site, the student may need to describe what occupational therapy is before talking about the project outcomes and limit professional language to reduce confusion among the audience. However, the capstone student would not need to describe occupational therapy if he or she were presenting at the AOTA conference because one assumes that those attending the presentation understand the professional language being used.

In preparing for any presentation, practicing is of utmost importance to reinforce that the delivery is robust and the time frame requirements are met. Ensuring that the presentation falls within allotted time constraints and allowing time for questions from audience are imperative. Planning ahead and preparing answers to questions that may be asked from audience members might reduce anxiety and allow for best preparation for professional discussion. Portraying a professional image by dressing appropriately in professional attire is critical as capstone students are representing themselves, the dissemination team, collaborating organization, and the university.

Journal Articles

A comprehensive, well-developed, well-written, and correctly referenced report of the capstone project might be an expectation of students' university to show that they have met the educational standards of the capstone project. Many students and their collaborators agree that it is well worth the extra time and effort to submit their capstone projects to various journals (either non–peer reviewed or peer reviewed, given the nature of the project). Non–peer-reviewed journals often do not have a process in place to ensure accuracy, quality, or rigor of the article; therefore, the publication time and also acceptance to the journal might be less. Peer-reviewed or refereed journals use a blinded process of multiple expert reviews to ensure article quality and rigor. An article that has been refereed may be accepted, considered accepted upon recommended revisions, or rejected. If revisions are necessary, keep in mind that it can take significant time to revise; multiple attempts may be necessary to correct the article for acceptance. When targeting a journal, the capstone student's timeline for dissemination will need to be considered for various reasons.

When considering which journal to submit work, the capstone student should keep in mind the type of articles the journal accepts (e.g., program development, research, expert opinion). Additionally, students should consider the target audience to which they would like to disseminate findings;

this will help guide students to possible journals. Some journals appropriate for dissemination of capstone students' work might not be in the profession of occupational therapy, especially if the project was interdisciplinary in nature. Considering the journal's mission is extremely important; when writing, students should ensure that the project's work aligns with the journal's focus.

Once students identify a journal, they will want to search articles that might be similar in nature to the project that have already been published. Find at least one article comparable to what the student intends to submit and review carefully how the authors structure their writing to organize and configure the submission similarly. Remember that space is limited, so concise writing is of utmost importance. Considering the audience may allow for either cutting information or suggest the need to elaborate on some concepts. For example, if a journal is within the occupational therapy profession, the student would not need to define or reference information on the profession's scope of practice because the audience will have this knowledge base.

Many journals have guidelines on writing document requirements, such as font and style, spacing and margins, headings, length, and preferred style for citations and referencing throughout paper and for tables and figures. It is the author's responsibility to understand and use the preferred style manual of the targeted journal (e.g., the manuals of the American Psychological Association and the American Medical Association). The style of the targeted journal might be different from the expectations of the university's final paper. If authors fail to submit work within the targeted journals specifications, they run the risk of immediate rejection.

CHAPTER SUMMARY

Where do you go from here? How can you leave your legacy to the DCE site? Completion of a DCE and dissemination of key findings is an important accomplishment for both the student and the profession of occupational therapy. As discussed earlier in this chapter and in other parts of this volume, capstone projects affect clients, families, societies, and health care professions. In addition, however, capstone experiences greatly influence the doctoral students who have completed them. New, in-depth knowledge will guide the future practice of an occupational therapy student who has completed a DCE. The mentorship, advocacy, program development, client interactions, and clinical skills built through a capstone experience may guide future clinical reasoning, career choices, and interactions with other clients and professionals. Therefore, it is worth spending time at the completion of a capstone project to reflect on the knowledge that has been gained and disseminated.

- What were the critical components and key findings of the capstone experience?
- How have they influenced you as a future occupational therapy practitioner?

- What impact did they have on the capstone site?
- What are the implications of findings obtained through the capstone project?
- How can they be carried forward?

In considering answers to these questions, capstone students may want to explore ways in which their work can be carried forward. Was a group protocol created that can be implemented by other practitioners when the student leaves? Were organization changes made, and if so, did the capstone student take measures to support the site's ability to maintain these changes? Did the capstone experience result in publications that will influence other practitioners' future clinical work or scholarship? Reflecting on these questions after project completion and dissemination can ensure that the efforts put forth during capstone experiences are sustained and that students take an active role in leaving behind a legacy that is the culmination of their hard work.

Learning Activities

1. The following case example illustrates how a doctoral capstone student answered the questions in Table 11-1 and how those answers brought focus to the project and assisted with determining scholarly deliverables.

Accessible: DCE took place in an urban public health safety-net hospital with an innovative collaborative care program designed to provide intensive primary care to community-dwelling individuals with brain care needs. The assessments for new patients were extensive and capture nuanced differences between clients; however, the neuropsychological diagnostic evaluation was not able to be interpreted for non–English-speaking individuals. Assessments were also lacking physical and functional components. The addition of physical and functional assessment components became the main focus of this DCE, but future projects may also address the occupational injustice of limited ability to evaluate non–English-speaking clients.

Collaborative: This site primarily aimed to achieve the following effective outcomes: improvements in behavioral and psychological symptoms of dementia, increased quality of life for patients and caregivers, maintenance of function (mental, physical, social, emotional), the ability to age in place, and decreased hospital admissions. Specific physical, functional, and social outcomes need more attention at this site.

Effective: At this site, initial home assessments were being performed by collaborative care team members. The individuals performing the home assessments were required to have a high school degree. During my capstone experience, I observed several home assessments and noted significant room for improvement. Changing this to an occupational therapy service would increase costs, but may reduce readmissions and improve outcomes, thus decreasing costs in the long run.

Leaders: Although it wasn't currently feasible for occupational therapy practitioners to complete home assessments at this site, they could provide education and consultative services to the collaborative care team members to increase quality.

Putting it all together: The primary needs identified by answering questions in Table 11-1 provided several ways in which the capstone experience could be focused. Through conversations with my site mentor and faculty advisor, it was clear that I wouldn't have time to adequately address all of the needs at the level I would like, so we decided to focus on adding important occupation-based functional outcome measures to the initial evaluation at the site. We educated clinicians about how occupational therapy practitioners could perform baseline evaluations to identify barriers to occupational performance, provide intervention, and reevaluate as needed and also promote mental, social, emotional, and physical health through various means to support aging in place and slow functional decline.

2.   Analyzing your impact: Questions to consider.

Who was/were the primary recipient(s) of your doctoral capstone project?

a.   Clients of the organization

b.   The organization as a whole or staff members of the organization; examples may include projects that:

   i.   Address clinician burnout within the organization

   ii.   Streamline intake processes or adapt other current procedures of the organization

   iii.   Provide clinical skills education

   iv.   Advocate for/educate on the role of occupational therapy to other clinicians and administrators

c.   Members of the community (an example of this is a project a student did with Title IX in a university setting; the recipients of the capstone project were students of the university who were offered free sexually transmitted infection testing)

d.   Other

What outcomes were measured?

a.   Client satisfaction, resulting life participation, wellness outcomes

b.   Staff burnout before and after an intervention, staff and client satisfaction with policies and procedures of the organization, clinician competence before and after a training, knowledge of occupational therapy within the organization

c.   Attendance at a community event, knowledge gained or satisfaction of attendees following a community event

d.   Other

Was a positive impact observed?

a.   Were significant or noteworthy outcomes observed? If so, at what level(s)? Other questions to consider here include:

   i.   Did you apply for institutional review board (IRB) approval?

   ii.   Was approval obtained?

   iii.   If IRB approval was not sought, do you now have deidentified data worth reporting via retrospective analysis?

   iv.   What is the best way to analyze the data you have collected?

b.   What were your outcome goals? Were goals met? See the resources section for a copy of the Goal Attainment Scale (Turner-Stokes, 2009; see also link provided in the Resources section at the end of the chapter), which may be helpful in determining the significance of your observed outcomes as they relate to the impact of your capstone experience.

In addition to considering the preceding questions, it is important to reflect on the knowledge you gained from the implementation process of your capstone experience. What lessons were learned through implementation? What went well? What might you do differently? Do you have information that would be helpful to future clinicians, administrators, or students following a similar path? Figure 11-1 depicts an example of an assessment of the impact resulting from a DCE that can guide you in writing a concise impact statement.

The figure depicts factors related to a student's doctoral capstone project. These factors were clarified by answering the preceding questions, and gave rise to the following example impact statement:

This capstone experience resulted in more than 100 community members being connected to new mental health resources. On average, attendees were "very satisfied" with the knowledge gained. In addition to the impact this project had on the community, individual clients benefited from occupation-based groups; clients on average were "very confident" with the new skills and knowledge learned in groups. Finally, qualitative feedback from the program director suggests that this project had an impact on the organization as a whole in the areas of quality of services and number of consumers reached.

REFERENCES

Agency for Healthcare Research & Quality. (2014). *Quick-start guide to dissemination for practice-based research networks.* Retrieved from https://pbrn.ahrq.gov/sites/default/files/AHRQ%20PBRN%20 Dissemination%20QuickStart%20Guide_0.pdf

Alexander, B. (2015). *Healing addiction through community: A much longer road than it seems?* Retrieved from http://brucekalexander.com/articles-speeches/healing-addiction-through-community-a much-longer-road-than-it-seems2

American Occupational Therapy Association. (2014). Occupational therapy practice framework: Domain and process (3rd ed.). *American Journal of Occupational Therapy, 68*(Suppl. 1), S1-S48.

American Occupational Therapy Association. (2018). Vision 2025. Retrieved from https://www.aota.org/Publications-News/AOTANews/ 2018/AOTA-Board-Expands-Vision-2025.aspx

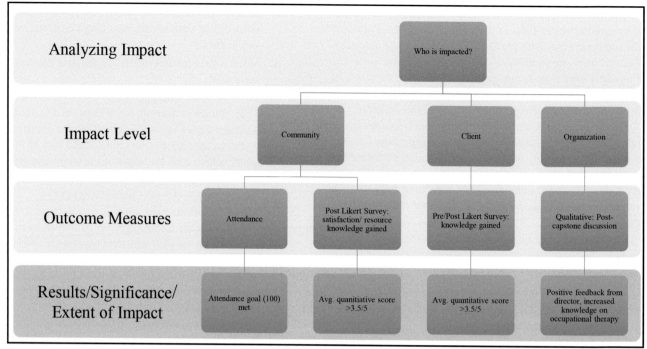

Figure 11-1. Analyzing impact of the capstone experience.

Dell, D. (2001). Regaining range of motion: Teach your patient exercises to help improve her range of motion and circulation. *Nursing, 31*(10), 50-52.

Harmsworth, S., Turpin, S., & the TQEF National Co-ordination Team. (2000). *Creating an effective dissemination strategy: An expanded interactive workbook for educational development projects.* Retrieved from https://ajpp-online.org/resources/downloads/06-CreatingAnEffective-DisseminationStrategy-AnExpandedWorkbook.pdf

James, S. E., Herman, J. L., Rankin, S., Keisling, M., Mottet, L., & Anafi, M. (2016). *The report of the 2015 U.S. transgender survey.* Washington, DC: National Center for Transgender Equality.

Kronenberg, F., Pollard, N., & Sakellariou, D. (Eds.). (2011). *Occupational therapies without borders: Volume 2. Towards an ecology of occupation-based practices* [e-book]. Elsevier.

Koblin, B. A., Husnik, M. J., Colfax, G., Huang, Y., Madison, M., Mayer, K., ... & Buchbinder, S. (2006). Risk factors for HIV infection among men who have sex with men. *AIDS, 20,* 731-739.

National LGBT Health Education Center. (n.d.). *Collecting sexual orientation and gender identity data in electronic health records: Taking the next steps.* Retrieved from http://www.lgbthealtheducation.org/wp-content/uploads/Collecting-SOGI-Data-in-EHRs-COM2111.pdf

Ostling, P. S., Davidson, K. S., Anyama, B. O., Helander, E. M., Wyche, M. Q., & Kaye, A. D. (2018). America's opioid epidemic: A comprehensive review and look into the rising crisis. *Current Pain and Headache Reports, 22*(5), 32. https://doi.org/10.1007/s11916-018-0685-5

Turner-Stokes, L. (2009). Goal attainment scaling (GAS) in rehabilitation: A practical guide. *Clinical Rehabilitation, 23,* 362-370.

Wasmuth, S., & Pritchard, K. (2016). Theater-based community engagement project for veterans recovering from substance use disorders. *American Journal of Occupational Therapy, 70,* 7004250020p1-7004250020p11.

World Health Organization. (2014). *Implementation research toolkit workbook: Disseminating the research findings.* Retrieved from http://www.who.int/tdr/publications/year/2014/9789241506960_workbook_eng.pdf

World Health Organization. (2018). *Knowledge translation.* Retrieved from http://www.who.int/ageing/projects/knowledge_translation/en/

RESOURCES

Link to Goal Attainment Scale: https://www.sralab.org/rehabilitation-measures/goal-attainment-scale

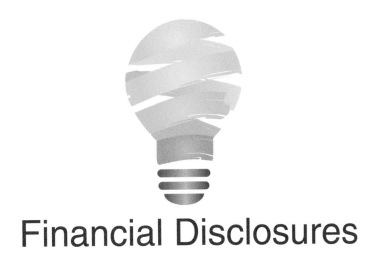

Financial Disclosures

Dr. Rebecca Barton has no financial or proprietary interest in the materials presented herein.

Dr. Julie A. Bednarski has no financial or proprietary interest in the materials presented herein.

Dr. Alison Bell has has no financial or proprietary interest in the materials presented herein.

Dr. Meghan Blaskowitz has no financial or proprietary interest in the materials presented herein.

Dr. Ann B. Cook has no financial or proprietary interest in the materials presented herein.

Dr. Elizabeth D. DeIuliis has no financial or proprietary interest in the materials presented herein.

Dr. Elena V. Donoso Brown has no financial or proprietary interest in the materials presented herein.

Dr. Tina DeAngelis has no financial or proprietary interest in the materials presented herein.

Dr. Amy M. Mattila has no financial or proprietary interest in the materials presented herein.

Dr. Katie M. Polo has no financial or proprietary interest in the materials presented herein.

Dr. Sally Wasmuth has no financial or proprietary interest in the materials presented herein.

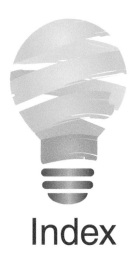

Index

Printed in the United States
by Baker & Taylor Publisher Services

Modeling, Simulation, and Control of AI Robotics and Autonomous Systems

Tanupriya Choudhury
Graphic Era University, India

Anitha Mary X
Karunya Institute of Technology and Sciences, India

Subrata Chowdhury
Sreenivasa Institute of Technology and Management Studies, India

C. Karthik
Jyothi Engineering College, India

C. Suganthi Evangeline
Sri Eshwar College of Engineering, India

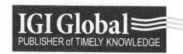

A volume in the Advances in Computational
Intelligence and Robotics (ACIR) Book Series

Published in the United States of America by
    IGI Global
    Engineering Science Reference (an imprint of IGI Global)
    701 E. Chocolate Avenue
    Hershey PA, USA 17033
    Tel: 717-533-8845
    Fax: 717-533-8661
    E-mail: cust@igi-global.com
    Web site: http://www.igi-global.com

Library of Congress Cataloging-in-Publication Data

CIP DATA PROCESSING

ISBN 9798369319628(hc) I ISBN 9798369347119(sc) I eISBN 9798369319635

This book is published in the IGI Global book series Advances in Computational Intelligence and Robotics (ACIR) (ISSN: 2327-0411; eISSN: 2327-042X).

British Cataloguing in Publication Data
A Cataloguing in Publication record for this book is available from the British Library.

For electronic access to this publication, please contact: eresources@igi-global.com.

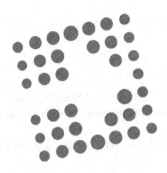

Advances in Computational Intelligence and Robotics (ACIR) Book Series

Ivan Giannoccaro
University of Salento, Italy

ISSN:2327-0411
EISSN:2327-042X

MISSION

While intelligence is traditionally a term applied to humans and human cognition, technology has progressed in such a way to allow for the development of intelligent systems able to simulate many human traits. With this new era of simulated and artificial intelligence, much research is needed in order to continue to advance the field and also to evaluate the ethical and societal concerns of the existence of artificial life and machine learning.

The **Advances in Computational Intelligence and Robotics (ACIR) Book Series** encourages scholarly discourse on all topics pertaining to evolutionary computing, artificial life, computational intelligence, machine learning, and robotics. ACIR presents the latest research being conducted on diverse topics in intelligence technologies with the goal of advancing knowledge and applications in this rapidly evolving field.

COVERAGE

- Neural Networks
- Computational Logic
- Natural Language Processing
- Cognitive Informatics
- Synthetic Emotions
- Evolutionary Computing
- Adaptive and Complex Systems
- Brain Simulation
- Heuristics
- Fuzzy Systems

IGI Global is currently accepting manuscripts for publication within this series. To submit a proposal for a volume in this series, please contact our Acquisition Editors at Acquisitions@igi-global.com or visit: http://www.igi-global.com/publish/.

Titles in this Series

For a list of additional titles in this series, please visit: http://www.igi-global.com/book-series/advances-computational-intelligence-robotics/73674

AI and IoT for Proactive Disaster Management
Mariyam Ouaissa (Chouaib Doukkali University, Morocco) Mariya Ouaissa (Cadi Ayyad University, Morocco) Zakaria Boulouard (Hassan II University, Casablanca, Morocco) Celestine Iwendi (University of Bolton, UK) and Moez Krichen (Al-Baha University, Saudi Arabia)
Engineering Science Reference • copyright 2024 • 299pp • H/C (ISBN: 9798369338964) • US $355.00 (our price)

Utilizing AI and Machine Learning for Natural Disaster Management
D. Satishkumar (Nehru Institute of Technology, India) and M. Sivaraja (Nehru Institute of Technology, India)
Engineering Science Reference • copyright 2024 • 340pp • H/C (ISBN: 9798369333624) • US $315.00 (our price)

Shaping the Future of Automation With Cloud-Enhanced Robotics
Rathishchandra Ramachandra Gatti (Sahyadri College of Engineering and Management, India) and Chandra Singh (Sahyadri College of Engineering and Management, India)
Engineering Science Reference • copyright 2024 • 431pp • H/C (ISBN: 9798369319147) • US $345.00 (our price)

Bio-inspired Swarm Robotics and Control Algorithms, Mechanisms, and Strategies
Parijat Bhowmick (Indian Institute of Technology, Guwahati, India) Sima Das (Bengal College of Engineering and Technology, India) and Farshad Arvin (Durham University, UK)
Engineering Science Reference • copyright 2024 • 261pp • H/C (ISBN: 9798369312773) • US $315.00 (our price)

Comparative Analysis of Digital Consciousness and Human Consciousness Bridging the Divide in AI Discourse
Remya Lathabhavan (Indian Institute of Management, Bodh Gaya, India) and Nidhi Mishra (Indian Institute of Management, Bodh Gaya, India)
Engineering Science Reference • copyright 2024 • 355pp • H/C (ISBN: 9798369320150) • US $315.00 (our price)

Machine Learning Techniques and Industry Applications
Pramod Kumar Srivastava (Rajkiya Engineering College, Azamgarh, India) and Ashok Kumar Yadav (Rajkiya Engineering College, Azamgarh, India)
Engineering Science Reference • copyright 2024 • 307pp • H/C (ISBN: 9798369352717) • US $365.00 (our price)

Intelligent Decision Making Through Bio-Inspired Optimization
Ramkumar Jaganathan (Sri Krishna Arts and Science College, India) Shilpa Mehta (Auckland University of Technology, New Zealand) and Ram Krishan (Mata Sundri University Girls College, Mansa, India)
Information Science Reference • copyright 2024 • 275pp • H/C (ISBN: 9798369320730) • US $320.00 (our price)

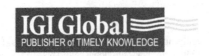

701 East Chocolate Avenue, Hershey, PA 17033, USA
Tel: 717-533-8845 x100 • Fax: 717-533-8661
E-Mail: cust@igi-global.com • www.igi-global.com

Table of Contents

Detailed Table of Contents

T. Preethiya, SRM Institute of Science and Technology, India
Priyanga Subbiah, SRM Institute of Science and Technology, India
T. Pandiarajan, Rajalakshmi Institute of Technology, India
Karthikeyan Subramanian, Birmingham City University, UAE
Prince Chelladurai, University College of Engineering, Villupuram, India
C. Selvalakshmi, Mangayarkarasi College of Engineering, India

Autonomous systems and AI have revolutionized industry automation and innovation. This abstract shows how this synergy changes our lives and work. AI has rapidly advanced autonomous systems like self-driving cars, drones, and robots. These systems can sense, make smart decisions, and adapt to changing environments with AI. They can navigate complex settings and interact with humans thanks to this superior sense Autonomous systems can make real-time judgments using AI methods like machine learning and deep learning. AI-driven decision-making assures adaptability and efficiency, whether a self-driving car chooses the safest route, or a drone optimizes its flying path. AI-assisted autonomous systems prioritize safety and reliability. These systems can detect anomalies and respond proactively to prevent accidents and failures through self-monitoring and diagnostics.

Elamathiyan A., Karpagam Academy of Higher Education, India
G. Dhivya, Karpagam Academy of Higher Education, India

A goal is to facilitate the recognition and segmentation of the route driven by autonomous vehicles through the use of machine learning (ML) models. The pixel-wise road detection task, the semantic segmentation architectures underwent training and comparison. By using XAI, the authors are able to interpret and read the predictions generated by these abstract models. They generated arguments for the recommended segmentation model for autonomous vehicle road detection using a range of XAI approaches. Supervised learning is enabled by KNN, Decision Tree, and Random Forest, which are the current algorithms used for comparison. On the other hand, the newly built K means clustering function best when paired for image processing since they are good with images. To display the results of computations for the evaluation parameters of each algorithm, including accuracy, sensitivity, recall and precision, tables, and the necessary features from the evaluation matrices are utilised. The k-means clustering system for explainable AI-based semantic object detection in automated cars achieves 94.58% accuracy on both train and test sets.

Chapter 3

Ajith K., Karpagam Academy of Higher Education, India
R. Sharmila, Karpagam Academy of Higher Education, India

Fully autonomous vehicles (FAVs) require internal monitoring in order to function without a human driver. The far-from-sufficient FAV, sufficient in-cabin monitoring is a prerequisite to ensure both people and vehicles. On public roadways, there are a lot of accidents that happen, most of them are the result of reckless driving. Modern driver monitoring systems evaluate driver behavior and, if necessary, highlight risky driving behaviours using special sensor technologies. The result accurately predicted bounding boxes and the real data show a considerable amount of overlap. Unlike most past efforts, the authors use a random forest to learn a template-based model. This way, forecast the object probability of a window in a sliding window technique and regress its aspect ratio using a single mode at the same time. Examined mobility services at increasing degrees autonomy, including the exercise caution and the best ways.

Chapter 4

Thirusudhan M., Karpagam Academy of Higher Education, India
Sasikumar S., Karpagam Academy of Higher Education, India

Real-time status monitoring and early defect diagnosis are becoming more and more necessary for modern industrial systems. Developing intelligent remote diagnostic technologies and integrating on-board and off-board diagnosis are two more unresolved research projects in the automotive industry. The automated transfer vehicle (ATV) equipment condition monitoring example in this chapter is part of a smart industrial use case. The suggested method successfully permits ATV fault scenarios to be seen in real time by expanding to a fleet of devices in an actual production plant. The application of a statistical threshold is the initial stage in creating a high-performance detection model for defect detection on stacked long short-term memory networks. For better computation speed, a second model trimming approach based on principal component analysis is suggested. The improved fault detection technique is ultimately applied by the airborne embedded computer platform with field-programmable gate arrays.

Chapter 5

Rajaram Vassudev Pai Kuchelkar, Liverpool John Moores University, India
Anupama Jawale, Narsee Monjee College of Commerce and Economics, India

One of the analyses is fatigue analysis which helps determine the durability of the product for its intended life. The fatigue analysis requires an input data from vehicle-road interaction obtained as vertical acceleration. The input data is then used in finite element analysis software or in a test rig instrumentation to perform a fatigue analysis. The focus of this study is about collecting the input data using a data acquisition device. OEM of the automobiles use proprietary data acquisition device for testing their vehicles for durability. However, the automotive body building companies or vehicle body builders which are 1-Tier companies below OEM have a limited budget for such an analysis and therefore they principally lag in advance analysis approach such as a fatigue analysis for the design of vehicle body. Instead, to sustain durability of vehicle, the design is made heavier. This research study is an effort to provide an affordable setup for data acquisition by making use of IoT and web technologies which are cost effective.

Chapter 6

Design and Fabrication of a Softrobotic Gripper for Involving Underwater Vehicles in Seaweed
Farming 95

Prabhakar Gunasekaran, Thiagarajar College of Engineering, India
Meenakshi S., Thiagarajar College of Engineering, India
Jainulafdeen A., K. Ramakrishnan College of Engineering, India
Ayyanar N., Thiagarajar College of Engineering, India
Rajalakshmi Murugesan, Thiagarajar College of Engineering, India

Seaweeds, crucial components of marine ecosystems, thrive in marine and coastal waters, notably in the Gulf of Mannar Biosphere. Despite their ecological importance, certain seaweed species pose a threat to coral reefs due to the release of hydrophobic allelochemicals. Fisherwomen, risking their lives in collecting seaweed seed stock from littoral zones, rocky shores, and deep-sea waters, encounter hazards such as sharp rocks, poisonous algae, cyanobacteria, and coral reefs. Societal research pinpoints risks, overexploitation, unorganized harvesting, and algal blooms as significant issues. The proposed solution involves integrating intelligent Soft Robotic Grippers into underwater vehicles for precise seaweed farming without harming coral reefs. Abacus FEA software aids in deformation analysis, guiding the gripper's design to safeguard fisherwomen and preserve coral reefs.

Chapter 7

Secure VANET Routing Protocols for Improved Vehicular Communication in Autonomous
Systems 109

Abarna S., National Engineering College, India
Naskath J., National Engineering College, India
Rathi Pathi R., National Engineering College, India
Jeyalakshmi C., Mohamed Sathak Engineering College, India

Vehicular ad hoc networks (VANETs) represent an advanced iteration of mobile ad hoc networks (MANETs) designed specifically for internet communication within vehicles. VANETs aim to enable vehicle-to-vehicle (V2V) communication, enhancing safety and convenience for drivers and passengers. However, the open nature of ad hoc networks and the absence of a well-defined line of defense make security a crucial concern for VANETs. Prior to deploying mobile ad hoc networks in hostile or sensitive areas, it becomes imperative to establish robust security services. This study addresses the need for a trusted VANET routing protocol that incorporates a diverse range of security services. The proposed approach implements a secure routing protocol based on the Dijkstra Algorithm to identify the secure and shortest path. For ensuring secure routing, the protocol employs route request (RREQ) and route reply (RREP) mechanisms to identify trustworthy nodes. Additionally, message authentication is utilized to provide end-to-end, hop-to-hop, and entire-route authentication. To transmit messages securely, the Diffie-Hellman Key Exchange Protocol is employed for message encryption, ensuring safe delivery to the intended destination. To assess the performance of the suggested protocol, the authors conducted simulations using NS2. These simulation results demonstrate that the proposed routing protocol outperforms existing methods, affirming its effectiveness in VANET environments.

Chapter 8

Autonomous Systems Revolutionizing Health Insurance Industry: Achieving Operational
Excellence in Services 131

Anupa Stanly, Karunya Institute of Technology and Sciences, India
K. Aruna, Karunya Institute of Technology and Sciences, India

Financial services, particularly the insurance service sector, are increasingly embracing technology. Autonomous systems, which include artificial intelligence (AI), machine learning, and automation, are driving a striking revolution in the health insurance industry. This research provides a comprehensive analysis of various facets, such as the use of autonomous systems, expediting claim processing, identifying, and preventing fraud, improving the customer experience, data-driven decision-making, and adherence to healthcare legislation. The study concludes by highlighting the sector's profound impact from autonomous systems and pointing to a promising future for health insurance that will be characterised by operational effectiveness and customer-centricity. This study sets out a thorough exploration of the dynamic world where autonomous systems are changing the laws governing health insurance. This investigation's main objectives are to achieve operational excellence and provide services that are utterly customer-centric.

The advent of artificial intelligence (AI) has had a profound impact on the realm of robotics, fundamentally altering the capabilities of self-governing devices. This abstract examines the significant influence of artificial intelligence (AI) on the field of robotics, emphasizing notable progress and practical implementations. Artificial intelligence (AI)-powered robots demonstrate improved capabilities in perception, decision-making, and adaptability, which allows them to thrive in a wide range of jobs across several domains such as industry, healthcare, space exploration, and autonomous vehicles. Machine learning methodologies, such as deep learning and reinforcement learning, enable robots to acquire aptitudes, enhance their performance, and engage in intelligent interactions with their surroundings. The ethical considerations, safety measures, and societal repercussions pertaining to AI-driven robots are also examined and analyzed.

The "synergistic swarm" investigates the incorporation of multi-robot systems in healthcare, introducing a fundamental change in patient care and medical operations. This abstract emphasises the collaborative synergy achieved by intelligently coordinating several robotic entities, resulting in improved efficiency, precision, and adaptability in healthcare environments. By utilising cutting-edge technology like artificial intelligence, robotics, and sensor networks, the system seeks to enhance many functions, including diagnostics and patient support, to their maximum efficiency. This chapter highlights the significant potential of combining different approaches to healthcare in order to improve the delivery of medical services. This could lead to more effective, patient-focused, and adaptable healthcare robotics in the changing healthcare industry.

Chapter 11

"Cogwheels of Care: Robotic Marvels in the Hospital Landscape" examines the incorporation of sophisticated robotics in contemporary healthcare. This abstract explores the profound influence of robots in hospitals, fundamentally changing patient care and enhancing medical capabilities. The chapter explores the ways in which these advanced robots enhance and simplify many jobs, ranging from surgical procedures to everyday activities, by maximising efficiency and accuracy. It emphasises the interdependent connection between technology and healthcare practitioners, focusing on the ethical considerations and societal consequences of this technological transformation. This research highlights the changing healthcare landscape, where the complex interaction between human expertise and robotic innovation is transforming the principles of compassionate and effective patient-centered care.

Chapter 12

Anshit Mukherjee, Abacus Institute of Engineering and Management, India
Gunjan Mukherjee, Brainware University, India

Cancer is one of the most serious threats to human health and life. Despite the advances in conventional therapies, such as surgery, chemotherapy, radiotherapy, and immunotherapy, there are still many challenges and limitations in achieving effective and precise cancer treatment. Nanorobots, inspired by natural biological nanomachines, offer a promising alternative for cancer diagnosis and therapy. Nanorobots are nanoscale devices that can perform various tasks under the guidance of external stimuli, such as magnetic fields, light, ultrasound, or chemical gradients. Nanorobots can be designed to target specific cancer cells or tissues, deliver drugs or genes, sense tumor biomarkers, perform minimally invasive surgery, or combine multiple functions for comprehensive treatment. In this chapter, the authors review the recent progress and applications of bio-inspired nanorobots for cancer diagnosis and therapy, with a focus on magnetic field-driven nanorobots. They also discuss the challenges and future perspectives of nanorobots in clinical translation.

Chapter 13

Ranjit Barua, Omdayal Group of Institutions, India

the bio-inspired compound continuum robot represents a groundbreaking innovation in the realm of minimally invasive surgery (MIS). Drawing inspiration from the flexibility and adaptability observed in nature, this robotic system employs a novel approach to navigating complex anatomical structures with enhanced precision. Mimicking the serpentine motion of snakes, the robot utilizes a compound continuum structure composed of interconnected segments. This design allows for unparalleled maneuverability, enabling the robot to navigate through confined spaces and intricate pathways within the human body. By emulating the biomechanics of natural organisms, the robot can reach anatomical locations that traditional rigid instruments might struggle to access. In this chapter, the authors will discuss the advanced biomimetic compound continuum robot for minimally invasive surgical applications.

Chapter 14

D. Raveena Judie Dolly, Karunya Institute of Technology and Sciences, India
D. J Jagannath, Karunya Institute of Technology and Sciences, India
J. Dinesh Peter, Karunya Institute of Technology and Sciences, India

Humans may encounter an arboviral illness through viruses transmitted by mosquitoes, commonly resulting in a fever known as breakbone fever. This term reflects the severity of muscle spasms and joint pains associated with the illness. While some cases are asymptomatic, others can be fatal. Dengue awareness often arises during seasonal changes. The integration of AI in dengue prediction becomes crucial for early diagnosis and treatment. Utilizing appropriate deep learning classifiers can aid in categorizing cases based on their severity. This article advocates for the implementation of an intelligent robotic fogger system in predicted areas. This approach employs interprofessional strategies to safeguard health workers and residents in regions prone to dengue outbreaks.

Preface

Welcome to *Modeling, Simulation, and Control of AI Robotics and Autonomous Systems*, edited by Tanupriya Choudhury, Anitha Mary X, Subrata Chowdhury, C. Karthik, and C. Suganthi Evangeline.

Intelligent Robotics and Autonomous Systems (IRAS) represent a confluence of robotics, artificial intelligence (AI), and control systems aimed at crafting intelligent machines capable of autonomous task execution. This edited volume delves into the intricate realms of system modeling, simulation, and control, elucidating their paramount significance in advancing the frontiers of IRAS.

System modeling, the foundational pillar, entails the creation of mathematical constructs that delineate the intricate dynamics of robotic systems. It encompasses a meticulous portrayal of kinematics, dynamics, sensors, actuators, and their interplay, thereby offering invaluable insights into system behaviors across diverse scenarios.

Simulation emerges as a pivotal tool, affording engineers the capability to scrutinize and refine their designs virtually, obviating the need for resource-intensive real-world testing. Leveraging software frameworks like MATLAB/Simulink or ROS, researchers can orchestrate a myriad of simulated environments and sensor inputs, gauging the efficacy of their designs under varying conditions.

Control, propelled by AI methodologies, assumes a central role in endowing robots with autonomous decision-making prowess. From reinforcement learning algorithms facilitating experiential learning to intricate control schemes orchestrating complex maneuvers, the amalgamation of AI and control theory augments the autonomy and efficacy of robotic systems manifold.

The applications of these methodologies reverberate across multifarious domains, exemplified vividly in the realm of autonomous driving systems and industrial automation. These technologies herald a paradigm shift, revolutionizing industries and augmenting human capabilities.

Moreover, the resurgence of research in autonomous systems underscores a transformative era characterized by unprecedented technological advancements. From chess-playing algorithms to self-driving vehicles and manufacturing line robots, the landscape of autonomous systems burgeons with innovation and promise.

As we embark on this journey through the realms of robotics and autonomous systems, this edited volume endeavors to furnish readers with a panoramic vista of cutting-edge breakthroughs, theoretical frameworks, and computational paradigms. It is our fervent hope that this compendium serves as a beacon, illuminating pathways towards the realization of intelligent, autonomous systems poised to redefine the contours of human endeavor.

ORGANIZATION OF THE BOOK

Chapter 1 delves into the symbiotic relationship between Autonomous Systems and Artificial Intelligence (AI), which has revolutionized industry automation and innovation. It explores how this synergy has transformed various aspects of our lives and work, particularly focusing on advancements in self-driving cars, drones, and robots. The chapter elucidates how AI empowers autonomous systems to sense, make intelligent decisions, and adapt to dynamic environments. Furthermore, it delves into AI-driven decision-making processes, emphasizing safety, reliability, and proactive anomaly detection to prevent accidents and failures.

Chapter 2 focuses on Explainable AI-Based Semantic Object Detection for Autonomous Vehicles, detailing machine learning models' applications in route recognition and segmentation. It explores various XAI approaches to interpret model predictions and evaluates their performance in autonomous vehicle road detection, emphasizing accuracy and efficiency.

Chapter 3 presents an AI-Based In-Cabin Monitoring System for Autonomous Vehicles, highlighting the importance of internal monitoring for fully autonomous vehicles. It discusses driver behavior evaluation, risky driving behavior detection, and the implementation of a Random Forest model to enhance object detection and user privacy.

Chapter 4 addresses Real-Time Fault Detection and Condition Monitoring for Industrial Autonomous Vehicles, emphasizing the necessity of early defect diagnosis in modern industrial systems. It proposes intelligent diagnostic technologies and on-board/off-board diagnosis integration, exemplified through an Automated Transfer Vehicle (ATV) equipment condition monitoring application.

Chapter 5 explores IoT in Day-to-Day Life, focusing on Vehicle Body Fatigue Analysis. It introduces an affordable IoT-based data acquisition setup for fatigue analysis in vehicle body design, aiming to bridge the gap between automotive manufacturers and vehicle body builders in durability testing.

Chapter 6 discusses the Design and Fabrication of a Softrobotic Gripper for Involving Underwater Vehicles in Seaweed Farming, highlighting the ecological importance of seaweeds and the hazards associated with manual harvesting. The chapter proposes integrating Soft Robotic Grippers into underwater vehicles for precise and eco-friendly seaweed farming.

Chapter 7 introduces Secure VANET Routing Protocols for Improved Vehicular Communication in Autonomous Systems, emphasizing security concerns in Vehicular Ad Hoc Networks (VANETs). It proposes a secure VANET routing protocol based on the Dijkstra Algorithm, incorporating message authentication and encryption for secure communication.

Chapter 8 explores Autonomous Systems' Revolutionizing Health Insurance Industry, focusing on operational excellence in health insurance services. It examines the impact of autonomous systems, including AI, machine learning, and automation, in expediting claim processing, fraud detection, and enhancing customer experience.

Chapter 9 delves into Artificial Intelligence in Robotics, emphasizing AI's transformative influence on robotic capabilities. It explores practical implementations of AI-powered robots in various domains, highlighting machine learning methodologies' role in enhancing perception, decision-making, and adaptability in robots.

Chapter 10 investigates Synergistic Swarm: Multi-Robot Systems in Healthcare, emphasizing the collaborative synergy achieved by coordinating multiple robotic entities in healthcare settings. It explores the applications of AI, robotics, and sensor networks in enhancing diagnostics, patient support, and medical operations.

Chapter 11 examines Cogwheels of Care: Robotic Marvels in the Hospital Landscape, exploring the profound influence of advanced robotics on patient care and medical capabilities. It discusses the ethical considerations and societal implications of integrating robots into healthcare, emphasizing the transformative potential of this technological evolution.

Chapter 12 introduces Bio-Inspired Nanorobots for Cancer Diagnosis and Therapy, exploring nanorobots' promising applications in cancer treatment. It discusses the recent progress and challenges in designing nanorobots for targeted drug delivery, sensing tumor biomarkers, and performing minimally invasive surgery, with a focus on magnetic field-driven nanorobots.

Chapter 13 presents Advanced Biomimetic Compound Continuum Robot for Minimally Invasive Surgical Applications, detailing a groundbreaking robotic system inspired by natural biomechanics. It explores the compound continuum robot's flexibility and adaptability in navigating complex anatomical structures, particularly in minimally invasive surgery.

Chapter 14 discusses An Intelligent Robotic Fogger System for Predicting Dengue Outbreaks, focusing on utilizing AI-driven robotic systems for disease prevention. It proposes implementing an intelligent robotic fogger system in predicted dengue outbreak areas, emphasizing interprofessional strategies to safeguard public health.

IN CONCLUSION

As we draw the curtains on this compendium, *Modeling, Simulation,* and *Control of AI Robotics and Autonomous Systems,* we reflect on the myriad facets of innovation, ingenuity, and interdisciplinary collaboration encapsulated within its pages. The journey through the realms of intelligent robotics and autonomous systems has been nothing short of exhilarating, unveiling a tapestry of cutting-edge research, transformative methodologies, and visionary perspectives.

From the revolutionary fusion of autonomous systems and AI, redefining industrial automation paradigms, to the advent of edge computing and machine learning heralding a new era in aerial autonomy, each chapter resonates with the collective pursuit of excellence and advancement. Proposals for intelligent bio-inspired autonomous underwater vehicles, explainable AI-based semantic object detection for autonomous vehicles, and real-time fault detection for industrial autonomous vehicles epitomize the relentless quest for innovation and progress.

Moreover, the exploration of human-robot interaction, synergistic swarm multi-robot systems in healthcare, and the integration of sophisticated robotics in the hospital landscape underscores the transformative potential of robotics in reshaping healthcare delivery and patient outcomes. The chapters on secure VANET routing protocols and autonomous systems revolutionizing the health insurance industry underscore the pivotal role of technology in enhancing safety, efficiency, and accessibility across diverse domains.

As we navigate the intricate landscapes of artificial intelligence, machine learning, and robotics, it becomes increasingly evident that our collective endeavors are not merely confined to the realms of academia or industry but resonate deeply with societal aspirations and challenges. The deployment of bio-inspired nanorobots for cancer diagnosis and therapy and the implementation of intelligent robotic fogger systems for predicting dengue outbreaks underscore the profound impact of robotics in addressing pressing global health challenges.

In conclusion, *Modeling, Simulation, and Control of AI Robotics and Autonomous Systems* serves as a testament to the indomitable spirit of human ingenuity and innovation. It is our fervent hope that this compendium not only serves as a comprehensive reference for researchers, engineers, and enthusiasts but also inspires future generations to push the boundaries of what is possible in the dynamic and ever-evolving field of robotics and autonomous systems.

Tanupriya Choudhury
Graphic Era University, India

Anitha Mary X
Karunya Institute of Technology and Sciences, India

Subrata Chowdhury
Sreenivasa Institute of Technology and Management Studies, India

C. Karthik
Jyothi Engineering College, India

C. Suganthi Evangeline
Sri Eshwar College of Engineering, India

Chapter 1
Autonomous System and AI

T. Preethiya
ⓘ https://orcid.org/0000-0003-3504-1884
SRM Institute of Science and Technology, India

Priyanga Subbiah
ⓘ https://orcid.org/0000-0002-2395-7492
SRM Institute of Science and Technology, India

T. Pandiarajan
ⓘ https://orcid.org/0009-0007-7808-8961
Rajalakshmi Institute of Technology, India

Karthikeyan Subramanian
Birmingham City University, UAE

Prince Chelladurai
University College of Engineering, Villupuram, India

C. Selvalakshmi
Mangayarkarasi College of Engineering, India

ABSTRACT

Autonomous systems and AI have revolutionized industry automation and innovation. This abstract shows how this synergy changes our lives and work. AI has rapidly advanced autonomous systems like self-driving cars, drones, and robots. These systems can sense, make smart decisions, and adapt to changing environments with AI. They can navigate complex settings and interact with humans thanks to this superior sense Autonomous systems can make real-time judgments using AI methods like machine learning and deep learning. AI-driven decision-making assures adaptability and efficiency, whether a self-driving car chooses the safest route, or a drone optimizes its flying path. AI-assisted autonomous systems prioritize safety and reliability. These systems can detect anomalies and respond proactively to prevent accidents and failures through self-monitoring and diagnostics.

DOI: 10.4018/979-8-3693-1962-8.ch001

INTRODUCTION

Systems that can operate independently of direct human assistance are known as autonomous systems. They have special traits that permit them autonomy, such as the ability to make judgments, perceive their surroundings through sense and perceptions, process data to make educated decisions, and execute actions or behaviors based on those conclusions. Systems with varying degrees of autonomy can do simple rule-based operations or more sophisticated decision-making powered by Artificial Intelligence (AI) algorithm.

Overview of Autonomous Systems

Autonomous systems come in many forms and are widely used in industries such as robotics and transportation. Self-driving cars, which use sensor data and AI algorithms to navigate roadways and make driving judgments, are a prominent example of the transportation industry. Additionally, a variety of industries, including delivery, disaster relief, and surveillance, have found use for unmanned aerial vehicles, or drones. Another important factor is robotics: service robots help humans with anything from housework to healthcare, while industrial robots streamline production processes (Aguirre & Rodriguez, 2017). Beyond these, there are more autonomous systems in industries such as agriculture and space exploration, each tailored to certain tasks and conditions.

Sensing devices for gathering environmental data and perception algorithms for interpreting it are essential parts of autonomous systems. To evaluate data and come to the right conclusions, these systems use AI-driven decision-making methods like machine learning and reinforcement learning. These systems can map out actions and govern their movements thanks to planning and control techniques. The last phase, known as actuator, is when choices are actually put into action. Examples of this include modifying a vehicle's course or moving a robot.

Although autonomous systems have a lot of potential, there are also a variety of obstacles and restrictions. Keeping these systems safe and dependable remains the top priority, particularly for vital uses like driverless cars and medical robotics (Tong et al., 2019). A number of ethical issues come up, including privacy concerns, decision-making procedures, and human-AI system interactions. Establishing frameworks for regulating new technologies and guaranteeing their appropriate deployment and use also requires addressing legal and regulatory obstacles.

Importance and Impact of AI in Autonomous Systems

The incorporation of Artificial Intelligence into Autonomous Systems represents a significant breakthrough, transforming their potential and influence across various sectors. The cornerstone that allows these systems to operate independently and intelligently is artificial intelligence. It is important because it enhances decision-making processes and enables systems to dynamically adjust to a variety of changing conditions. Through the utilization of AI techniques such as deep learning and machine learning, autonomous systems are capable of processing large volumes of data in real-time and deriving actionable insights. This combination increases the efficiency, accuracy, and adaptability of these systems by enabling them to maneuver through complicated environments, make snap decisions, and continuously learn from their experiences. AI in autonomous systems is having a broad impact on various industries. For example, self-driving cars are revolutionizing transportation, robotic automation is streamlining manufacturing, and surgical robots and diagnostic AI are improving healthcare. Additionally, AI-driven autonomy opens up new avenues for innovation, pushing industries to rethink procedures and discover uncharted territory in terms of technological incorporation while leading to progress in a variety of fields. To fully realize the transformative potential of AI within autonomous systems, however, and to address societal concerns and ensure responsible deployment and usage, strong regulatory frameworks are required, along with ethical considerations, safety assurances, and other issues.

UNDERSTANDING AUTONOMOUS SYSTEMS

Autonomous Systems exhibit distinctive traits, chiefly autonomy in decision-making, perception of their surroundings through sensors, sophisticated data analysis, and execution of actions based on these assessments. This autonomy can range from basic rule-based operations to complex, AI-driven decision-making processes. These systems often comprise a network of sensors—such as cameras, LIDAR, radar, or other environmental detectors—enabling them to gather data crucial for their operations (Cui et al., 2019; Hodge et al., 2021). Subsequently, these data inputs undergo processing and interpretation using AI algorithms, including machine learning and neural networks, to generate informed decisions and actions.

Autonomous systems comprise a broad range of technologies intended to function autonomously, across various domains, without continual human supervision. Autonomous vehicles are a standout system among the others. The future of mobility will be drastically altered by self-driving cars, which integrate a sophisticated network of sensors, artificial intelligence algorithms, and mapping technologies to navigate roads and make decisions in real time. In addition, unmanned aerial vehicles, also known as drones (Mehta et al., 2021), have become incredibly useful instruments in a variety of fields, including disaster relief, logistics, surveillance, and agriculture. These vehicles use AI and sensors to carry out tasks on their own. Another important category that is applicable to both the industrial and service sectors is robotics. Industrial robots increase productivity by performing repetitive, precise tasks, which optimizes manufacturing processes. On the other hand, service robots help people in a variety of contexts, such as healthcare and housework. demonstrating how flexible and useful autonomous technology can be to enhance daily tasks. Beyond their use on land, autonomous underwater and aerial vehicles also contribute to atmospheric research, space exploration, underwater exploration, and research and maintenance, all of which further the frontiers of scientific knowledge. These various kinds of autonomous systems, each customized to particular environments and tasks, use sensor technology, AI algorithms, and actuation mechanisms to operate independently. They support a range of industries and are revolutionizing the execution and management of tasks in multiple domains.

Autonomous Vehicles

Autonomous vehicles, which integrate cutting-edge technology to navigate and operate without constant human intervention, represent a transformative innovation in transportation that will revolutionize mobility. Leading this category are self-driving cars, which are outfitted with a complex web of sensors, cameras, radar, LIDAR, and GPS, allowing them to sense and understand their surroundings instantly. These cars analyze enormous volumes of data using AI algorithms and machine learning models, making snap judgments regarding their speed, direction, and interactions with their surroundings. Self-Driving Cars seek to improve efficiency and safety on the roads by continuously assessing and responding to shifting traffic patterns, road conditions, and unforeseen obstacles. They may also help reduce accidents that result from human error (Cui et al., 2019; Hodge et al., 2021; Tong et al., 2019).

Drones and Robotics

Drones and robotics are two important subcategories in the field of autonomous systems that have been applied in a wide range of industries. Unmanned aerial vehicles (UAVs), or drones, are small, unmanned aircraft that are outfitted with sophisticated sensors and artificial intelligence capabilities. These aerial vehicles are used for a variety of tasks, such as delivery and logistics, aerial photography, and surveillance. Drones have shown to be extremely useful in a variety of industries, including entertainment, infrastructure inspection, agriculture monitoring, disaster response, and entertainment (Hodge et al., 2021; Mehta et al., 2021). This is because they can fly independently and maneuver through a variety of environments. They are essential tools in many industries because of their small size, agility, and effective access to dangerous or remote areas.

Simultaneously, robotics has advanced significantly, with sophisticated machines capable of performing intricate tasks with precision and efficiency. For example, industrial robotics has become an integral part of manufacturing processes, streamlining production lines and performing tasks such as welding, assembly, and quality control. These self-driving robots are guided by AI algorithms and sensor feedback, increasing productivity and ensuring consistent quality. Robots designed as companions or assistants in healthcare, hospitality, and household chores have demonstrated adaptability in service-oriented domains, assisting humans in tasks ranging from assisting surgeons in operating rooms to assisting the elderly with daily activities.

Drones and robotics have a lot in common: they are both autonomous beings powered by AI algorithms that use sensor technology to understand their surroundings and carry out preprogrammed tasks (Aouf et al., 2019). But they serve different environments and uses; robotics functions in terrestrial environments, while drones are primarily used in aerial spaces. Research is still being done on both categories to improve their capabilities, give them more autonomy, and integrate them into new domains. Despite the wide range of potential uses for drones and robotics, there are still many unanswered questions in these fields, including those pertaining to safety, legal requirements, morality, and public opinion. All things considered, their integration promises greater productivity, safety, and innovation in a variety of operational environments, signifying a paradigm shift in a number of industries.

Industrial Automation

One of the most important uses of autonomous systems is industrial automation, which integrates cutting-edge technology to transform manufacturing processes and increase productivity and efficiency in industrial environments. Fundamentally, industrial automation is the use of robotics, AI-driven systems, and autonomous machinery to carry out tasks that have historically been performed by humans. These self-contained systems use sensors, actuators, and AI algorithms to carry out precise, repetitive tasks at different production stages.

Industrial robots are a key component of industrial automation because they are designed to complete certain tasks quickly and precisely. Numerous tasks are carried out by these robots, such as welding, painting, assembling, handling materials, and quality assurance. They increase production output, maintain consistent quality, and decrease operational errors whether they work independently or in tandem with human labor.

Moreover, autonomous mobile robots (AMRs) and guided vehicles (AGVs) traverse factory floors while moving supplies and products between various workstations. These cars optimize logistics and reduce manual handling by navigating safely in dynamic environments through the use of sensors and AI-based navigation systems (Aguirre & Rodriguez, 2017).

Predictive maintenance has advanced thanks to the integration of AI and machine learning in industrial automation. In order to anticipate equipment breakdowns or maintenance requirements, AI-driven algorithms evaluate sensor data. This allows for proactive interventions, lowers unscheduled downtime, and increases Overall Equipment Effectiveness (OEE).

There are several advantages to industrial automation. These include higher productivity, lower operating expenses, better-quality products, safer workplaces thanks to automated dangerous tasks, and quick response to shifting consumer demands.On the other hand, there are still some drawbacks which includes the upfront costs associated with implementation, the requirement for specialized knowledge to oversee and maintain automated systems, worries about employment displacement, and the necessity of strong cybersecurity defenses to shield linked systems from possible attacks.

ROLE OF AI IN AUTONOMOUS SYSTEMS

Artificial Intelligence plays a fundamental role in Autonomous Systems, acting as the cognitive engine that allows these systems to operate autonomously and decide for themselves. Artificial Intelligence serves as the central nervous system of autonomy, enabling the processing of sensor data and directing subsequent actions accordingly.

Data Processing and Analysis: The enormous volumes of data gathered by sensors integrated into autonomous systems are processed in large part by AI algorithms. These algorithms sort through intricate datasets, finding pertinent information, interpreting the surrounding context, and extracting patterns. AI algorithms effectively process data, regardless of the type—visual data from cameras, spatial data from GPS systems, or other sensory inputs.

AI-Powered Decision-Making: AI powers autonomous systems' decision-making. These systems can learn from data and experiences through deep learning, reinforcement learning, machine learning models, and other AI techniques, gradually strengthening their decision-making capabilities. Whether it is navigating a road for an autonomous vehicle, identifying objects in the path of a drone, or figuring out the best course of action for an industrial robot on a manufacturing line, they analyze the interpreted data to make informed decisions or take actions.

Adaptability and Learning: Adaptability is a key component of artificial intelligence in autonomous systems. These systems are always picking up new skills and adjusting to their ever-changing surroundings. They can improve their performance and responsiveness by honing their decision-making through continuous learning processes based on historical data, real-time data, and feedback loops.Increasing Efficiency and Autonomy: High levels of autonomy are made possible for Autonomous Systems to function by AI algorithms. AI greatly improves these systems' efficacy and efficiency by automating decision-making procedures and lowering the need for continual human intervention. Their independence allows them to operate in a range of situations and surroundings, which makes them flexible and able to adjust to different circumstances.

Increasing Efficiency and Autonomy: High levels of autonomy are made possible for Autonomous Systems to function by AI algorithms. AI greatly improves these systems' efficacy and efficiency by automating decision-making procedures and lowering the need for continual human intervention. Their independence allows them to operate in a range of situations and surroundings, which makes them flexible and able to adjust to different circumstances.

Safety and Risk Mitigation: AI helps to improve autonomous systems' safety. These systems can improve overall safety in applications like drones, industrial automation, and autonomous vehicles by analyzing potential risks, predicting outcomes, and making decisions to mitigate risks.

AI Algorithms and Techniques

AI algorithms play a pivotal role in automation by enabling machines and systems to perform tasks, make decisions, and adapt to changing circumstances without constant human intervention. In automation, artificial intelligence algorithms are what power the intelligence and decision-making that are built into systems. Together, these algorithms provide a broad toolkit that makes automation possible in a number of sectors (Da Silva Assis et al., 2016). The foundation of artificial intelligence, Machine Learning (ML) algorithms, makes automation easier by enabling systems to learn from data patterns and make predictions or decisions without explicit programming. Supervised learning algorithms in ML facilitate automation by training models on labeled data to predict or classify outcomes. This is an essential component in automating processes like manufacturing predictive maintenance or image recognition for quality control. Furthermore, unsupervised learning algorithms find hidden structures or patterns in data, which helps automate the process of grouping related data points. An advanced subset of machine learning called deep learning (DL) uses neural networks to process large amounts of data and perform tasks like computer vision, natural language processing, and autonomous decision-making in industrial settings. In order to automate sequential decision-making processes, Reinforcement Learning (RL) algorithms enable systems to learn optimal behaviors through interactions with an environment. By handling repetitive tasks, streamlining workflows, and enabling systems to learn and adapt to changing conditions, these AI algorithms collectively empower automation and revolutionize efficiency, accuracy, and adaptability in automated workflows across industries.

Deep Learning and Neural Networks

Neural networks and deep learning (DL) are sophisticated subsets of machine learning that are essential to the development and operation of autonomous systems. These technologies have allowed Autonomous Systems to perform sophisticated tasks and make judgments based on complex patterns and data, revolutionizing their capabilities.Using artificial neural networks with several layers, Deep Learning is a branch of machine learning. From enormous volumes of data, these deep neural networks are able to identify patterns, extract features, and make predictions or classifications. Because this technique can handle unstructured data like text, audio, and images, it has had a significant impact on autonomous systems.

Neural Networks use linked nodes, or neurons, arranged in layers to simulate the composition and operations of the human brain. These networks can process complex information in a hierarchical manner because of their input, hidden, and output layers. Numerous neural network architectures, including generative adversarial networks (GANs), recurrent neural networks (RNNs), and convolutional neural networks (CNNs), have proven useful in a range of autonomous systems applications. CNNs are excellent at analyzing images and videos, which enables Autonomous Systems to carry out activities like segmentation, object detection, and image classification. They're widely used in applications like lane markings, traffic signs, and pedestrian detection in autonomous vehicles. Recurrent neural networks, or RNNs, are utilized in situations where temporal dependencies are present because they are efficient at processing sequential data.

Natural Language Processing and Perception

Natural Language Processing (NLP) and perception stand as pivotal components in the realm of Autonomous Systems, playing integral roles in facilitating communication with humans and understanding the surrounding environment. NLP techniques empower these systems to comprehend, process, and generate human language, encompassing tasks such as speech recognition, language understanding, text generation, and dialog systems. By interpreting spoken or written language, NLP enables autonomous vehicles to respond to voice commands, chatbots to engage in conversations, and systems to analyze textual data for insights or decision-making. Simultaneously, perception in Autonomous Systems involves the fusion of data from various sensors like cameras, LIDAR, and radar, enabling the systems to comprehend their environment. Computer vision algorithms decode visual information, aiding in object recognition, scene understanding, and environment interpretation, vital for autonomous vehicles to navigate safely or for robots to interact seamlessly in dynamic settings. The integration of NLP and perception empowers Autonomous Systems to communicate effectively with humans and gain insights from their surroundings, fostering advancements in applications like autonomous vehicles, robotics, and smart environments, paving the way for more intelligent and intuitive interactions between machines and humans.

APPLICATIONS OF AUTONOMOUS SYSTEMS AND AI

Autonomous Systems integrated with Artificial Intelligence applications have permeated diverse industries, reshaping operations and introducing unprecedented efficiency, precision, and innovation. Within transportation, the emergence of self-driving cars and autonomous vehicles powered by AI algorithms has redefined mobility, promising safer and more efficient travel. Healthcare has seen a revolution with AI aiding in diagnostics, personalized treatment plans, and even drug discovery, improving patient care and outcomes.

AI in Automobiles

Industries have embraced AI-driven automation, transforming manufacturing processes in Industry 4.0 by optimizing production lines, predictive maintenance, and smart logistics. Agriculture benefits from precision farming techniques, employing drones and IoT sensors to monitor crops and resources, maximizing yields sustainably. Financial services utilize AI for fraud detection, risk assessment, and algorithmic trading, enhancing operational efficiency and security. Retail experiences AI-driven advancements with personalized customer service, recommendation systems, and inventory management. Smart city initiatives harness AI for traffic management, energy optimization, and public safety enhancement. Even in scientific exploration and space missions, AI supports navigation, data analysis, and robotics, enabling groundbreaking discoveries. These applications underscore the breadth of AI-driven Autonomous Systems, catalyzing advancements across industries and significantly impacting how we live, work, and explore the world around us.

Self-Driving Cars

Self-Driving Cars, which aim to transform transportation by enabling vehicles to navigate and operate autonomously without constant human intervention, represent the convergence of cutting-edge technology, artificial intelligence, and automotive engineering. These vehicles are fundamentally equipped with an advanced array of sensors, cameras, radar, LIDAR, and GPS systems to enable real-time perception and interpretation of the surrounding environment. The data gathered from these sensors is processed by AI algorithms, specifically machine learning and deep learning models, which allow the car to make decisions instantly about navigation, route planning, object detection, and reacting to changing traffic conditions (Brown, 2016; Da Silva Assis et al., 2016; Kumar et al., 2019; Preethiya et al., 2018; Preethiya et al., 2019a; Preethiya et al., 2020).

Advanced Driver-Assistance Systems (ADAS)

Modern cars are equipped with advanced driver-assistance systems (ADAS), which are an intermediate step toward complete autonomy. ADAS features include automatic emergency braking, adaptive cruise control, and lane-keeping assistance.

Perception systems that interpret sensor data, mapping technologies that offer a digital depiction of the surroundings, decision-making algorithms that evaluate data and choose the best course of action for driving, and actuation mechanisms that convert decisions into movements of the vehicle are important parts that enable these vehicles to operate autonomously.

When it comes to the development and application of self-driving cars, safety is still the top priority. For these cars to be safe and dependable, rigorous testing, simulations, and ongoing AI algorithm development are essential. Significant obstacles that must be overcome include liability issues, regulatory frameworks, public acceptance, and ethical considerations.

The implications of self-driving cars on society could be extensive. They promise to improve road safety by lowering human error-related accidents, streamline traffic, make transportation more accessible to people with limited mobility, and possibly even change the look of cities by rearranging transportation infrastructure (Amrutkar et al., 2024; Koubaa et al., 2021).

AI in Healthcare and Medicine

The application of artificial intelligence to medicine and healthcare promises ground-breaking discoveries and breakthroughs that will change treatment regimens, patient care, diagnosis, and healthcare delivery systems. Artificial intelligence, which is distinguished by its capacity to evaluate enormous volumes of data, spot patterns, and forecast outcomes, has shown itself to be a potent ally in enhancing medical procedures and resolving enduring issues in the healthcare sector.

Fundamentally, artificial intelligence in healthcare spans a wide range of uses, utilizing deep neural networks, computer vision, natural language processing, and machine learning algorithms to extract knowledge from complicated medical data. Healthcare practitioners can now extract actionable insights from a variety of sources, including genomic sequencing, medical imaging, electronic health records (EHRs), and real-time patient monitoring.

Furthermore, remarkably accurate diagnosis of conditions such as neurological disorders, cancer, and cardiovascular diseases has been demonstrated by AI-powered medical imaging systems, helping radiologists to interpret imaging results more precisely. Through the extraction of valuable information from unstructured medical texts, natural language processing aids in clinical decision-making and promotes more effective documentation (Bajwa et al., 2021).

The application of AI in healthcare has great potential, but there are drawbacks as well, including the need for transparent and understandable AI models, regulatory compliance, data privacy, and ethical issues with AI-driven decision-making in patient care.

Robotics in Surgery

Robotics in surgery is a game-changing development in medical technology that combines advanced technology and surgical techniques to improve accuracy, dexterity, and patient outcomes. In contrast to conventional surgical techniques, robotic surgery uses robotic systems under the control of surgeons to carry out minimally invasive procedures with increased accuracy and control (Chopra et al., 2022).

Surgical robots, which are operated by surgeons via a console and furnished with cutting-edge technology like robotic arms and specialized instruments, are the foundation of robotic surgery. These systems include micro-scale instruments that can perform complex movements and maneuvers that are difficult for human hands to perform alone, as well as high-definition cameras that provide three-dimensional views of the surgical site.

AI in Diagnosis and Treatment

With the use of cutting-edge algorithms and data analytics, artificial intelligence in diagnosis and treatment has become a ground-breaking area in healthcare, revolutionizing patient care, diagnosis, and treatment approaches. Artificial Intelligence technologies employ machine learning, deep learning, and natural language processing to analyze large datasets that include genetic data, clinical research findings, medical images, and electronic health records. Through the analysis of imaging scans, laboratory results, and patient histories, these sophisticated algorithms provide healthcare providers with enhanced diagnostic capabilities, assisting in the early detection of diseases with remarkable accuracy. Additionally, by incorporating patient-specific data, AI-driven systems facilitate the development of individualized treatment plans, enabling the use of customized drugs and therapies that maximize efficacy while minimizing side effects.

AI in Industrial Automation

Artificial Intelligence (AI) is a key player in the transformation of industrial automation through the advancement of conventional manufacturing processes (Kautish et al., 2024). AI algorithms bring about the era of smart factories by optimizing efficiency, improving precision, and enabling predictive maintenance in industrial settings. Large-scale sensor and machine datasets are analyzed by AI-powered systems, which enable real-time decision-making to maximize efficiency, minimize errors, and cut down on downtime. By identifying patterns in production lines, machine learning algorithms optimize workflows, anticipate equipment failures, and proactively schedule maintenance, thereby averting expensive disruptions. AI-enabled collaborative robots, or cobots, operate alongside people to accomplish complex tasks safely and precisely. AI-powered computer vision systems supervise quality control, checking goods to make sure they meet strict requirements. While AI increases productivity, there are still issues that need to be addressed, including workforce adaptation to AI-integrated environments, cybersecurity threats, and ensuring ethical AI deployment. Notwithstanding these obstacles, artificial intelligence's (AI) incorporation into industrial automation is redefining manufacturing and holding out the prospect of greater productivity, affordability, and innovation in the industrial sector.

Other Applications

AI algorithms are essential for fraud detection, risk assessment, and trading decision automation in the banking and finance industries. Healthcare uses AI for medical image analysis, treatment optimization, and illness diagnosis, while retail uses AI for personalized recommendations, inventory control, and chatbots for customer service. AI is having an impact on education through chatbots for student support, adaptive tutoring systems, and personalized learning experiences. In addition, AI improves cybersecurity protocols, transforms the way utilities distribute energy, and maximizes agricultural yield through precision farming methods. AI is being used by the entertainment sector for content creation, personalization, and recommendation. AI also has an impact on human resources, logistics, transportation, and other areas. It makes things easier for autonomous cars, automated hiring, predictive maintenance, and route optimization. The fact that AI is being widely used in these fields demonstrates how it can spur innovation, improve operations, and bring about revolutionary changes that have a significant impact on a wide range of businesses and daily life (Mohan et al., 2023; Preethiya et al., 2019b; Venkat et al., 2023).

Real-Time Case Studies

Waymo, a subsidiary of Alphabet Inc., is developing autonomous driving technology, with plans for commercial deployment. However, a 2018 collision in Arizona raised concerns about safety and readiness. Amazon's warehouse robots have improved efficiency but have also caused accidents, including collisions with human workers and inventory damage. The integration of AI and robotics in warehouse automation raises concerns about workplace safety, human-robot collaboration, and job displacement. IBM Watson, an AI-powered platform used in healthcare, has faced criticism for its accuracy, scalability, and integration with existing systems. Despite its potential to improve clinical decision-making and patient outcomes, data quality, interoperability, and trust remain significant barriers to adoption. Amazon Go Stores use AI and sensor fusion technology to provide cashier-less shopping experiences, but face challenges such as technical reliability, accuracy in tracking, job displacement, privacy concerns, and surveillance. Autonomous drones are being developed for agricultural applications, but face technical issues like flight stability, obstacle avoidance, and data processing. Regulatory hurdles and socio-economic impacts on traditional farming practices and rural communities are also a concern. Robotic Process Automation (RPA) in finance automates repetitive tasks like data entry, reconciliation, and report generation, mimicking human interactions with computer systems. Challenges include ensuring accuracy in complex financial processes, integrating RPA with existing systems, and addressing security risks. Additionally, there are concerns about job displacement and the need for upskilling finance professionals to work effectively with RPA systems.

ETHICAL AND SOCIAL IMPLICATIONS

The rapid integration of Artificial Intelligence into various facets of daily life brings forth a spectrum of ethical and social implications that warrant careful consideration. One primary concern lies in the potential bias embedded within AI algorithms, leading to unfair treatment or discrimination. Biased datasets might perpetuate societal prejudices, reflecting in AI decisions across sectors such as hiring, lending, and criminal justice. The opacity of some AI models poses challenges in understanding their decision-making processes, raising questions about accountability and transparency. Privacy breaches and data security vulnerabilities arise from the extensive collection and utilization of personal data by AI systems, necessitating stringent safeguards to protect sensitive information. Additionally, the potential for job displacement due to automation and shifts in workforce dynamics triggers discussions about retraining programs and equitable access to opportunities in an AI-driven economy (Daniel, 2023; Vesnic-Alujevic et al., 2020).

Autonomous agriculture and precision farming revolutionise food production, improving efficiency, resource use, and crop yields. However, autonomous systems in agriculture create challenges and ethical issues. Because autonomous machinery collects vast data on crop conditions, soil health, and agricultural processes, data ownership and privacy are major considerations. Farmers must handle data ownership, usage, and exploitation. AI-driven decision-making also raises algorithm transparency and accountability concerns. Farmers seek independent, reliable, and in their best interests autonomous machinery algorithms. Autonomous agricultural technology may replace conventional farming practices and influence rural communities, which might have socioeconomic effects. Technical innovation, ethical values, regulatory supervision, and stakeholder interaction are needed to deploy autonomous farm systems properly. Farmers, researchers, legislators, and industry stakeholders must collaborate to use autonomous farming for sustainable food production.

The maritime industry is developing autonomous ships with AI-driven navigation systems to improve productivity and reduce human error. Autonomous vessels in busy waterways and their ability to adapt to unexpected environmental conditions pose safety risks. Diverse strategies are needed to address these concerns. First, create robust sensor systems that can recognise and manoeuvre around barriers to prevent collisions. Coordination and collision avoidance need good communication with other boats. Safe and lawful operation requires international marine standards. Establishing public trust in autonomous maritime technology requires fail-safe techniques to intervene in crises and avert tragedies. To tackle these complexities, reliable communication systems and extensive testing are essential. By proactively addressing these issues and prioritising safety, the maritime sector can safely deploy autonomous ships and develop trust in this revolutionary technology.

Delivery drones might change urban logistics as Amazon and Google lead attempts to deliver things in congested areas. Drone integration into cities is difficult. Due to the rising number of drones, airspace management is a major concern, raising questions about safety legislation and accidents with other aircraft or people. Safe and ethical delivery drone deployment requires overcoming technology difficulties like collision avoidance systems. Navigating air traffic control and privacy laws is vital. To establish urban drone operations guidelines, local authorities, communities, and aviation groups must collaborate. Collaboration and coordination are needed to achieve delivery drones' transformative potential while prioritising safety and public welfare.

Automotive innovations like Tesla's Autopilot and Full Self-Driving (FSD) capabilities assist drivers with lane-keeping and autonomous parking. Despite promised safety and convenience gains, these features have been challenging to implement. Multiple crashes have occurred due to drivers overusing Tesla's self-driving technologies. Tesla's autonomous driving strategy is challenged by the accidents. The degree of human supervision needed for these duties and the system's capabilities and constraints have been questioned. Concerns remain concerning driver complacency while using semi-autonomous features, which may diminish concentration and hinder reaction. Tesla and other companies struggle to promote advanced capabilities while ensuring customer comprehension and proper use. Continuous refinement of autonomous systems, honest disclosure of their powers, and aggressive misuse prevention are needed to address these issues. Tesla and other innovators may enhance autonomous driving by solving safety and user awareness issues.

CONCLUSION

Autonomous systems and artificial intelligence have the potential to completely transform industries in the future, but they also face a number of obstacles that must be addressed for responsible and successful integration. The advancement of deep learning and natural language processing will be the main focus of AI's future development, opening up new possibilities for analysis and communication. However, ethical issues with AI decision-making transparency, bias reduction, and accountability present serious difficulties that call for careful regulation and moral frameworks. Though moral and legal challenges still exist, autonomous systems, particularly in the transportation sector, will prioritize infrastructure development and safety improvement. The impending difficulty is adjusting to AI's impact on the workforce, which calls for significant work redefinition and reskilling. Strong security measures to protect AI systems and user data will be required in tandem with cybersecurity threats and the requirement for data privacy regulations. Furthermore, proactive policies and international cooperation will be necessary to address societal effects like bias perpetuation and socioeconomic disparities as well as ensure equitable AI accessibility. The future of AI and Autonomous Systems depends on proactive ethical thinking, legal frameworks, and cooperative efforts to fully realize their potential while reducing the inherent difficulties for a tech future that is both responsible and inclusive.

REFERENCES

Aguirre, S., & Rodriguez, A. (2017). *Automation of a Business Process Using Robotic Process Automation (RPA): A Case Study*. Springer. . doi:10.1007/978-3-319-66963-2_7

Amrutkar, C., Satav, A., Sonawwanay, P. D., & Pawar, A. H. (2024). Overview of Autonomous Vehicle and Its Challenges. Techno-Societal 2022. *ICATSA*, *2022*, 243–251. doi:10.1007/978-3-031-34648-4_25

Aouf, A., Boussaid, L., & Sakly, A. (2019). Same fuzzy logic controller for two-wheeled mobile robot navigation in strange environments. *Journal of Robotics*, *2019*, 2465219. doi:10.1155/2019/2465219

Bajwa, J., Munir, U., Nori, A., & Williams, B. (2021, July). Artificial intelligence in healthcare: Transforming the practice of medicine. *Future Healthcare Journal*, *8*(2), e188–e194. doi:10.7861/fhj.2021-0095 PMID:34286183

Brown, B. (2016). The social life of autonomous cars. *MIT Technology Review, 50*(2).

Chaurasia, A., Parashar, B., & Kautish, S. (2024). Artificial Intelligence and Automation for Industry 4.0. In S. Kautish, P. Chatterjee, D. Pamucar, N. Pradeep, & D. Singh (Eds.), *Computational Intelligence for Modern Business Systems. Disruptive Technologies and Digital Transformations for Society 5.0*. doi:10.1007/978-981-99-5354-7_18

Chopra, H., Baig, A. A., Cavalu, S., Singh, I., & Emran, T. B. (2022, August 17). Robotics in surgery: Current trends. *Annals of Medicine and Surgery (London)*, *81*, 104375. doi:10.1016/j.amsu.2022.104375 PMID:36051814

Cui, Q., Wang, Y., Chen, K.-C., Ni, W., Lin, I.-C., Tao, X., & Zhang, P. (2019). Big data analytics and network calculus enabling intelligent management of autonomous vehicles in a smart city. *IEEE Internet of Things Journal*, *6*(2), 2021–2034. doi:10.1109/JIOT.2018.2872442

Da Silva Assis, L., da Silva Soares, A., Coelho, C. J., & Van Baalen, J. (2016). An evolutionary algorithm for autonomous robot navigation. *Procedia Computer Science*, *80*, 2261–2265. doi:10.1016/j.procs.2016.05.404

Daniel, T. (2023). Autonomous AI Systems in Conflict: Emergent Behavior and Its Impact on Predictability and Reliability. *Journal of Military Ethics*, *22*(1), 2–17. doi:10.1080/15027570.2023.2213985

Gupta, S., Upadhyay, D., & Dubey, A. K. (2019). Self-Driving Car Using Artificial Intelligence. In M. Kumar, R. Pandey, & V. Kumar (Eds.), *Advances in Interdisciplinary Engineering. Lecture Notes in Mechanical Engineering*. Springer. doi:10.1007/978-981-13-6577-5_49

Hodge, V. J., Hawkins, R., & Alexander, R. (2021). Deep reinforcement learning for drone navigation using sensor data. *Neural Computing & Applications*, *33*(6), 2015–2033. doi:10.1007/s00521-020-05097-x

Khamis, A., Patel, D., & Elgazzar, K. (2021). Deep Learning for Unmanned Autonomous Vehicles: A Comprehensive Review. In A. Koubaa & A. T. Azar (Eds.), *Deep Learning for Unmanned Systems. Studies in Computational Intelligence* (Vol. 984). Springer. doi:10.1007/978-3-030-77939-9_1

Mehta, P. L., Kalra, R., & Prasad, R. (2021). A Backdrop Case Study of AI-Drones in Indian Demographic Characteristics Emphasizing the Role of AI in Global Cities Digitalization. *Wireless Personal Communications*, *118*(1), 301–321. doi:10.1007/s11277-020-08014-6 PMID:33424130

Mohan, P., Sabarwal, T., & Preethiya, T. (2023). Indian Sign Language Character Recognition System. *2023 4th International Conference on Electronics and Sustainable Communication Systems (ICESC)*. IEEE. 10.1109/ICESC57686.2023.10193309

Preethiya, T., Muthukumar, A., & Durairaj, S. (2018) Providing Secured Data Aggregation in Mobile Wireless Sensor Network. *Proceedings of 4th IEEE International Symposium on Robotics and Manufacturing Automation*. IEEE. 10.1109/ROMA46407.2018.8986735

Preethiya, T., Muthukumar, A., & Durairaj, S. (2019a). Double Cluster Head Heterogeneous Clustering for Optimization in Hybrid Wireless Sensor Network. *Wireless Personal Communications. Wireless Personal Communications*, *110*(4), 1751–1768. doi:10.1007/s11277-019-06810-3

Preethiya, T., Muthukumar, A., & Durairaj, S. (2019b). Mobility Handling in Cluster based Mobile Wireless Sensor Network. *Proceedings of 2019 IEEE International Conference on Clean Energy and Energy Efficient Electronics Circuit for Sustainable Development (INCCES)*. IEEE. 10.1109/INCCES47820.2019.9167692

Preethiya, T., Muthukumar, A., & Durairaj, S. (2020). An energy efficient clustering and multipath routing for mobile wireless sensor network using game theory. *International Journal of Communication Systems*, *33*(7), 1–18.

Tong, W., Hussain, A., Bo, W. X., & Maharjan, S. (2019). Artificial intelligence for vehicle-to-everything: A survey. *IEEE Access : Practical Innovations, Open Solutions*, *7*, 10823–10843. doi:10.1109/ACCESS.2019.2891073

Venkat, Y., Chand, K. P., & Preethiya, T. (2023). An intrusion detection system for the Internet of Things based on machine learning. *2023 International Conference on Recent Advances in Electrical, Electronics, Ubiquitous Communication, and Computational Intelligence (RAEEUCCI)*. IEEE. 10.1109/RAEEUCCI57140.2023.10134432

Vesnic-Alujevic, L., Nascimento, S., & Pólvora, A. (2020). Societal and ethical impacts of artificial intelligence: Critical notes on European policy frameworks. *Telecommunications Policy*, *44*(6), 2020. doi:10.1016/j.telpol.2020.101961

Chapter 2
Explainable AI–Based Semantic Object Detection for Autonomous Vehicles

Elamathiyan A.

Karpagam Academy of Higher Education, India

G. Dhivya

(iD) https://orcid.org/0000-0001-7058-7917

Karpagam Academy of Higher Education, India

ABSTRACT

A goal is to facilitate the recognition and segmentation of the route driven by autonomous vehicles through the use of machine learning (ML) models. The pixel-wise road detection task, the semantic segmentation architectures underwent training and comparison. By using XAI, the authors are able to interpret and read the predictions generated by these abstract models. They generated arguments for the recommended segmentation model for autonomous vehicle road detection using a range of XAI approaches. Supervised learning is enabled by KNN, Decision Tree, and Random Forest, which are the current algorithms used for comparison. On the other hand, the newly built K means clustering function best when paired for image processing since they are good with images. To display the results of computations for the evaluation parameters of each algorithm, including accuracy, sensitivity, recall and precision, tables, and the necessary features from the evaluation matrices are utilised. The k-means clustering system for explainable AI-based semantic object detection in automated cars achieves 94.58% accuracy on both train and test sets.

INTRODUCTION

Autonomous car technology has advanced significantly in the last few years, changing the way people travel and paving the way for more efficiency, convenience, and safety in the future. Securing the reliable and transparent detection of objects in the vehicle's surrounds is a major problem in the development of

DOI: 10.4018/979-8-3693-1962-8.ch002

autonomous vehicles, and integrating state-of-the-art technologies is a crucial part of this transformative journey. According to Tyagi, A. K., &Aswathy, S. U. (2021), in this perspective, the intersection of semantic object recognition and explainable artificial intelligence appears as a vital frontier, where advances are paving the way for autonomous systems that are safer and easier to understand.

In order to sense and manoeuvre through their surroundings, autonomous cars depend on complex sensor arrays, such as radar, LiDAR, and cameras. This perceptual framework is centred on semantic object detection, which is the process of identifying and categorising items according to their semantic meaning.But in safety-critical applications like autonomous driving, questions have been raised regarding the interpretability of some deep learning models' decisions due to their opaque nature. Presenting Explainable AI, a paradigm that improves prediction accuracy while demystifying decision-making by offering explanations for why a given object was recognised or a specific action was performed.

Antoniadi, A. M., et al (2021), for autonomous vehicles to be widely used, trust must be developed among users, authorities, and the general public. Acceptance may be hampered by the opacity of conventional deep learning models. Explainable AI promotes trust in the technology by providing transparency, allowing consumers to understand how the car interprets its environment and makes judgements.

The above figure 1 described the general architecture of object detection. The ability of an artificial intelligence system to give clear and intelligible justifications for its choices and behaviours is known as explainable artificial intelligence, or XAI. Semantic object detection is the process of locating and categorising things in a scene or image according to their semantic significance. The use of XAI with semantic object detection in autonomous cars is important in order to maintain the transparency and reliability of the system. Autonomous vehicles have developed so quickly because of artificial intelligence (AI), which has the potential to significantly change the transportation landscape.

As these vehicles venture into ever-more complex and dynamic environments, the synergy between Semantic Object Detection and Explainable AI (XAI) represents a critical frontier that promises not only

Figure 1. Architecture of object detection

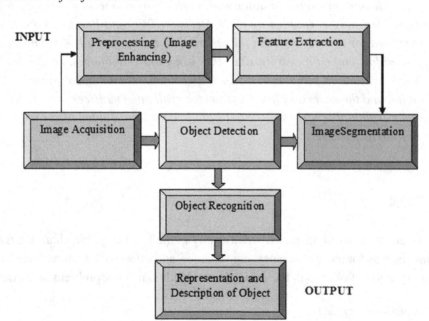

technological advancement but also a paradigm shift in how we view, trust, and incorporate autonomous systems into our daily lives.Using input from input image acquisition, pre-processing, also known as picture enhancement, is carried out first. For object identification, the output of this stage is delivered. The feature extraction is notified simultaneously with the preprocessed image output. In order to segment the image that needs to be identified, the segmentation stage gets the output from these two steps. These procedures are the fundamental and main ones used to identify parts of images. the object identified in the subsequent object detection step. Forwarded to the representation and description step is the input from object recognition. Upon completion, the outcome is presented in an easy-to-understand format according to the specifications.

Semantic Object Detection, an essential part of autonomous vehicle perception, broadens the car's understanding of its surroundings beyond simple identification. This sophisticated ability, according to Zhao, J., et al. (2021), comprises assigning semantic importance to objects in the visual field in addition to their recognition. Traffic signs, people, cars, and other contextually significant entities enable the automobile to make decisions based on its perception of the scene's semantic content. These entities are more than just pixels on a screen.

Object Detection in Neural Network

Object detection networks give the bounding box with the object's coordinates and the kind of object that can be found in the picture. Similar to image classification networks, object detection networks utilize convolution layers to identify visual features. These basic procedures should be followed in order to develop a neural network for object detection: Start by compiling a range of topic-representative pictures. Next, label and provide a name to every picture. After that, a neural network is constructed by Google Colab using these pictures, which are referred to as a "training set".

Explainable AI-based Semantic Object Detection works with humans and autonomous systems in addition to models and algorithms. Designing user-friendly and instructive human-machine interfaces becomes essential. The interface should provide succinct explanations in addition to communicating the AI's decisions in order to facilitate successful collaboration between the automobile and its human operators.

With the convergence of Semantic Object Detection and Explainable AI, the development trajectory of autonomous cars is being fundamentally altered. Its implications extend beyond the fine technical specifics of algorithms and models, into the fields of safety, trust, and societal integration. We must investigate the transparent possibilities of a future where autonomous vehicles live in harmony with humans, given the complex landscape of self-driving cars. This confluence becomes a societal responsibility that goes beyond technology. This goes beyond simply a convergence of technologies since it also represents a convergence of understanding, transparency, and the possibility of a safer and more comprehensible autonomous travel experience, Zablocki, E., et al (2022).

Autonomous vehicles (AVs) have advanced significantly in the last several years, thanks in large part to advances in artificial intelligence (AI).Wang, J., et al (2022), Autonomous driving relies heavily on object detection, which is the process of identifying and classifying objects in the vehicle's surroundings. Autonomous cars are becoming more and more dependent on reliable and safe object detection as they maneuver through complex and dynamic environments. This work aims to investigate the issues, possible remedies, and significance of explainable AI-based semantic object identification for driverless vehicles.

Autonomous vehicles, often known as self-driving cars, sense their surroundings using a range of sensors, including cameras, radar, and lidar. The cornerstone of the perception system, object recognition, enables the vehicle to recognize and respond to a wide range of items, including bikes, pedestrians, cars, and obstructions. Recent breakthroughs in artificial intelligence (AI), particularly in deep learning, have revolutionized traditional object recognition approaches, with a focus on computer vision algorithms. Recurrent neural networks (RNNs) and convolutional neural networks (CNNs), two deep learning models, have demonstrated superior performance over other models in object detection tests. However, because these models are opaque and difficult to understand how they make decisions, it is difficult to trust and employ them in safety-critical applications such as autonomous driving. As a result, the explainable AI paradigm has emerged, focusing on building models whose conclusions are understandable and interpretable by people. Semantic object detection is not only capable of identifying objects; it can also give those descriptive labels such as "car," "pedestrian," or "traffic light." This semantic knowledge is essential for the car to make sensible decisions and navigate safely in a range of environments. Arrieta, A. B., et al (2020), Explain ability combined with semantic object recognition ensures that decisions made by AI models are transparent and provide justifications for how an object was recognized and classified.

To solve the issues with semantic object detection in autonomous automobiles, engineers and researchers are looking into a variety of approaches. One way is to use complex deep learning networks designed specifically for object detection tasks. Models like the You Only Look Once (YOLO) and Single Shot MultiBox Detector (SSD) have gained popularity because to their accuracy and real-time performance. Another crucial strategy to employ is multi-sensor fusion. Autonomous vehicles have many sensors fitted, each of which records a different aspect of their environment. Data from cameras, lidar, radar, and other sensors are combined to improve overall perception capability, leading to more reliable and strong object detection, as assessed byAziz, L., et al (2020).

Explain ability is achieved by integrating interpretable machine learning models with post-hoc explanation techniques. Interpretable models, such as rule-based systems or decision trees, require transparent decision-making processes at their core. Post-hoc explanation techniques, on the other hand, aim to explain the decisions made by complex models after they have been trained. Simple, locally relevant explanations for specific model predictions are generated by methods like LIME (Local Interpretable Model-agnostic Explanations).For semantic object detection in autonomous automobiles, explain ability integration offers a number of benefits. To begin with, it allays concerns regarding the mystery surrounding deep learning algorithms by enhancing the legitimacy of AI models. Autonomous vehicle acceptance is likely to increase as manufacturers, regulators, and end users are able to understand and trust the AI's decision-making process. Secondly, systems are easier to troubleshoot and improve when they have explanation capability. By understanding how the model reacts to different scenarios, developers can identify and fix potential biases or weaknesses in the system. This repeated feedback loop is crucial for the creation of trustworthy object detection systems as well as continuous improvement.Explainable AI also helps with regulatory compliance. As the usage of autonomous vehicles spreads, regulatory frameworks are being developed to ensure safety and accountability, Omeiza, D., et al (2021), legal criteria are met by explainable AI, which offers a transparent framework that is auditable and validateable.

There are five parts to this paperwork. The introductionportion work that was covered in Section I. The shortcomings and restrictions of the current systems are examined in Section II. In Section III, we explained our recently proposed system design work for explainable AI-based semantic object detection for autonomous vehicles. The explanation and thorough output result for our recently built system are provided in Section IV. The end of this study is covered in Section V.

LITERATURE REVIEW

This literature review explores the rapidly evolving field of autonomous vehicle technologies, with a focus on integrating XAI concepts to improve transparency and interpretability in semantic object identification algorithms. Understanding the methods, challenges, and advancements in explainable AI is crucial as the demand for prudent and astute decision-making in self-driving cars grows. This survey aims to illustrate the crucial relationship between state-of-the-art technology and the crucial need for transparency in autonomous systems by analyzing the major contributions, strategies, and emerging patterns in the field of explainable AI-based semantic object identification.

Mankodiya et al., (2022), describes a method for semantic object detection in autonomous cars using explainable AI (XAI). The authors propose a method called OD-XAI to enhance the interpretability of object detection algorithms in autonomous vehicles. The goal of this work is to demonstrate that autonomous vehicles (AVs) can identify and segment their path using deep learning (DL) models. Three semantic segmentation architectures were trained and evaluated with the goal of pixel-wise road detection. The maximum IoU scores on the test and train sets were 0.9621 and 0.9459, respectively. These deep learning algorithms are referred to as "black box models" due to the difficulty in understanding their exceedingly intricate design.With XAI, they can interpret and comprehend the predictions of these abstract models. Using a range of XAI methods, they produced justifications for the proposed segmentation model for road detection in autonomous vehicles.

Ponn, et al (2020),uses cameras to tackle problems with automated vehicle object detection. Finding and comprehending the difficult situations that come up during this process is the primary objective of the study. In this study, these additional variables that impact camera-based object detection accuracy are thoroughly investigated for the first time. To make matters worse, it is challenging to appropriately characterize the detection performance and explain specific detection findings because the existing algorithms are based on artificial intelligence. In order to evaluate and explain the detection performance of various object detection techniques, a modeling technique based on the examined effect variables is provided, and the recently developed SHapley Additive exPlanations (SHAP) methodology is utilized.The findings demonstrate that, independent of the detection technique, many factors affecting detection performance always have the same impact. Two examples of these parameters are the object's positioning inside the image and its relative rotation toward the camera. The findings demonstrate that, irrespective of the detection technique employed, a number of significant parameters, such as an object's location on the picture or its relative rotation towards the camera, significantly impact the detection performance. Specifically, the vulnerabilities found in the analyzed object detectors could be leveraged to create important and demanding situations for automated car testing and type certification processes.

Thakker et al (2020) detailed in the paper, which offers a novel approach utilizing Semantic Web technologies and is demonstrated with a smart cities flood monitoring application inside the context of an EU-funded project. Overviewing "explainable deep learning" as a subset of the "explainable AI" challenge, the paper provides an outline of the concept. Monitoring of drainage and gullies in strategic areas that are vulnerable to flooding issues should be a component of any flood monitoring system. Cameras are used to display the impacted areas in real-time after a DL-based classifier is often developed to detect things such as leaves, plastic bottles, and other objects. The existence and coverage of these objects in the input data are then used to train the classifier to identify blockages. They inventively provide an Explainable AI solution in this article by combining DL and Semantic

Web technologies to build a hybrid classifier. In this hybrid classifier, the DL component determines item existence and coverage level, while the semantic rules, developed in close collaboration with experts, do categorization. Our hybrid classifier makes use of expert knowledge specifically linked to flooding, providing flexibility in classifying the image based on elements and their coverage links. The experimental findings, shown with a real-world use case, showed that the hybrid approach to image classification performed 11% better on average (F-Measure) than the DL-only classifier. Another noteworthy advantage is that it applies experts' knowledge in developing guidelines for decision-making to account for complex circumstances.

Atakishiyev et al. (2021), makes intelligent decision-making entirely intelligible to humans, yet current autonomous vehicles lack a component that accomplishes this. As a result, society views technology less favorably. Because of this, AI systems for driverless cars need to be able to defend its conclusions in real time and make safe decisions while still adhering to international rules and regulations. This research provides important insight into the process of developing explainable artificial intelligence (XAI) solutions for self-driving cars. In specifically, they offer the following contributions. The most recent XAI research for autonomous driving is first given in-depth overview form. They continue by offering a XAI paradigm that considers the social and legal conditions necessary for autonomous driving systems to be rational. Lastly, they provide a range of XAI methodologies as prospective research topics for later work that can improve operational safety and transparency to assist regulators and other stakeholders in embracing autonomous driving technology.

Moradi et al. (2023) emphasizes model-independent explainable AI techniques for object recognition in image data. By using a unique masking methodology for AI-based object identification systems, we propose and implement a black-box explanation approach called Black-box Object identification Explanation by Masking (BODEM). To generate several versions of an input image, we advise using both local and remote masking techniques. Distant masks measure the impact of disturbing pixels outside of an object on the detection model's conclusions, whereas local masks perturb pixels inside a target item to see how the object detector responds to these changes. A saliency map is subsequently produced, indicating the relative importance of each pixel based on the comparison of the detection output pre- and post-masking. To show how important each pixel in the original image is in relation to the objects that were located, a heatmap is then constructed. Experiments on different models and datasets of object detection have demonstrated that BODEM is a useful tool for interpreting object detector behavior and identifying shortcomings. This enables BODEM to be used in settings such as black-box software testing to evaluate and explain AI-based object detection methods. Data augmentation tests also conducted by BODEM suggest that the local masks generated by the system might be utilized to further train the object detectors and enhance the robustness and precision of their detection services.

Hussain et al. (2021), eXplainable Artificial Intelligence (XAI) is defined as a collection of approaches and procedures for turning so-called "black-box" AI algorithms into "white-box" algorithms, which produce results that are transparent and explicable and provide information about the parameters, factors, and steps the algorithm used to arrive at those results. The authors of this work take a `engineering' approach to illustrate the principles of XAI, adding to the body of previous research on the subject. They go over the stakeholders in XAI while providing an engineering viewpoint on the mathematical structure of the system. After that, we use an autonomous car as a case study to discuss the numerous uses of XAI for its various components, including perception, object recognition, control, action decision-making, and so on.

Olszewska (2022) the paper "Snakes in Trees: An Explainable Artificial Intelligence Approach for Automatic Object Detection and Recognition" is presented, outlining a novel explainable system that makes use of snakes that reside inside trees to sense and identify objects automatically. The suggested approach uses recursive snake computation, or parametric active contours. This results in multi-layered snakes, with the first layer representing the main object of interest and the subsequent levels defining the various foreground sub-parts. These snakes divide the world into areas based on visual clues that they interpret into semantic notions. Decision trees are generated based on these attributes, which leads to efficient semantic categorization of the pieces and automatic scene annotation. In relation to smart cities,

Dong, J.,et al(2023)aims to develop explainable Deep Learning (DL) models that will improve the dependability of autonomous driving systems by looking into the literature. The work expresses the decision-making process of the AV system as an image-based language creation (or image captioning) problem, as opposed to the conventional classification objective. To provide human-understandable explanations, the suggested method creates textual descriptions of the driving events before making any driving decisions. This results in the suggestion of a revolutionary multi-modal deep learning architecture that can mimic the correlation between an image (driving state) and a language (descriptions) at the same time. The Transformer-based structure of its complete system allows it to effectively simulate the learning processes of human drivers and perform worldwide attention.The results show that, in addition to producing appropriate driving judgments for autonomous vehicles (AVs), the suggested model can also produce coherent and valid words to explain specific driving scenarios. Additionally, it is noted that the suggested model performs noticeably better in terms of creating explanations and motivating actions than many baseline models. Given that the suggested model explains the behavior of an antivirus program, it may help boost end-user confidence.

Fujiyoshi, H., et al (2019),discusses deep learning for image recognition in the context of autonomous cars. It provides insights on the development and challenges of using deep learning models to recognize and interpret visual data—which is crucial for self-driving cars—and specializes in complex computational techniques. The purpose of the paper "Deep learning-based image recognition for autonomous driving" is to provide light on the advancements and challenges in the field of autonomous driving by utilizing deep learning techniques for picture recognition.

Muhammad, K.,et al(2022)the paper's conclusions are as follows as a consequence: Scene recognition for vision-sensor-based autonomous vehicles is still a field that requires significant work. That's why the majority of the scene understanding research that is now being done involves computationally sophisticated deep learning models. This assessment defines, examines, and assesses the current state of the area. We also look at state-of-the-art performance and temporal complexity studies of state-of-the-art modeling alternatives, in addition to covering the fundamental scene understanding pipeline. Not to add, distinguished achievements as well as noteworthy shortcomings of current research projects are emphasized. Furthermore, the paper offers an extensive summary of the datasets that are currently available along with an analysis of the difficulties that researchers continue to encounter despite their late achievements.Finally, to welcome researchers and practitioners to this exciting area, our work suggests directions for future study.

Bourdon, P., et al. (2021),Together with the details of the broader medical imaging background, Explainable Artificial Intelligence (XAI) is used to evaluate these types of imaging-related challenges. They also go over the rise in popularity of deep learning in this field and examine machine learning techniques created for breast cancer diagnosis. In actuality, despite the encouraging outcomes of the past few years, cutting edge research indicates that deep learning systems confront numerous significant hurdles. Talk about the latest developments and solutions to these problems as well.

Shen et al. (2022) examines how semantic AI may affect security in the setting of autonomous cars. In the rapidly developing field of semantic artificial intelligence (AI) security studies, they conduct the first thorough knowledge organization. 53 of these publications are collected, examined, and arranged by them according to important study facets for the security field. Based on quantitative comparisons between security works from closely comparable areas and current AD AI securities works vertically, they have compiled a list of the six most significant scientific gaps that we have found. These could offer perceptions and possible paths for the community, research purpose, methodology, and design in addition to design.They take the lead in bridging the largest methodology-level gap in science by creating PASS, an open-source, standard, and extensible system-driven evaluation platform for the semantic AD AI security research community. They moreover use representative semantic AD AI assaults on our created platform prototype to illustrate the capabilities and benefits of such a platform.

SYSTEM DESIGN

This chapter assessed the K-Means clustering algorithm for object segmentation against the other system segmentation and classification approaches currently in use in order to establish the most efficient method for explainable AI-based object identification of driverless autos. Figure 2 below the architecture displays the general block diagram for analysis. The stage that comes after the initial image pre-processing is called image enhancement. The process of segmenting photos is then initiated with the finished output. This stage's output is sent to the categorization phase. After this is done, the total performances are compared with the existing methods.

Explainable Artificial Intelligence

It is important to comprehend the decision-making process behind a particular item detector detection in order to provide context. Yet, due to their numerous trainable weights and hierarchical nonlinear struc-

Figure 2. Proposed system design

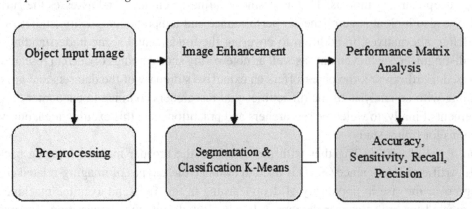

ture, deep neural networks—the foundation of all currently available object detectors—are inherently opaque. Therefore, developing methods that improve decision transparency and provide understandable explanations for individual actions is the aim of the recently established field of research known as eXplanatory Artificial Intelligence (XAI). In recent years, numerous methods have been proposed for this goal. The so-called model-agnostic interpretation method is explained in this section. Next, a K-Means is displayed, allowing for a quicker and easier approximation of the explanation.

K-Means Clustering Algorithm

K-means clustering is a simple, unsupervised technique for segmentation item discovery. Using this K-means approach, the total number of clusters and cluster centers is computed using the following image. It is necessary to choose cluster locations that maintain a safe distance from the cluster core in order to achieve effective clustering. Once the connecting of pixels in several clusters is finished, the pixels are prematurely aggregated. Next, based on distance measurements, new cluster centers are found and data points are assigned to them.

The pseudocode for K-Means clustering algorithm is shown in the above figure 3. New pixels are added or removed from each cluster throughout each iteration phase, which also affects the cluster's centroid. This iteration 75 procedure is repeated until there is no variance in the cluster centers. The final image shows the clustered output of the K-means algorithm. The K-means algorithm is used iteratively in two steps to minimize the distance between a data point and its centroid. This technique determines whether the image has any naturally occurring clusters by compiling a set of data characteristics from the vector space. It divides the pixels into a preset number of clusters using relatively straightforward processes.

The iterative two-step K-means technique can be used to reduce the distance between data points and the centroid of k-clusters. In the first step, the c centroid is calculated, and in the second phase, each data point is assigned to the cluster whose centroid is closest to that specific data point. The Euclidean distance is one of the methods most frequently used to determine the distance to the nearest centroid. Following grouping, the cluster points are assigned to the Euclidean distance that minimizes the distance between each center and each data point based on the centroid, and each cluster's new centroid is recalculated. The clusters of a partition are defined by its centroid and member items. The point at which all of the

Figure 3. Pseudocode for K-means algorithm

Algorithm 4: K-means Clustering

Step 1: Input image

Step 2: Get the values of k and choose the cluster centers

Step 3: Calculate the distance between pixels and cluster centers

Step 4: Assign each pixel to the nearest cluster center

Step 5: Compute the mean i.e. Cluster for each cluster

Step 6: Check whether there is any variation in cluster centers

Case1: If yes, then set the new mean as cluster centers and follow step 3

Case2: If no, then compute the statistics and separable information items in a cluster are separated from one another by their total distance is known as the cluster's centroid. The centroid-based technique is an iterative procedure that minimizes the overall distances between each item and its cluster centroid across all clusters. Assuming a collection of centers, V = {v1,v2,....,vc}, and a set of data points, X = {x1,x2,x3,.....,xn}.

1.   Choose "c" cluster centers at random.
2.   Determine how far apart each data point is from the cluster centers.
3.   Assign the data point to the cluster center that has the shortest distance between it and the other cluster centers.
4.   4. Utilizing, recalculate the new cluster center:

$$vi = (1ci) \sum xci\,j=1\ j \qquad\qquad (1)$$

Where the number of data points in the ith cluster is denoted by "ci".

5.   Compute the distances between every data point and the recently discovered cluster centers once more.
6.   Stop if no data point is reassigned, and then go back to step 3 if not.

If the original cluster center is chosen wrongly and the method converges to local minima, the resulting cluster will be erroneous. Typically, the first cluster centers are chosen at random from the incoming photographs. Throughout the clustering process, it is imperative to take into account the local link between the data points. Using the histogram approach, the mean intensity value for each tissue class is initialized.

Diagram 4 illustrates the pre- and post-K-means clustering algorithm operation. Image intensities are re-distributed inside the cluster upon the convergence of the cluster means recalculation. This means

Figure 4. K-means clustering

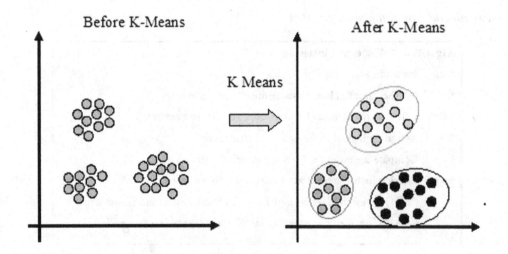

Figure 5. Flowchart of K-means clustering algorithm

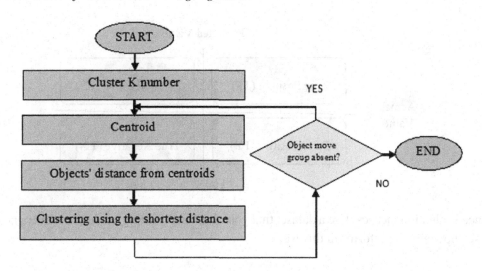

that the output mask contains tissue class labels ranging from one to K. The K-means algorithm has a disadvantage despite being a straightforward clustering technique.

The ideal centroid is attained by resolving a difficult optimization issue, and its initial position dictates the quality of the ultimate solution. Although randomization is the most popular initialization, other techniques can be applied depending on the situation to choose the initial centroid.The K-means clustering model algorithm is displayed in Figure 5. The following part covered the overall comparison result between the suggested system and the current system.

RESULT AND DISCUSSION

In addition to presenting contemporary object detectors, this section gives an overview of several assessment metrics. Images from the automated driving domain must be gathered for the continuing research. The performance of the object detectors will be analyzed, modeled, and explained using this data set. The production process demands a large time and resource commitment because the data set needs to be as large as feasible and every item in the pictures needs to be tagged. Thus, the most relevant data set is chosen after looking through those that are available to the general publicKang, Y.; et al (2019). Additionally, a large number of the relevant data sets for automated driving that have been released into the public domain for research are also somewhat recent. When applying K-Means techniques for object detection, Random Forest, Decision Tree, and KNN algorithms are used. The recently proposed K-Means study makes use of MATLAB 2013A to calculate a classifier mean's efficacy.

Performance Metrics

Figure 6, the confusion matrix, provides an example and synopsis of a categorization technique's efficacy. The performance analysis of the K Means machine learning classification models can be evaluated using

Figure 6. Confusion matrix

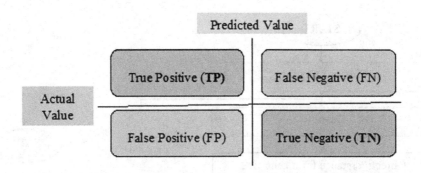

performance evaluation metrics. Use a dataset that your machine learning model has never encountered before to see how well it performs in this way.

Accuracy

A figure representing an error rate that deviates from 100% is displayed by the accuracy formula. Prior to assessing accuracy, the error rate must be evaluated. Error rate as a percentage can also be obtained by dividing the observed value by the actual value.

Accuracy = (TP+TN)/(TP+TN+FN+FP)

Refer to figure 7 above and table 1 for the accuracy result using the recommended and current technologies. By comparing the K Means with other existing systems, they are 94.58% accurate.

Sensitivity

By dividing the total number of positives by the number of precise positive forecasts, one can calculate sensitivity.

Sensitivity = TP/(TP+FN)

Table 1. Accuracy

Algorithm	Accuracy (%)
KNN	83.36
DT	84.46
RF	86.35
K Means	94.58

Figure 7. Accuracy graph

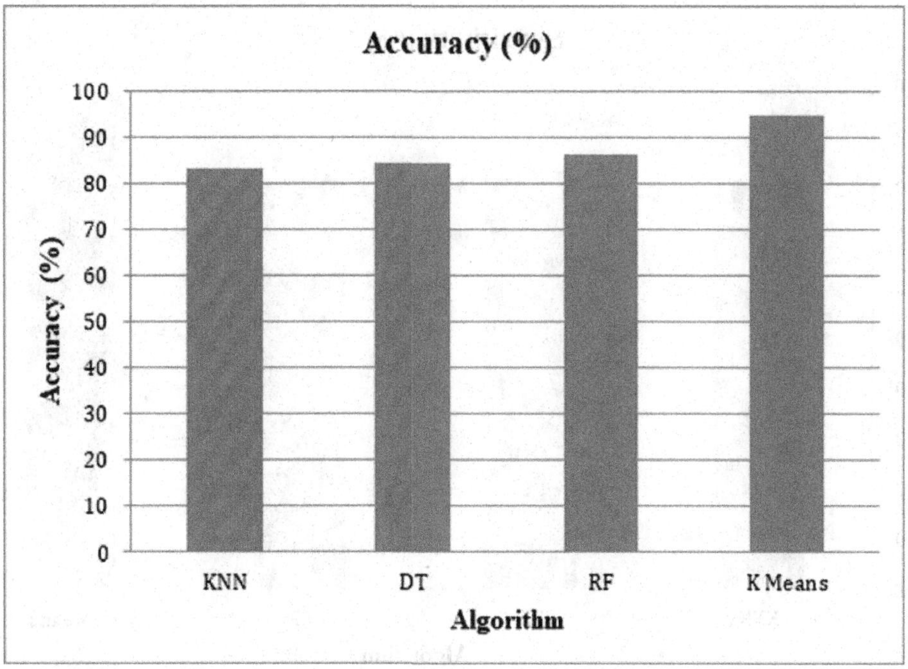

Table 2. Sensitivity

Algorithm	Sensitivity (%)
KNN	81.17
DT	83.52
RF	85.76
K Means	92.14

Table 2 yields the sensitivity results with the current and recommended systems, which are shown in the previously described figure 8. It shows that the K Means produces a higher sensitivity result of 92.14%, which is better than the comparative existing approaches.

Recall

Recall provides information about the model's ability to identify true positives. This instance shows how few patients with the condition were actually found because there are no genuine positives. There are two false negatives accessible.

Recall = (TP) / (TP+FN)

The results of the recall utilizing the recommended and current systems are shown in Figure 9, which was previously addressed and is derived from Table 3. According to the plotted graph, our

Figure 8. Sensitivity graph

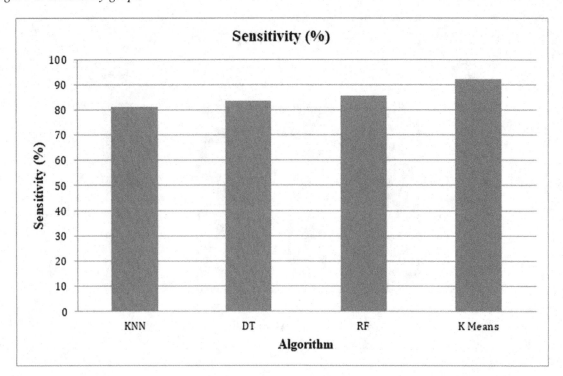

Table 3. Recall

Algorithm	Recall (%)
KNN	80.45
DT	82.36
RF	86.24
K Means	90.36

newly constructed K Means system offers a recall of 90.36% higher than the previously described current systems.

Precision

The accuracy level indicates how well many measures agree with one another. You can evaluate precision by computing the average deviation, which sums together the measurement errors.

Precision =TP/((TP+FP))

A screenshot taken from Table 10 is shown in Figure 10, which shows how precise the recommended and available technologies are. Plotting the results shows that our newly designed K Means system outperforms the previously described existing approaches with a precision of 93.69%.

Figure 9. Recall graph

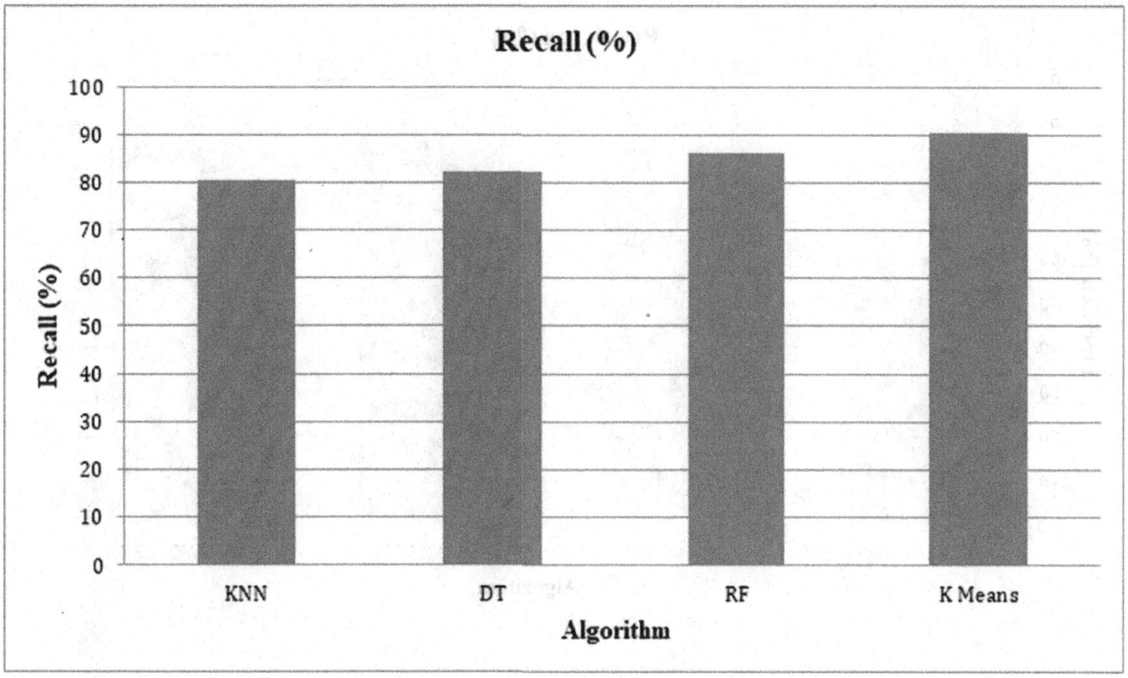

Table 4. Precision

Algorithm	Precision (%)
KNN	84.52
DT	87.18
RF	89.72
K Means	93.69

CONCLUSION

This work provides a comprehensive, interpretable performance analysis of object detectors used in automated driving using AI. Then, a unique method is shown that enables the modeling and even explanation of the behavior of machine learning-based object detectors using simple models (K-Means). The very high accuracy shown by the trained K-Means for forecasting the detection performance supports the assumption that an object's detection result may normally be connected to its presented information. Therefore, a simple K-Means algorithm might replicate the detection ability of an object detector with high accuracy by combining data about the object's characteristics and the surrounding environment from a large collection of autonomous vehicles.By modeling and explaining the object detectors using AI data, it will be feasible to discover challenging scenarios for automated vehicle testing in the future. An further use for these models is in virtual simulation. The established K-Means methodology may be used to any type of object detector and achieves 94.58% accuracy, as demonstrated by the nearly similar

Figure 10. Precision graph

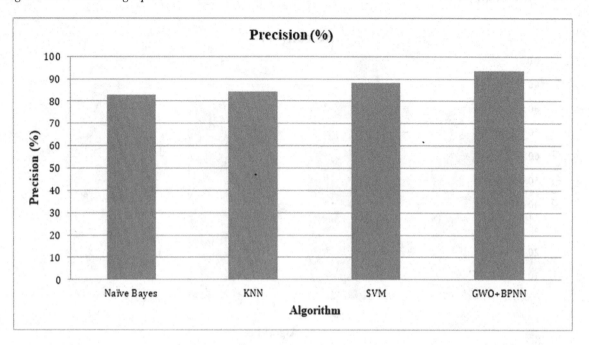

results for all object detectors studied. Eventually, other algorithms will be added to the XAIsystem to provide textual explanations to users.

REFERENCES

Antoniadi, A. M., Du, Y., Guendouz, Y., Wei, L., Mazo, C., Becker, B. A., & Mooney, C. (2021). Current challenges and future opportunities for XAI in machine learning-based clinical decision support systems: A systematic review. *Applied Sciences (Basel, Switzerland)*, *11*(11), 5088. doi:10.3390/app11115088

Arrieta, A. B., Díaz-Rodríguez, N., Del Ser, J., Bennetot, A., Tabik, S., Barbado, A., & Herrera, F. (2020). Explainable Artificial Intelligence (XAI): Concepts, taxonomies, opportunities and challenges toward responsible AI. *Information Fusion*, *58*, 82–115. doi:10.1016/j.inffus.2019.12.012

Atakishiyev, S., Salameh, M., Yao, H., & Goebel, R. (2021). Explainable artificial intelligence for autonomous driving: A comprehensive overview and field guide for future research directions. *arXiv preprint arXiv:2112.11561*.

Aziz, L., Salam, M. S. B. H., Sheikh, U. U., & Ayub, S. (2020). Exploring deep learning-based architecture, strategies, applications and current trends in generic object detection: A comprehensive review. *IEEE Access: Practical Innovations, Open Solutions*, *8*, 170461–170495. doi:10.1109/ACCESS.2020.3021508

Bourdon, P., Ahmed, O. B., Urruty, T., Djemal, K., & Fernandez-Maloigne, C. (2021). Explainable ai for medical imaging: Knowledge matters. *Multi-faceted Deep Learning: Models and Data*.

Dong, J., Chen, S., Miralinaghi, M., Chen, T., Li, P., & Labi, S. (2023). Why did the AI make that decision? Towards an explainable artificial intelligence (XAI) for autonomous driving systems. *Transportation Research Part C, Emerging Technologies, 156*, 104358. doi:10.1016/j.trc.2023.104358

Fujiyoshi, H., Hirakawa, T., & Yamashita, T. (2019). Deep learning-based image recognition for autonomous driving. *IATSS Research, 43*(4), 244–252. doi:10.1016/j.iatssr.2019.11.008

Hussain, F., Hussain, R., & Hossain, E. (2021). Explainable artificial intelligence (XAI): An engineering perspective. *arXiv preprint arXiv:2101.03613*.

Kang, Y., Yin, H., & Berger, C. (2019). Test Your Self-Driving Algorithm: An Overview of Publicly Available Driving Datasets and Virtual Testing Environments. [Google Scholar] [CrossRef]. *IEEE Transactions on Intelligent Vehicles, 4*(2), 171–185. doi:10.1109/TIV.2018.2886678

Mankodiya, H., Jadav, D., Gupta, R., Tanwar, S., Hong, W. C., & Sharma, R. (2022). Od-xai: Explainable ai-based semantic object detection for autonomous vehicles. *Applied Sciences (Basel, Switzerland), 12*(11), 5310. doi:10.3390/app12115310

Moradi, M., Yan, K., Colwell, D., Samwald, M., & Asgari, R. (2023). Model-agnostic explainable artificial intelligence for object detection in image data. *arXiv preprint arXiv:2303.17249*. doi:10.2139/ssrn.4429462

Muhammad, K., Hussain, T., Ullah, H., Del Ser, J., Rezaei, M., Kumar, N., & de Albuquerque, V. H. C. (2022). Vision-based semantic segmentation in scene understanding for autonomous driving: Recent achievements, challenges, and outlooks. *IEEE Transactions on Intelligent Transportation Systems, 23*(12), 22694–22715. doi:10.1109/TITS.2022.3207665

Olszewska, J. I. (2022, February). Snakes in Trees: An Explainable Artificial Intelligence Approach for Automatic Object Detection and Recognition. In ICAART (3) (pp. 996-1002).

Omeiza, D., Webb, H., Jirotka, M., & Kunze, L. (2021). Explanations in autonomous driving: A survey. *IEEE Transactions on Intelligent Transportation Systems, 23*(8), 10142–10162. doi:10.1109/TITS.2021.3122865

Ponn, T., Kröger, T., & Diermeyer, F. (2020). Identification and explanation of challenging conditions for camera-based object detection of automated vehicles. *Sensors (Basel), 20*(13), 3699. doi:10.3390/s20133699 PMID:32630350

Shen, J., Wang, N., Wan, Z., Luo, Y., Sato, T., Hu, Z., & Chen, Q. A. (2022). Sok: On the semantic ai security in autonomous driving. *arXiv preprint arXiv:2203.05314*.

Thakker, D., Mishra, B. K., Abdullatif, A., Mazumdar, S., & Simpson, S. (2020). Explainable artificial intelligence for developing smart cities solutions. *Smart Cities, 3*(4), 1353–1382. doi:10.3390/smartcities3040065

Tyagi, A. K., & Aswathy, S. U. (2021). Autonomous Intelligent Vehicles (AIV): Research statements, open issues, challenges and road for future. *International Journal of Intelligent Networks, 2*, 83–102. doi:10.1016/j.ijin.2021.07.002

Wang, J., Li, Y., Zhou, Z., Wang, C., Hou, Y., Zhang, L., & Chen, S. (2022). When, where and how does it fail? A spatial-temporal visual analytics approach for interpretable object detection in autonomous driving. *IEEE Transactions on Visualization and Computer Graphics*. PMID:36040948

Zablocki, É., Ben-Younes, H., Pérez, P., & Cord, M. (2022). Explainability of deep vision-based autonomous driving systems: Review and challenges. *International Journal of Computer Vision*, *130*(10), 2425–2452. doi:10.1007/s11263-022-01657-x

Zhao, J., Zhao, W., Deng, B., Wang, Z., Zhang, F., Zheng, W., & Burke, A. F. (2023). Autonomous driving system: A comprehensive survey. *Expert Systems with Applications*, 122836.

Chapter 3
AI–Based In–Cabin Monitoring System for Autonomous Vehicles

Ajith K.
Karpagam Academy of Higher Education, India

R. Sharmila
Karpagam Academy of Higher Education, India

ABSTRACT

Fully autonomous vehicles (FAVs) require internal monitoring in order to function without a human driver. The far-from-sufficient FAV, sufficient in-cabin monitoring is a prerequisite to ensure both people and vehicles. On public roadways, there are a lot of accidents that happen, most of them are the result of reckless driving. Modern driver monitoring systems evaluate driver behavior and, if necessary, highlight risky driving behaviours using special sensor technologies. The result accurately predicted bounding boxes and the real data show a considerable amount of overlap. Unlike most past efforts, the authors use a random forest to learn a template-based model. This way, forecast the object probability of a window in a sliding window technique and regress its aspect ratio using a single mode at the same time. Examined mobility services at increasing degrees autonomy, including the exercise caution and the best ways.

INTRODUCTION

Systems for intelligent surveillance and monitoring are commonly employed to guarantee security and safety. Closed-circuit television (CCTV) and video surveillance cameras are common forms of public monitoring. Intelligent transportation systems also use video monitoring for tasks like road traffic and in-cab monitoring. Public visual information is also necessary for driving automation to do various duties. However, these AVs may be operated by the driver a human if necessary. The cars meant solely for passenger use; they lack drivers. As a result, nobody is responsible for such AVs. Moreover, the occupants of shared and public transportation (such ridesharing, car-sharing, and car-full services in

DOI: 10.4018/979-8-3693-1962-8.ch003

autonomous vehicles) are unfamiliar with each other. Therefore, it's imperative to ensure each individual sat in such AVs is secure and healthy. The vehicle should also be protected from external dangers and/ or any malicious behavior on the part of its occupants. As a result, FAVs essentially need a complex, real-time in-cabin monitoring task.

In-Cabin Monitoring

Bosch et al. have proposed visible light camera's eye-tracking. The works that the authors have reviewed have shown signs of anger, fear, melancholy, curiosity, humiliation, urgency, boredom, annoyance, and other emotions. In level 4 autonomous vehicles, driver monitoring plays a major role in advanced driving (ADAS). In the authors, Yifang, et al (2020) have examined problems to developments linked automobiles several efforts and the AI techniques employed to guarantee the safety of AVs within the cabin. Popular AI techniques for three distinct tasks driving assistance, takeover preparedness, and driver status monitoring have been enlisted. Emotion, tiredness, distraction, and attention detection are all included in driver status monitoring. Intention analysis and warnings about driving risks are features of driver assistance, while evaluation of takeover preparation is a feature of takeover readiness. They have included several works using AI for these tasks in their survey. There has been an evaluation of the driving monitoring and assistance systems. They investigated driving while taking the driver, the vehicle, and the road environment into consideration. This review focuses on the following factors: driver distraction, driver weariness, and aggressive driving style.

Safety and Security in Level Four and Beyond AVs

Protecting someone or something from harm, risk, or danger is what it means to be safe. Protection of people and property against outside dangers and illegal activity is referred to as security. Security and safety measures must be included in an antivirus program. Ensuring the security of an individual or object from inadvertent mishaps is known as safety. In a similar vein, security is defence against intentional harm by Mallaboyev, N. M., et al (2022). When it comes to the main issues about vehicle needs from being mishandled, but the occupants also need safety.

Occupants and Objects

Many categories seen inside the AV's cabin are taken into account when creating the database. Passengers, kids, pets, smoking materials, mobile phones, car seats, drinks, luggage, personal possessions, and hazardous or destructive objects are among them by Rathi, B. Senthil et al (2021). Volunteers were observed doing one activity at a time and sporadically executing numerous activities while their photographs were being taken.

Cellular and Electronic Devices

It's possible that the car's interior has electronic and cell phone devices. These could be tablets, laptops, cell phones, or any combination of these. Nonetheless, require identification in order trace misplaced or lost device since they can identify certain images that include gadgets and cell phones.

Smoking Items

Since smoking is harmful to your health, it should not be allowed in public areas. Public transportation should be applied to vehicles that are shared or utilized for transportation. As a result, smoking is not allowed within this kind of vehicle. Therefore, smoking item detection needs to be a part of the IMS for the security and safety of drivers and passengers. We have separated out smoking products into four categories: cases, lighters, e-cigarettes, and cigarettes.

Food and Beverages

To maintain the cleanliness and safety of the in-cabin, detection is crucial when it comes to shared vehicle food and beverages. A passenger's eating or drinking during the voyage could annoy other passengers. For instance, spilling on others can occur from negligent eating or drinking. Additionally, the lingering food and drink debris could pose a risk to the subsequent occupants of the car. Additionally, this kind of litter can interfere with car controls, seriously impairing vehicle safety. In order to alert passengers in the event that using food or beverages within a car causes any issues.

Harmful Objects

Weapons, dangerous equipment, and harmful items must be identified in order prevent stop any acts of violence or vandalism to protect the higher-end autonomous driving vehicles. Tools including screwdrivers, scissors, baseball bats, knives, and so on have been confiscated as potentially hazardous materials. Here are a handful of these pictures.

Face Anonymization

For public surveillance systems, privacy is a major concern. As an open monitoring system, IMS experiences the same issue. Many nations have placed stringent limitations on the use of facial recognition technology in public spaces in order to protect personal data. By protecting, facial anonymization effectively resolves this problem. An effective approach for the face anonymization of the inhabitants has been proposed in our earlier studies. For face swapping and re-enactment, GAN is employed. We advise utilizing the virtual human faces produced by GANs as the source image. By doing this, improved anonymization is guaranteed. Preserving the face features of the target image is important.

Face Detection

The majority of object detection research in static pictures has been on face and person detection. These domains were chosen because face and person detection are critical steps in most systems involving human-computer interaction. Basic forms and constraints are used by the majority of early face detection programs. Kumar, Ashu et al (2019) developed a technique that can recognize face components by using local restrictions on an image pyramid. It explains an analogous rule-based approach. Rule-based approaches are beneficial in terms of processing cost and work well for faces due to their regular internal structure. By storing a human face as a set of binary relationships between the mean intensities of eleven distinct regions, the concept of the "template ratio" was extended. The template ratio method worked on the assumption that these correlations would hold true in the face of significant changes in illumination direction and intensity.

AI Camera Positioning

There are two primary issues with FAVs and two primary issues with the front-facing cameras that are placed for external influences. Besides, it's hard to watch the second row from the front of the car because of obstructions in your line of sight. Two front-facing cameras are required to fully monitor the in-cabin entertainment system in FAVs, as depicted in these drawings Mishra, Ashutosh et al (2022). Outside, it will also double the difficulty of the same challenge. There will be similar issues with every other AI camera. That being said, the recommended position place powerful IMS activates something strange it becomes necessary to conduct thorough observation or surveillance in addition to obtaining evidence.

Comparison of Popular Object Detection Models

We have compared several AI algorithms to determine which strategy is optimal item identification methods are enumerated and surveyed. One example is "you only look once (YOLO or yolo)", which classification for one of them. An example of a two-stage detector is R-CNN. Even though there are many variations of both types, the algorithms' effectiveness depends on how they are implemented. Regarding inference delay, one-stage techniques are considered, and in terms of accuracy, two-stage detectors are thought to be suitable explain by Faniadis, Efstathios, and Angelos Amanatiadis (2020). These methods' retrained weights are currently accessible for a wide range of object categories. However, using the pre trained weights of these algorithms directly was producing false results. This failure can be related to the viewing angle of the AI camera.

In-Cabin Measurement

This technique gauges the concentration of pollutants within the cabin in particular environmental conditions. Depending on ISO 16000-6:2011 requirements, either a Summa canister, Tedlar bag, or Tenax-TA tube is used for this. SVOCs are examined using GC/MS utilizing a polyurethane foam (PUF) sample used by Lan, Hangzhen (2020). Volatile carbonyls, such as formaldehyde, are sampled using DNPH cartridges and evaluated using high-performance liquid chromatography (HPLC), following ISO 16000-3:2011. When it comes to the identification and measurement of VOCs SVOCs, on-site monitoring method may be suitable in addition to the off-site analysis. For instance, portable tools such typically used the field to detect the PM concentrations in-cabin. Because they are simple to use in the field, in-cabin measurements are frequently utilized.

Machine Learning

A key characteristic that unites a wide variety of techniques, heuristics, and algorithms is machine learning: they somehow endow a system with the capacity to carry out a certain task by means of a collection of cases. By giving the system a collection of example patterns from both classes from a set of training data, we hope to automatically teach the system the characteristics that distinguish one class from the other within the context of our pattern classification problem. The positive and negative instances have labels of +1 and -1, respectively. The degree of performance that the trained system attains on a collection of instances that were absent from the training set, or test set, is the objective and a key indicator of success. By using the test set to assess performance, we are able to ascertain the system's ability to generalize to data that it has never seen before.

A model of the domain, or an input/output mapping, is what is meant to be extracted by the system from a set of training examples. This is the definition of the task of learning from examples. This kind of tactic appeals to me especially for several reasons. Most importantly, we can learn a problem's attributes via instances, which spares us from having to explicitly build a solution. A customized solution may suffer when a user imposes what he considers to be the essential components or characteristics of a decision problem by Greener, Joe G., et al (2022). A learning-based approach abstracts away the important components and relationships in a decision problem automatically as a trained model. However, learning-based techniques may have the issue of poor generalization due to overfitting, in which the model has "too well" mastered the decision problem and is unable to generalize to new data.

The five sections of this essay are listed below: Session 2 of the current system shows its shortcomings in object detection using kaggle datasets and other machine learning and artificial learning techniques. The third session was a demonstration of the suggested sentiment analysis method. It blends Random Forest (HCSO RF) with Hybrid Chicken Swarm Optimization concepts. The outcomes of the anticipated system are shown in Session 4. An examination of the recommended approach for object detection in vehicle cabins rounds off Session 5.

RELATED WORKS

Artificial and machine learning approaches are covered in this section. A summary of pertinent literature is provided prior to using this evaluation to pinpoint knowledge gaps and make clear particular research goals.

Several businesses have lately revealed that their in-cabin surveillance systems use deep learning models like YOLO versions to track driver behavior in an effort to improve passenger safety and security. The car owners have also been surveyed regarding the AI methods employed for in-cabin surveillance. They claim that services applications car is made feasible by artificial intelligence (AI). The release of an in-car monitoring dataset enables interior vehicle monitoring byKatrolia, Jigyasa Singh, et al (2021). A hardware implementation for monitoring a car's occupants and driver has been completed. Poon, Yen-Sok, et al (2022) developing a driver monitoring system with deep learning and in-cabin surveillance; they have also gathered a dataset of telemetry and video data for this use.

Person Identification

Among the multipurpose objectives of facial recognition technology are classification, discrimination, and recognition. Urbanization and smart cities demand facial recognition for a multitude of purposes. Consequently, a range of person-identifying facial recognition systems have been given by earlier researchers. Three types of face recognition methods exist: local, holistic, and hybrid. While holistic approaches use the full face, including the background, local methods only use a subset of the features on the face for facial identification. Hybrid approaches integrate both local and comprehensive techniques, as their name suggests. With the advent of artificial intelligence (AI) that makes use of CNNs and DL, facial recognition algorithm performance has grown. Dixit, Priyanka, and Sanjay Silakari (2021) made public DeepFace, a deep neural network-powered facial recognition system. Furthermore, multiple further enlarged forms of DeepFace have been verified by independent investigations. Thorough examination of face recognition techniques, comparative analysis, and prospective uses in the future were conducted. Common facial recognition techniques were divided into three categories: hybrid, holistic, and local techniques. Different approaches were compared for accuracy, complexity, and robustness. The advantages and disadvantages of each tactic were also examined. Wang et al. successfully reviewed deep learning-based facial recognition techniques in their work. They investigated in detail a number of popular DL-based techniques, including autoencoder-, CNN-, and GAN-based methods have produced a summary of the primary technology roadblocks and emerging real-world issues with deep facial recognition.

In-cabin monitoring was used in an experiment to examine how drivers interacted with automated driving. This study aimed to apply a similar methodology with FAVs. The detection of violence in vehicles is reviewed by an Authors Saxena, Anvita et al (2020) have investigated a range of research papers and artificial intelligence techniques for emotional recognition in cars in order to identify violent situations in carpooling services. An analysis of the in-vehicle monitoring system (IVMS) revealed the need for in-cabin passenger anomaly detection in order to curb unsafe driving behaviors. Their system included a camera and a computer, according to a patent filing, and it was deemed appropriate for a modern car. Among its responsibilities were identifying the seat, the individuals occupying it, their orientation, and the orientation of the seat itself. To avoid foreign objects like bottles, cans, electronic devices, keys, books, etc. from interfering with car controls or breaking them down, an in-cabin safety and cleaning issue has been considered. Similarly, numerous studies and works of literature have been published in the past about the monitoring of a car's interior. Safety and averting hazardous conditions in the event of an accident become critical at high degrees of autonomous driving. Due to the limitations and restrictions found inside the vehicle's interior, Priyadarshi, Rahul (2020) found it can be challenging to decide which sensor placement is best for them. Artificial data was produced in order to assess person position in cabin environment with specific people' postures to create photorealistic scenes. On the other hand, their generated dataset contains scenes when people are looking forward. The safety of the occupants in the case of an accident has been their main concern. They produced a synthetic dataset with many scenes in order to comply with European safety rules. In-cabin monitoring systems have lately been developed by numerous companies and sectors.

It consists of many AI-assisted intelligent monitoring cameras that draw attention to an important point about where these cameras should be placed inside the AV's cabin. It contrasts the in-cabin monitoring experiences that result from different camera placements. The surveillance camera records both inside and outside of the cabin when it is installed in front-facing (FF) mode by Ramos-Sorroche, Emilio, et al (2023). Consequently, the person outside the car is mistakenly identified by the object detector algorithm as the car's occupant. The installation of rooftop (RT) cameras, however, makes it simple to avoid such circumstances. The only thing captured by the camera in the middle of the rooftop is the AV's inside.

Passenger Discomfort and Health Issues

The cabin of an airplane is much more airtight than a building and can accommodate considerably more people per square foot. Another problem is the discomfort patients experience from decreased cabin pressure. These changes may have an effect if the body contains trapped air. Ascending altitude causes air to escape from the sinuses and middle ear, which is why many travellers describe feeling like their ears are popping. This is generally not thought to be a problem. Pressure equilibrium must be restored to the middle ear and sinuses during the aircraft's altitude decrease before to landing Milledge, James (2020). In the event that this doesn't happen, discomfort could feel like your ears or sinuses are closed. It not only makes your ears pop, but it also severely harms the sinuses in your nasal canal. In order to investigate these aspects of human comfort, state-of-the-art computational fluid dynamics technologies are required. A non-invasive method for assessing how lower pressure affects the sinuses cabin and ear lobes and for helping find a way to reduce discomfort is the use of CFD.

Multi-Scale Feature Representations

Representing and processing multi-scale data efficiently is one of the primary challenges in object detection. Previous detectors frequently use the pyramidal feature hierarchy that is taken from backbone networks to make predictions directly. Feature Pyramid Network (FPN) is one of the first papers that suggests a top-down method for combining features from different scales. More recently, feature network topology is automatically designed by NAS-FPN using neural architecture search. Performance-wise, NAS-FPN is more effective, but the search process requires hundreds not coherent erratic. In this research, we aim to improve the principled and intuitive aspects. In a recent study, outstanding model efficiency for image categorization is demonstrated by simultaneously increasing network width, depth, and resolution.

The deformable part-based model is the most well-known example and one of the object detection paradigms that has been studied the most. This method integrates several discriminatively learnt components by using a star model called pictorial structure. The components model is the top layer, while the star model is the bottom layer. This paradigm can be conceptualized as having two layers. However, DNNs' general layers, the work by Trewartha, Amalie, et al (2022) takes advantage of domain knowledge the sections are structured with a cinematic aesthetic and are based on personally created Histogram of Gradients (HOG) descriptors.

Deep Architectures

Compositional models are deep models for object detection and parsing that express the object as a layered composition of image primitives. Part-based models serve as an inspiration for these models. The And/or graph is a well-known example that uses a tree to represent an item, and nodes to represent separate pieces, and or nodes to show alternative modes of the same part. Similar to DNNs, the And/or graph consists of several layers, with the lowest layers representing tiny generic picture primitives and the uppermost levels representing object components. These compositional models are easier to interpret than DNNs used by Tarnawski, Jakub M., et al. (2020). On the other hand, they require deduction, while the DNN models that are studied in this work are merely feed-forward and do not need latent variable deduction. Segment-based compositional models for detection are also examples, whereas primitives focus on shape and use Gabor filters or larger HOG filters. These solutions are usually hindered by the complexity of training and use specially designed learning mechanisms. Additionally, they combine bottom-up and top-down methods for drawing conclusions.

Neural Networks

Neural networks (NNs) are compositional models with less interpretable and broader nodes than the models previously stated. It has been several years since NNs of which convolutional NNs are the most well-known example were originally used to vision-related problems. Until recently, few people were aware of how effective these models known as DNNs were for large-scale picture categorization applications used by Tian, Yongqiang, et al. (2021). However, their usefulness for detection is limited. A more complex type of detection called scene parsing has been attempted with multi-layer convolutional neural networks.

Medical image segmentation has been investigated using DNNs. However, the NNs are used in all approaches as super pixel-level, pixel-by-pixel local, or semi-local classifiers. Our localization technique is regression, but it requires the full image as input. As a result, using NNs in this way is more efficient. This is maybe the closest answer to ours; it makes use of a much smaller network, different characteristics, and a different loss function to distinguish between numerous instances of the same class.

SYSTEM DESIGN

This section explains the recommended research architecture and technique. The hybrid machine learning strategy uses data from the vehicle interior camera covering a wide range of activities, including different doing so, to train the system using Google's Kaggle dataset (Human, bag, pet, etc.). In order to integrate and use the suggested methods practically and improve the results, a set of activities that allow drivers to predict a specific person's car with increased sensitivity, specificity, accuracy, and precision must be established. Because they have different budgets and preferences, scientists also employ machine learning techniques that are more effective and less costly. An outline of the suggested methodology is provided in Figure 1.

Training

Segmentation instances are used to generate data on the observed shape variance. This data is encoded by the shape model such that the shape-variant Hough transform can use it. The established border appearance model provides a measure of the probability given is part of sought-after defining the boundaries with precision in a training set, the user establishes the segmentation task. The primary variations in object shape and local border appearance that may arise during segmentation must be captured in the training set's images. In addition to borders, landmarks are used show the relationship boundaries various items.

Pre-Processing (Mean Filter)

The median filter in image processing is most frequently used to remove noise, such as salt and pepper. Median filters have several applications in image processing. On the other hand, median filters struggle to remove heavy-tailed noise, obliterate fine details like lines and crisp edges, as well as perform badly when noise that is dependent on the input is present. The investigation into nonlinear median-based filters has produced excellent findings and opened up some exciting new research directions. Because versatility, ability to preserve edges, and resistance to spurious noise, the traditional median filter continues to be

Figure 1. Flow chart for the proposed techniques

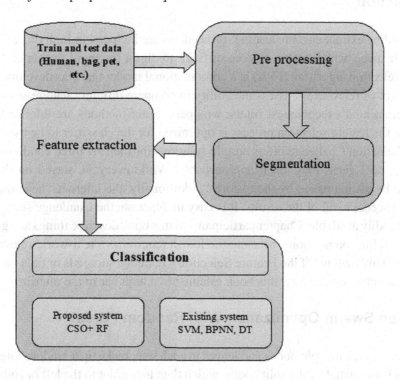

the standard in applications including image processing. However, little elements in the image, like tiny lines and borders, are frequently lost when using the median filter. More median-type filters, including stack and weighted filters, have become accessible in recent years.

Segmentation (Edge Detection)

When transitioning from image processing to picture analysis, image segmentation is a crucial step. On the one hand, it forms the basis of the target expression and has a major impact on the feature measurement. On the other hand, by means of segmentation, feature extraction, and parameter measurement, it serves as the intended expression, reducing the original image to a more abstracted and simplified form. Consequently, high-level visual analysis and comprehension are enabled. Real-world production uses image segmentation extensively, and it has essentially taken over all related image processing fields.

The accuracy of edge detection is critical to many applications of vision systems. The reason for this is because edges aid in defining the form and placement of the objects being studied. Edge-based methods are widely used for image segmentation because they provide the data needed for image analysis and pattern recognition processes carried out during high level image processing. Edge identification is a challenging problem, especially when dealing with low contrast, noisy, and fuzzy images. Consequently, scholars discussed it in great detail over time. Although several edge detection methods have already been proposed, most of them belong to one of two categories: moment-based methods or image-based methods.

Feature Extraction

Features that could be extraneous, misleading, or needless are included in high dimensional data. This widens the search space, which makes it more difficult to digest the input further and impedes learning. The feature selection algorithm (FSA) is a computational model that was developed in response to a particular concept of relevance. Possess the ability to compare different feature selection techniques empirically different kind's techniques: filters, wrappers. Filter methods are inferior to wrapping approaches because the feature selection process is optimized for the classifier to be used.

The Feature Selection Challenge offers simple solutions for the first three conditions. Seventy-five teams showed up, so I guess they felt it approachable. While everyone stayed on the scale, the top performers could be distinguished by their scores. Additionally, the internet, the companion CD, and this book provide access to all of the results. It is easy to duplicate the Challenge since all the data and Matlab code are readily available. Chapter participants in this book describe things at a greater level than in previous comparable competitions. Meeting the fourth requirement real-world relevance may be the most challenging. Time will tell if the Feature Selection Challenge succeeds or fails on this one. As the public record of an intriguing rivalry, this book establishes a high bar in the interim.

Hybrid Chicken Swarm Optimization With Random Forest

A collection of trees, Tt, with split nodes and leaves in each tree, make up a random forest. Every image patch that arrives is evaluated by the split nodes, which then forward it to the left or right child based on how the patch appears. During training, the picture patches' statistics are stored in each leaf L.

Chicken Swarm Optimization

The suggested approach uses the chicken swarm optimization (CSO) technique in conjunction with a limited number of carefully chosen characteristics to identify feature combinations that optimize classification accuracy. With respect to training and validation sets, the CSO's fitness function seeks to optimize maintaining fewest amount chosen in below Figure 2.

This allows each chicken to be described by its position. Each of the three has a unique position update formula: a hen, a chick, and a rooster. Based on the swarm's fitness function values, identify the position of the chickens with this equation:

$$X_{i,j}(t+1)=X_i \cdot r_{Num-hNum,j}^{(t)} \tag{1}$$

Procedure for Removal and Distribution The following are the possible contents of the concrete, where the eggs are dispersed around the search area Pop do if i=(rNum+hNum +1). If then.

$$X_{i,j}(t+1)=lb+(ub-lb)Xrand \tag{2}$$

In this context, pop refers to population size. The search range's lower and upper bounds are represented by the symbols lb and ub, respectively. Here is a description of the primary steps:

Figure 2. Algorithm for chicken swarm optimization

```
Initialize RN, HN, CN, M N, G;
Randomly initialize each chicken in the swarm
Xi(i = 1, 2, ..., N ).;
Initialize the max numbers of iteration Tmax;
whileT <Tmax do for each iteration
        ifT % G equals 0 then
end

        foreachchicken Xi in the swarm do
                ifXi is a roster then
                        Update Xi's location using equation 1;
                end
                ifXiis a henthen
                        Update Xi's location using equation 3;
                end
                if Xi is a chick then
                        Update Xi's location using equation 6;
                end
                Evaluate the new solution using equation 7;
        end
end
```

1. Setting the population's initial value. The first individual determination between the CSO and PSO algorithms and parameter parameters is the main topic of discussion.
2. An evaluation of fitness. Splitting up into smaller groupings. The two halves of the original population that are divided using the same scale are known as subgroups 1 and 2.
3. To determine the global optimum value, we simulate a swarm of chickens foraging by allocating responsibilities to subgroup 1 using the CSO technique. Figure 3 below describes the CSO optimization flow diagram.

The PSO method adjusts the particle's position and velocity in subgroup 2 in order to determine subgroups 1 and 2 in order to share information while updating the optimal swarm value. The revised Subgroup ideal values are computed and used to determine the allotted accomplished and desired obtained.

Figure 3. CSO flow diagram

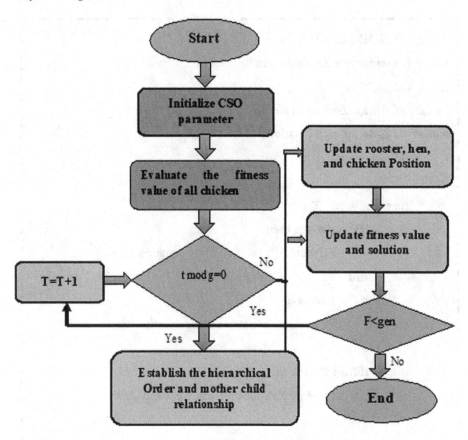

Random Forest-RF

It is the likelihood for each class c in a classification issue, denoted by the symbol p(c|L). The distribution that one wants to estimate in a regression job is over the continuous parameter x ∈ RH. To achieve both objectives, random forests for object identification must be trained to identify and classify patches that belong to an object as well as use those patches to regress the location and scale of the object.

Depending on whether the sample should move left or right, a binary-valued function decides which internal node in the tree should receive it. The set of decision trees is represented by T dt given any sample of data, the elements in Y will reach the tree's leaf. For this (admittedly simple) tree, let the notation be LF (Q) ∈ T td. If this is not present, a decision tree consists of a node that has a left and a right subtree. A data sample x ∈ X is split function φ: X → {0, 1} determines whether it is routed to the left decision sub-tree tl∈ T dt (if φ(x) = 0) or the right one tr∈ T dt (if φ(x) = 1). ND (φ, tl, tr)∈ T td is one technique to depict such a tree. Finally, to generate a prediction about a data sample, a decision forest is an ensemble F ⊆ T td of decision trees that averages the individual forecasts obtained from each tree. Figure 4 shows the pseudo code for the random forest algorithm.

Uncertain Regression Forests often represent a non-linear mapping M: RM → RK, where an example x is mapped to a goal prediction y. A portion of the training set is used to train each binary decision tree in the ensemble, {Tt} T t=1 (where T is the number of trees), in order to get this mapping. To lower the

Figure 4. Pseudo code for the random forest algorithm

Algorithm 1: Pseudo code for the random forest algorithm

To generate c classifiers:

for i=1 to c do

    Randomly sample the training data D with replacement to produce D_i

    Create a root node, N, containing D_i

    Call BuildTree(N_i)

end for

BuildTree(N):

if N contains instances of only one class then

    return

else

    Randomly select x% of the possible splitting features in N

    Select the feature F with the highest information gain to split on

    Create f child nodes of $N, N_1,...,N_f$ where F has f possible values $(F_1,...,F_f)$

for i=1 to do

    Set the contents of N_i to D_i, where D_i is all instances in N that match F_l

    Call BuildTree(N_i)

    end for

end if

uncertainty of the target variables in the resulting subsets, the given training data is recursively divided into two divisions using a single decision tree Tt.

More specifically, the data is divided into two distinct subsets, L and R, by the splitting functions $\varphi(x)$, from which a random sample is taken by each node in a tree. We measure the information gain first, and then evaluate all splitting functions. By using the splitting function $\varphi*(x)$ that produces largest information gain L and R subsets. All samples that fall within this leaf are used to estimate a density model p(y), which is then used leaf node target if any these conditions are met. Taking target and obtaining is the simplest method for estimating the probability distribution p(y). But there are even more complex variations, such as nonparametric densities or using a Gaussian kernel density estimate.

RESULT AND DISCUSSION

In this presentation, the findings of the suggested system, Hybrid Chicken Swarm Optimization with Random Forest (HCSORF), are explained. The recently built classification algorithm—which uses datasets from the Kaggle website is validated and introduced using object detection in the cabin of a single vehicle. In the training raw dataset, there are many characteristics for both letters and integers. MATLAB 2013a is used in study recommended system with HCSORF in object detection in the cabin. A 13th generation Intel i3 CPU with 16GB RAM and 512GB ROM powers the machine. The SVM, BPNN, DT, and recently constructed CSO with RF are compared in terms of sensitivity and accuracy metrics.

Confusion Matrix

To summarise the performance ML, a confusion matrix employed this method employed categorization matrix shows how much TP, TN, FP, and FN the model generated using the test set of data. Picture 6 above shows the structure of the confusion matrix for performance evaluation.

Accuracy

Accuracy is calculated only a small percentage of patients may have cancer in an unbalanced dataset such as the cancer dataset, accuracy is misleading and cannot be used to assess a model's performance.

Accuracy = (TP+TN)/(TP+TN+FN+FP)

Examining Figure 6, Table 1 shows that the correctness of the suggested system, determined by HCSORF, is 88.16, 1.82 times greater than the accuracy of the existing system, determined by 86.34.

Sensitivity

Sensitivity (SN) is calculated as the ratio of accurately predicted positives to all positives. The ratio of correctly predicted actual yeses to all actual yeses is the definition of sensitivity.

Sensitivity = TP/(TP+FN)

Figure 5. Confusion matrix

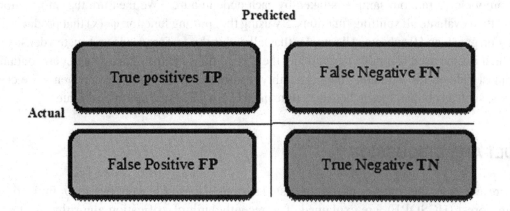

Table 1. Result values for accuracy with proposed and existing system

Algorithm	Accuracy
SVM	82.31
BPNN	84.65
DT	86.34
HCSORF	88.16

Figure 6. Accuracy graph of the proposed and current systems as a result

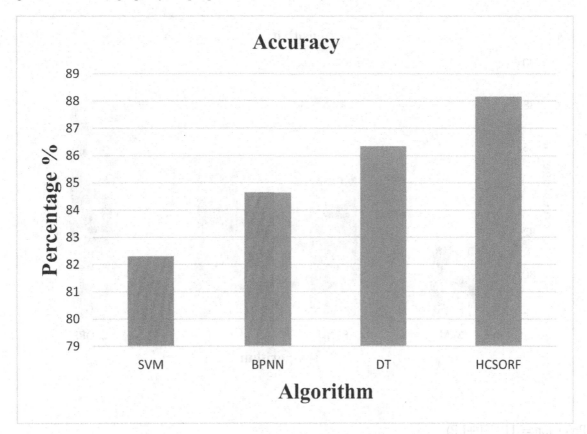

Based on Table 2's findings and with reference to Figure 7, the suggested system's HCSORF-determined sensitivity is 87.98, 2.43 times higher than the current system's 85.55 sensitivity.

Precision

A class's accuracy was defined instances that classifier identified as belonging to that specific class to categorized in that class purpose spam filtering and web search results, precision a measure of relevance or exactness matters. Decrease the amount of legitimate emails that are labeled as spam using the spam filtering algorithm.

Table 2. Result values for sensitivity with proposed and existing system

Algorithm	Sensitivity
SVM	81.36
BPNN	84.65
DT	85.55
HCSORF	87.98

Figure 7. Result sensitivity graph for proposed and existing system

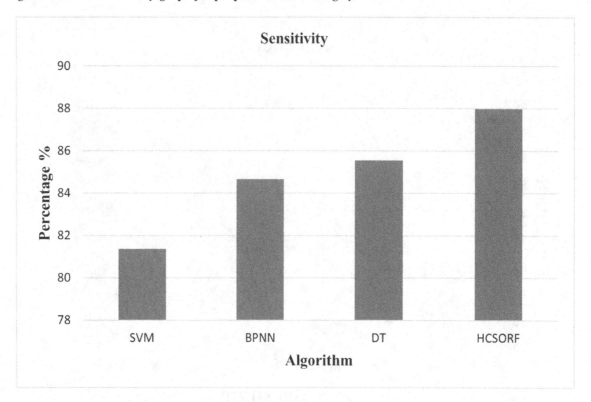

Precision = TP/(TP+FP)

The results in Table 3 show that the recommended system's precision, based on HCSORF assessment, is 90.65. This is 4.46 times more exact than the current system, according to the 86.19 evaluation of Figure 8.

F1 Score

Recall and precision are its harmonic means. Recall and precision scores for a model are aggregated. Over the course of the dataset, the accuracy statistic documents how frequently a model has produced accurate predictions.

Table 3. Result values for precision with proposed and existing system

Algorithm	Precision
SVM	84.16
BPNN	85.43
DT	86.19
HCSORF	90.65

Figure 8. Result precision graph for proposed and existing system

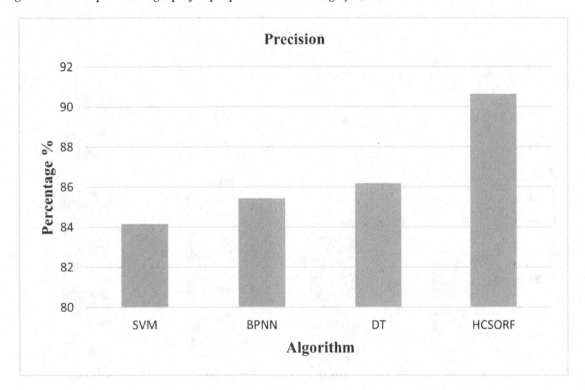

F1-score = 2 * (percision*recall)/(precision+recall)

In Figure 10, the F1 score of the proposed system is 88.23, which is 3.27 times higher than the F1 score of the current system, which is 84.96, according to HCSORF. Table 5 displays these outcomes.

Specificity

The specificity indicator is the ratio of all real nodes to precisely anticipated actual nodes. To calculate SP, divide the entire amount of negatives divided by the total amount of successfully anticipated. It is also known as TNR.

Specificity = TN/(TN+FP)

Table 4. Result values for F1-score with proposed and existing system

SVM	F1-score
SVM	82.06
BPNN	83.15
DT	84.96
HCSORF	88.23

Figure 9. Result F1-score graph for proposed and existing system

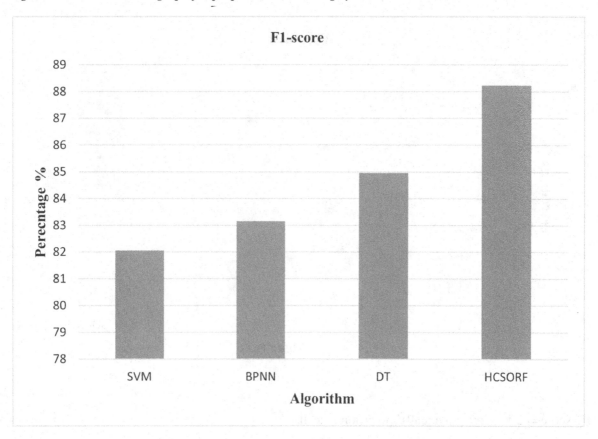

Based on Table 5's results, the suggested system's Specificity (91.65) is 4.4 times higher than the current system's Specificity (87.25) in reference to Figure 10. This is based on HCSORF data.

The graph below and the Tables 1, 2, 3, 4, and 5 above show that the performance of the suggested system is significantly better than the present system's. The results for Specificity are shown in the previous Figures (6, 7, 8, 9, 10). This means that the suggested method works better when the HWODT technique is applied to Drug Analysis for the Healthcare method. According to this, the recommended tactics performed better in the object detection system in vehicle cabin.

Table 5. Result values for specificity with proposed and existing system

Algorithm	Specificity
SVM	83.57
BPNN	85.87
DT	87.25
HCSORF	91.65

Figure 10. Result specificity graph for proposed and existing system

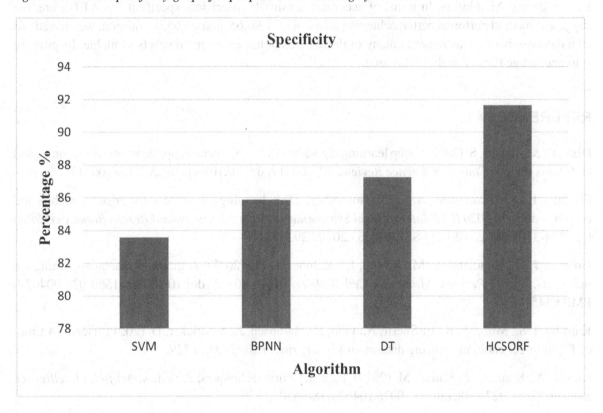

CONCLUSION

In this research, propose ML strategy add learning component to the current system so that it can be tailored to the specific needs of each driver. Long-term goals include learning from the gathered data and adjusting the previously strict thresholds to greater flexibility. This will be accomplished by gaining new insights and establishing correlations between the observed behavior and the underlying data using machine learning techniques. To improve the performance of each driver in accurately identifying potentially risky situations, these findings ought to be assessed and subsequently included into the threshold-based system. Extensive experiments were conducted using the data to establish how an implementation may be done in order to match this need. Businesses and academic institutions want a reliable IMS and a large enough database. A wide range of potential outcomes, including preferred variants for AV in-cabin monitoring, are included in our database. An RT camera is used in the first level to carry out routine monitoring tasks, while further monitoring is required in the second level to hunt down the offender and victim and gather any remaining pieces of evidence. Regarding private AVs, privacy is not a big concern; in public AVs, on the other hand, privacy is crucial. On-device AI, on the other hand, is the foundation of the proposed IMS and has information security advantages built in. In addition, communication of only insignificant details like the number of passengers, occupancy, etc., is required during the travel. It is possible to identify privacy threats that arise in unusual circumstances. We have suggested using facial anonymization to protect people's privacy. Users' privacy has been enhanced by our suggested Hybrid Chicken Swarm Optimization with Random Forest (HCSO RF) on-device AI solution. In terms of accuracy, sensitivity, precision, specificity, and F1-score, the suggested method performs better, achieving 88.16, 87.98, 90.65, and 91.65.In addition, we created our own database because there aren't many of these kinds of use cases and datasets available. Its purpose is to encourage further study in this area.

REFERENCES

Dixit, P., & Silakari, S. (2021). Deep learning algorithms for cybersecurity applications: A technological and status review. *Computer Science Review*, *39*, 100317. doi:10.1016/j.cosrev.2020.100317

Faniadis, E., & Amanatiadis, A. (2020, November). Deep learning inference at the edge for mobile and aerial robotics. In *2020 IEEE International Symposium on Safety, Security, and Rescue Robotics (SSRR)* (pp. 334-340). IEEE. 10.1109/SSRR50563.2020.9292575

Greener, J. G., Kandathil, S. M., Moffat, L., & Jones, D. T. (2022). A guide to machine learning for biologists. *Nature Reviews. Molecular Cell Biology*, *23*(1), 40–55. doi:10.1038/s41580-021-00407-0 PMID:34518686

Katrolia, J. S., Mirbach, B., El-Sherif, A., Feld, H., Rambach, J., & Stricker, D. (2021). Ticam: A time-of-flight in-car cabin monitoring dataset. *arXiv preprint arXiv:2103.11719*.

Kumar, A., Kaur, A., & Kumar, M. (2019). Face detection techniques: A review. *Artificial Intelligence Review*, *52*(2), 927–948. doi:10.1007/s10462-018-9650-2

Lan, H., Hartonen, K., & Riekkola, M. L. (2020). Miniaturised air sampling techniques for analysis of volatile organic compounds in air. *Trends in Analytical Chemistry*, *126*, 115873. doi:10.1016/j.trac.2020.115873

. Ma, Y., Wang, Z., Yang, H., & Yang, L. (2020). Artificial intelligence applications in the development of autonomous vehicles: A survey. *IEEE/CAA Journal of AutomaticaSinica, 7*(2), 315-329.

Mallaboyev, N. M., Sharifjanovna, Q. M., Muxammadjon, Q., & Shukurullo, C. (2022, May). INFORMATION SECURITY ISSUES. In Conference Zone (pp. 241-245). IEEE.

. Milledge, J. (2020). Hypobaria: high altitude, aviation physiology, and medicine. *Cotes' lung function*, 615-637.

Mishra, A., Cha, J., & Kim, S. (2022). Privacy-preserved in-cabin monitoring system for autonomous vehicles. *Computational Intelligence and Neuroscience, 2022,* 2022. doi:10.1155/2022/5389359 PMID:35498178

Poon, Y. S., Lin, C. C., Liu, Y. H., & Fan, C. P. (2022, January). YOLO-based deep learning design for in-cabin monitoring system with fisheye-lens camera. In *2022 IEEE International Conference on Consumer Electronics (ICCE)* (pp. 1-4). IEEE. 10.1109/ICCE53296.2022.9730235

Priyadarshi, R., Gupta, B., & Anurag, A. (2020). Deployment techniques in wireless sensor networks: A survey, classification, challenges, and future research issues. *The Journal of Supercomputing, 76*(9), 7333–7373. doi:10.1007/s11227-020-03166-5

Ramos-Sorroche, E., Rubio-Aparicio, J., Santa, J., Guardiola, C., & Egea-Lopez, E. (2023). In-cabin and outdoor environmental monitoring in vehicular scenarios with distributed computing. *Internet of Things : Engineering Cyber Physical Human Systems,* 101009.

Rathi, B. S., Kumar, P. S., & Vo, D. V. N. (2021). Critical review on hazardous pollutants in water environment: Occurrence, monitoring, fate, removal technologies and risk assessment. *The Science of the Total Environment, 797,* 149134. doi:10.1016/j.scitotenv.2021.149134 PMID:34346357

Saxena, A., Khanna, A., & Gupta, D. (2020). Emotion recognition and detection methods: A comprehensive survey. *Journal of Artificial Intelligence and Systems, 2*(1), 53–79. doi:10.33969/AIS.2020.21005

Tarnawski, J. M., Phanishayee, A., Devanur, N., Mahajan, D., & Nina Paravecino, F. (2020). Efficient algorithms for device placement of dnn graph operators. *Advances in Neural Information Processing Systems, 33,* 15451–15463.

Tian, Y., Ma, S., Wen, M., Liu, Y., Cheung, S. C., & Zhang, X. (2021). To what extent do DNN-based image classification models make unreliable inferences? *Empirical Software Engineering, 26*(5), 84. doi:10.1007/s10664-021-09985-1

Trewartha, A., Walker, N., Huo, H., Lee, S., Cruse, K., Dagdelen, J., Dunn, A., Persson, K. A., Ceder, G., & Jain, A. (2022). Quantifying the advantage of domain-specific pre-training on named entity recognition tasks in materials science. *Patterns (New York, N.Y.), 3*(4), 100488. doi:10.1016/j.patter.2022.100488 PMID:35465225

Chapter 4
Real–Time Fault Detection and Condition Monitoring for Industrial Autonomous Vehicles

Thirusudhan M.

Karpagam Academy of Higher Education, India

Sasikumar S.

Karpagam Academy of Higher Education, India

ABSTRACT

Real-time status monitoring and early defect diagnosis are becoming more and more necessary for modern industrial systems. Developing intelligent remote diagnostic technologies and integrating on-board and off-board diagnosis are two more unresolved research projects in the automotive industry. The automated transfer vehicle (ATV) equipment condition monitoring example in this chapter is part of a smart industrial use case. The suggested method successfully permits ATV fault scenarios to be seen in real time by expanding to a fleet of devices in an actual production plant. The application of a statistical threshold is the initial stage in creating a high-performance detection model for defect detection on stacked long short-term memory networks. For better computation speed, a second model trimming approach based on principal component analysis is suggested. The improved fault detection technique is ultimately applied by the airborne embedded computer platform with field-programmable gate arrays.

INTRODUCTION

The manufacturing industry domains have seen significant changes since the advent of the Industry 4.0 concept. The sophistication of conventional manufacturing plans and procedures has increased as a result of industrialization and information technologies including robotics, big data, the Internet of Things (IoT), and intelligent measuring techniques. Automating and integrating these technologies into industrial processes makes production setups more sustainable and manageable. These advancements increased productivity and adaptability but decreased the amount of human interaction on production

DOI: 10.4018/979-8-3693-1962-8.ch004

sets. However, automation and artificial intelligence (AI) shouldn't take the place of workers on the manufacturing floor; instead, man-hours from these technologies should be applied to more difficult jobs with thoughtful solutions.Intelligent technologies such as autonomous robots are usually assigned repetitive jobs in smart industrial settings, with people being assigned more complex and creative activities by Verma, Amar Kumar, et al (**2021**). In today's sophisticated industrial environments, a lot of autonomous machinery performs routine tasks like patrolling or the cautious and secure transfer of supplies and parts without the need for human assistance. They can also work in areas where labor laws and safety standards are in effect. That manner, they can ensure the safety of workers even when they are carrying out dangerous jobs.

Since autonomous equipment has become a vital part of the fleets of equipment used in industrial facilities, high uptime and continuous operation are needed. This means that your car can now run on its own. Over twenty years have gone by since reality replaced science fiction. This is made possible by recent developments in the fields of radars and microprocessors10. There has also been a notable advancement in the creation of portable and lightweight technologies. This has led to the development of ultra-light technology, which enables quick decision-making in emergency scenarios.

Concepts of Autonomous Driving

Over the past decade, a lot of progress has been made in the field of autonomous vehicles. Autonomous vehicles, or simply AVs for short, are self-driving cars. They may follow preprogrammed instructions, perform automated chores, and observe their surroundings. Systems for autonomous cars serve a variety of functions. an exhaustive list of all the jobs and functions an autonomous system is capable of doing. Three main components make up the strategy.

- Sensing and perception,
- Planning,
- Control.

Every system needs sensors to collect and process the ambient data needed for it to work, which makes them an indispensable part of the system. In order to give the system a safe and sensible course, the sensed data is employed in planning. Actuator: The actuator is guided by the control component of the system along the intended, practical path. Every single one of these components needs to be arranged while building an AV system. With or without assistance from a human driver, an autonomous vehicle (AV) system can park a car on its own thanks to a feature by Van Wyk, Franco, et al (**2019**). Two major factors have led to the increased interest in autonomous parking in recent times. First of all, it provides a high level of safety for novice drivers who could find parkingurban planners and managers are particularly concerned about the second issue, which is the scarcity of parking spaces, because of the traffic. For this reason, creating an automated parking system for smart cars has become imperative. Table 1 shows the Universe of faults and list of monitoring variables.

Artificial Intelligence

Computers and robots with artificial intelligence can do tasks that are normally done by humans. These include the ability to recognize speech, translate between languages, analyze visual stimuli, and make

Table 1. Universe of faults and list of monitoring variables

Fault List		Monitored Variables	
Name	**Notation**	**Name (Units)**	**Notation**
Air Flow Sensor Fault (F1)	AFS	Air Pressure (KPa)	Pm
Leakage in AIS (F2)	AIS_leak	Amount of Fuel Injected (mg)	FC
Blockage of Air Filter (F3)	AF_blockage	Air to Fuel Ratio	A/F
Throttle Angle Sensor Fault (F4)	TAS	Engine Speed (rpm)	NE
Less Fuel Injection (F5)	LFI	Vehicle Speed (km/h)	SPD
Added Engine Friction (F6)	AEF	Throttle Angle (deg)	TA
Air/Fuel Sensor Fault (F7)	AFuel_S	Air Flow Meter (Volts)	VG2
Engine Speed Sensor Fault (F8)	ESS		

decisions. Presently, artificial intelligence can be classified into three categories: artificial general intelligence (AGI), artificial super intelligence (ASI3), and restricted AI. Strong AI, or AGI, is machine intelligence that is able to do all tasks at a level almost equivalent to human intellect, as opposed to ASI, which is machine intelligence that is always more intelligent than human cognition. Artificial intelligence is often generated in the current world in order to accomplish the task needed.Having said that, it's plausible that certain companies are secretly researching AI. In many aspects, artificial intelligence (AI) has changed our lives significantly throughout the years. With enough training, it can now do tasks that humans were previously unable to accomplish by Cai, Yingfeng, et al (**2021**).

Intelligent machines in an industrial setting, such as robots, are physical systems with varying degrees of independence that collaborate in a range of dynamic physical situations. The intrinsic capability of these autonomous robots to operate in a variety of unforeseen conditions makes them susceptible to a variety of mechanical and operational issues. Maintaining operations and minimizing unscheduled downtime for these equipment necessitates fast fault detection, diagnosis, and monitoring. Because of advancements in deep learning (DL), hardware system processing power, and advanced measurement technologies, data-driven defect detection approaches have immense potential in production contexts. Utilizing data-driven fault detection methods that extract features from recorded sensor inputs, equipment operational irregularities are identified. A diagnosis is established in relation to a reference.Smart sensors can be used to carry out intricate measurements that yield precise information on the operating environment of the devices. This is why proper analysis of such data produces useful information that allows human operators to track the current status of the devices in real time and monitor component levels said by Yao, Lei, et al. (**2020**).

Machine Learning

Mathematical and analytical models and algorithms are developed and automated using machine learning (ML) to improve system performance for a given task. Uncovering hidden insights in data requires the application of machine learning (ML), which uses methods from operations research, statistics, and heuristic procedures but does not provide explicit guidance on what to look for or how to proceed. The three primary subfields of machine learning are unsupervised learning, supervised learning, and reinforcement learning by Chen, Zhenpeng (**2019**). These are explained in the section below.

Unsupervised Learning

Understanding data that is generated solely from input data is known as unsupervised learning. Data points are arranged according to a set of criteria in a process called clustering, which is a method for unsupervised learning. All data sets can be grouped into groups using the clustering approach by Liu, Ze, et al (**2021**).

Supervised Learning

Supervised learning (SL) is used to build an output and input prediction model. Among SL approaches, regression analysis is the subgroup that searches for a relationship between variables. By utilizing the correlation between variables gathered from the dataset, machine learning uses this to predict the outcome of an event. A classifier that accurately determines which category a new observation falls into and forecasts the target class for each data category by Yao, Lei, et al (**2021**).

Reinforcement Learning

Artificial intelligence (AI) will progress faster into machine learning in the real world thanks to a new technique called reinforcement learning (RL), which focuses on decision-making. We present a quick comparison of reinforcement learning, unsupervised learning, and supervised learning.

Effective diagnostics and monitoring are possible when all of the equipment is networked with all of the other industrial operational systems and equipment. Or, to put it another way, every component of the industrial environment must be viewed as an Internet of Things (IoT) device and connected to other nearby IOT devices. Because of this, these gadgets are linked together and use virtual networks like the cloud to continuously and quickly exchange data. In many scenarios, however, where real-time data transfer and analysis are essential, bottlenecks may result from the volume of data, the computational load on the centralized cloud, and the bandwidth utilized by several devices.It is consequently impractical to transfer all of the raw data to the centralized cloud server for processing needs. One potential remedy for the aforementioned obstacles is edge artificial intelligence, or edge computing combined with artificial intelligence said by Deng, Wanghua, and Ruoxue Wu (**2019**). Using smart sensors attached to Internet of Things devices, Edge AI does preprocessing or inference at the edge nodes, near to the source, before data is transferred to the central cloud. This approach provides lower latency, quicker responses, data security, and scalability even if it transfers less data. Therefore, Edge AI offers beneficial solutions for industrial Internet of things devices, including automated transfer vehicles (ATVs), which depend on fast data rates and low transmission latency to monitor their condition in real time.

An open-source FIWARE-based data distributor middleware platform, an industrial ATV, an edge AI accelerator, a data storage unit, a visualization tool, and other components have been combined into a freshly constructed testbed. The suggested method is widely applicable and can be modified for any production tool that has Internet of Things connection protocols and sensors installed by Gupta, Abhishek, et al. (**2021**). We have customized our ATV use case to fit the robot fleet condition monitoring platform solution. Notable conclusions drawn from this research include:

- A general-purpose Edge AI framework that provides defect diagnostics and real-time status tracking has been unveiled.
- Assessing the design and identifying operational issues is aided by the use of industrial ATV use cases.
- Sensor fusion and the data-driven DL algorithm are used for inference by edge AI accelerator hardware.
- Real-time inference results from edge AI devices are sent to the data storage via a data pipeline powered by the open-source middleware platform FIWARE.

The five sections of this essay are listed below: Session 2 of the current system shows its shortcomings in data prevention in IoT and other techniques. The third session was a demonstration of the suggested System for data security in vehicle. The outcomes of the anticipated system are shown in Session 4. An examination of the recommended approach for vehicle data in IoT rounds off Session 5.

LITERATURE REVIEW

The Internet of Things, smart measurement technologies, and the Internet can all be used to connect physical environments or equipment into the digital world. Because of their different hardware and other components, these settings and devices frequently have problems interacting and communicating with one another. Standards and software have been created to enable this kind of transformation. The author Ouyang, Zhenchao, et al (**2019**) platform FIWARE, for example, has components that allow for effective communication between Internet of Things devices.

The researcher Bakdi, Azzeddine, et al (**2021**) FIWARE platform is a great tool for creating smart environments, according to a number of studies in the literature. For instance, consider developing cloud- and Internet-of-things (IoT)-based health system applications and services that interface with FIWARE platform components via a range ofUtilizing a platform that integrates data from the FI-WARE platform, Internet of Things technologies, and port measurement equipment, an architecture for monitoring and decision-making for seaport settings was highlighted. The FIWARE platform was utilized for irrigation operations to test the design of precision agriculture software in an authentic agricultural setting. The efficacy of the FIWARE platform for smart city applications is demonstrated by building a new testbed and modeling huge IoT installations. Based on preliminary studies conducted in multiple areas, a variety of Internet of Things devices can safely and efficiently connect with one another using the FIWARE platform and its components. FIWARE was utilized to give this project a flexible and all-inclusive base.

A author Yaqoob, Ibrar, et al (**2019**) central server processes the environmental data collected by Internet of Things (IoT) sensors in the environment that most data-centric smart solutions offer. However, this approach can have certain drawbacks with regard to data security, network resource usage, and latency. Numerous studies that circumvent these limits are reported in the literature, making use of edge AI technologies. Edgent is an edge AI system designed to operate at low latency by utilizing deep neural networks for edge differencing, based on a digital twin architecture for anomaly detection and industrial system condition monitoring. The edge processing methods based on single-shot multi box detectors for real-time video smart parking surveillance applications were evaluated in terms of detection accuracy, adaptability, and system dependability.An innovative artificial intelligence (AI) system utilizing lightweight convolutional neural networks (CNNs) and multi-sensor data fusion techniques for real-time event recognition is being tested on the LiBr absorption chiller, a typical air conditioner component. Two distinct deep learning models and a reference air quality dataset were used to evaluate the proposed structure. Extensive research has been conducted on edge AI frameworks and approaches; however, most of the studies are either domain-specific or lack real-world testing environments.

According to Sun, Lei, et al(2020) Universe of Watched Variables and Engine Failures Eight different engine failures are being looked into, including one black actuator fault, three blue plant faults, and four red sensor faults. Three steady-state operational conditions are used in order to replicate the model: The range of pedal angle (PA) is 15 to 20 degrees. The tracked data contained seven variables that were monitored by the engine. Using a 3-D plot of engine speed, throttle angle, and air pressure signals, pre- and post-fault data is gathered for 10 seconds, with the fault on-set time set at 2.5 seconds. This allows for the separation of the nominal data's operational domains. To replicate all of the 10 severity levels (6 to 15%) for each operational scenario, a 1% step size variation is utilized.

The author Bae, Il at al(**2019**) outlines the procedure for identifying and diagnosing a problem, regardless of the operating region in which it occurs. Industrial equipment may work better and last longer thanks to developments in sensor and measuring technologies. The data gathered from a range of sensors is then examined using signal processing techniques to enable further uses, such as equipment failure detection and condition monitoring during operation. Since machine learning is widely used in many academic domains, data-driven modeling approaches are used in industrial environments for defect classification and detection. Deep learning (DL) techniques are mostly beneficial for these applications due to their ability to produce high-capacity models through direct learning from raw data. Various papers describe the use of data from sensors and deep learning algorithms to identify anomalies, diagnose issues, and track the health of Internet of Things (IoT) devices. Another study uses time/frequency domain sound data with DL to diagnose gear breakdowns. For instance, they suggest using the wavelet transform of vibration signals from acceleration sensors as the input for the DL model to determine the failure states of a planetary gearbox. Integrating several signals can aid in a more accurate and dependable diagnostic and health monitoring of industrial machinery since different sensors can detect the environment with different attributes.

Robot Operating

The researcher Simon, Martin, et al (**2019**) majority of mobile robots, such as ATVs and other Internet of Things gadgets, are composed of numerous physical parts, such as wheels, engines, cameras, and other sensors. Building flexible and efficient software interfaces for utilizing and operating robots is more challenging due to the variety of these components. Furthermore, these limitations might make communication between IoT components more difficult. Robot hardware is made up of many sensors and actuator elements. To make controlling this hardware easier, ROS middleware provides a standardized development environment with common sensor drivers and interface techniques. The ROS ecosystem makes it possible for several robots with similar parts to use the same code blocks with very little modification.Robots can be controlled and operated by a suite of software applications known as the Robot Operating System (ROS). Nodes, services, messages, and topics are the four main ideas that ROS provides. Nodes are software components that communicate and perform computations together. A node can publish messages over a topic and receive published messages from other nodes that are subscribed to the same subject. Similar to standard web services, the service paradigm is composed of requests from client nodes and responses from server nodes. Moreover, all nodes on a ROS platform must be linked to the master node, which controls and coordinates all communication.

Edge Computing

A network resource or machine that sits between cloud servers and a system's data sources is called an edge. In general, edge devices are located close to data sources due to their compact, decentralized, and power-efficient nature. Together, edge computing and artificial intelligence create edge artificial intelligence. A good example of this combination is the local application of machine learning or deep learning algorithms to data collected from physical devices via edge node computer capabilities said by Chiu, Yu-Chen, et al. (**2020**). Edge AI achieves this by bringing processing power and artificial intelligence closer to data sources. There is a difference in the amount of raw data that is moved to centralized cloud servers from Internet of Things device hardwareAll inference models running on edge nodes generate it as their only output. Decentralized processing of received data at edge nodes reduces the amount of computing power and network bandwidth needed for centralized servers. Hence, implementing edge AI techniques reduces latency and transmission costs while enhancing data security, privacy, scalability, and dependability.

FIWARE Platform

A middleware that facilitates the development of smart manufacturing solutions is called a Generic Enabler (GE) on the FIWARE platform. Generic Entires (GEs) are software components designed to work with several applications and/or architectures. Arranging suitable GEs based on a system's needs is the platform's concept. A context broker is at the heart of any FIWARE system. Processing, analyzing, and displaying context information, as well as interacting with robotics and the Internet of Things, are just a few of the tasks that specific GEs are made to perform explained by Liu, Liangkai, et al (**2020**). API and context data management are also under their purview. The foundational components of the FIWARE platform are a CB and a database that stores context data. In Internet of Things scenarios, CB is responsible for the context entities, which consist ofto enable FIWARE CBs to use and publish NGSI v2 entities generated by ROS messages, an additional GE known as FIROS establishes a communication channel between the robotic domain and cloud.

The Six Levels of Automation

With the increasing prevalence of autonomous vehicles (AVs) across the globe, it is necessary to assess our progress in realizing the vision of AVs by assessing their performance on their dynamic driving task (DDT) through the use of an extensive hierarchical table. SAE's comprehensive taxonomy (Level 0–Level 5) covers the six automation steps. Below is a list of them:

Level 0 (No Automation)

Almost all cars on the road belong to this class. Whoever supplies the DDT has complete influence over them. Mechanisms to provide the driver with temporary support in an emergency might exist. Since human involvement is necessary to operate the emergency systems, the vehicle cannot be termed auto-mated by Langarica, Saúl (**2019**).

Level 1 (Driver Assistance)

This one has the least automation. In some situations, the car's electronics might provide the driver with some temporary assistance. Because it allows the human driver to focus on other driving-related tasks like steering and braking, adaptive cruise control, which allows an automobile to maintain a safe distance from the vehicle in front of it, may be regarded as Level 1 by Li, Da, et al (**2020**).

Level 2 (Partial Driving Automation)

Advanced driving assistance systems (ADAS) are similar to Level 2, which allows steering and speed control of an automobile remotely but still requires a human driver to be present. The term "self-driving" is misleading, even if a person can still operate an automobile at any time. Tesla Autopilot enables cer-tification up to level two by Guo, Ningyuan, et al. (**2020**).

Level 3 (Conditional Driving Automation)

Compared to Level 2 vehicles, the car can now operate with greater autonomy. They are equipped with several sensors that allow them to sense their environment and make choices for themselves. However, a human driver needs to be prepared to take over in the unlikely event that the technology malfunctions. A few other features that aren't included in Level 2 cars are automated emergency braking (AEB), driver monitoring (DM), and traffic jam assistance (TJA) by Manoharan, Dr Samuel. (**2019**).

Level 4 (High Driving Automation)

In the case of a problem or system failure, Level 4 cars are equipped to take control. There is a distinc-tion between cars classified as Level 4 and Level 3. Even though they can function independently, they are now limited to a low-speed, geofenced metropolitan area. This will result from any future changes made to the infrastructure and laws. Human drivers usually do not need help from others, however they always have the option to intervene and take over by Carranza-García, Manuel, et al (**2021**).

Level 5 (Full Driving Automation)

With this, the dream of driverless vehicles has come true. Dynamic driving is not necessary since Level 5 cars totally do away with the need for human interaction. There won't be any kind of accel-erator or brake pedal or steering wheel. These will be capable of doing all driving maneuvers that a typical human driver can. A level 5 vehicle is exempt from geo-fencing since it is autonomous and able to move anywhere. Even though Level 5 vehicles have already undergone a great deal of world-wide study and testing, it will take some time before they are made available to the general public by Rohan, Ali et al (**2019**).

Infeasible Sensing

However, the author Yin, Shen(**2019**) due to their basic characteristics, embedded sensors usually have very limited perception capabilities and are unable to sense their surroundings. The primary drawback of using visual-based object detection as the primary sensing technique is that the inference's success is usually dependent on the caliber of the collected photos. The image quality can be affected by a number of factors, including brightness, weather, distance of the camera from the subject, and image resolution. Neither the road lighting nor the bicycle lights quickly lit the affected section of the path. Due to erroneous assumptions on the pedestrian, the pre-trained deep learning model initially misclassified them as an unknown entity, a car, and finally a bicycle.This experience has demonstrated that decisions made solely on the basis of one kind of sensor can often lead to disastrous outcomes. One viable potential approach to stop this is to combine different sensing modalities for perception, such as those from Li-DAR sensors, sensors placed at intelligent traffic signals, and sensors from other cars. Such technique is referred to as "sensor fusion".

Trade-Off Between Reliability and Latency

Usually, the researcher Jabbar, Rateb, et al. (**2020**) explain an inference's performance includes both correctness and delay. Because the accuracy of the model mostly depends on the caliber of the input data and the model's competency, shallow neural network models and "bad quality" data can both reduce the inference accuracy of a pre-trained deep learning model. A further communication delay is caused by moving the workload from the mobile device to a more powerful edge server using a more advanced neural network model. On the other hand, the offloading could sometimes become inefficient due to the channel dynamics. Some apps may not be able to handle the additional latency, even if it didn't exist.The trade-offs between latency and inference accuracy must therefore be carefully considered while developing edge intelligence. Achieving an appropriate trade-off between increased latency and dependability requires minimizing the wireless transmission delay between the devices and the edge server.

Limited Resources

In contrast to a large number of strong GPUs and CPUs integrated at the cloud, edge servers sometimes cannot handle a high rate of device offloading requests due to restrictions in computation, cache, and power resources, as well as limitations in connection bandwidth. In particular, cooperative resource allocation and optimal offloading decisions on the limited resources at the edge server are critical for edge intelligence said by Hong, Yuanduo, et al (**2021**).

Data Security and Privacy

In many edge intelligence application domains, data security and privacy considerations are crucial since it is likely that the mobile device data needed for processing and inference contains private and sensitive information that the user may not have wanted to be collected. Using autonomous driving as an example, consider the sheer number of images the AVs take, many of which contain sensitive personal data used by Muhammad, Khan, et al (**2020**). A direct transfer of this type of data to the edge server for processing could jeopardize user privacy. This problem usually occurs during the training and inference phases of the model. This problem can be fixed by uploading the intermediate features to the edge server after the device has processed the fundamental data (or training).

SYSTEM DESIGN

The efficacy of the proposed architecture is assessed in conditions similar to an actual industrial workstation. However, the proposed technique has not yet been applied in real production. Integration can be accomplished using the current architecture without necessitating major modifications to the system's constituent parts.

Proposed System Architecture

This work proposes an architecture for a real-time defect detection and condition monitoring system that is edge AI-based and general-purpose. There are five primary layers in the architecture:

- The IoT layer,
- The edge layer,
- The FIWARE layer,
- The data storage layer
- The visualization layer.

ROS-installed devices comprise the Internet of Things layer. For data collection, some devices have installed sensors. After the ROS topic publication system receives information from the master node on certain topics, relevant messages are disseminated. Part of the edge layer are edge AI devices that have deep learning algorithms for inference. All these little decentralized devices are placed close to one other in the IoT layer. The chosen IoT device is connected to each edge device via an Ethernet wire. The IoT device releases topics, and the edge device uses ROS to subscribe to them.

The results, acquired through the use of real-time sensor data collected from subjects by the DL-based defect detection algorithm, are disseminated over another topic on the master node. FIROS, a database, and GEs acting as a CB make up the FIWARE layer. FIROS transforms the message comprised in the topics broadcast by the master node into NGSI v2 entities before it is sent from IoT devices to the CB. After these entities and attributes are published from the CB, they are kept up to date in the database. The primary components of the data storage layer are those related to data persistence, specifically a database server and processing engine capable of transforming data delivered by CB into the appropriate format for database storage.

Device Components

The system should scale for a fleet of ATV equipment and a myriad of other IoT devices for status monitoring, even if the trials are conducted with a single ATV. It should be easy for any hardware running ROS to communicate with the system. Additionally, there isn't a built auto-model updating mechanism in the system, and the DL model utilized at the edge for inference is assumed to be static. As such, it is assumed that an operator may manually update the edge model as necessary, and the edge model's long-term resilience to equipment state drifts is not explored.

Fault Diagnosis of Battery Cells

Battery cells can malfunction due to four main reasons: overcharging, overdischarging, overcurrent, and overtemperature. The battery cells could sustain irreversible harm from them. They are included in the problem diagnosis since these fault scenarios are connected to the battery's properties. Batteries must go through complex chemical and physical processes in order to charge and discharge. That being said, the cells may explode and catch fire if they are overcharged, overdischarged, or overcurrent. Battery charging and discharging voltages must be continuously and in real-time monitored to avoid these issues. Using the over-charged/over-discharged/over-current protection, the system controller will halt charging or discharging the battery cells if the current or the upper or lower cut-off voltage approaches the maximum value.

In the same vein, overheating is an additional error that must be prevented. The prototype 12S system makes use of six thermistors, which are fastened to the spaces between each pair of batteries, to track the temperature within each battery cell. Two-level reporting and protection mechanism and temperature-window self-recovery strategy are proposed. The controller will not automatically shut off or charge in order to warn users if the temperature rises above 50 °C. However, the controller will initiate the second-level protection as soon as the cell temperature over 60 °C, thereby halting the charging and discharging procedure. If the temperature of each cell falls below 40 oC, the controller will initiate the self-recovery procedure immediately. The faults listed above can be found using the flowchart.

Robot Operating System

Mobile robots, including ATVs and other Internet of Things devices, often include a large number of components in their hardware, including wheels, engines, cameras, and other sensors. The multiplicity of these elements makes it challenging to design software interfaces for robot operation and control that are both efficient and adaptable. Furthermore, these kinds of limitations might affect how well-integrated IoT entities are. To overcome these difficulties, ROS middleware offers a standardized development platform with shared sensor drivers and interface solutions, which simplifies the use of robot hardware with a variety of sensors and actuator elements. With very small changes, numerous robots with comparable components can use the same code blocks thanks to the ROS ecosystem.Robot control and operation are made easier by a group of software applications known as ROS. ROS comprises four primary concepts: nodes, messages, topics, and services. Nodes are software elements that interact with one another and do calculations.

Any node can receive published messages by having the capacity to subscribe to and post messages over a topic. The service model's client node requests and server node answers are comparable to those of conventional web services. On a ROS platform, all nodes also need to be connected to the master node, which manages and plans out all communication.

Edge Artificial Intelligence

"Edge" describes any network or computational device positioned in between cloud servers and system data sources. Edge devices are often tiny, distributed, and low-power devices that are situated in close proximity to data sources. The fusion of artificial intelligence and edge computing is known as edge AI. The utilization of edge node computing resources for local machine learning or deep learning algorithm processing of hardware device data explains this combination. In other words, edge AI brings processing power and artificial intelligence closer to the data. The outcome of inference models operating on edge nodes is provided to centralized cloud servers instead of all the raw data collected from the hardware of IoT devices. The amount of data that is obtained will increase, so the processing power and network of centralized servers.

FIWARE Platform

The middleware FIWARE platform and its generic enabling components facilitate the building of smart industrial systems. Software components referred to as GEs are designed for various applications and/or architectures. The idea behind the platform is to compile relevant GEs according to system requirements.

A context broker is the central component of any FIWARE system (CB). Application-specific GEs manage context data/API, process, evaluate, and display context information, and communicate with robots and the Internet of Things, among other tasks. The FIWARE platform's most basic version consists of the CB and database that store context information. In IoT settings, context entities are managed by CB and are where the data generated by IoT devices is kept. Moreover, a distinct GE known as FIROS establishes the link between the robotic domain and cloud in order to transform ROS messages into NGSI v2 entities that FIWARE CBs may use and publish.

On-line Module

There is constant system monitoring for the online FDD module. The generalized likelihood ratio test, or GLRT, is a method used to process the sensor data in order to identify problems in real time. The reference feature set from training across a moving window of data is recovered once the issue has been identified. The following blocks, the severity estimations and the classification blocks, use training parameters to categorize defects and estimate severity levels, respectively. The name of the failing component, the problem's on-set time, its severity, and the required repair action are all provided to the user via the fault diagnostic decision block. To facilitate their use in the online and offline modules.

RESULT AND DISCUSSION

This section presents the experiment results related to the use of the ATV in different fixed-to-the-ground barriers that could result in low- or high-level anomalies. First, a detailed explanation of the testing setup and real-time inference findings is provided. The data storage interface is then shown. The dashboards and built-in monitoring system are finally shown. A comprehensive analysis of the collected data is provided in the conclusion.

Testing Environment and Real-Time Inference

The previously mentioned pre-trained DL model is used by the edge AI unit to infer information about the ATV's state while it performs a predetermined load-carrying task over a route. In the simulated testing environment, the Python client code designed for the ATV edge AI unit is used to execute the DL model and draw conclusions. It also subscribes to the ROS topics, which supply the sound and vibration data transmitted by the ROS master node from both motors. After being tagged, the ATV moves across the first three metal objects in this environment, which are known to produce high-level anomalies when the offline model is being trained.Next, by drawing a rectangle on the ground and following it until it reaches the starting point's coordinates, the ATV path planning task directs the vehicle to continue along the path. While traveling to the terminal, the ATV also crosses three copper cables that are known to cause low-level irregularities for ATV operating circumstances shows in figure 1.

Most notably, the high- and low-level abnormalities in this study can be tailored by the end users to fit any behavior that occurs within particular production environment settings. The ATV uses sound and vibration sensors near the DC motors to collect data while it completes the preprogrammed duty. The Edge AI unit then uses these data to filter and process them in order to make decisions about the ATV's status in real time.

Interface of the Data Storage

FIWARE is the middleware platform that is used to implement data transfers. Elastic search data persistence stack maintenance and backups then take place. Within the data storage, each subject released by the ATV and to which the FIWARE platform subscribes has its own index pattern. In our testing environment, the Kibana tool is used to find and refine the data captured in Elastic search. It displays the results obtained when the ATV performs a specific load-carrying operation four times. When the ATV is found to be in normal operating condition, the chart's first row displays the time-stamps corresponding to those hits on the x-axis and the quantity of hits on the y-axis.Examples of

Figure 1. ATV operating circumstances of vehicle

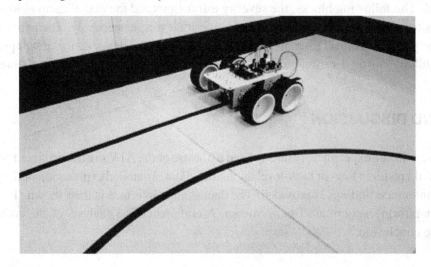

low-level anomalies found in the ATV are shown in the center graph. Time stamps that correspond to the high-level abnormalities detected by the ATV are plotted on the x-axis of the bottom graph. For the most part, the trials are conducted in open, unobstructed locations using the ATV. The bulk of data input results in the dashboard show healthy hits, indicating that the fused data acquired by sensors accurately depicts the state of the field in figure 2. After the data is examined, a high-level abnormal state is discovered when the metal bumpers that are fastened to the ground come into touch with the ATV's primary wheels.

Moreover, since this physical state was included in the model as a low-level anomaly, it appears that the ATV crosses copper cables more frequently, increasing low-level anomaly hits. Along with anomalous cases, the time axis displays the DL model's high model capacity. The experimental verification ensures that the timestamp data displayed in the dashboard is accurate and represents actual, physical occurrences of the anomaly events, even with slight delays caused by network latency. High and low anomalous strike times are influenced by turning velocity, ATV pace, and physical separation between cables.

Data Visualization and Alert Tool for Condition Monitoring

Dashboards for inferred conditions and real-time condition monitoring are generated based on the findings and the data utilized for the inference. Grafana is used to visualize elastic search data and to provide real-time email alerts to end-user stakeholders in the case that data alterations are made accidentally. Grafana's versatility makes it an easy tool to set up for a range of data formats. It can also be used by end-user operators to develop dashboards that show information from monitored environments and outcomes from Edge AI inference. This page displays the most recent, real-time statistics on ATV operations. The data is refreshed every five minutes. Two-dimensional graphs provide the raw vibration and sound data from both motors, while a gauge-style chart shows the ATV's current

Figure 2. Fused data acquired by sensors accurately

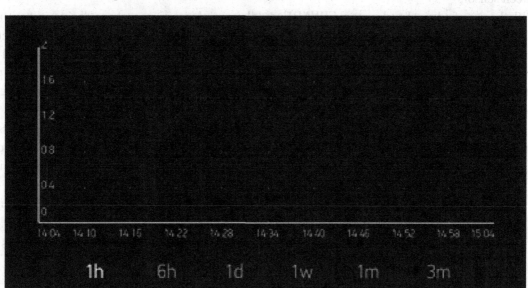

Figure 3. Dashboard is updated

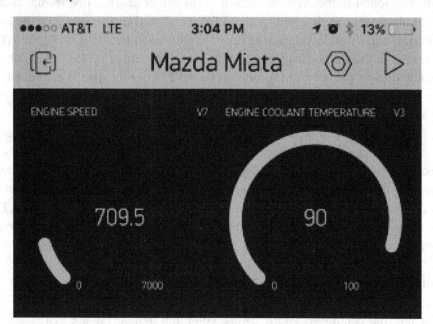

state.Every 5 mi, 30,000 data points are added to each graph, and 100 Hz is the frequency at which the data are collected.

Every time the dashboard is updated, the 500 most recent data points are added to the right side of each graph, and the 500 oldest data points are taken out of the left shows in figure 3. The 512 data points are represented by the findings of the DL model, thus the changes in anomaly hits exactly match the additional 512 data points. Consequently, each motor's sound and vibration data are displayed in the graphs below, which also serve to illustrate the differences between the data from anomalous and healthy samples. These graphs are useful tools for tracking the system's hardware condition thirteen of seventeen sensors

With the use of edge AI and custom FIWARE middleware, this project seeks to design and evaluate a real-time fault diagnosis and condition monitoring system. Since the suggested system architecture is broad in nature, it can be readily scaled and configured for various use cases, enabling several IoT devices to be status monitored at the same time. Furthermore, the potential power benefits of processing data using edge resources have been demonstrated using experimental data employing edge AI technology.

In terms of latency, privacy, communication costs, and storage costs, using the edge processing technique yields significant performance advantages. The benefits offered by edge AI are measured using a variety of criteria. The computation of these metrics takes into account two distinct scenarios:

- All raw vibration and audio data obtained from the sensors is transmitted to a central server for processing;
- The centralized server only stores and visualizes the DL model inference results following the data's filtering and processing at the edge AI unit.

For every scenario, the table presents three more metrics that are computed and presented: average bandwidth use, data transmission latency, and average duration for inference. The strain resulting from the transfer and processing of all the vibration and audio data collected from sensors to the central server is shown in the raw sensor data column. The outcomes of moving the data to the central server for archiving and visualization, however, are displayed in the "processed data at the edge AI unit" column. When numerous autonomous devices and human operators need to collaborate in the same space, real-time, safety-critical systems compute these performance indicators.

CONCLUSION

In addition to an in-house, specially designed middleware solution built on the FIWARE platform, this study demonstrated a comprehensive real-time defect detection and condition monitoring architecture utilizing edge AI. A wide range of use cases, such as logistics, agricultural, health applications, and security systems, can make use of the architecture's adaptability. As part of a smart manufacturing solution, we used an ATV condition monitoring use case to show off the system. The architecture is adaptable enough, even with ROS, to work with a range of IoT devices that can be used with various kinds of generic enablers and data adapters. Based on data from its numerous sensors, the ATV's edge AI gadget makes inferences.

When tested using offline ATV data, the deep learning method produces very high test accuracy, averaging 99.94% over 25 trials. The collected information and findings are then added to the data archive. The middleware system's customizing option for sensor subscriptions makes it simple to discontinue transferring raw sensor data over the network. After that, the data visualization tool generated dashboards and informed administrators as needed. To demonstrate the efficiency of the installed system, trials were conducted in a model industrial environment with a variety of operational irregularities, using ATVs to perform predetermined load-carrying activities. The developed system tracked and diagnosed ATV issues in real time using the data that was observed. Also, when the suggested edge AI solution is applied, the ATV use case requires 43 times less network traffic. Furthermore, the total data transfer time is reduced by a factor of 37 in comparison to conventional central server systems. The middleware layer may be readily expanded to handle other IoT devices, even if the experiments and system viability are shown with a single ATV. This is because different FIROS platform instances may be configured to run on different ATV units. However, there are trade-offs between the number of ATV units that are available and the cost of equipment. In order to improve operational efficiency in a smart manufacturing context, the system may therefore be integrated into actual problems. In subsequent work, we'll take a number of actions to extend the study's scope. We will provide a dynamic edge AI model training and update mechanism in the event that the DL model's performance deviates. Adding Auto ML integration and a dynamic model approach will help us improve our architecture. Model auto-update scenarios can be more easily created by integrating Auto ML techniques into the suggested architecture. Furthermore, since the suggested design incorporates a variety of equipment monitoring interface types, our upcoming work will also concentrate on extensive testing.

REFERENCES

Bae, I., Moon, J., & Seo, J. (2019). Toward a comfortable driving experience for a self-driving shuttle bus. *Electronics (Basel)*, *8*(9), 943. doi:10.3390/electronics8090943

Bakdi, A., Bounoua, W., Guichi, A., & Mekhilef, S. (2021). Real-time fault detection in PV systems under MPPT using PMU and high-frequency multi-sensor data through online PCA-KDE-based multivariate KL divergence. *International Journal of Electrical Power & Energy Systems*, *125*, 106457. doi:10.1016/j.ijepes.2020.106457

Cai, Y., Luan, T., Gao, H., Wang, H., Chen, L., Li, Y., Sotelo, M. A., & Li, Z. (2021). YOLOv4-5D: An effective and efficient object detector for autonomous driving. *IEEE Transactions on Instrumentation and Measurement*, *70*, 1–13. doi:10.1109/TIM.2021.3065438

Carranza-García, M., Torres-Mateo, J., Lara-Benítez, P., & García-Gutiérrez, J. (2021). On the performance of one-stage and two-stage object detectors in autonomous vehicles using camera data. *Remote Sensing (Basel)*, *13*(1), 89. doi:10.3390/rs13010089

Chen, Z., Liu, Q., & Lian, C. (2019, June). Pointlanenet: Efficient end-to-end cnns for accurate real-time lane detection. In 2019 IEEE intelligent vehicles symposium (IV) (pp. 2563-2568). IEEE.

Chiu, Y. C., Tsai, C. Y., Ruan, M. D., Shen, G. Y., & Lee, T. T. (2020, August). Mobilenet-SSDv2: An improved object detection model for embedded systems. In *2020 International conference on system science and engineering (ICSSE)* (pp. 1-5). IEEE. 10.1109/ICSSE50014.2020.9219319

Deng, W., & Wu, R. (2019). Real-time driver-drowsiness detection system using facial features. *IEEE Access: Practical Innovations, Open Solutions*, *7*, 118727–118738. doi:10.1109/ACCESS.2019.2936663

Guo, N., Lenzo, B., Zhang, X., Zou, Y., Zhai, R., & Zhang, T. (2020). A real-time nonlinear model predictive controller for yaw motion optimization of distributed drive electric vehicles. *IEEE Transactions on Vehicular Technology*, *69*(5), 4935–4946. doi:10.1109/TVT.2020.2980169

Gupta, A., Anpalagan, A., Guan, L., & Khwaja, A. S. (2021). Deep learning for object detection and scene perception in self-driving cars: Survey, challenges, and open issues. *Array (New York, N.Y.)*, *10*, 100057. doi:10.1016/j.array.2021.100057

Hong, Y., Pan, H., Sun, W., & Jia, Y. (2021). Deep dual-resolution networks for real-time and accurate semantic segmentation of road scenes. *arXiv preprint arXiv:2101.06085*.

Jabbar, R., Shinoy, M., Kharbeche, M., Al-Khalifa, K., Krichen, M., & Barkaoui, K. (2020, February). Driver drowsiness detection model using convolutional neural networks techniques for android application. In *2020 IEEE International Conference on Informatics, IoT, and Enabling Technologies (ICIoT)* (pp. 237-242). IEEE. 10.1109/ICIoT48696.2020.9089484

Langarica, S., Rüffelmacher, C., & Núñez, F. (2019). An industrial internet application for real-time fault diagnosis in industrial motors. *IEEE Transactions on Automation Science and Engineering*, *17*(1), 284–295. doi:10.1109/TASE.2019.2913628

Li, D., Zhang, Z., Liu, P., Wang, Z., & Zhang, L. (2020). Battery fault diagnosis for electric vehicles based on voltage abnormality by combining the long short-term memory neural network and the equivalent circuit model. *IEEE Transactions on Power Electronics*, *36*(2), 1303–1315. doi:10.1109/TPEL.2020.3008194

Liu, L., Lu, S., Zhong, R., Wu, B., Yao, Y., Zhang, Q., & Shi, W. (2020). Computing systems for autonomous driving: State of the art and challenges. *IEEE Internet of Things Journal*, *8*(8), 6469–6486. doi:10.1109/JIOT.2020.3043716

Liu, Z., Cai, Y., Wang, H., Chen, L., Gao, H., Jia, Y., & Li, Y. (2021). Robust target recognition and tracking of self-driving cars with radar and camera information fusion under severe weather conditions. *IEEE Transactions on Intelligent Transportation Systems*, *23*(7), 6640–6653. doi:10.1109/TITS.2021.3059674

Manoharan, D. S. (2019). An improved safety algorithm for artificial intelligence enabled processors in self driving cars. *Journal of Artificial Intelligence and Capsule Networks*, *1*(2), 95–104. doi:10.36548/jaicn.2019.2.005

Muhammad, K., Ullah, A., Lloret, J., Del Ser, J., & de Albuquerque, V. H. C. (2020). Deep learning for safe autonomous driving: Current challenges and future directions. *IEEE Transactions on Intelligent Transportation Systems*, *22*(7), 4316–4336. doi:10.1109/TITS.2020.3032227

Ouyang, Z., Niu, J., Liu, Y., & Guizani, M. (2019). Deep CNN-based real-time traffic light detector for self-driving vehicles. *IEEE Transactions on Mobile Computing*, *19*(2), 300–313. doi:10.1109/TMC.2019.2892451

Rohan, A., Rabah, M., & Kim, S. H. (2019). Convolutional neural network-based real-time object detection and tracking for parrot AR drone 2. *IEEE Access : Practical Innovations, Open Solutions*, *7*, 69575–69584. doi:10.1109/ACCESS.2019.2919332

Simon, M., Amende, K., Kraus, A., Honer, J., Samann, T., Kaulbersch, H., & Michael Gross, H. (2019). Complexer-yolo: Real-time 3d object detection and tracking on semantic point clouds. In *Proceedings of the IEEE/CVF Conference on Computer Vision and Pattern Recognition Workshops* (pp. 0-0). IEEE. 10.1109/CVPRW.2019.00158

Sun, L., Yang, K., Hu, X., Hu, W., & Wang, K. (2020). Real-time fusion network for RGB-D semantic segmentation incorporating unexpected obstacle detection for road-driving images. *IEEE Robotics and Automation Letters*, *5*(4), 5558–5565. doi:10.1109/LRA.2020.3007457

Van Wyk, F., Wang, Y., Khojandi, A., & Masoud, N. (2019). Real-time sensor anomaly detection and identification in automated vehicles. *IEEE Transactions on Intelligent Transportation Systems*, *21*(3), 1264–1276. doi:10.1109/TITS.2019.2906038

Verma, A. K., Nagpal, S., Desai, A., & Sudha, R. (2021). An efficient neural-network model for real-time fault detection in industrial machine. *Neural Computing & Applications*, *33*(4), 1297–1310. doi:10.1007/s00521-020-05033-z

Yao, L., Fang, Z., Xiao, Y., Hou, J., & Fu, Z. (2021). An intelligent fault diagnosis method for lithium battery systems based on grid search support vector machine. *Energy*, *214*, 118866. doi:10.1016/j.energy.2020.118866

Yao, L., Xiao, Y., Gong, X., Hou, J., & Chen, X. (2020). A novel intelligent method for fault diagnosis of electric vehicle battery system based on wavelet neural network. *Journal of Power Sources, 453*, 227870. doi:10.1016/j.jpowsour.2020.227870

Yaqoob, I., Khan, L. U., Kazmi, S. A., Imran, M., Guizani, N., & Hong, C. S. (2019). Autonomous driving cars in smart cities: Recent advances, requirements, and challenges. *IEEE Network, 34*(1), 174–181. doi:10.1109/MNET.2019.1900120

Yin, S., Rodriguez-Andina, J. J., & Jiang, Y. (2019). Real-time monitoring and control of industrial cyberphysical systems: With integrated plant-wide monitoring and control framework. *IEEE Industrial Electronics Magazine, 13*(4), 38–47. doi:10.1109/MIE.2019.2938025

Chapter 5
IoT in Day-to-Day Life:
Vehicle Body Fatigue Analysis

Rajaram Vassudev Pai Kuchelkar
Liverpool John Moores University, India

Anupama Jawale
ⓘ https://orcid.org/0000-0002-9982-5218
Narsee Monjee College of Commerce and Economics, India

ABSTRACT

One of the analyses is fatigue analysis which helps determine the durability of the product for its intended life. The fatigue analysis requires an input data from vehicle-road interaction obtained as vertical acceleration. The input data is then used in finite element analysis software or in a test rig instrumentation to perform a fatigue analysis. The focus of this study is about collecting the input data using a data acquisition device. OEM of the automobiles use proprietary data acquisition device for testing their vehicles for durability. However, the automotive body building companies or vehicle body builders which are 1-Tier companies below OEM have a limited budget for such an analysis and therefore they principally lag in advance analysis approach such as a fatigue analysis for the design of vehicle body. Instead, to sustain durability of vehicle, the design is made heavier. This research study is an effort to provide an affordable setup for data acquisition by making use of IoT and web technologies which are cost effective.

INTRODUCTION

The term fatigue in this context means the cyclic loading of material. The principle of fatigue is based on the material S-N curve, which is material strength (S) versus the number of load cycles (N). As the number of load cycles increases, the material strength weakens. A fatigue analysis is conducted to determine the durability and life of the component. A lab setup with test rigs and instrumentation is a conventional technique used for conducting fatigue analysis. In the modern world of digitization, finite element-based approaches are commonly used. The finite element approach is

DOI: 10.4018/979-8-3693-1962-8.ch005

considered the best approach due to savings in time and resources over the conventional approach. To conduct fatigue analysis for the vehicle body using a finite element approach, the inputs from vehicle-road interaction such as vertical acceleration and number of cycles are necessary. The vehicle is instrumented with data acquisition devices and the vehicle-road response is captured. The road surface quality equally influences fatigue behaviour. If the road is rough or undulated, the vertical acceleration is more intense, which results in reduced fatigue life. If the road is good, fatigue life is longer. Vehicles travel mostly on concrete or asphalt types of roads during their life span. The seasonal changes like monsoon rains and floods spoil the road surface, and this in turn influences fatigue. Therefore, study of fatigue is necessary on type of roads intended for the design of the vehicle. The fatigue analysis is used by Original Equipment Manufacturer (OEM) for fully built bodies like cars, utility vehicles, truck cabins, and chassis whereas hardly ever used by vehicle body builders for body building applications like buses, truck load bodies, containers etc. This is due to the lack of road load input data for benchmark vehicles, the high cost of proprietary data acquisition equipment to generate own data, and time constraints for body building development activity required by customers. In the Indian market, vehicle body builders are facing stiff competition from their peers in terms of product pricing, weight, mileage, and payload carrying efficiencies. Vehicle body builders must make constant efforts on light weighting of vehicle body to gain leverage over their competitors and therefore may consider a proper analytical approach such as fatigue analysis for durability confirmation. This research study focuses on the way of capturing and recording the vehicle-road response using low-cost data acquisition methods, making it affordable for the vehicle body builders to conduct vehicle body fatigue analysis.

The data acquisition instruments are required for recording the vehicle-road response. The proprietary data acquisition instruments available on the market are expensive as they are designed for robust usage like measuring the leaf springs or vehicle axle components which have high vertical acceleration values. The vehicle body has a lower operating range of vertical acceleration as compared to vehicle components below vehicle suspension which makes it feasible to use low-cost IoT components for data acquisition. The vehicle body builders cannot afford the cost of proprietary data acquisition instrumentation. As a result, as a first step, there is a need to suggest an affordable tool for data acquisition and a method for preparing input data for fatigue analysis, which are discussed in this research study.

The main aim of this research is to propose an affordable solution to the vehicle body builders on data acquisition for vehicle body fatigue analysis. With this affordable solution, the body builders will incur low expense on the data acquisition instrument and can focus on the analysis part. The research objectives are formulated based on the aim of this study which are as follows:

- To study the recent developments in the tools and techniques used for data acquisition of vehicle-road interaction.
- To propose a low-cost data acquisition device using IoT for acquiring the parameters for fatigue analysis.
- To acquire a dataset practically using the proposed data acquisition instrument.
- To analyse the acquired dataset and prepare input test cases for fatigue analysis.

The research questions are as follows.

- What are the modern tools and techniques used for vehicle-road data acquisition?
- How to build simple IoT based circuit and a tool for data acquisition for fatigue analysis?
- How to acquire a dataset for fatigue analysis using a simple data acquisition?
- How to analyse and post-process the acquired data and prepare input test cases for fatigue analysis?

Vehicle body fatigue analysis is conducted with inputs of vertical acceleration and number of cycles. The analysis is then performed using a finite element analysis approach. The scope of the study is about the data acquisition of vertical acceleration and devising methods for the determination of the number of cycles and test cases for finite element analysis. The scope excludes performing a finite element analysis. As the vehicle bodies operate in the lower vertical acceleration range described in the problem statement, the scope of the study is applicable to all types of vehicle bodies only. On the other hand, a vehicle chassis is subjected to a higher range of vertical acceleration from the vehicle-road response. As this needs a higher degree of accuracy and precision on data acquisition instruments fulfilled by proprietary instruments, the vehicle chassis is excluded from the scope of study. The scope of the study is to devise affordable data acquisition instrumentation using IoT technologies in the field of computer science.

This study will provide a cost-effective method for the vehicle body builder and guide them to create their own data acquisition device and road test database using low-cost electronics and open-source IDE platforms for programming microcontrollers. This study will also show how to process the collected data and prepare the input test cases for fatigue analysis.

BACKGROUND

Introduction

In this section, we will explore the literature on fatigue analysis studies conducted by researchers and the data acquisition methods using IoTs that can be adopted for capturing the vehicle-road response. The literature study is broadly classified based on Fatigue Analysis, Data Acquisition Process, Data Acquisition Devices and Data Analysis as tabulated in Table 1,2,3 and 4 respectively.

Inputs for Fatigue Analysis

From the above review, it can be summarised that the inputs principally needed for fatigue analysis are a data acquisition system for collection of vehicle-road response, sensors connected to vehicle body, and a data recording device such as a SD card or a computer system/smart phone. Optionally, GPS, time module, and Wi-Fi modules may be used to record the location of the vehicle, record the time of the capturing event, and transmit the data wirelessly.

Various Approaches to Collecting Inputs for Fatigue Analysis

From the above literature, the various approaches used for collecting input data are as below.

Table 1. Literature review based on fatigue analysis

Reference	Description
(Xuewen et al., 2020)	In this research study, the finite element method was used to find out the S-N curve of the structure. The load spectrum was determined based on empirical data. The load spectrum is fatigue load and the number of cycles per hour. With the above load spectrum and S-N curve of the structure, the linear Palmgren-Miner cumulative damage model was used to calculate the fatigue life. The topology optimization technique is used for the improvement of structural design.
(Polat, 2017)	In this research study, the CAD model of the subject frame was done in the Solid Works CAD software. The Ansys Static Programmer software was used for the finite element analysis model. A static analysis was performed using the on-vehicle weight method. The fatigue analysis is performed using Ncode Design Life software using the test track data and then the fatigue life of the parts on the model is examined. Three important steps are mentioned for fatigue analysis, such as selection of fatigue methods, selection of installation methods, and selection of a curve for material fatigue (S-N curve).
(Salokhe et al., 2016)	In this research study, the damage detection of a structure is studied, which is like fatigue. The technique used here is based on dynamic response collected from the structure under study. A technique called Singular Value Decomposition (SVD) is used to predict the damage of the structure.
(Ogunoiki, 2015)	This research study has discussed three methods of data acquisition: the empirical method, the analytical method, and the semi-analytical method. The empirical method consists of a customer survey and proving ground. The analytical method consists of finite element analysis and multi-body dynamics. The semi-analytical method consists of a combination of analytical and empirical methods. A lab setup is used here with a quarter vehicle test rig. Transducers such as Piezoelectric Accelerometer, load cell, and linear variable differential transformer are used in the equipment for measurement of signals. A hydraulic power unit is used to apply the road input excitations to the test rig. Different computer software such as Cubus, QanTiM, and LabVIEW are used to acquire the data from the test rig. The above experiment is also done in CAD and SIMPACK multi-body dynamics and the results are compared in this study. Machine Learning aspects are also studied in this paper.
(Shafiullah & Wu, 2013)	In this research study, an Accelerated Durability test is modelled. A conjugative approach consisting of finite element analysis and fatigue analysis for a specific durability life is used. Instead of a time-based technique, a frequency-based technique is used to accelerate the fatigue analysis. For fatigue analysis, Ncode Design Life software is used.
(Dongpo & Xuhui, 2011)	This research study follows a CAE-based approach. The data for the virtual proving ground is verified using MATLAB software. The durability analysis is carried out using explicit finite element code using LSDYNA, a proprietary CAE software package.
(Mo et al., 2000)	This research study uses a different technique for durability study (or fatigue analysis) using a virtual proving ground. A virtual proving ground is a laboratory test with finite element analysis. From the analysis, fatigue life is predicated on the stress magnitude and load history. Fatigue life results of the vehicle components from the computer simulation are compared with physical test results.
(Sener, n.d.)	This research study applies to the fatigue analysis of automatic transmission shafts. The design of shafts requires a service history or load history of the shaft. The process of capturing service history and load history is done with a data acquisition system. The amount of service history data needed is huge, so a 12-bit data acquisition system is used. A high sampling rate such as 4KHz is used, which generates a data rate of 20MB per hour. In this study, proprietary data acquisition systems are referred to as expensive equipment. Therefore, an innovative approach to cost-effective data acquisition technique with data compression is studied.
(Ilic et al., n.d.)	This research study was carried out in Turkey. Around fifty Turkish roads were studied to capture the characteristics of fatigue and define a load spectrum. A leaf spring of a test vehicle was studied for equivalent fatigue damage caused by an accelerated test method. Fatigue analysis and estimated fatigue life were calculated using a finite element analysis approach and verified by using the Palmgren-Miner rule. Two types of methods have been used in this study. One is the questionnaire method, and the second is the black box method. The questionnaire method is used to survey the types of roads and types of loads. After getting the questionnaire results, a road test is programmed with a vehicle equipped with transducers to run on several types of roads with different load cases. The measured data is analysed and processed for spikes and is filtered. Frequency analysis and arithmetic manipulations are done to generate inputs for fatigue analysis. As the road signals are formed from random vibrations, the data is processed with approaches such as range pair, rain flow level crossing, and counting methods to compare the signals in a meaningful manner.

- Collecting data on different types of road surfaces.
- Collecting data at different speeds.
- Collecting data on proving grounds.
- Using a CAE tool such as multi-body dynamics on virtual proving ground.

*Table 2. **Literature** review based on data acquisition process for fatigue analysis*

Reference	Description
(Xuewen et al., 2020)	In this research study, the load spectrum was determined using empirical data. The S-N curve of the structure was determined using finite element analysis.
(Wang et al., 2019)	In this research study, a pressure sensor is used in the air spring circuit to sense the vertical loads. The data acquisition of pressure signals is done using the Agilent Digital Signal Acquisition System.
(Polat, 2017)	In this research study, the acceleration data was collected from four different test tracks. The length of the test track is about 3 km. These acceleration values are converted to gravitational acceleration format, which is in terms of g.
(Salokhe et al., 2016)	In this research study, the data acquisition of acceleration is done by applying a heavy-duty sensor to the subject structure.
(Ogunoiki, 2015)	In this research study, data acquisition is done on a test rig setup using multi-body dynamics Finite Element Analysis tools.
(Shafiullah and Wu, 2013)	In this research study, data acquisition is done by a proprietary tool, somat eDAQ, and accelerations and strains are captured in this process. An extremely high sampling rate of 2500 Hz was used in this study.
(Mo et al., 2000)	In this research study, the data acquisition of the acting forces takes place within the finite element analysis. The vehicle model runs on the digital proving track developed in the form of finite elements. There is no physical equipment or device used for data acquisition in this study. The kind of data acquisition device used on a physical test vehicle is not described in this study.
(Sener, n.d.)	A stand-alone real-time data acquisition system was used in this research study. The system is attached to a single-board-based computer. This system is 12bit and offers a high sampling rate of 100KHz and has a storage capability of 1 GB.
(Ilic et al., n.d.)	In this research study, the data acquisition was done by deploying a load transducer and two strain gauges on the leaf spring of the suspension system, one strain gauge on the transmission shaft, and one strain gauge on the steering shaft. The vertical loads created by road roughness, manoeuvres, and acceleration were measured by two half-bridge strain gauges.

- Mounting sensors at different locations on the vehicle body.
- Using different types of chassis platforms for same type body application.

Conventional Methods versus Modern Methods of Data Acquisition

It has been discovered that conventional approaches use proprietary data acquisition devices, which are both expensive and accurate when used for high data sampling rates. The researchers have discovered low-cost data acquisition techniques that use smartphones, inexpensive sensors, and open platforms like Arduino to produce findings that are comparable to those of more traditional instruments. In situations when accuracy is crucial, like with dynamic machinery or high-speed applications, conventional approaches should be employed. While using modern methods, it is important to be aware of the appropriate sampling rate and measurement range.

Data Processing and Analysis Techniques

Fourier transforms and related approaches, including windowed Fourier transforms, are frequently used to process data for vibration signals with a sinusoidal component. However, additional methods, such as range pair, rain flow, and counting procedures, are used to process the random vibration signals from the vehicle-road (Ilic et al., n.d.).

Table 3. Literature review based on data acquisition devices

Reference	Description
(Ur Rehman et al., 2021)	This research study uses IoT for monitoring and control of substations to provide safe electricity to consumers. The equipment used is a Microcontroller ESP32 with the Cayenne IoT platform. It uses different types of sensors, namely current sensors, voltage sensors, frequency sensors, humidity sensors, temperature sensors, and oil level sensors. The Cayenne platform is useful for real-time monitoring, data logging, and control.
(Shuai et al., 2021)	In this research study, the data was acquired with sensors which include acceleration sensors, pull-type displacement sensors, strain flowers, and GPS with the help of a video auxiliary system. The collection equipment consisted of an eDAQ system and NCode Design Life analysis software.
(Pal Singh & Singh, 2021)	In this research study, a low-cost data acquisition system consisting of an Arduino Uno is used for vehicle-road interaction. The accelerometer ADXL345 is used for capturing acceleration factors, and the GPS receiver Ublox Neo 6M is used for capturing the location coordinates. The Arduino Uno uses an 8-bit ATmega328P microcontroller.
(Jamaludin, 2021)	The Arduino based board is used in this research study. The different modules used in the circuit are a current and voltage sensor unit, a real-time clock module, a power supply module, and a secure digital card module. The type of microcontroller on the Arduino board is the Atmega328P type.
(Moreno et al., 2020)	This research study states that the configuration is required for measurement of high-frequency-based vehicular applications. The sensors required for the study are displacement sensors, acceleration sensors, and speed sensors. The different kinds of sensors make the price of data acquisition equipment skyrocket. This study proposes a low-cost data acquisition, 'Arduino Due', with enhancement of its limitations on the speed of data transfer. By using some programming techniques, the 'Arduino Due' is made compatible with the requirements of high-frequency vehicular applications. The paper compares various Arduino boards and selects the 'Arduino Due' as the most relevant board for this application.
(Amestica et al., 2019)	The researcher studied different types of digital platforms and programmed using the Arduino IDE platform, which is used for data acquisition applications and performing digital controls. The three types of Arduino boards studied in this research paper were Arduino Uno, Arduino Mega, and Arduino Due. ESP-based boards, that is, ESP8266 and ESP32 boards, were also used in this study. Comparison is made for execution time with the above boards in this study. ESP boards can be connected to a Wi-Fi network.
(Wong et al., 2019)	In this research study, a data logger is prepared using Arduino. The 1Sheeld Android Application is used, which connects to the timestamp, accelerometer, and Bluetooth of the smartphone.
(González et al., 2018)	This research study uses an Arduino-based system along with low-cost accelerometers. The accelerometer ADXL345 and MPU6050 are used. Vehicle dynamics applications are being studied. A comparison of the performance of the Arduino-based data acquisition is made with professional data acquisition systems. A professional data acquisition system with 4 channels connected to piezoelectric accelerometers has been used. The study concludes that the low-cost system is suitable for data acquisition for vehicle dynamics applications.
(Chellaswamy et al., 2018)	This research study is about road surface monitoring. The road surface deformities, such as the potholes are studied. The data acquisition equipment used in this study consists of the following: Arduino Uno with ESP8266, Ultrasonic Sensor, MEMS Accelerometer, GPS Receiver, and Access Point. A layered architecture has been used, starting from top level to bottom level, as Cloud Server, Edge Server, Node IoT, and Sensors.
(Wali & Areeb, 2018)	In this research study, Proposed data acquisition equipment consists of an Arduino Mega 2560 and a Raspberry Pi. Different types of proprietary data acquisition are compared with Arduino board-based data acquisition in terms of cost.
(Wu et al., 2018)	This research study is about a massive data collection of driving events. An on-board device in the vehicle was used in this study. The on-board device is made of the MT662 chip, which contains a Wi-Fi/Bluetooth transceiver and an FM receiver. The sensing data on acceleration and angular velocity is generated by a built-in chip called the BMI120. The BMI120 chip is a low-powered 3-axis low-g accelerometer and 3-axis gyroscope. It produces 50 sets of data per second.
(Monterrey, 2018)	In this research study, road load data acquisition on heavy trucks is studied. A proprietary data acquisition device is used. Accelerometers and strain gauges are used for acquiring road signals. LabVIEW software is used to read, process, store, and analyse the information.
(Gonzalez et al., 2017)	The researcher studies road anomalies using a smart phone. The smart phone's inbuilt sensor accelerometer is used for the purpose of capturing acceleration in (m/s^2). The dataset collected in this study is made available to the public.
(Agrawal et al., 2016)	In this research study, the data acquisition system uses the Arduino Uno board, an MPU 6050 accelerometer, and a temperature sensor. The analysis is performed on MATLAB software.
(Du et al., 2016)	In this research study, a ZigBee module is used to collect accelerations. The acceleration is measured in the Z-axis. An embedded 3G/4G module is used to transmit the data to an FTP server. A micro controller (MCU) (type TC12C5608AD) is used. An accelerometer (type MMA8451Q) is used.

continued on following page

Table 3. Continued

Reference	Description
(Mohamed et al., 2014)	In this research study, smart phones are used for data acquisition. Accelerometer, Gyroscope and GPS inside the smart phone are used to collect data and the data is stored in the form of file. The file is dumped into micro-SD card in the smartphone. This paper studies capturing events for a speed bump. From the acceleration data, the features for speed bump are extracted using the conditions for acceleration in Z axis and X axis. This data is further classified and studied for machine learning.
(Of & Signal, 2013)	In this research study, various components of data acquisition are explained. Single channel, multi-channel and pc-based data acquisition are described. LabVIEW software is used for controlling of data acquisition. Noise filter is applied.
(Perttunen et al., 2011)	This research study is about road roughness measurement. Smart phones are used to collect data. (The smartphone model used is the Nokia N95 8GB). The sampling rate is 38Hz for the accelerometer and 1Hz for GPS readings. The data collection tool is written in Java. The position of the smart phone was on the rack of the windscreen. The test drive was 25km in 40 minutes. A camera was attached to capture the drive. Cobblestone data was filtered out. The data was classified based on types of road anomalies based on feature extraction and selection techniques, and the statistics of the findings were plotted.
(Chen, 2009)	In this research study, a remote-controlled signal analyser (HP3560A) is used in this study and controlled over the internet using LabVIEW.
(Junnila & Niittylahti, 2003)	This research study discusses various worldwide open standards for wireless communications. These include Bluetooth, ZigBee module, WLAN, Wireless USB, Spike, Nanonet, RF-232, UWB, RF Transceivers.

Table 4. Literature review based on data analysis or signal processing

References	Methodology used for processing of signals
(Men et al., 2018)	This research study discusses processing vibration signals. It says relative mean square (RMS) is an important index for the study of vibrations. Further, this paper discusses certain problems with the computation of RMS value and therefore proposes an improved method called the time domain filtering method in this study.
(P. Wang, 2017)	In this research study, the acceleration signal is studied. The signal consists of noise, which is removed using the Fourier transform. The wavelet analysis is applied, which achieves the noise removal. A wavelet analysis is a time-frequency analysis used for de-noising signals. A Fourier transform is used to convert the signal from the time domain to the frequency domain. The displacement signal is calculated in this study from the acceleration signal.
(U et al., 2015)	The limitations of Fast Fourier Transform (FFT) are discussed in this research study. The study discusses that if the measured signals have high sensitivity and many times invariant harmonics, then it is difficult to extract fault-related signals. Hence, a Windowed Fourier Transform (WFT) approach is used. This study was applied to the study of bearing vibrations and finding out the fault frequencies of the bearing.
(Baoquan, 2011)	A blasting vibration signal is studied in this research. The Fast Fourier Transform (FFT) is used in conjunction with the Short-time Fourier Transform (STFT).
(Hu et al., 2011)	In this research study, time domain sea maps with windowed Fourier transformation are examined.
(Q. Wang et al., 2009)	In this research study, MATLAB software is used to do frequency domain analysis to identify motor noise. Power spectrum analysis combined with holographic spectrum analysis is conducted to find the abnormal vibration of the motor more precisely.

Related Datasets for Fatigue Analysis

(Gonzalez et al., 2017) freely publishes data sets of the data collected on various types of roads for analysis. The acceleration data is collected in the X, Y, and Z axes. The researcher has collected the data on asphalt bump roads, potholed roads, metal bump roads, and regular roads. This data can be studied for fatigue analysis inputs.

Highlights of Literature Review

According to the literature evaluation, a vehicle's fatigue analysis can also be referred to as its durability analysis. There are several different approaches, including lab-based and finite element-based approaches. The cost of using lab-based procedures makes them unsuitable for our target users, Vehicle Body Builders (VBB), who operate as lean businesses with little resources for research and development. The optimum approach is a combination of realistic, low-cost data acquisition of vehicle-road on a chosen road track defined by the vehicle body designer and employing a finite element analysis tool for fatigue analysis. This ought to be the most affordable solution for vehicle fatigue analysis.

In the different reviews of literature on vehicle fatigue analysis, the open-source, low-cost data acquisition system known as Arduino has been offered and demonstrated as a low-cost alternative. For gathering data, sensors like the MCU6050 and the ADXL3XX series have been developed. For remotely acquiring or monitoring the signals, web technologies including cloud servers, client servers, and Wi-Fi modules like ESP8266 and ESP32 have also been employed. Road roughness has been measured using the aforementioned technologies. The built-in accelerometers and other sensors of smartphones have been extensively used by researchers to collect data. Researchers have utilised rain-flow or counting methods to study random vibrations, while Fourier transform techniques have been used to study dynamic machinery and vibration signals with cyclic patterns.

FATIGUE ANALYSIS

Introduction

The methodology for vehicle body fatigue analysis using IoT broadly covers the following steps as depicted in Figure 1.

- The vehicle-road interaction leads to vertical acceleration.
- The vertical acceleration is captured using a data acquisition instrument sampled for a short duration of about 3 to 5 minutes.
- The sampled data is analysed for a frequently occurring pattern of acceleration values.
- The frequency of occurrences is extrapolated to desired life span of the vehicle.
- Finally, the number of cycles is computed which serves as input test case for fatigue analysis.

Methodology for Data Acquisition

- A data acquisition device shall be deployed in the vehicle as per the vehicle designer's requirement.
- The accelerometer of the data acquisition device shall be attached to a hard point on the vehicle body, such as a seat mounting or over the front or rear wheels.
- The accelerometer's Z axis shall be aligned parallel to the vertical axis as shown in Figure 2, which is also perpendicular to the ground plane.

Figure 1. Flow chart for fatigue analysis study

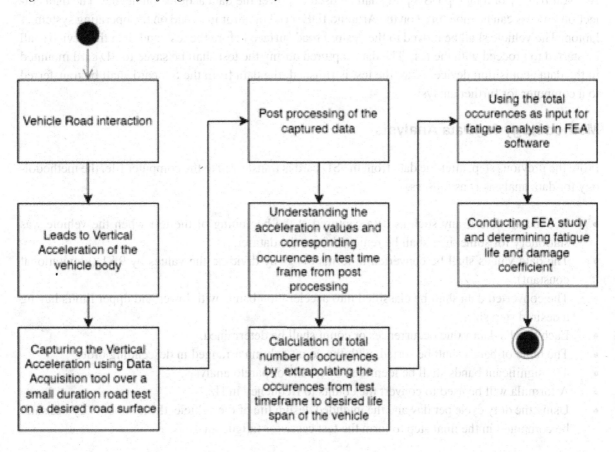

Figure 2. Vehicle layout showing ground plane and vertical axis

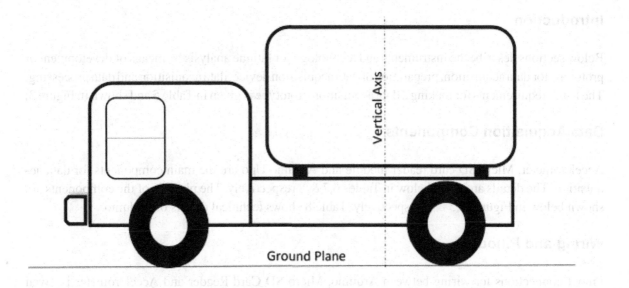

A 5-volt battery or a laptop USB port shall be used to power the data acquisition device. The data collection process can be monitored on the Arduino IDE serial monitor installed on the operating system of laptop. The vehicle shall be moved to the desired road surface before the test, and then the device shall be started to proceed with the test. The data captured during the test shall be saved to SD card mounted in the data acquisition device. After the test is finished, the data from the SD card shall be transferred to a computer for further analysis.

Methodology for Data Analysis

From the previous step, after the data from the SD card is transferred to the computer file, the methodology for data analysis is as follows.

- Redundant data if any such as data captured at the beginning of the test when the vehicle was stationery for some time shall be removed from the dataset.
- The data values shall be converted in terms of 'g' by dividing the values by 9.81 (gravitational constant).
- The converted data shall be classified into acceleration bands with lower and upper limits having a desired step size.
- Each band's data value occurrences or count shall be determined.
- The table of bands shall be sorted, with the count column arranged in descending order.
- The significant bands shall be identified by means of pareto analysis.
- A formula will be used to convert the counts to frequency in Hz.
- Using the duty cycle per day and the intended design life of the vehicle, the number of cycles shall be computed in the final step to form the test cases for fatigue analysis.

INSTRUMENTS AND TECHNOLOGY FOR FATIGUE ANALYSIS

Introduction

Below sections describe the instruments and technology for fatigue analysis by means of development of prototype for data acquisition, preparation of data acquisition device, data acquisition and data processing. The list of requirements for making a data acquisition prototype is given in Table 5 and shown in Figure 3.

Data Acquisition Components

Accelerometer, Micro SD card reader module and Arduino Uno are the main components for data acquisition. The details are given below in Tables 6,7 & 8 respectively. The pictures of the components are shown below in Figures 4,5 & 6 respectively. Table 8 shows technical details of Arduino.

Wiring and Pinout

Pinout connections for wiring between Arduino, Micro SD Card Reader and Accelerometer is given below in Table 9 and 10. Wiring layout is given in Figure 7.

Table 5. Requirements for Prototype data acquisition

Sn	Description	Qty
1	Arduino Uno Board	1
2	ADXL 345 Accelerometer	1
3	Micro SD Card Reader Module	1
4	Jumper Wires	10
5	USB Power Cable for Arduino Uno	1
6	Laptop installed with Arduino IDE	1
7	Object Vehicle	1
8	Adhesive Tape	20 centimetres
9	Micro SD Card	1

Figure 3. Layout of data acquisition device

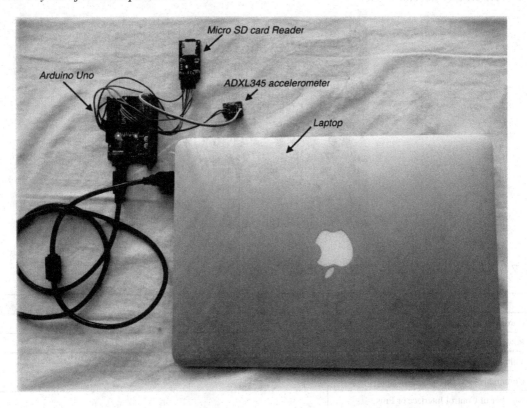

The data acquisition device preparation is done by uploading a code (also known as a sketch) to the Arduino Board microcontroller. The code for the data acquisition device is written in C++ using the Arduino IDE software. For uploading the code, the code is opened in the Arduino IDE on the laptop connected to the Arduino board of data acquisition, and the code is uploaded by the upload button on the IDE. The data acquisition device is ready for deployment. (LastMinuteEngineers.com, 2022), PiMyLife(2022), (Mechatronics, 2022; PiMyLife, 2022; toptechboy.com, n.d.) provide coding referrals.

Table 6. Technical data of ADXL345 accelerometer (Analog Devices Inc. and Inc., 2008)

Sn	Description	Values
1	Sensitivity range	+/- 2g to +/- 16g
2	Input voltage supported	5V / 3.3V
3	Output data rate (Measurement rate)	0.1 to 3200 Hz
4	Number of pins	8
5	Axes	3 (X-axis, Y-axis and Z-axis). X and Y axis are in plane of the board. Z axis is perpendicular to the plane of the board.
6	Pin configuration and description	GND, VCC, CS, INT1, INT2, SDO, SDA, SCL GND to ground, VCC to power supply, CS to chip select, INT 1: interrupt, INT2: interrupt, SDO: serial data output, SDA: serial data (I2C), SCL: serial communications clock

Note. In this study, we will use the Z axis to measure vertical acceleration.

Figure 4. ADXL354 accelerometer

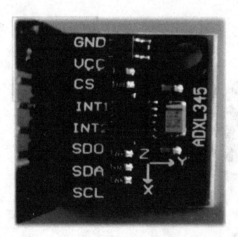

Table 7. Technical data of micro-SD card reader module

Sn	Description	Values
1	Card type & capacity	Micro sd card (<=2GB) and micro sdhc card (<=32GB)
2	Power Supply or Input Supply Voltage (VDC)	4.5~5 Volts
3	Voltage regulator	3.3 Volts
4	Communication Protocol	SPI
5	Number of Control Interface or Pins	6
6	Control Interface	GND, VCC, MISO, MOSI, SCK, CS GND to ground, VCC is the power supply, MISO, MOSI, SCK is the SPI bus, CS is the chip select signal pin
7	PCB Size (L x W) mm	40 x 24

Figure 5. Micro SD card reader module
Courtesy: www.robu.in

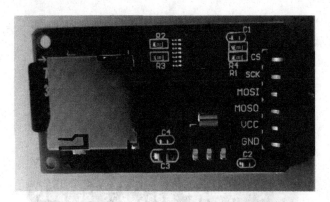

Table 8. Technical data of Arduino uno

Sn	Description	Values
1	Input Voltage (Recommended)	7-12V
2	Analog I/O Pins	6
3	Digital I/O Pins	14 (of which 6 provide PWM output)
4	PWM Digital I/O Pins	6
5	Clock Speed	16 MHz
6	Flash Memory	32 KB
7	SRAM (KB)	2
8	EEPROM	1 KB (ATmega328P)
9	DC Current for 3.3V Pin (mA)	50
10	DC Current per I/O Pin (mA)	20
11	On Board LEDs	Yes
12	Operating Temperature (C)	-10 to 60
13	Weight (gm)	25
14	Length (mm)	68.6
15	Width (mm)	53.4
16	Height (mm)	12.5

Data Acquisition

An asphalt road consisting of average roughness was selected as shown in Figure 8. The prototype data acquisition device was installed on the vehicle body. The accelerometer sensor of the data acquisition device is deployed at the co-driver seat mounting hard point as shown in Figures 9. The Z axis of the accelerometer is ensured to be perpendicular to the plane of the road surface. A road test was taken at vehicle speed 30 Kilometres per hour for 3-5 minutes duration. Vertical acceleration data was acquired

Figure 6. Arduino Uno
Courtesy: www.electronicscomp.com

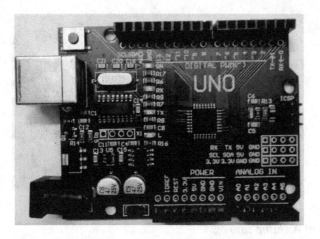

Table 9. Pinout connection for Arduino uno and micro SD card reader

Micro SD Card Reader Pin	Arduino Uno Pin	Remarks
+5	5V	Power Supply
CS	4	Chip Select
MOSI	11	SPI Data
SCK	13	clock
MOSO	12	SPI Data
GND	GND	Ground

Table 10. Pinout connection for Arduino uno and ADXL 345 accelerometer

Arduino	ADXL345
A4 PIN(SDA)	SDA PIN
A5 PIN(SCL)	SCL PIN
GND PIN	GND
5V	VCC

during the test drive at a sampling rate of 2 Hertz (Hz). The test was monitored on a laptop by a co-driver using Arduino IDE serial monitor.

Data Processing and Results

The dataset collected in this study has 384 data points at a sampling rate of 2Hz. Higher sampling rates may also be selected by the designer, such as 5Hz, 10Hz etc. The accelerometer has a maximum capacity of 3200Hz. The total time duration of the test = number of data points/sampling rate

Figure 7. Writing diagram of data acquisition circuit preparation of data acquisition device

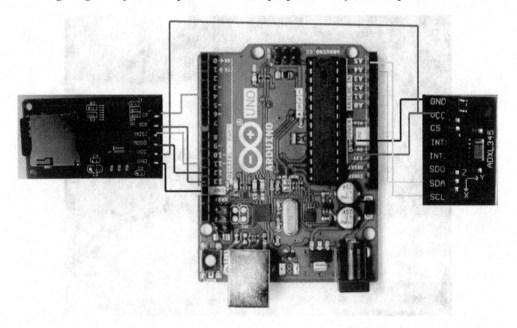

Figure 8. Road surface

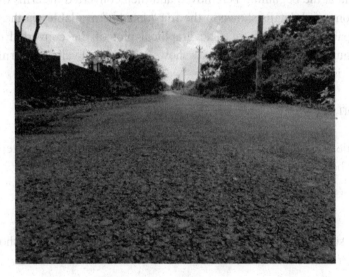

= 384 / 2

= 192 seconds

= 3 minutes, 12 seconds

The dataset collected in this study can be downloaded from GitHub link https://github.com/rajaram-pai-kuchelkar/daq.git. File name: roadtest_24.05.2022.csv .

Figure 9. Deployment of data acquisition at vehicle seat mounting

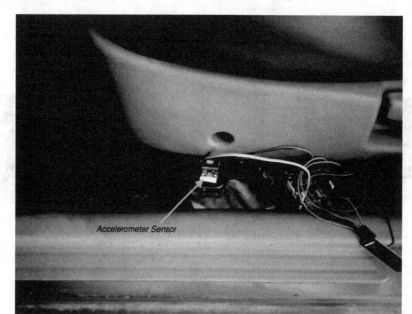

The redundant data at the beginning is removed and then converted in terms of g by dividing each value by 9.81. The converted data is shown in the file "data.txt" available via the GitHub link https://github.com/rajaram-pai-kuchelkar/daq.git. The graphical plot of the converted dataset against data points is shown in Figure 10 as below. The y-axis shows acceleration values in terms of g (gravitational constant) and the x-axis shows the data points.

Data Classification

The converted data file is classified in the form of bands of accelerations, with step size taken as 0.25g as shown in Table 11 below. A histogram is plotted as shown in Figure 11.

Data Sorting

The classified data is sorted based on count values field in descending order as shown in Table 12.

Figure 10. Dataset plot of road test

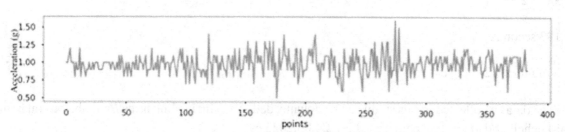

Table 11. Test sample classification of data

Acceleration Range (g)		count
lower limit	upper limit	
0	0.25	0
0.25	0.5	0
0.5	0.75	13
0.75	1	142
1	1.25	201
1.25	1.5	25
1.5	1.75	3
1.75	2	0

Figure 11. Histogram plot of test sample classification

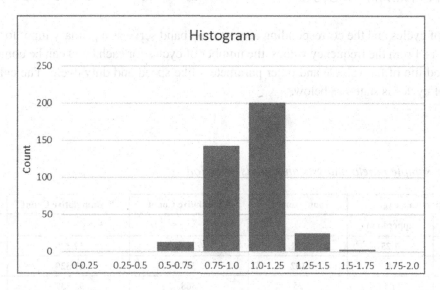

Table 12. Test sample sorted data

Acceleration Range		count (sorted)
lower limit	upper limit	
1	1.25	201
0.75	1	142
1.25	1.5	25
0.5	0.75	13
1.5	1.75	3
0	0.25	0
0.25	0.5	0
1.75	2	0

Pareto Analysis and Selection of Bands

The cumulative count and percentage cumulative count is determined as shown in Table 13. Pareto rule 80:20 is applied and the percentages up to 80% are selected.

Calculation of Frequency

The frequency is determined by dividing the number of occurrences (count) for each acceleration band by the total duration in seconds given by the below formula and shown in Table 14.

   n is the total number of points
   s is the sampling rate in Hz
   o_i is the occurrence for i^{th} band
   f is the frequency in Hz for i^{th} band, $f = oxs/n$

Calculation of Number of Cycles

The number of cycles and the corresponding acceleration band serve as a primary input for conducting fatigue analysis. From the frequency values, the number of cycles for each band can be computed based on the required life of the vehicle and other parameters like speed and duty cycle. The calculation for the number of cycles is stated as below.

Table 13. Test sample pareto analysis and bands selection

Acceleration Range (g)		count (sorted)	Cumulative Count	% Cumulative Count	Remarks
low limit	upper limit				
1	1.25	201	201	52.34%	selected
0.75	1	142	343	89.32%	selected
1.25	1.5	25	368	95.83%	discarded
0.5	0.75	13	381	99.22%	discarded
1.5	1.75	3	384	100.00%	discarded
0	0.25	0	384	100.00%	discarded
0.25	0.5	0	384	100.00%	discarded
1.75	2	0	384	100.00%	discarded

Table 14. Test sample frequency determination

Acceleration Range (g)		Count (o) (sorted)	Frequency (f) Hz
lower limit	upper limit		
1	1.25	201	1.05
0.75	1	142	0.74

f is the frequency of occurrence of an acceleration in a particular band in Hz.

D is the duty cycle in kilometres (kms) per day.

v is the average speed in kms per hour.

L is the life in years.

N is number of cycles, calculated as per below formula: N = (fxLxDx1.314e+6)/v

Where, the value 1.314e+6 is obtained by converting speed v in kms per second and life L in days i.e. 365x60x60 = 1.314e+6.

Considering, L = 15 years, D = 200 kms / day, v = 50 kms/ hour

The number of cycles calculated for sample data is shown in Table 15.

Results

From Table 15, the average acceleration range and number of cycles forms the input test cases for fatigue analysis as shown in Table 16.

SUMMARY

The findings of the research study showed that inexpensive Arduino-based IoT devices were the most recent breakthroughs in tools and approaches for data acquisition. The expense of proprietary data acquisition devices was the primary reason for this research study on utilising low-cost IoT for data acquisition. In this study, the authors constructed a prototype data acquisition device using open-source software, Arduino IDE, and low-cost IoT hardware, comprising Arduino Uno, an accelerometer ADXL345 and a MicroSD Card reader. The cost of components was within INR 2000. The prototype data acquisition device was used to collect real-world data of a vehicle driving through a road test. The vehicle-road

Table 15. Test sample number of cycles

Acceleration Range (g)		Value (sorted)	Frequency Hz	No. of Cycles
lower limit	upper limit			
1	1.25	201	1.05	8.25E+07
0.75	1	142	0.74	5.83E+07

Table 16. Results: Test cases for fatigue analysis

Test Case	Acceleration (g)	No of Cycles
1	1.125	8.25E+07
2	0.875	5.83E+07

response was acquired and analysed using dataset classification, sorting, pareto technique, and formulae to get the number of cycles for fatigue analysis.

REFERENCES

Agrawal, S., Kumar, V., Anand, N., Agarwal, V. K., & Islam, A. (2016). *Development of Data Acquisition System and Data Analysis Technique for Automotive Applications. 50*(Ic), 3–6.

Amestica, O. E., Melin, P. E., Duran-Faundez, C. R., & Lagos, G. R. (2019). An Experimental Comparison of Arduino IDE Compatible Platforms for Digital Control and Data Acquisition Applications. *IEEE CHILEAN Conference on Electrical, Electronics Engineering, Information and Communication Technologies, CHILECON 2019*, (pp. 1–6). IEEE. 10.1109/CHILECON47746.2019.8986865

Baoquan, G. (2011). *Time-domain Analysis and Research on blasting vibration signals Based on Fourier I °.* Research Gate.

Chellaswamy, C., Famitha, H., Anusuya, T., & Amirthavarshini, S. B. (2018). *IoT Based Humps and Pothole Detection on Roads and Information Sharing.* Research Gate.

Chen, E. N. (2009). Remote analysis of mechanical vibration based on client/server architecture. *ICEMI 2009 - Proceedings of 9th International Conference on Electronic Measurement and Instruments*, (pp. 10–13). IEEE. 10.1109/ICEMI.2009.5274399

Dongpo, L., & Xuhui, M. (2011). *Virtual Proving Ground.*

Du, Y., Liu, C., Wu, D., & Li, S. (2016). Application of Vehicle Mounted Accelerometers to Measure Pavement Roughness. *International Journal of Distributed Sensor Networks, 2016*(6), 8413146. doi:10.1155/2016/8413146

González, A., Olazagoitia, J. L., & Vinolas, J. (2018). A low-cost data acquisition system for automobile dynamics applications. *Sensors (Basel), 18*(2), 366. doi:10.3390/s18020366 PMID:29382039

Gonzalez, L. C., Moreno, R., Escalante, H. J., Martinez, F., & Carlos, M. R. (2017). Learning Roadway Surface Disruption Patterns Using the Bag of Words Representation. *IEEE Transactions on Intelligent Transportation Systems, 18*(11), 2916–2928. doi:10.1109/TITS.2017.2662483

Hu, F., He, Q., & Kong, F. (2011).. . *Time-Frequency Vibration Representation for Steel Mill Condition Monitoring., 1,* 1–5.

Ilic, S., Katupitiya, J., & Tordon, M. (n.d.). *In-vehicle data logging system for fatigue analysis of drive shaft.*

Jamaludin, W. A. W. (2021). *Photovoltaic-Thermoelectric Generator Monitoring System using Arduino Based Data Acquisition system Technique.*

Junnila, S., & Niittylahti, J. (2003). Wireless technologies for data acquisition systems. *Proceedings of the 1st International Symposium on Information and Communication Technologies*, (pp. 132–137). IEEE.

LastMinuteEngineers.com. (2022). *Interfacing Micro SD Card Module with Arduino.* Last Minute Engineers.

Men, X., Liu, H., Chen, N., & Li, F. (2018). *A new time domain filtering method for calculating the RMS value of vibration signals. 51605191*, 2016–2019.

Mo, K., Suh, K., & Hong, S. (2000). New Approach in Vehicle Durability Evaluation, Virtual Proving Ground. *Test*, (March), 1–5.

Mohamed, A., Fouad, M. M. M., & Elhariri, E. (2014). *RoadMonitor: An Intelligent Road Surface Condition Monitoring System RoadMonitor: An Intelligent Road Surface Condition Monitoring System.* Springer. doi:10.1007/978-3-319-11310-4

Monterrey, C. (2018). *Road Load Data Acquisition system with SAE-J1939 Communications Network: Integration and Laboratory Test.* [Thesis, Instituto Tecnológico y de Estudios Superiores de Monterrey].

Moreno, C., González, A., Olazagoitia, J. L., & Vinolas, J. (2020). The acquisition rate and soundness of a low-cost data acquisition system (LC-DAQ) for high frequency applications. *Sensors (Basel)*, *20*(2), 524. doi:10.3390/s20020524 PMID:31963552

Of, A., & Signal, V. (2013). *A LabVIEW BASED DATA ACQUISITION SYSTEM FOR MONITORING Sunita Mohanta Department of Electronics and Communication Engineering National Institute of Technology Rourkela, Odisha-769008 Sunita Mohanta Dr. Umesh Chandra Pati Department of Electronics and Co.*

Ogunoiki, A. O. (2015). *University of Birmingham Research Archive.* University of Birmingham.

Pal Singh, H., & Singh, R. (2021). Low Cost Data Acquisition System for Road-Vehicle Interaction Using Arduino Board. *Journal of Physics: Conference Series*, *1831*(1), 012031. doi:10.1088/1742-6596/1831/1/012031

Perttunen, M., Mazhelis, O., Cong, F., Ristaniemi, T., & Riekki, J. (2011). Distributed Road Surface Condition Monitoring. Lecture Notes in Computer Science. Springer. doi:10.1007/978-3-642-23641-9

PiMyLife. (2022). *Arduino Accelerometer using the ADXL345.*

Polat, F. (2017). *Journal of Engineering Research and Applied Science. Dece.*

Salokhe, N., Thakre, P., Awale, R. N., & Kambale, S. (2016). *Vibration Based Damage Detection using Overall Frequency Response and Time Domain.*

Sener, A. S. (n.d.). *Determination Of Vehicle Components Fatigue Life Based On Fea Method And Experimental Analysis Determination Of Vehicle Components Fatigue Life Based On Fea Method And.* 2(Lcv), 133–146.

Shafiullah, A. K. M., & Wu, C. Q. (2013). Generation and validation of loading profiles for highly accelerated durability tests of ground vehicle components. *Engineering Failure Analysis*, *33*, 1–16. doi:10.1016/j.engfailanal.2013.04.008

Shuai, J., Heng, S., Jing, Y., Feng, Y., Han, N., & Mengqin, Y. (2021). *Load Spectrum Acquisition, Analysis and Application of The Electric Bus in Road Simulation Test Based on*. 479–483. toptechboy. com. (n.d.). *ARDUINO LESSON 21: LOG SENSOR DATA TO AN SD CARD*.

Ur Rehman, S., Mustafa, H., & Larik, A. R. (2021). IoT Based Substation Monitoring Control System Using Arduino with Data Logging. *Proceedings - 2021 IEEE 4th International Conference on Computing and Information Sciences, ICCIS 2021*. IEEE. 10.1109/ICCIS54243.2021.9676384

Wali, S., & Areeb, M. (2018). Development of Low-Cost DAQ for Power System Signals Using Arduino. *2018 IEEE 21st International Multi-Topic Conference (INMIC)*, (pp. 1–5). IEEE. 10.1109/INMIC.2018.8595519

Wang, J., Zhao, Y., Yang, Y., & Yang, J. (2019). *Fatigue Analysis for Bogie Frame of Urban Transit Rail Vehicle under Overload Situation. Qr2mse*. Research Gate.

Wang, Q., Yan, K., & Li, H. (2009). *Motor Noise Source Identification Based on Frequency Domain Analysis*. Research Gate.

Chapter 6
Design and Fabrication of a Softrobotic Gripper for Involving Underwater Vehicles in Seaweed Farming

Prabhakar Gunasekaran
Thiagarajar College of Engineering, India

Meenakshi S.
Thiagarajar College of Engineering, India

Jainulafdeen A.
K. Ramakrishnan College of Engineering, India

Ayyanar N.
 https://orcid.org/0000-0002-4452-5293
Thiagarajar College of Engineering, India

Rajalakshmi Murugesan
 https://orcid.org/0000-0001-8532-2452
Thiagarajar College of Engineering, India

ABSTRACT

Seaweeds, crucial components of marine ecosystems, thrive in marine and coastal waters, notably in the Gulf of Mannar Biosphere. Despite their ecological importance, certain seaweed species pose a threat to coral reefs due to the release of hydrophobic allelochemicals. Fisherwomen, risking their lives in collecting seaweed seed stock from littoral zones, rocky shores, and deep-sea waters, encounter hazards such as sharp rocks, poisonous algae, cyanobacteria, and coral reefs. Societal research pinpoints risks, overexploitation, unorganized harvesting, and algal blooms as significant issues. The proposed solution involves integrating intelligent Soft Robotic Grippers into underwater vehicles for precise seaweed farming without harming coral reefs. Abacus FEA software aids in deformation analysis, guiding the gripper's design to safeguard fisherwomen and preserve coral reefs.

DOI: 10.4018/979-8-3693-1962-8.ch006

INTRODUCTION

Underwater robots has advanced significantly, opening up new avenues for industrial applications, research, and exploration in aquatic environments. Rigid grippers are widely used in traditional underwater robotic systems. Although they work well in some situations, they have significant drawbacks. Underwater environments present significant challenges for rigid grippers due to their severe conditions, which include changing pressure, unexpected currents, and complex topography (Wei et al., 2016). A study conducted in (Bao et al., 2020; Fischell et al., 1806; Stenius et al., 2022) looked at the opportunities and difficulties of using autonomous underwater vehicles (AUVs) for seaweed farming. Prior research has brought to light the challenges associated with implementing autonomous systems in maritime settings, especially when it comes to tasks like navigation and farm localization. Scholars have underscored the significance of creating resilient technologies to tackle these obstacles and maximize AUV functioning in seaweed farms. Primary focus areas in the literature are sidescan sonar data collection, dead-reckoning navigation techniques, and early farm localization methods. The development and application of AUV systems for efficient seaweed farming techniques has benefited greatly from the insightful information these studies have offered. These obstacles make it harder to manage delicate and accurate interactions with marine creatures, handle breakable items, and maneuver in small areas. Furthermore, because of their limited adaptability and chance of unexpected accidents, inflexible grippers may unintentionally disrupt the surrounding marine habitat (Hughes et al., 2016). These soft grippers present a viable path for developing the capabilities of underwater robotic systems because they provide improved compliance, adaptability, and the capacity to negotiate challenging underwater terrains more effectively (Soft Robotics Toolkit, n.d.). Soft grippers' increased versatility makes them ideal for a variety of applications, including environmental monitoring, marine exploration, and conservation. It also allows for effective navigation through intricate underwater environments. The effective use of soft robotic grippers as we explore the ocean's depths is a sign of our dedication to comprehending and protecting the delicate balance of underwater ecosystems, in addition to being a technological accomplishment (Chen & Xu, 2023). The structural behavior of soft robotic grippers is evaluated with the use of Finite Element Analysis (FEA). This simulation method helps with gripper design optimization by enabling a thorough analysis of deformations, stresses, and performance under varied circumstances (Huang, 2021). To ensure the effectiveness and dependability of soft robotic grippers in their intended applications, FEM plays a critical role in bridging theoretical design concepts with practical implementation (Nordin et al., 2013; Soft Robotics Toolkit, n.d.; Xavier et al., 2021).

PROBLEM STATEMENT

Red seaweed called Kappaphycus alvarezii is also referred to as "cottonii" or "cottonii seaweed as shown in figure 1(c). " It is widely grown for commercial purposes and is a member of the Solieriaceae family. Carrageenan is a type of hydrocolloid that is used in many different industries. Seaweeds are macroscopic algae growing in the marine and shallow coastal waters and on rocky shores. It plays a major role in marine ecosystems and abundantly available in the region of Gulf of Mannar Biosphere. However, some species of seaweed clash coral reefs and damage them severely due to the release of hydrophobic allelochemicals. Therefore, the ecological balance is required in seaweed growth, otherwise it results in algal bloom, which is shown in figure 1(e). This factor induces the Indian government to promote the seaweed cultivation to a greater extent. Over the years, fisherwomen in Ramanathapuram district of Tamilnadu are engaged in collecting the Seed stock of seaweeds from littoral zones, rocky shores and deep-sea waters for economic gain. It endangers their lives due to presence of sharp rocks, poisonous algae's, cyanobacteria, coral reefs which is shown in figure 1(f) and other species in the ocean. They are staying in the seabed lined with slippery coral for more than 7 hours to search and collect the considerable number of seaweeds without any proper safety materials.

The risks associated with seaweed collection, human seeking effort, overexploitation of sea resources (continuous, indiscriminate, and unorganized harvesting of seaweeds), and algal bloom have been identified as significant problems by this societal research. The figure 1(d) depicts fisherwomen engaged in the traditional method of seaweed harvesting. In the illustration, fisherwomen are shown wading in shallow waters, meticulously handpicking seaweed from underwater vegetation. Traditional harvesting techniques are labor-intensive because they frequently require manual labor. Harvesting can be labor-intensive and require specialized personnel. The underwater robot currently employing the Newton Sea Gripper, as depicted in Figure 1a and 1b is specifically designed for seaweed farming, representing a rigid approach. When using hard grippers or any equipment in delicate marine environments, there is a serious risk of damaging coral reefs. Coral reefs are vulnerable to physical harm because they are delicate ecosystems that offer vital habitats for a wide variety of marine species. Current R&D projects are investigating novel farming methods, cutting-edge monitoring systems, and environmentally friendly seaweed farming techniques in an attempt to solve some of these problems. Resilience and efficiency in seaweed farming systems can be increased by taking a more comprehensive and technologically-aware approach. Underwater operations can be carried out with less risk to coral reefs and other delicate marine ecosystems by combining these factors with developments in soft robotics and responsible operational procedures. Underwater robotics must prioritize environmental conservation if our oceans are to remain healthy in the long run.

An important step toward environmental sustainability in the seaweed farming sector has been taken with the introduction of soft robotic grippers. These grippers minimize disturbances to fragile marine habitats, like coral reefs, while preserving biodiversity and reducing environmental risks because they provide a gentler alternative to traditional harvesting methods. Soft robotic grippers ensure the long-term health and resilience of marine ecosystems by utilizing sustainable harvesting practices. This helps the ecosystems adapt to climate change. By giving ecological factors top priority, this proactive strategy promotes a more sustainable future for both coastal communities and marine life.

The Indian government took many initiatives to enhance the livelihood of fisherwomen.

Among them, seaweed cultivation is one of the initiatives to gain marginal income. Coastal fisher families, especially fisherwomen in Self Help Groups (SHG) are actively involved in collecting the seaweeds from the deep-sea waters and rocky shores. It seems to be risking their lives for occupation. Therefore, the difficulties are faced by the fisherwomen in coastal areas of Tamilnadu, where the seaweeds are abundantly available. So, it is important to save the lives of fisherwomen involved in seaweed collection.

Figure 1. a. Underwater robot, b. Hard gripper, c. Kappaphycus alvarezii (seaweed), d. seaweed farming, e. Algal bloom f. Coral reef

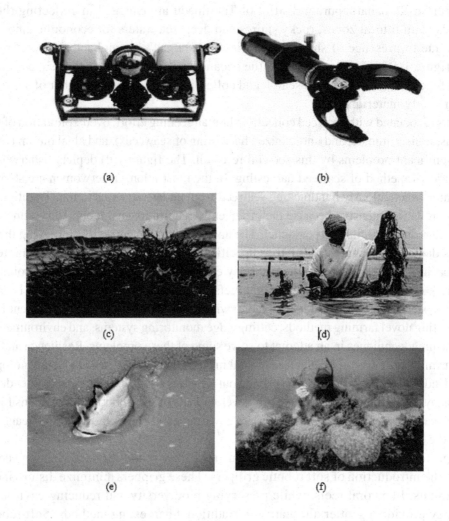

ACTUATION TECHNOLOGIES FOR SOFT ROBOTIC GRIPPERS AND MANIPULATORS

Pneumatic Actuation

Pneumatic systems and compressed air enable controlled and gentle manipulation in an unpressurized soft robotic gripper intended for seaweed grabbing. Because it is made of materials that are both flexible and water-resistant, the gripper can flex and conform to the irregular shapes of seaweed, deforming compliantly under pressure and fitting the curves of the underwater environment. Using soft pneumatic actuators, like bellows or chambers, the soft robotic gripper gently and non-intrusively grasps seaweed without causing damage. The actuators expand or contract in response to air pressure. Control valves precisely adjust the grip force by controlling the flow of compressed air. A pressure regulation system keeps the pressure at just the right levels to allow for efficient seaweed harvesting without endangering

Figure 2. Pneumatic Actuation

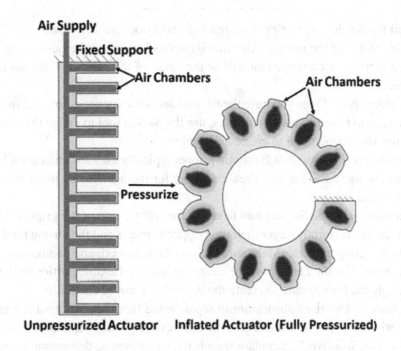

the delicate marine flora. In underwater applications, safety features such as pressure relief valves add to the dependability of the gripper.

A control unit incorporates automation into the soft robotic gripper, coordinating the deflation and inflation cycles to manipulate seaweed with grace. This technology is especially useful for jobs requiring a soft and adaptable grip to prevent harming fragile marine ecosystems, such as environmental monitoring or underwater harvesting. The ability of soft robotics to facilitate sustainable and non-intrusive interactions with marine environments is exemplified by the seaweed-grabbing gripper. The soft robotic gripper for seaweed grabbing operates through a carefully designed process, as illustrated in the accompanying Figure 2.

Hydraulic Actuation

In soft robotics, hydraulic actuation is a ground-breaking method that offers robotic systems unparalleled accuracy, adherence, and flexibility (Chen & Xu, 2023). This technology can be used to create soft robotic structures that can easily interact with delicate objects, navigate through complex environments, and dynamically adjust their stiffness for optimal performance. Because of its high force transmission, modular design, and capacity for complex deformations, hydraulic actuation is an essential element in the development of bioinspired and flexible soft robotic solutions. Applications for hydraulic actuation can be found in many different domains, such as enhancing dexterity in manipulating objects and ensuring safety in human-robot interactions. This emphasizes how important hydraulic actuation will be in determining how soft robotics develops in the future.

SOLIDWORKS DESIGN

The steps outlined for developing a gripper design in SolidWorks are as follows:

Sketch the basic shape of the gripper: Use the Sketch tool to create the basic shape of the gripper. Start by drawing a rectangle or a shape that will be then base of the gripper. Then use the Extrude tool to create a 3D object.

Add details to the gripper: Once you have the basic shape, add any necessary details. For example, if you want your gripper to have fingers or tentacles, use the Sketch tool to create the shape of the finger or tentacle, then use the Extrude tool to create a 3D object.

Create a cavity for the actuator: A soft robotic gripper typically uses an actuator such as a pneumatic or hydraulic system to move the fingers. Create a cavity for the actuator by using the Extrude tool to create a void in the base object.

Use the Surface tool: Use the Surface tool to create the soft portion of the gripper. This can be done by creating a surface that is slightly larger than the gripper's fingers and then using the Loft tool to connect the surface to the gripper's base. Make sure the surface is smooth and continuous.

Use the Flex feature: Use the Flex feature to create the soft and flexible portion of the gripper. Select the Surface and apply the Flex feature to create the desired amount of flexibility.

Use the Split feature: Use the Split feature to separate the flexible portion of the gripper from the base object. This will allow you to test and analyze the flexible portion separately from the base.

Test the design: Use SolidWorks Simulation tools to test the stress, deformation, and motion of the flexible portion of the gripper. You can apply various loads and boundary conditions to test the gripper's behavior.

Make any necessary changes: Based on the results of your testing, make any 21 necessary changes to the design until you are satisfied with the functionality of the gripper.

Finalize the design: Once you have made all necessary changes, finalize the design and save it as a 3D file that can be used for manufacturing.

Figure 2a, 2b, 2c and 2d displays the developed gripper model in SolidWorks with different design views. These illustrations provide a thorough examination of the gripper's design and attributes from several perspectives.

FINITE ELEMENT MODELING

Finite element modeling simulation in Abaqus involves creating a digital model of a physical structure or system, dividing it into small, finite elements, and then applying boundary and loading conditions to simulate real-world scenarios. The software then uses numerical methods to solve the equations governing the behavior of the system, and provides information on stress, deformation, temperature distribution, fluid flow, and other variables of interest. The following steps are used to simulate the gripper in Abaqus using finite element modelling:

Create the model: Import the 3D model of the soft robotic gripper that was designed in SolidWorks into Abaqus. Make sure the model is properly meshed.

Create a step: In Abaqus, create a new step and name it something like "Pressure Load." This step will be used to apply the pressure to the gripper.

Figure 3. 3D view

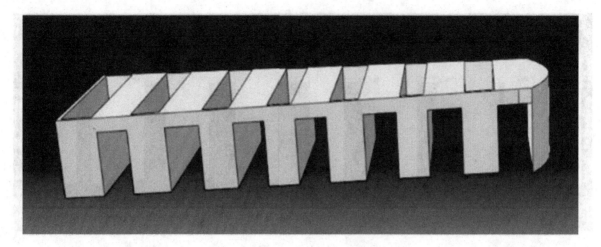

Figure 4. Top view

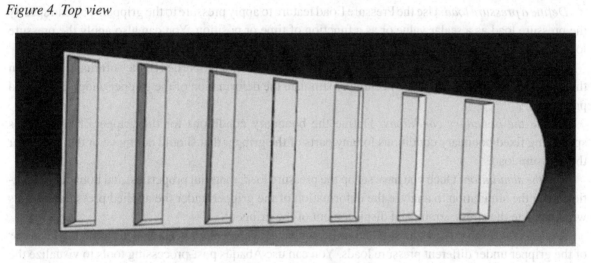

Figure 5. Bottom view

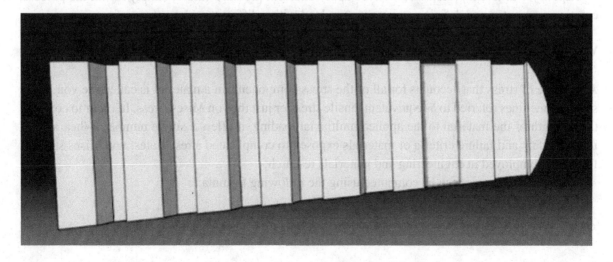

Figure 6. Side view

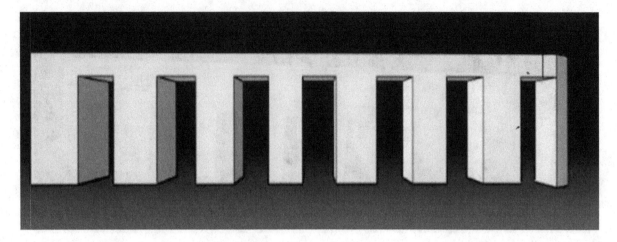

Define a pressure load: Use the Pressure Load feature to apply pressure to the gripper. You can specify the pressure load as a scalar value or as a function of time or position. You can also apply the pressure load to a specific set of nodes or to a region of the gripper.

Define the material properties: In Abaqus, define the material properties of the soft material used in the gripper. This will allow you to accurately simulate the deformation of the gripper under the applied pressure.

Define the boundary conditions: Define the boundary conditions for the gripper. This includes specifying fixed boundary conditions for any parts of the gripper that should not move or deform under the pressure load.

Run the simulation: Once you have set up the pressure load, material properties, and boundary conditions, run the simulation to analyze the deformation of the gripper under the applied pressure. Abaqus will calculate the stress, strain, and displacement of the gripper.

Analyze the results: After the simulation is complete, analyze the results to determine the behavior of the gripper under different pressure loads. You can use Abaqus post-processing tools to visualize the results, including deformation and stress contours.

Repeat for different pressure values: To apply different pressure values, simply repeat the process, creating a new step and defining a new pressure load with a different scalar value or function.

Von-Mises Stress Analysis

A measure of stress that accounts for all of the stress components in a material is called the von Mises stress, sometimes referred to as equivalent tensile stress or just the von Mises stress. In order to compare the strength of the material to the applied multiaxial loading, it offers a single number. When assessing the safety and failure criteria of materials exposed to complicated stress states, von Mises stress is frequently employed in engineering and materials research.

The von Mises stress can be computed using the following formula:

$$\sigma_{von-mises} = \sqrt{(\tilde{A}_x^2 + \tilde{A}_y^2 + \tilde{A}_z^2 - \sigma_x \sigma_y - \sigma_y \sigma_z - \sigma_z \sigma_x + 3\left(\tau_{xy}^2 + \tau_{yz}^2 + \tau_{zx}^2\right))}$$

where,

$\sigma v_{on\text{-}mises}$ is the von Mises stress.

σx σy, and σz a_re the normal stresses in the x, y, and z directions, respectively.

$\tau x Y$, $_\tau yz$ a_{nd} τzx ar_e the shear stresses on the xy, yz and zx planes, respectively.

MOULDING PREPARATION

Ecoflex Silicone 00-30mm is a type of two-part platinum-cure silicone rubber that is commonly used for mold making and casting applications. It has a Shore A hardness of 00, which means it is extremely soft and flexible, making it ideal for creating molds of delicate or intricate object.

De*sign the mould:* Create a 3D model of the mould using CAD software, such as SolidWorks or AutoCAD. The mould should be designed to the exact specifications of the desired soft robotic gripper, with the correct size, shape, and features.

Choose the moulding material: Select a suitable material for the mould, such as silicone or polyurethane. The material should be able to withstand the heat and pressure of the moulding process without degrading or deforming.

Prepare the moulding surface: Prepare the surface of the mould by applying a release agent, such as silicone spray or wax, to prevent the moulding material from sticking to the surface.

Mix the moulding material: Mix the chosen moulding material according to the manufacturer's instructions. This typically involves mixing a base material with a curing agent in a specific ratio.

Pour the moulding material: Pour the mixed moulding material into the mould cavity, making sure to fill it completely and evenly. Cure the moulding material: Allow the moulding material to cure for the recommended amount of time. This may involve leaving it at room temperature or applying heat to accelerate the curing process.

Demould the soft robotic gripper: Once the moulding material is fully cured, demould the soft robotic gripper by carefully removing it from the mould. Be careful not to damage the gripper during the demoulding process. Trim and finish the soft robotic gripper: Trim any excess material from the gripper and finish the surface as desired. This may involve sanding, polishing, or applying a coating or paint.

RESULTS AND DISCUSSION

ABAQUS software was used to perform a Finite Element Analysis (FEA) to evaluate a modeled soft robotic gripper's performance at different pressure values. The 3D model considered the hyperelastic properties of soft materials, and a finely detailed mesh accurately captured deformation. Pneumatic actuation was simulated by applying pressure loads, and boundary conditions were designed to mimic actual operating conditions. The selection of nonlinear static or dynamic analyses was based on the magnitude of deformation. Post-processing provided information about pressure distribution, displacement, strain, and stress. The goal of the simulation was to gain insight into the gripper's behavior and deformation under various pressure conditions, which would aid in design optimization and practical application.

Figure 7. Working prototype of soft robotic gripper fabricated by Embedded lab of Thiagarajar college of engineering

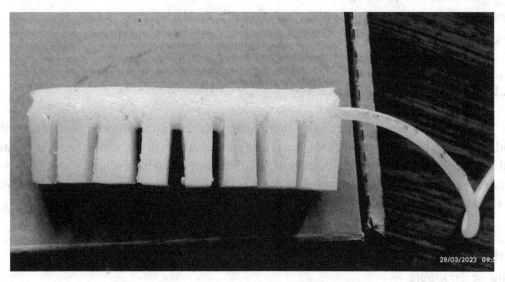

The von Mises stress distribution and gripper deformation were calculated for pressure values of 30 kPa, 40 kPa, and 50 kPa as illustrated in figures 5a, 5b, 5c and corresponding deformation magnitudes were tabulated in table1. The maximum magnitude of bending deformation of 57.4mm was found to occur at 50 kPa. This result suggests a relationship in which the gripper's ability to bend in the desired direction increases with pressure. The findings imply that manipulating the pressure levels may be a useful strategy for managing and enhancing the gripper's bending behavior in certain situations.

CONCLUSION

Soft robotic grippers have emerged as a promising technology for seaweed farming. Unlike traditional hard grippers, soft grippers can manipulate delicate and irregularly shaped seaweed without damaging it. This makes them ideal for tasks such as harvesting, sorting, and transporting seaweed. It can be designed to mimic the way that natural organisms manipulate objects. For example, researchers have developed grippers that use suction to attach to the seaweed, or that wrap around the seaweed like a vine. These grippers are perfect for use in underwater environments because they can be controlled remotely. Soft robotic grippers have the potential to revolutionize seaweed farming by making it more efficient, cost-effective, and environmentally friendly. They could enable farmers to harvest more seaweed with less labor, and to process the seaweed more quickly and efficiently. This could make seaweed farming more economically viable and help to meet the growing demand for sustainable food and fuel sources.

This initial study of the soft robotic gripper's bending behavior represents a significant step toward understanding its deformable properties and flexibility. The study's sophistication is highlighted by the use of ABAQUS software for Finite Element Analysis (FEA).

Figure 8. For 30KPa

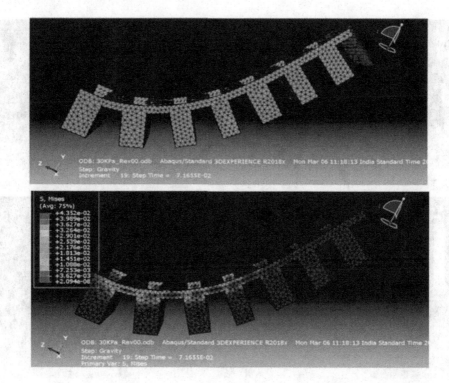

Figure 9. For 40KPa

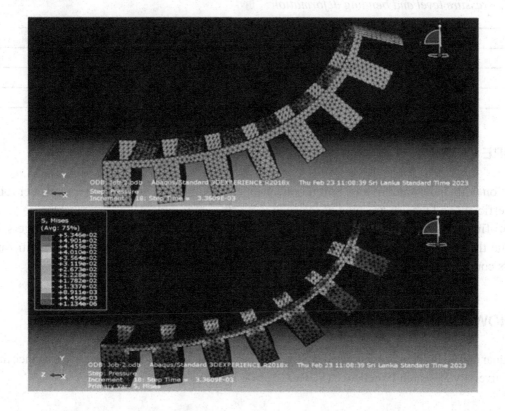

Figure 10. For 50KPa

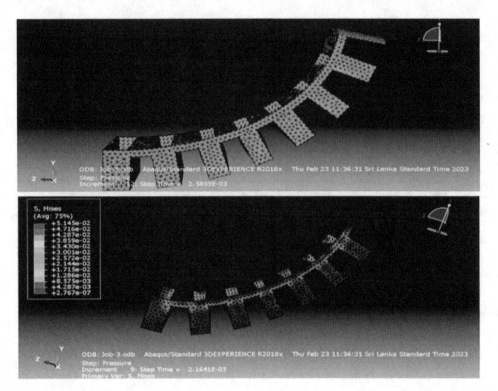

Table 1. Pressure level and bending deformation

Pressure Level (KPa)	Bending deformation(mm)
30	36.2
40	46.5
50	57.4

FUTURE WORK

Integration with underwater robots: Soft robotic grippers could be integrated with underwater robots to enable efficient and precise grasping of seaweed in marine environments.

Multi-fingered grippers: Current soft robotic grippers typically have only one or two fingers, which may limit their ability to grasp irregularly shaped objects such as seaweed. Developing multi-fingered grippers could increase the versatility and efficiency of seaweed grasping.

ACKNOWLEDGMENT

N. Ayyanar and G. Prabhakar acknowledge SERB SURE, India, for providing financial assistance through State University Research Excellence (SURE/2022/003424).

S. Meenakshi expresses her gratitude to Thiagarajar College of Engineering (TCE) for their support in conducting this research work. Additionally, she acknowledges the financial assistance provided by TCE under the Thiagarajar Research Fellowship scheme (File.no: TRF/Jul-2023/4) with heartfelt appreciation.

REFERENCES

Bao, J., Li, D., & Qiao, X. (2020). Integrated navigation for autonomous underwater vehicles in aquaculture: A review. *Information Processing in Agriculture, 7*(1).

Chen, S., & Xu, H. (2023). A pneumatic–hydraulic hybrid actuator for underwater soft robot swimming and crawling. *Sensors and Actuators A: Physical, 356.* doi:10.1016/j.sna.2023.114284

Fischell, E., Stanton, T. K., Kukulya, A., & Andone, C. (1806). Lavery, Monitoring of macroalgae (kelp) farms with autonomous underwater vehicle-based split-beam sonar, September 2018. *The Journal of the Acoustical Society of America, 144*(3).

Huang, W. (2021). Modeling soft swimming robots using discrete elastic rod method. *Proc. Bioinspired Sensing, Actuation, Control Underwater Soft Robotic Syst.*

Hughes, J., Culha, U., Giardina, F., Guenther, F., Rosendo, A., & Iida, F. (2016). Soft manipulators and grippers: A review. *Frontiers in Robotics and AI, 3*, 1–12. doi:10.3389/frobt.2016.00069

Nordin, I. N. A. M., Razif, M. R. M., & Natarajan, E. (2013). 3-D finite-element analysis of fiber-reinforced soft bending actuator for finger flexion. IEEE/ASME international conference on advanced intelligent mechatronic, Wollongong, Australia.

Soft Robotics Toolkit. (n.d.). Modeling and Design Tool for Soft Pneumatic Actuators. Soft Robotics Toolkit. https:// softroboticstoolkit.com/book/modeling-soft-pneumatic-actuators

Stenius, I., Folkesson, J., Bhat, S., Sprague, C. I., Ling, L., Özkahraman, Ö., Bore, N., Cong, Z., Severholt, J., Ljung, C., Arnwald, A., Torroba, I., Gröndahl, F., & Thomas, J.-B. (2022). A System for Autonomous Seaweed Farm Inspection with an Underwater Robot. *Sensors (Basel), 22*(13), 5064. doi:10.3390/ s22135064 PMID:35808560

Wei, Y., Chen, Y., Ren, T., Chen, Q., Yan, C., Yang, Y., & Li, Y. (2016). A novel, variable stiffness robotic gripper based on integrated soft actuating and particle jamming. *Soft Robotics, 3*(3), 134143. doi:10.1089/soro.2016.0027

Xavier, M. S., Fleming, A. J., & Yong, Y. K. (2021, February). Finite element modeling of soft uidic actuators: Overview and recent developments. *Advanced Intelligent Systems, 3*(2), 2000187. doi:10.1002/ aisy.202000187

APPENDIX

Solid Works Design Parameters

By using the following values, gripper is designed in solidworks software.

Number of Chambers: 8

Total height:115mm

Height of the chamber: 30mm

Gap between two chambers: 10mm

Thickness of the gripper: 5mm

Commercial tools for FEM analysis:

- ABAQUS
- ANSYS
- COMSOL
- MARC etc.

Chapter 7
Secure VANET Routing Protocols for Improved Vehicular Communication in Autonomous Systems

Abarna S.
ⓘ https://orcid.org/0000-0001-6574-6821
National Engineering College, India

Naskath J.
National Engineering College, India

Rathi Pathi R.
National Engineering College, India

Jeyalakshmi C.
Mohamed Sathak Engineering College, India

ABSTRACT

Vehicular ad hoc networks (VANETs) represent an advanced iteration of mobile ad hoc networks (MANETs) designed specifically for internet communication within vehicles. VANETs aim to enable vehicle-to-vehicle (V2V) communication, enhancing safety and convenience for drivers and passengers. However, the open nature of ad hoc networks and the absence of a well-defined line of defense make security a crucial concern for VANETs. Prior to deploying mobile ad hoc networks in hostile or sensitive areas, it becomes imperative to establish robust security services. This study addresses the need for a trusted VANET routing protocol that incorporates a diverse range of security services. The proposed approach implements a secure routing protocol based on the Dijkstra Algorithm to identify the secure and shortest path. For ensuring secure routing, the protocol employs route request (RREQ) and route reply (RREP) mechanisms to identify trustworthy nodes. Additionally, message authentication is utilized to provide end-to-end, hop-to-hop, and entire-route authentication. To transmit messages securely, the Diffie-Hellman Key Exchange Protocol is employed for message encryption, ensuring safe delivery to the intended destination. To assess the performance of the suggested protocol, the authors conducted simulations using NS2. These simulation results demonstrate that the proposed routing protocol outperforms existing methods, affirming its effectiveness in VANET environments.

DOI: 10.4018/979-8-3693-1962-8.ch007

INTRODUCTION

Today's world has seen a rise in the use of wireless technology, which may be applied in a variety of contexts at any time. Wireless networks provide communication between nodes via wireless data links, whereas ad hoc networks rely on nodes banding together to route and forward messages. Vehicle ad hoc networks (VANETs) are the most popular and pertinent uses of ad hoc mobile networks. VANETs connect nodes automatically and don't require any pre-existing infrastructure. According to (Nidhal M et al, 2015), the main goals of VANET networks are to improve road safety and offer convenience services to drivers. Because it directly affects passenger lives, protecting VANETs from potential threats is essential. Vehicle connectivity to the internet and service access is made possible by VANETs (Lai W K et al, 2015). Vehicular Ad hoc Networks allow for communication between stirring cars in a limited region. Vehicles can interact directly with one another in Vehicle-to-Vehicle (V2V) communication, but they can also communicate with infrastructure components like roadside units (RSUs) in vehicle-to-infrastructure (V2I) communication (Rehman et al, 2013). Researchers have recently concentrated on a variety of VANET-related issues, such as broadcasting, routing, security, architectures, applications, and protocols; as well as Quality of Service (QoS). Cities are experiencing an increase in accidents and traffic congestion as a result of the growing number of automobiles on the road. To solve these problems, vehicles must communicate effectively and securely (Rehman et al, 2013). VANETs are networks that use a variety of routing protocols, which can be broadly classified into five categories: topology-based, position-based, cluster-based, geocast, and broadcast (Kamboj S et al, 2014).

When compared to conventional wireless networks, Vehicle Ad-Hoc Networks (VANETs) include a number of distinctive features. Above all, VANETs are extremely dynamic and fast-changing ecosystems. The network topology is always changing, as vehicles travel in different directions and at different speeds. VANET protocols must be flexible and able to handle sudden changes in network connectivity due to this dynamism. Fig 1 depicts the different characteristics of VANET which are most commonly known. The fact that VANETs depend on wireless communication is another important feature. Since cars interact wirelessly with other cars and with the infrastructure along the road, they are vulnerable to a number of problems with wireless communication, including fading, attenuation, and interference from other signals (Saini M et al, 2016). Time-sensitive applications such as traffic signal coordination and collision avoidance necessitate low-latency answers for communication in VANETs (Kumar V et al, 2013). Furthermore, because of the constant data interchange between vehicles, VANETs produce enormous amounts of data, which calls for effective data processing and management systems.

Commercial Applications of VANETs Commercial applications have a plethora of potential thanks to Vehicle Ad-Hoc Networks (VANETs). Among the most well-known is location-based marketing and advertising. Businesses are able to target potential customers with relevant adverts depending on their location and interests thanks to VANETs' connectivity and data exchange capability (Hamdi M M et al, 2020). For example, a coffee shop could entice passing vehicles to stop for a cup of coffee by sending them a special discount voucher. Furthermore, fleet management systems are made possible by VANETs, which help businesses save a lot of money by monitoring vehicle performance, optimizing routes, and enhancing fuel efficiency. Figure 2 Describes the application of VANET in different areas such as safety purpose, commercial and convenience purpose.

Convenient Services with VANETs Living in an urban environment has never been more convenient thanks to VANETs. Smart parking is among the most concrete instances. By having access to real-time information regarding parking spots that are accessible nearby, drivers can spend less time and get less

Figure 1. VANET characteristics

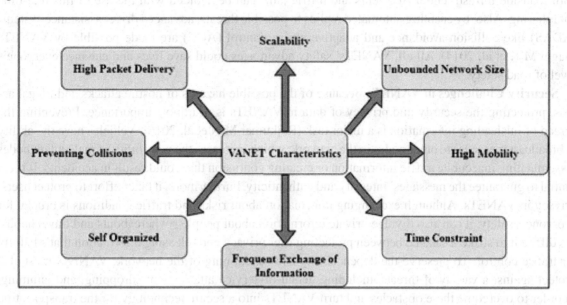

Figure 2. VANET applications

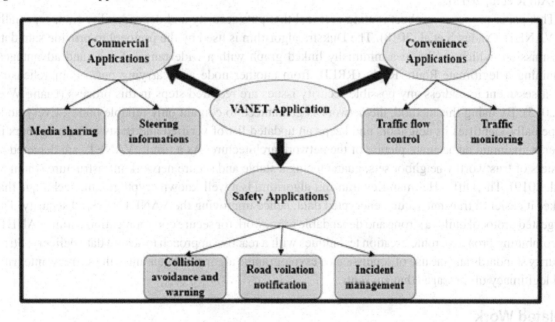

frustrated looking for a place to park. Additionally, ride-hailing and car-sharing services can be made easier for consumers to utilize without the inconvenience of owning a car thanks to VANETs. Dynamic routing and traffic congestion alerts are further advantages for commuters, since they enable them to bypass traffic bottlenecks and get at their destinations more quickly.

Safety Enhancements through VANETs The fact that VANETs improve road safety is among its most important features. In order to share information on traffic patterns, potential hazards on the road, and emergency scenarios, vehicles outfitted with VANET technology can connect with one another and with roadside infrastructure. Accidents and traffic jams can be avoided with the use of this real-time data sharing. Also, by enabling automated replies to possible threats, advanced driver assistance systems (ADAS) like collision avoidance and adaptive cruise control (ACC) are made possible by VANETs (Saggi M K et al, 2014). All all, VANETs' safety advantages could save lives and enhance everyone's level of road safety.

Security Challenges in VANETs Because of the possible hazards of hostile attacks and illegal access, protecting the security and privacy of data in VANETs is of utmost importance. Preventing the spread of misleading information is a major task (Rajkumar M N et al, 2016). Vehicles have the ability to broadcast messages to other nodes in the network, which increases the possibility of malevolent nodes disseminating inaccurate traffic information or creating confusion that could result in accidents. It is essential to guarantee the messages' integrity and authenticity. Furthermore, it takes effort to protect users' privacy in VANETs. Although exchanging information about risks and traffic conditions is crucial for everyone's safety, it can also divulge private information about people's whereabouts and travel habits. It's difficult to strike a balance between protecting user privacy and releasing information that's helpful for traffic control. To preserve the dependability and functioning of the network, VANETs must also protect against a variety of threats, including denial-of-service attacks, eavesdropping, and jamming. In order to overcome these obstacles and turn VANETs into a secure technology for the transportation of the future, it is imperative that strong security measures and encryption protocols be implemented (Al-Ani R et al, 2018).

This paper proposes a robust routing protocol that puts security and dependability first, especially for VANETs (Yadav S et al, 2018). The Dijkstra algorithm is used by the protocol to provide safe data transmission, which results in a minimally linked graph with a wide range of uses and advantages. Obtaining a legitimate Route Reply (RREP) from another node and carrying out a comprehensive self-assessment to address any possible security issues are required steps in this process (Liang W et al, 2015). By using this method, the network is guaranteed to contain only reliable nodes. Every node perpetually identifies its neighbors and keeps an updated list of verified and trustworthy neighbors in order to maintain an accurate picture of the network architecture. As a result, VANETs are depicted as clusters of trustworthy neighbor sets, guaranteeing a stable and secure network infrastructure (Inam M et al, 2019). The Diffie-Hellman Key transmit algorithm is a well-known cryptographic technique that makes it easier to transmit secure, encrypted data, hence improving the VANET's overall security. The suggested protocol builds a strong and dependable framework for secure communication within VANETs by combining proactive route creation techniques with a reactive approach to secure data delivery. Strict security standards and the use of sophisticated cryptographic algorithms guarantee the secrecy, integrity, and legitimacy of messages that are sent.

Related Work

Numerous researchers have dedicated their efforts to developing secure and efficient routing algorithms for VANETs. The aim is to enhance energy utilization and ensure secure routing, thereby eliminating network vulnerabilities and improving overall network performance. Routing protocols in VANETs can be categorized as topology-based and operation-based protocols (Singh R et al, 2018). Various secure routing protocols have been proposed to counteract attacks and enhance security. One such protocol is based on a game theory algorithm (Paramasivan B et al, 2015), which utilizes perfect Bayesian equilibrium and signaling to establish a secure routing protocol. This approach effectively reduces attacks from malicious nodes and incorporates neighbor reporting to enhance security. Another protocol, known as Secure B-MFR (Patil C et al, 2014), focuses on finding efficient routing paths with minimal hops while encrypting messages using secret keys.

The Trust Allocation Certificate (TAC) plays a significant role in establishing a trusted communication path (Charusheela M et al, 2014). TAC helps identify malicious behavior such as trust falsification and packet dropping, enhancing security. Additionally, the use of the elliptic curve digital signature algorithm (ECDSA) and digital verification with a certificate authority (Sarma A H K D et al, 2011) further improves performance. A hybrid routing protocol based on minimal spanning trees has been proposed, incorporating the Diffie-Hellman key exchange and certificate authority (Ghosh U et al, 2014). This protocol employs secure techniques for authentication and message verification. LETSRP (Biswas A K et al, 2020) utilizes the Winternitz One-Time Signature Scheme to authenticate transmitted data, ensuring secure communication in wireless sensor networks.

Position-Based Secure Routing Protocol (Singh G et al, 2019) combines elements from Most Forward within Radius protocols, while incorporating a security module using station-to-station key agreement. Machine learning and deep learning algorithms (Zhao L et al, 2016) have also been applied to derive routing protocols based on packet flow datasets, optimizing the routing environment to satisfy QoS and trust requirements.

Misbehavior detection is crucial for secure routing protocols, and a stacking approach utilizing classification techniques (Sonker A et al, 2020) can be employed. Secure routing protocols such as SE-AODV (Rajdeep S et al, 2014) and Energy-optimized Secure Routing (EOSR) (Yang T et al, 2018) address the identification and isolation of malicious nodes, taking into account factors such as trust level, remaining energy, and path length to optimize routing decisions. In summary, secure VANET routing protocols focus on overcoming attacks and ensuring trustworthiness, while considering parameters such as packet loss and malicious node detection. These protocols employ various techniques, including game theory, encryption, certificate authorities, and machine learning, to establish secure and efficient routing paths in VANETs.

In the area of VANETs, researchers have made significant strides in developing secure and efficient routing algorithms to enhance energy utilization and ensure secure routing. These efforts are aimed at eliminating network vulnerabilities and improving overall network performance. Routing protocols in VANETs can be broadly categorized as topology-based and operation-based protocols. Several secure routing protocols have been introduced to combat attacks and bolster security. For instance, a game theory-based protocol employs perfect Bayesian equilibrium and signaling to establish secure routing, effectively mitigating malicious node attacks. Secure B-MFR focuses on finding efficient routing paths with minimal hops while encrypting messages using secret keys. Trust Allocation Certificate (TAC) plays a vital role in identifying malicious behavior and enhancing security, further strengthened by techniques like the elliptic curve digital signature algorithm (ECDSA) and digital verification with a certificate authority. Additionally, a hybrid routing protocol utilizes minimal spanning trees, the Diffie-Hellman key exchange, and certificate authorities to ensure secure authentication and message verification. The use of the Winternitz One-time Signature Scheme in LETSRP guarantees secure data authentication in wireless sensor networks (Bangotra D K et al, 2018). The Position-Based Secure Routing Protocol combines various routing elements and security modules, including station-to-station key agreements, while machine learning and deep learning algorithms optimize routing based on packet flow datasets to meet Quality of Service (QoS) and trust requirements. Misbehavior detection, essential for secure routing, can be implemented using stacking approaches and classification techniques (Mejri M N et al, 2016). Secure routing protocols such as SE-AODV and Energy-optimized Secure Routing (EOSR) identify and isolate malicious nodes, considering factors such as trust levels, path length, and remaining energy to optimize routing decisions. In conclusion, secure VANET routing protocols aim to address attacks, ensure trustworthiness, and consider parameters like packet loss and malicious node detection. These protocols utilize a range of techniques, including game theory, encryption, certificate authorities, and machine learning, to establish secure and efficient routing paths in VANETs.

To address these issues, the protocol employs the Dijkstra algorithm to establish a minimally connected graph, ensuring efficient and reliable routing paths. This (Gadkari M. Y et al, 2012) introduces a stringent security process where nodes must obtain a valid Route Reply (RREP) and undergo self-assessment, guaranteeing that only trustworthy nodes are allowed into the network. Continuous neighbor detection and verified neighbor lists are used to create reliable clusters, enhancing network integrity and stability.

This work presents a robust VANET-specific routing protocol emphasizing security and reliability by employing the Dijkstra algorithm to establish a minimally connected graph. Nodes must acquire a valid RREP and undergo self-assessment for security, ensuring only trustworthy nodes join the network. Continuous neighbor detection and verified neighbor lists create reliable clusters, maintaining network integrity. The Diffie-Hellman Key Exchange enhances message security. The protocol blends proactive route construction with reactive data transmission, forming a dependable communication framework in VANETs, guaranteeing message confidentiality, integrity, and authenticity through advanced cryptographic techniques and stringent security protocols.

Proposed Work

In this section, we present a comprehensive description of a robust routing protocol designed specifically for Vehicular Ad Hoc Networks (VANETs). The protocol ensures a high level of security by allowing nodes to autonomously construct routes and transmit data securely using the Dijkstra algorithm. This innovative approach greatly contributes to the establishment of a minimally connected graph, opening up various applications and benefits. Prior to joining a VANET, each participating node undergoes a critical validation process. This involves acquiring a valid Route Reply (RREP) from another node and conducting a thorough self-assessment to address any potential security concerns. By adhering to these stringent security measures, the protocol guarantees that only trustworthy nodes become part of the network. Figure 3 depicts the formulation of VANET architecture.

To maintain an accurate understanding of the network topology, each node continually detects its neighboring nodes and maintains an up-to-date list of verified and trusted neighbors. Consequently, a

Figure 3. Formulation of VANET

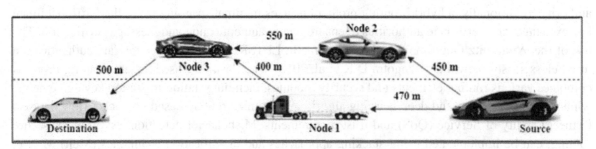

VANET can be represented as an amalgamation of multiple sets of reliable neighbor clusters, ensuring a dependable and secure network environment. To facilitate the transmission of secure messages, the protocol employs the renowned Diffie-Hellman Key Exchange algorithm. This cryptographic technique enables the exchange of trustworthy and encrypted messages, enhancing the overall security of the VANET. By combining the proactive measures of route construction and the reactive approach to secure data transmission, our protocol establishes a robust and reliable framework for secure communication within VANETs. Its utilization of advanced cryptographic algorithms and adherence to strict security protocols further ensures the confidentiality, integrity, and authenticity of the exchanged messages (Sampoornam K P et al, 2020). Figure 4 is a system diagram of VANET.

Identifying Trustworthy Neighbors and Forming of Safe Route

The process of identifying trustworthy neighbors and establishing safe routes within a network involves the utilization of Dijkstra's algorithm. Originally developed to address the single-source shortest route problem in static graphs, this approach offers an effective solution. It initiates from the source node and systematically explores the entire network to determine the shortest path between nodes. It's important to note that for a given transportation network, an upper bound on the distance between any two nodes can be precomputed. The proposed Dijkstra algorithm incorporates an Efficient Graph (EG) array, which contains a comprehensive list of vehicles and their corresponding reliability values. To commence the algorithm, the reliability value of the source vehicle, denoted as EG(source), is set to 0, while the reliability values of other unvisited vehicles are initialized as null (EG(unvisited)). Subsequently, unvisited vehicles stemming from the source node are evaluated to determine their journey reliability values. Overall workflow of proposed algorithm is shown in figure 5.

Once all the neighbors of a particular vehicle have been considered, that vehicle is marked as visited, and its journey reliability value is set as final. This iterative process continues until all nodes have been visited, and their final reliability values have been established. The accompanying pseudocode for the Dijkstra algorithm is presented below. Figure 4 illustrates the step-by-step execution of the Dijkstra algorithm, leading to the identification of the shortest and most efficient path. The algorithm generates a formulated graph that meticulously tracks the records of each node, facilitating the determination of the optimal route.

The provided pseudocode represents the Dijkstra algorithm, which is commonly used to get the shortest route in a graph. In the context of a VANET (Vehicular Ad Hoc Network), this algorithm can be applied to identify an efficient path between a given source vehicle and its destination. Digikstra work flow depicted in figure 6. Let's walk through the steps of the algorithm:

Initialization:
Set the distance of each node in the VANET formulated graph to infinity.
Mark all nodes as unvisited.
Set the distance of the source vehicle to 0.
Main Loop:
Repeat the following steps until the algorithm terminates.
Select the node (curr) with the lowest distance among the unvisited nodes in the graph.
Mark curr as visited.
Neighbor Evaluation:
Iterate through each neighbor (nxt) of the current node (curr).

Figure 4. Overall Process Flow Diagram

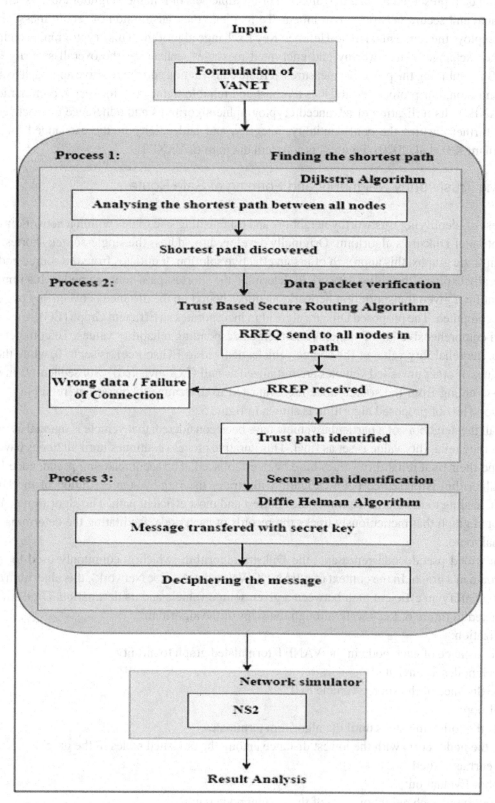

Figure 5. Algorithm flow diagram

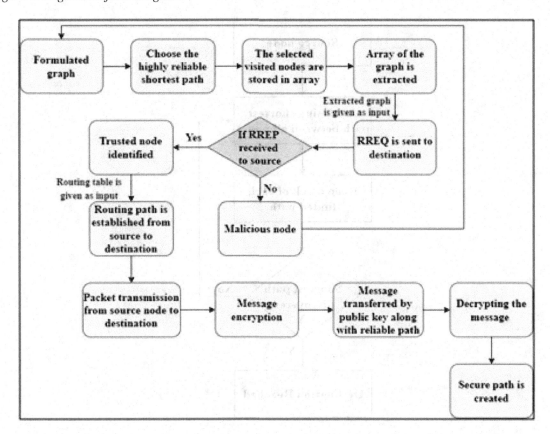

If nxt has not been visited:

Calculate the new distance (newdist) from the source node (curr) to nxt.

If the new distance is smaller than the current distance of nxt:

Update nxt's distance to newdist.

Set nxt's routeToNode as curr (the node that leads to nxt with the shortest distance).

Destination Reached:

If the current node (curr) is the destination (dest), return the path from the resource to the end.

No Valid Path:

If the node with the lowest score (distance) in the graph has a distance of infinity, it indicates that there is no valid path from the source to the destination.

The algorithm continues to iterate until either the destination is reached, in which case the optimal path is returned, or it determines that there is no valid path between the source and destination. The algorithm's efficiency lies in the fact that it progressively explores nodes with lower distances, updating their distances and routes as necessary. Note that the "calc(curr, nxt)" function in the pseudocode represents a calculation to determine the distance between the current node (curr) and its neighboring node (nxt). The specific calculation will depend on the characteristics of the VANET and the metrics used for evaluating distances.

Figure 6. Dijkstra algorithm working

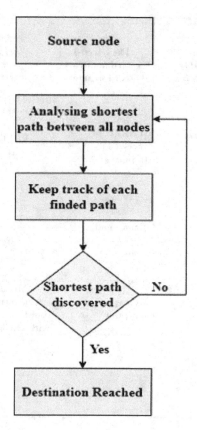

Trusted Node Identification

The process of identifying trusted nodes within the VANET involves a series of steps to ensure the reliability and security of communication along the efficient route. Let's elaborate on these steps:

Recording Heard Vehicles: As the efficient route is discovered, each vehicle encountered along the route receives a Route Request (RREQ) message. The receiving vehicle records information about the transmitting vehicle, specifically which vehicle is heard. This step allows for the establishment of a comprehensive record of the vehicles encountered during the routing process.

Forwarding RREQs: Upon receiving an RREQ, the vehicle determines the next hop based on the data updated by the RREQ extension. The RREQ message is then forwarded to the next hop along the route. It's important to note that intermediate vehicles along the route are not authorized to send a Routing Reply (RREP) message back to the source vehicle, even if they possess a valid route to the destination. This limitation ensures that only trusted nodes, specifically the destination vehicle, can initiate the response.

Dynamic Reliability Values: Due to the dynamic nature of the VANET, where vehicles are constantly moving, the reliability values at intermediate vehicles may become outdated over time. This is particularly relevant as the routing process incorporates the time domain, taking into account the changing positions and movements of vehicles. Therefore, the reliability values associated with intermediate vehicles need to be regularly updated and validated to maintain accurate trustworthiness assessments.

Algorithm

Algorithm:Dijkstra

Input: A Vanet formulated graph and a source vehicle (source),Destination of vehicle(des).
Output: An efficient path.
for each node in graph do:
node.dist=infinity
node.visited=false
end
source.dist=0
while true do:
curr=nodeWithLowestDistance(graph)
curr.visited=true
for nxt in curr.n do:
if nxt.visited==false then:
newdist=calc(curr,nxt)
if new.dist<nxt.dist then:
nxt.dist=newdist
nxt.routeToNode=curr
end
end
end
if curr==dest then:
return path(dest)
if nodeWithLowestScore(graph).dist==infinity then:
not correct path
end
end

Destination Vehicle Response: Once the RREQ reaches the destination vehicle, an appropriate response, namely the Routing Reply (RREP), is generated and sent back to the source vehicle. This RREP serves as the starting point for data transfer between the source and destination vehicles, initiating a secure and reliable communication session (Hu F et al, 2020).

Figure 7 visually represents the process of trusted node identification. By sending RREQ messages to each node encountered along the efficient route and receiving RREP responses, it becomes possible to assess whether a particular node can be considered trusted or potentially malicious (Patil C et al, 2014). This method ensures that only reliable and secure nodes are involved in the communication process, enhancing the overall security of the VANET. The provided pseudocode outlines the Trust Node Identification algorithm, which aims to determine the most reliable path from a source to a target vehicle in a given graph. Let's go through the steps of the algorithm:

Broadcast RREQ Packet: The algorithm starts by broadcasting a Route Request (RREQ) packet from the source vehicle, initiating the process of finding a reliable path to the destination.

RREP Reception Loop: A loop is initiated with the variable i set to 0. The loop continues until i reaches a value greater than or equal to 3 or until no Routing Reply (RREP) packet is received.

Path Comparison: If the ID of the source vehicle is less than the ID of the next node along the path, a break statement is executed, indicating that the current path is the most reliable and no further iterations are necessary. However, if the source vehicle's ID is greater than or equal to the next node's ID, the path is updated.

Path Update and RREQ Broadcast: If a node finds an updated path, it sends an RREQ packet to continue the process of identifying the most reliable path. Data packets are then sent from the source vehicle to the destination vehicle using the updated path.

Figure 7. Trust node identification protocol

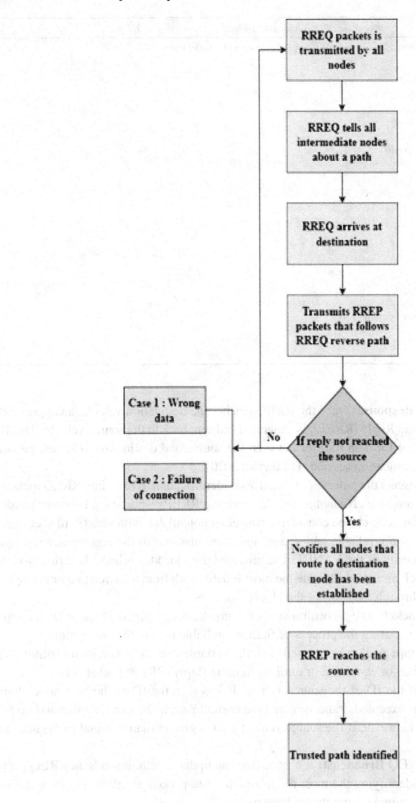

RREQ Update and Broadcast: If a node does not find an updated path, the previous ID is updated, and a check is performed. If the ID of the source vehicle's RREQ is greater than the next node's RREQ ID, the RREQ is updated, and a new RREQ packet is broadcast from the destination vehicle to the source vehicle. This step allows for further exploration of alternative paths.

RREP Reception and Data Transmission: If an RREP packet is received, it is used to update the routing table. Subsequently, data packets can be sent from the source to the target vehicle using the established reliable path.

Destination Not Reached: If an RREP packet is not received within the loop or the destination is not reached, it indicates that a reliable path to the destination could not be found.

The Trust Node Identification algorithm combines the use of RREQ and RREP packets to iteratively explore and update the path towards the destination vehicle, ensuring that the most reliable and secure route is identified.

Data Transfer Security

Ensuring the security of data transfer is paramount in any communication system. In this context, the proposed approach employs symmetric encryption to safeguard the data packets during transmission. The source node takes the data packets intended for transfer and encrypts them symmetrically using a secret key, denoted as K. Symmetric encryption algorithms, such as AES (Advanced Encryption Standard), are commonly used for this purpose. By applying the same secret key for encryption and decryption, the confidentiality and integrity of the data are preserved. In step 3 of the process (not explicitly mentioned in the provided context), a route is established for data transmission. (Lazrag H et al, 2018) This could involve the use of routing protocols, such as the Dijkstra algorithm, to get the optimal path from the source node to the target node. The route ensures that the encrypted data packets are sent along a reliable and efficient path. Upon receiving the encrypted data packets, the destination node decrypts them using the same secret key, K. By employing the corresponding decryption algorithm, the target node successfully retrieves the original valid message contained within the data packets.

Figure 8, which is not explicitly described in detail, illustrates the operation of the Diffie-Hellman algorithm in the context of message transfer from the source to the target node. The Diffie-Hellman algorithm allows two ends to share a secret key over an insecure communication channel (Pandit C M et al, 2014). While the algorithm itself is not directly mentioned in the provided context, it likely plays a crucial role in the secure exchange of the secret key K, ensuring that only authorized parties can decrypt the data packets.By combining symmetric encryption for data confidentiality and integrity and possibly incorporating the Diffie-Hellman algorithm for secure key exchange, the proposed approach ensures the security of data transfer from the source node to the destination node.

The provided pseudocode represents the Diffie-Hellman algorithm, which is a key exchange protocol used to produce a shared secret key between two end nodes over an insecure communication channel. Let's go through the steps of the algorithm:

- Global Public Elements: The algorithm begins by initializing the global public elements (q, a), which are known to both the source and destination nodes. These elements are typically prime numbers and generator values chosen in advance.
- Key Generation for the Source Node: The source node generates its private key, Xsrc, which is a randomly selected integer less than the value of q. Then, it computes its public key, Ysrc, using the

formula Ysrc = a^Xsrc mod q. Here, '^' denotes exponentiation and 'mod' represents the modulo operation.

- Key Generation for the Destination Node: Similarly, the destination node generates its private key, Xdst, and computes its public key, Ydst, using the same formulas as the source node.
- Calculation of Secret Key by the Source: The source node calculates the secret key by raising the destination node's public key, Ydst, to the power of its own private key, Xsrc. This is done modulo q. The resulting value represents the shared secret key.
- Calculation of Secret Key by the Destination: The destination node performs the same calculation as the source node, but using its private key, Xdst, and the source node's public key, Ysrc. Again, the calculation is performed modulo q.
- Shared Secret Key: The final step results in both the source and destination nodes having computed the same shared secret key. This shared secret key can now be used for various purposes, such as symmetric encryption or message authentication.

This algorithm helps two people share secret information safely without sending it directly over an unsecured channel.The algorithm relies on the computational complexity of calculating discrete logarithms to ensure the secrecy of the shared key.

Performance Evaluation and Simulation Setup

Simulation parameters play a crucial role in setting up and running simulations to study and analyze various aspects of a system or network. In the provided table, several simulation parameters are listed along with their corresponding values. The coverage area specifies the geographical extent of the simulated network. In this case, it is defined as 500 meters by 500 meters, indicating that the simulation focuses on a specific area of that size. The simulation time determines the duration of the simulated scenario. In this case, it is set to 350 milliseconds, indicating that the simulation captures events and activities within that time frame. The parameter has a minimum value of 50 and a maximum value of 100, indicating that the simulation considers scenarios with different node densities. In this case, it is set to "High" for traffic intensity and "Highway" for road type, indicating a scenario with high traffic load and highway-like road characteristics.

The transmission ranges are set as for On-Board Units (OBUs), the range is set to 50 meters, while for Roadside Units (RSUs), it is set to 100 meters. These values determine the communication coverage and connectivity between nodes. The packet size is set to 512 bytes, and a total of 100 packets are considered. These values affect the data transfer and transmission efficiency within the simulated network moreover the nodes can move at speeds up to 70 kilometers per hour. The proposed routing protocol ETBSRP parameter specifies the algorithm or protocol used for routing decisions in the simulated network. The chosen mobility model, manhattan suggests that the nodes move in a random manner along the street network. The MAC (Media Access Control) layer parameter specifies the protocol used for controlling access to the shared communication medium. The algorithms Dijkstra is used for identifying the shortest path in the network, next Trust Routing Protocol is used to detect trust nodes in the routing process and finally Diffie-Hellman used for secure message transmission by establishing shared secret keys.

Figure 8. Diffie Hellman key exchange protocol working

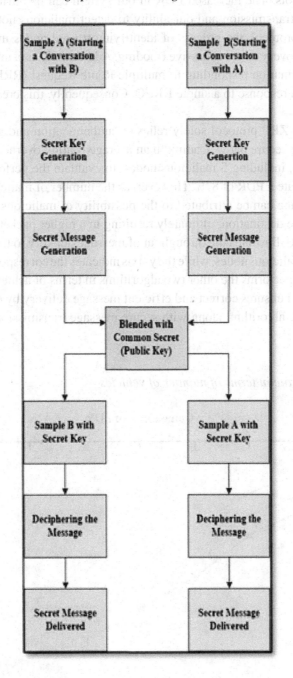

Performance Analysis

Packet delivery Rate:Figure 9 displays a graph depicting the number of nodes on the X-axis and the Packet Delivery Ratio (PDR) on the Y-axis. The graph demonstrates that our proposed protocol, the Emphasized Trust-Based Secure Routing Protocol (ETBSRP), achieves a higher PDR compared to the

AOMDV and ZRP protocols. The increased PDR in our system can be attributed to our selection of secure paths for message transmission and our ability to detect malicious nodes before sharing information. In the AOMDV protocol, the process of identifying trusted nodes incurs additional message overhead during route discovery due to excessive flooding. Additionally, as a multipath routing protocol, AOMDV leads to the destination responding to multiple Route Request (RREQ) packets, resulting in longer overhead packets in response to a single RREQ. Consequently, this creates a significant amount of control overhead.

On the other hand, the ZRP protocol solely relies on authentication and signatures to share information without employing secure paths, leading to an average routing overhead. In this study, focused a network with 100 nodes, including 5 malicious nodes, to evaluate the performance of our proposed protocol. The results indicate a PDR of 87%. However, as the number of malicious nodes increases, the PDR decreases. This decline can be attributed to the possibility of malicious nodes causing delays in forwarding messages to the destination, ultimately resulting in a higher packet loss ratio.

Throughput: Figure 10 illustrates the throughput of message delivery to the destination. The x-axis represents the number of malicious nodes, while the y-axis indicates the corresponding throughput values. The proposed protocol outperforms the other two algorithms in terms of achieving a higher throughput rate. The proposed protocol ensures correct and efficient message delivery by employing a shortest and most efficient path-finding algorithm, along with secure message transmission that minimizes routing

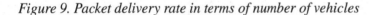

Figure 9. Packet delivery rate in terms of number of vehicles

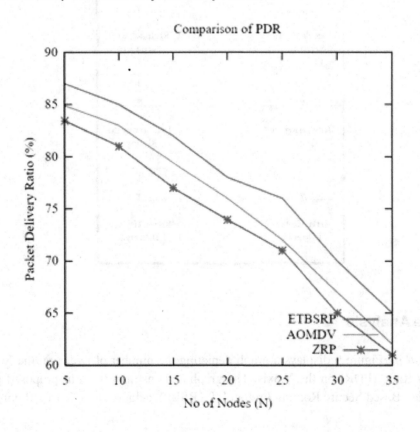

Figure 10. Throughput in terms of number of malicious vehicles

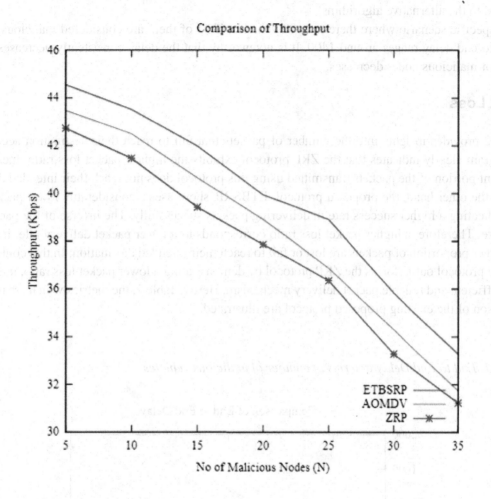

overhead compared to the other algorithms. This efficient routing strategy contributes to the improved throughput observed in the proposed protocol.

In the AOMDV algorithm, slight changes in throughput are observed compared to the proposed protocol. When a link split occurs in the present network topology, AOMDV attempts to discover alternative routes from available backup routes between the end to end node pairs. This process adds to the packet delivery time, resulting in a slightly reduced throughput. On the other hand, the ZRP algorithm prioritizes message security through encryption with signatures. While this enhances the security of message delivery, it sacrifices throughput as it does not prioritize finding the most efficient path. In this evaluation, the presence of malicious nodes was limited to a range of 35, with a difference of 5 between each range. In this scenario, the throughput achieved was 44.5. However, as the number of malicious nodes increases beyond this range, the throughput decreases accordingly.

End to End Delay : In this scenario, we examine different propagation models along with fixed routing protocols and changing node counts. Among the models, the Emphasized Trust-Based Secure Routing Protocol (ETBSRP) demonstrates the shortest end-to-end latency, as depicted in Figure 11. During comparison process of the proposed protocol, it exhibits superior performance than the other two protocols. The proposed protocol achieves slightly faster message delivery with reduced delays compared to the alternative algorithms.

In a specific scenario where there are 100 vehicles, if 35 of them are considered malicious nodes, the end-to-end delay ranges around 1400. It is noteworthy that the delay consistently decreases as the number of malicious nodes decreases.

Packet Loss

Figure 12 provides insights into the number of packets that fail to reach their destination accurately. The diagram clearly indicates that the ZRP protocol exhibits the highest packet loss ratio, meaning a significant portion of the packets transmitted using this protocol does not reach their intended destination. On the other hand, the proposed protocol, ETBSRP, showcases a considerably lower packet loss ratio, indicating a higher success rate in delivering packets successfully. The inverse of the packet delivery rate. Therefore, a higher packet loss ratio corresponds to a lower packet delivery rate, implying that a larger proportion of packets are lost or fail to reach their intended destination. In this context, the ETBSRP protocol outperforms the ZRP protocol by demonstrating a lower packet loss ratio, indicating a more efficient and reliable packet delivery mechanism. Here in table 2, the metrics which are used for comparison of the existing proposed protocol are illustrated.

Figure 11. End to End Delay in terms of number of malicious vehicles

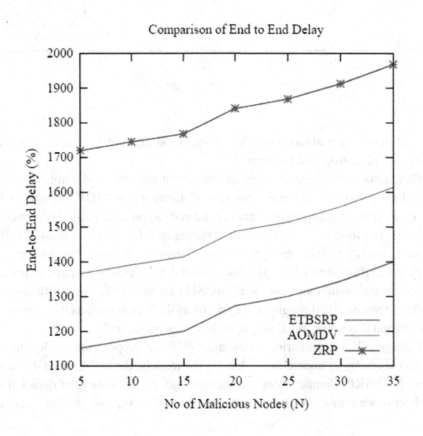

Figure 12. Packet Loss in terms of number of malicious vehicles

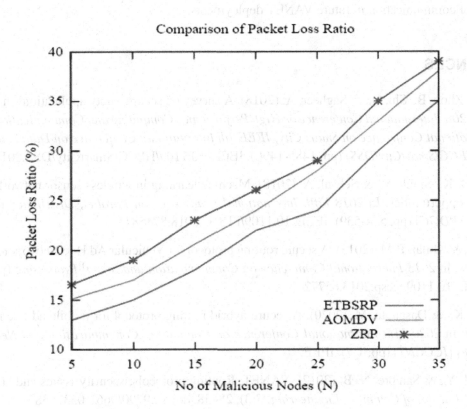

CONCLUSION

This paper introduced a secure and efficient routing protocol for message delivery in Vehicular Ad-Hoc Networks (VANETs). The proposed protocol, called Emphasized Trust-Based Secure Routing Protocol (ETBSRP), employs the Dijkstra algorithm to establish routes by creating a formulated graph to determine the most optimal path. To verify trusted nodes, we utilize RREQ and RREP requests, updating the routing table with the final values. Additionally, we ensure secure message transmission by employing the Diffie-Hellman key exchange algorithm for message encryption. Through this research, ETBSRP has been used as a routing protocol to enhance the quality of service (QoS) in VANETs. This protocol is well-suited for larger networks and considers various parameters such as configuration, node trust levels, and node battery life throughout the routing process. As a result, it improves speed and reduces overhead. Moreover, the proposed protocol incorporates multipath routing, which reduces unnecessary control messages during route formation in scenarios involving congestion or node failure. By identifying hostile nodes, ETBSRP ensures secure connections within the network. Through simulation experiments, we have demonstrated that the ETBSRP protocol outperforms existing routing strategies in terms of packet delivery ratio (PDR), packet loss ratio (PLR), average end-to-end time, and throughput. The results highlight the effectiveness of the proposed ETBSRP in enhancing the QoS of VANETs while ensuring secure communication. Looking ahead, we emphasize the implementation of advanced security algorithms, including encryption, decryption, and blockchain approaches, to provide even higher levels of security to VANETs. By incorporating these measures, we aim to further enhance the protection and reliability of communication in future VANET deployments.

REFERENCES

Al-Ani, R., Zhou, B., Shi, Q., & Sagheer, A. (2018). A survey on secure safety applications in vanet. In *2018 IEEE 20th International Conference on High Performance Computing and Communications; IEEE 16th International Conference on Smart City; IEEE 4th International Conference on Data Science and Systems (HPCC/SmartCity/DSS)* (pp. 1485-1490). IEEE. 10.1109/HPCC/SmartCity/DSS.2018.00245

Bangotra, D. K., Singh, Y., & Selwal, A. (2018). Machine learning in wireless sensor networks: Challenges and opportunities. In *2018 Fifth International Conference on Parallel, Distributed and Grid Computing (PDGC)* (pp. 534-539). IEEE. 10.1109/PDGC.2018.8745845

Bhoi, S. K., & Khilar, P. M. (2013). A secure routing protocol for Vehicular Ad Hoc Network to provide ITS services. In *2013 International Conference on Communication and Signal Processing* (pp. 1170-1174). IEEE. 10.1109/iccsp.2013.6577240

Biswas, A. K., & Dasgupta, M. (2020). A secure hybrid routing protocol for mobile ad-hoc networks (MANETs). In *2020 11th International Conference on Computing, Communication and Networking Technologies (ICCCNT)* (pp. 1-7). IEEE.

Gadkari, M. Y., & Sambre, N. B. (2012). VANET: Routing protocols, security issues and simulation tools. *IOSR Journal of Computer Engineering*, 3(3), 28–38. doi:10.9790/0661-0332838

Ghosh, U., & Datta, R. (2014). SDRP: Secure and dynamic routing protocol for mobile ad-hoc networks. *IET Networks*, 3(3), 235–243. doi:10.1049/iet-net.2013.0056

Hamdi, M. M., Audah, L., Rashid, S. A., & Alani, S. (2021). VANET-based traffic monitoring and incident detection system: A review. *International Journal of Electrical & Computer Engineering (2088-8708), 11*(4).

Hamdi, M. M., Audah, L., Rashid, S. A., Mohammed, A. H., Alani, S., & Mustafa, A. S. (2020). A review of applications, characteristics and challenges in vehicular ad hoc networks (VANETs). In 2020 international congress on human-computer interaction, optimization and robotic applications (HORA) (pp. 1-7). IEEE.

Hu, F., Chen, B., Shi, D., Zhang, X., & Pan, H. Z. (2020). Secure Routing Protocol in Wireless Ad Hoc Networks via Deep Learning. In 2020 IEEE Wireless Communications and Networking Conference (WCNC) (pp. 1-6). IEEE. doi:10.1109/WCNC45663.2020.9120545

Inam, M., Li, Z., Ali, A., & Zahoor, A. (2019). A novel protocol for vehicle cluster formation and vehicle head selection in vehicular ad-hoc networks. *International Journal of Electronics and Information Engineering*, 10(2), 103–119.

Kamboj, S., & Chawla, S. (2014). Geocast routing in vehicular Ad Hoc networks: A survey. [IJCSIT]. *International Journal of Computer Science and Information Technologies*, 5(4), 5365.

Kumar, K. R. (2010). VANET parameters and applications: A review. *Global Journal of Computer Science and Technology*, *10*(7), 72–77.

Kumar, V., Mishra, S., & Chand, N. (2013). Applications of VANETs: present & future. *communications and network, 5*(01), 12-15.

Lai, W. K., Lin, M. T., & Yang, Y. H. (2015). A machine learning system for routing decision-making in urban vehicular ad hoc networks. *International Journal of Distributed Sensor Networks*, *11*(3), 374391. doi:10.1155/2015/374391

Lazrag, H., Chaibi, H., Saadane, R., & Rahmani, M. D. (2018). An optimal and secure routing protocol for wireless sensor networks. In *2018 6th International Conference on Multimedia Computing and Systems (ICMCS)* (pp. 1-5). IEEE. 10.1109/ICMCS.2018.8525911

Liang, W., Li, Z., Zhang, H., Wang, S., & Bie, R. (2015). Vehicular ad hoc networks: Architectures, research issues, methodologies, challenges, and trends. *International Journal of Distributed Sensor Networks*, *11*(8), 745303. doi:10.1155/2015/745303

Mejri, M. N., & Ben-Othman, J. (2016). GDVAN: A new greedy behavior attack detection algorithm for VANETs. *IEEE Transactions on Mobile Computing*, *16*(3), 759–771. doi:10.1109/TMC.2016.2577035

Pandit, C. M., & Ladhe, S. A. (2014). Secure routing protocol in MANET using TAC. In *2014 First International Conference on Networks & Soft Computing (ICNSC2014)* (pp. 107-112). IEEE. 10.1109/CNSC.2014.6906693

Paramasivan, B., Prakash, M. J. V., & Kaliappan, M. (2015). Development of a secure routing protocol using game theory model in mobile ad hoc networks. *Journal of Communications and Networks (Seoul)*, *17*(1), 75–83. doi:10.1109/JCN.2015.000012

Patil, C., & Nataraj, K. R. (2014). A Secure Routing Protocol for VANET. *International Journal of Engine Research*, *3*(5).

RadhaKrishna Karne, D. T. (2021). Review on vanet architecture and applications. [TURCOMAT]. *Turkish Journal of Computer and Mathematics Education*, *12*(4), 1745–1749.

Rajkumar, M. N., Nithya, M., & HemaLatha, P. (2016). Overview of VANETs with its features and security attacks. *International Research Journal of Engineering and Technology, 3*(1).

Rehman, S. U., Khan, M., Zia, T., & Zheng, L. (2013). Vehicular ad-hoc networks (VANETs): an overview and challenges. *Journal of Wireless Networking and communications, 3*(3), 29-38.

Saggi, M. K., & Sandhu, R. K. (2014). A survey of vehicular ad hoc network on attacks and security threats in VANETs. In *International Conference on Research and Innovations in Engineering and Technology (ICRIET 2014)* (pp. 19-20). IEEE.

Saini, M., & Singh, H. (2016). VANET its characteristics attacks and routing techniques: A survey. *International Journal of Scientific Research*, *5*(5), 1595–1599.

Sampoornam, K. P., Saranya, S., Vigneshwaran, S., Sofiarani, P., Sarmitha, S., & Sarumathi, N. (2020). A comparative study on reactive routing protocols in VANET. In *2020 4th International Conference on Electronics, Communication and Aerospace Technology (ICECA)* (pp. 726-731). IEEE. 10.1109/ICECA49313.2020.9297550

Sarma, A. H. K. D., Kar, B. A., & Mall, C. R. (2011). Secure routing protocol for mobile wireless sensor network. In *2011 IEEE Sensors Applications Symposium* (pp. 93-99). IEEE. 10.1109/SAS.2011.5739778

Shaktawat, R. S., Singh, D., & Choudhary, N. (2014). An efficient secure routing protocol in MANET Security-Enhanced AODV (SE-AODV). *International Journal of Computer Applications*, 97(8). Advance online publication. doi:10.5120/17030-7329

Singh, G., Rohil, H., Rishi, R., & Ranga, V. (2019). LETSRP: A secure routing protocol for MANETs. *Int J Eng Adv Technol (IJEAT). ISSN*, 9(1), 2249–8958.

Singh, R., Kathuria, K., & Sagar, A. K. (2018). Secure routing protocols for wireless sensor networks. In *2018 4th international conference on computing communication and automation (ICCCA)* (pp. 1-5). IEEE. 10.1109/CCAA.2018.8777557

Sonker, A., & Gupta, R. K. (2020). A new combination of machine learning algorithms using stacking approach for misbehavior detection in VANETs. *International Journal of Computer Science and Network Security*, 20(10), 94–100.

Yadav, N., & Chug, U. (2019). Secure Routing in MANET: A Review. In *2019 International Conference on Machine Learning, Big Data, Cloud and Parallel Computing (COMITCon)* (pp. 375-379). IEEE.

Yadav, S., Rajput, N. K., Sagar, A. K., & Maheshwari, D. (2018). Secure and reliable routing protocols for VANETs. In *2018 4th International Conference on Computing Communication and Automation (ICCCA)* (pp. 1-5). IEEE. 10.1109/CCAA.2018.8777690

Yang, T., Xiangyang, X., Peng, L., Tonghui, L., & Leina, P. (2018). A secure routing of wireless sensor networks based on trust evaluation model. *Procedia Computer Science*, 131, 1156–1163. doi:10.1016/j.procs.2018.04.289

Zhao, L., Li, Y., Meng, C., Gong, C., & Tang, X. (2016). A SVM based routing scheme in VANETs. In *2016 16th International Symposium on Communications and Information Technologies (ISCIT)* (pp. 380-383). IEEE. 10.1109/ISCIT.2016.7751655

Chapter 8
Autonomous Systems Revolutionizing Health Insurance Industry:
Achieving Operational Excellence in Services

Anupa Stanly

(iD) https://orcid.org/0009-0003-7374-8618

Karunya Institute of Technology and Sciences, India

.

K. Aruna

Karunya Institute of Technology and Sciences, India

ABSTRACT

Financial services, particularly the insurance service sector, are increasingly embracing technology. Autonomous systems, which include artificial intelligence (AI), machine learning, and automation, are driving a striking revolution in the health insurance industry. This research provides a comprehensive analysis of various facets, such as the use of autonomous systems, expediting claim processing, identifying, and preventing fraud, improving the customer experience, data-driven decision-making, and adherence to healthcare legislation. The study concludes by highlighting the sector's profound impact from autonomous systems and pointing to a promising future for health insurance that will be characterised by operational effectiveness and customer-centricity. This study sets out a thorough exploration of the dynamic world where autonomous systems are changing the laws governing health insurance. This investigation's main objectives are to achieve operational excellence and provide services that are utterly customer-centric.

INTRODUCTION

The integration of autonomous systems is driving a seismic upheaval in the health insurance sector. Artificial intelligence and machine learning are powering these cutting-edge technologies, which are

DOI: 10.4018/979-8-3693-1962-8.ch008

completely changing how insurers handle claims, control risks, and communicate with policyholders. Insurers are under tremendous pressure to improve efficiency, accuracy, and customer experience as healthcare costs continue to rise and regulatory requirements get more intricate. In this context, autonomous systems show promise as never before seen, providing previously unheard-of chances to boost productivity, enhance judgement, and spur industry innovation.

The health insurance industry is entering a new era of efficiency and efficacy with the integration of autonomous systems. Insurance companies may speed workflows, minimise administrative hassles, and minimise risks by using these technologies to automate regular tasks like fraud detection and claims processing. Furthermore, insurers can use massive volumes of data to customise services, allocate resources more efficiently, and make data-driven decisions that spur strategic expansion and innovation thanks to autonomous systems. Insurance companies are well-positioned to provide more value to policyholders, improve operational resilience, and succeed in a market that is becoming more and more competitive as they adopt these game-changing technologies.

LITERATURE REVIEW

The relentless pace of technological advancement is pushing the health insurance sector towards a significant shift. Autonomous systems, a fusion of artificial intelligence (AI), machine learning, and automation, are at the centre of this metamorphosis and are poised to revolutionise how health insurance is created, provided, and experienced (*The Impact of Big Data and Artificial Intelligence (AI) in the Insurance Sector*, 2020). The development of autonomous systems shines as a beacon of hope in a field frequently plagued by bureaucratic delays, rising prices, and the persistent search for operational efficiency. Increased enrollment in insurance, particularly among low-income households, can be facilitated by digital health insurance management systems and an increase in new digital mediators in the insurance sector is indicative of technology's immediate impact (Stoeckli et al., 2018). The expert interviews have unambiguously shown that organizational culture, technology policy, and strategic philosophy do affect how widely health insurance companies are utilizing autonomous systems (Akter et al., 2022; *Technology and Innovation in the Insurance Sector*, n.d.). Health insurers should concentrate on raising their service standards and come up with ways to preserve the tacit base of knowledge generated by wearable technology for long-term competitive advantage (Nayak et al., 2019).

The history of health insurance is replete with difficulties, from the difficulty of claims processing to the consistently rising price of healthcare. These ongoing problems have long hindered the industry's ability to deliver services that are easily accessible, effective, and client-focused. Health insurers, however, are now in a position to overcome these obstacles and usher in a new era of operational excellence due to the integration of autonomous systems. The insurance firms, not investing in new technology may not seem like a realistic option and should let the future digital business be performed as new or separate divisions that are evolved from concept to completion without legacy applications if it desires to survive into the next few decades (Eling & Lehmann, 2018). By mandating quick reaction times, these new rivals encourage innovation and hasten industry transition. They go beyond simply digitizing the business model to anticipate consumers' demands and offer intelligent solutions and services rather than traditional products and services (Cappiello, 2018). Incumbents work with Insurtechs and digital platforms to start making the best use of the opportunity, as these alliances have the potential to enable more customized online distribution, predictive underwriting, and much more effective management of insurance claims and significantly boost the insurance penetration in India (Alpesh Shah et al., 2021). Regulators need to realize how technologies function to facilitate innovations that the policyholder stands to benefit. Technologies that enable easier business for both the insured and the insurer enhances more scientific pricing and helps both parties should be encouraged (Report on InsurTech in the Context of Risk Assessment, Product Design and Pricing, n.d.).

THE CURRENT LANDSCAPE OF THE HEALTH INSURANCE INDUSTRY

Many important reasons have influenced the dynamic landscape that the health insurance sector is navigating today. More and more people are facing financial hardship as a result of rising health-care expenditures that are outpacing inflation. Insurance companies have to deal with increased administrative costs in addition to rising medical costs, which are partly caused by the complexity of processing claims and the need for regulatory compliance. Insurance companies now face an even more challenging operating environment as a result of the introduction of new rules and mandates intended to increase access to treatment and improve quality, such as the Affordable treatment Act in the United States.

Further, policyholders' expectations are changing, and they now want their insurers to provide them with more ease, transparency, and personalised service. Digitalization and technological advancements have given customers access to resources and information, empowering them to compare insurance plans, look for alternative care, and take a more active role in managing their health and insurance coverage. Insurance companies face pressure to innovate and set themselves apart in this more competitive market by offering value-added services, boosting customer happiness, and increasing consumer engagement.

The COVID-19 pandemic has highlighted the value of adaptability, resiliency, and creativity in the health insurance sector amidst these difficulties. The pandemic has changed how healthcare services are provided and used, hastening the use of telehealth and virtual care solutions. In order to satisfy the evolving needs of policyholders, insurers are adjusting their products and business practices. At the same time, they are managing the financial effects of the pandemic, which include rising claim volumes and unstable healthcare utilisation trends.

Insurance companies that want to increase productivity, accuracy, and customer satisfaction in this situation must strategically integrate autonomous technologies into their claims processing operations. Insurance companies may improve their decision-making powers, streamline processes, and lower administrative costs by utilising cutting-edge technology like artificial intelligence, machine learning, and data analytics.

Autonomous Systems in the Health Insurance Industry

The health insurance sector uses a variety of autonomous technologies to improve operational efficiency overall, expedite operations, and improve consumer experiences. These autonomous systems make use of data analytics, automation, machine learning, and artificial intelligence (AI). The major autonomous systems frequently used in health insurance are:

- **AI-Powered Chatbots:**

The application of AI-powered chatbots, which improve customer relationships, expedite processes, and raise overall efficiency, is highly advantageous to the health insurance industry. Artificial intelligence (AI)-driven chatbots have become indispensable resources in the health insurance industry, dramatically altering both client relations and operational effectiveness (Eling et al., 2022). These sophisticated chatbots offer several advantages that improve user experience and expedite certain business operations.

The capacity of AI-powered chatbots to provide immediate and reachable 24/7 customer service is one of their main advantages in the health insurance market. These chatbots, which are always on and available to policyholders, guarantee that they can always get support and information, making the experience more responsive and user-friendly. This is especially important in the healthcare industry, as prompt assistance and information might be vital.

When it comes to promptly answering commonly requested questions concerning policy details, managing claims, paying premiums, and other common difficulties, these chatbots thrive. Because chatbots answer frequently asked questions automatically, they reduce the need for customers to wait for assistance or negotiate complex phone interfaces, which improves both the efficacy and pleasure of customer care.

In the claims processing sector, chatbots equipped with artificial intelligence (AI) functionalities are indispensable for aiding users. They provide claim status updates, simplify the required paperwork, and generally improve the efficiency of the claims process. Customer satisfaction is increased and the claims process is sped up by keeping policyholders informed and participating.

Additionally, policyholders' general health literacy is increased by employing these chatbots. They can communicate complicated insurance plans, coverage details, and exclusions in an easy-to-understand manner. Chatbots assist customers in making informed decisions about their coverage by translating complex insurance jargon.

Artificial intelligence (AI)-powered chatbots are crucial for automatically reminding and informing policyholders (Akter et al., 2022). These reminders may include dates that are significant for future renewals, premium payment deadlines, and other events. This proactive approach guarantees that insurance is up to date and that policyholders are advised of important actions they need to take.

Chatbots that use AI can provide personalized wellness and health recommendations in addition to answering queries. These chatbots can analyze individual health data to provide tailored advice, encourage healthy living choices, and offer information on wellness programs supported by insurance companies. This fosters care for the well-being of policyholders and enhances long-term health outcomes.

In short, Artificial intelligence (AI)-driven chatbots are revolutionizing the health insurance sector by optimizing customer support, streamlining the claims process, and supporting wellness and health-related programs. These chatbots have a significant potential to improve customer experiences and boost the effectiveness of health insurance operations as technology develops.

- **Predictive Analytics and Machine Learning Models:**

In the health insurance sector, predictive analytics and machine learning models have emerged as indispensable instruments, providing features that improve risk assessment, decision-making, and overall efficiency in operation. These technologies' capacity to evaluate and forecast health concerns is one of its main advantages. Insurance companies can predict the possibility of certain health problems in their policyholders by using predictive analytics, which can evaluate large datasets to find patterns and trends linked to particular medical disorders. These models use past data to help create more precise risk profiles for individuals, which enables insurers to adjust rates and policies accordingly.

A subset of artificial intelligence called machine learning models plays a major role in the underwriting procedures used in the health insurance industry. These models may independently assess a wide range of variables, including medical history, lifestyle decisions, and demographic data, to ascertain if a prospective policyholder is insurable. This reduces the possibility of human bias and speeds up the underwriting process while ensuring a more complex and data-driven assessment of risk. Predictive analytics is also essential for spotting fraud in the health insurance market. These models can detect potentially fraudulent activity by analysing claim trends and spotting anomalies, which enables insurers to take preventative action (Yaneva, n.d.). This preserves the financial interests of insurance companies and upholds the integrity of the insurance system as a whole.

Machine learning models simplify the examination of insurance claims in the field of claims processing. By automatically comparing claims to pre-established standards, these models can streamline the procedure and reduce the chance of inaccuracy. Furthermore, they aid in the identification of anomalies or discrepancies, enhancing the precision of choices made about the approval or rejection of claims.

Initiatives for personalised health and wellbeing are also revolutionised by the application of machine learning and predictive analytics. With the use of these technologies, insurers may evaluate policyholders' specific health data and deliver them personalised suggestions. This proactive strategy can result in fewer claims and lower expenses for the insurance company, in addition to cultivating a healthier clientele. Additionally, these technologies support health insurance firms' overall financial viability. Insurers can more effectively plan and distribute resources by precisely forecasting patterns of healthcare utilisation and related costs. They may then optimise premium pricing, properly manage risk, and guarantee the long-term profitability of their offers as a result.

- **Automated claims processing:**

In the health insurance sector, automated claims processing is a crucial development that has completely changed the way insurance claims are managed and greatly increased productivity. This creative method uses automated technologies and processes to expedite the whole claims process, from filing to settlement. Accelerated claim adjudication is one of the main advantages of automated claims processing. Automated systems evaluate claims based on predetermined standards using algorithms, allowing for quick and precise decision-making (Guzmán-Ortiz et al., 2020). This guarantees that valid claims are handled quickly and speeds up the policyholders' compensation procedure.

Moreover, the danger of errors resulting from manual data entry and evaluation is reduced by automated claims processing. These systems can identify discrepancies, errors, or perhaps fraudulent activity in claims submissions by utilising machine learning and data analytics. This helps to maintain the claims adjudication process's general integrity and correctness.

Policyholders benefit from a more smooth and open experience as a result of the automation of claims processing. Electronic documentary submission is available to claimants, who can also get automated updates on the status of their submissions and monitor the status of their claims in real-time. Policyholders value the convenience and openness provided by automated systems, and this increased visibility helps to build their trust and transparency provided by automated frameworks (Eckert et al., 2022). Additionally, automated techniques for processing claims help health insurance providers save money.

Insurers can maximise their operating costs by eliminating the need for a great deal of physical labour and minimising the likelihood of errors. This cost-effectiveness is especially important in an industry where total financial performance can be greatly impacted by administrative costs.

The adoption of automated claims processing not only saves money but also fits in with the larger industry trend towards digital transformation. Health insurance firms can maintain their competitiveness by adopting technology innovations that enhance their operational efficiency and establish them as modern, user-friendly service providers. For sensitive health data to be protected, strong cybersecurity safeguards must be in place when implementing automated claims processing, even with these benefits. Safeguarding patient privacy and security during the claims process necessitates strict adherence to healthcare standards, including the Health Insurance Portability and Accountability Act (HIPAA). In short, automated claims processing is a revolutionary development in the health insurance industry that brings advantages including faster processing, lower error rates, more cost-effectiveness, and higher customer satisfaction. The incorporation of automated technologies is probably going to be a major factor in determining how claims administration in the health insurance sector develops in the future.

- **Fraud Detection Algorithms:**

Through the identification and prevention of fraudulent activity, fraud detection algorithms are essential in preserving the financial stability of health insurance systems. Within the realm of health insurance, fraud can take many different forms, such as fraudulent claims, identity theft, and policyholder-provider cooperation. In addition to addressing these issues, the use of sophisticated fraud detection algorithms has other important advantages. Pattern and anomaly analysis within big datasets is one of the main purposes of fraud detection systems. These algorithms detect possibly fraudulent actions by looking at past claim data and highlighting anomalies. These algorithms can adjust and change over time, picking up new information and increasing in accuracy thanks to machine learning techniques. These algorithms support a proactive strategy for reducing the likelihood of fraud. Detecting fraud in real-time is possible because to fraud detection algorithms, which highlight questionable behaviours as they happen. This is preferable to depending just on post-claim audits, which can be laborious and resource-intensive. This prompt action safeguards policyholders and insurers by preventing money from being paid out for fraudulent claims. Furthermore, fraud detection algorithms support health insurance companies' broader efforts to control costs. Insurance companies can lessen the financial losses brought on by paying out on inflated or fraudulent claims by spotting and stopping fraudulent claims. As a result, insurance programmes continue to be financially viable, which may result in more consistent premium prices for policyholders.

The advanced algorithms used for fraud detection enable them to take into account a wide range of parameters. These could include patient demographics, provider behaviour, geographic trends, and claim history. These algorithms can improve their ability to detect fraud by developing a sophisticated knowledge of what defines normal or suspicious behaviour by looking at a large number of data points. Successful fraud detection requires industry-wide collaboration. Information concerning fraudulent activity and anonymised data are frequently shared by insurance firms. The ability of the industry to fight fraud on a larger scale is improved by this collaborative approach, which makes it possible to develop more reliable fraud detection algorithms that can spot patterns that may affect several insurers. Striking a balance between thorough fraud detection and quick processing of valid claims is crucial, though. Inadvertently flagging legitimate claims by overly aggressive algorithms might cause delays and problems for policyholders (Gellweiler & Krishnamurthi, 2020). To maintain accuracy while reducing false positives, fraud detection algorithms must be continuously improved and adjusted. Algorithms for detecting fraud are essential resources for the health insurance sector, as they aid in the detection and prevention of fraudulent activity. Their flexibility, suppleness, and capacity to take into account a wide range of factors render them indispensable for preserving the fiscal soundness of health insurance schemes and cultivating policyholder confidence. These algorithms will need to be continuously improved in order to keep up with changing fraud techniques as technology develops.

- **Data Analytics Platforms:**

The health insurance industry has evolved to rely extensively on data analytics tools, which enable providers to glean insights from large and intricate datasets that may be put to use. These platforms offer several benefits in terms of decision-making, risk management, and operational efficiency. They do this by utilising cutting-edge analytics tools and technologies to analyse, interpret, and visualise data. Finding relevant patterns and trends in a variety of datasets is one of the main functions of data analytics platforms in the health insurance industry. These insights can be used by insurers to improve pricing tactics, customise policy offerings, and adjust to shifting market conditions. These systems facilitate a data-driven approach to business decisions by utilising real-time and historical data, which eventually improves the competitiveness and sustainability of health insurance products.

Another crucial area where data analytics tools come in handy is risk management. Through the analysis of vast amounts of policyholder, healthcare provider, and healthcare trend data, these platforms assist insurers in recognising possible hazards and forecasting upcoming difficulties. These platforms' predictive analytics make it possible to identify high-risk individuals or groups, allowing insurers to proactively carry out focused interventions and preventive actions (Ostrowska, 2021). Data analytics tools greatly simplify the process of managing claims. These platforms can examine past claim data to spot trends, evaluate the veracity of claims, and spot possible fraud. By lowering reimbursements linked to inflated or fraudulent claims, this helps with cost control efforts in addition to speeding up the claims processing workflow. Additionally, in the health insurance sector, data analytics systems are crucial to improving customer experience. Insurers can obtain knowledge about preferences, behaviours, and expectations by examining client data and interactions. In order to increase customer satisfaction and retention rates, this data can be used to improve service offerings, personalise communications, and optimise customer interaction methods.

A new field where data analytics tools are having a big influence is population health management. Large-scale data aggregation and analysis capabilities of these systems enable insurers to see patterns, use resources effectively, and create focused interventions aimed at enhancing population health as a whole. In addition to helping policyholders, this proactive strategy also helps ensure the long-term viability of health insurance programmes (Flückiger & Duygun, 2022). Adopting data analytics platforms in the health insurance industry is closely linked to privacy and data security concerns. To protect the confidentiality and integrity of patient data, insurers must prioritise strong cybersecurity measures and adherence to laws like the Health Insurance Portability and Accountability Act (HIPAA). This is because health-related information is sensitive. By utilising data to support decision-making, improve risk management, expedite claims processing, enhance customer experience, and support population health management, data analytics systems play a critical role in transforming the health insurance market.

The use of data analytics in health insurance is anticipated to grow as technology develops, spurring additional advancements and enhancements in the sector.

- **Blockchain for Claims Management:**

Blockchain technology is revolutionising the health insurance industry by providing a safe and decentralised method of managing claims. In this case, the entire claims processing procedure is made more transparent, efficient, and secure by using blockchain technology. Dispersed ledger technology, which is the foundation of blockchain, allows transactions to be recorded securely and transparently over a network of computers. Blockchain technology is used in health insurance to produce an unchangeable, tamper-proof record of each stage in the claims handling procedure. This will allow all relevant parties, including policyholders, healthcare providers, and insurers, to have access to a single version of the truth.

The increased transparency that blockchain offers is among the main advantages of using technology for health insurance claims processing. Every claim-related transaction or modification is documented in a block, which is then connected chronologically. Because there is a shared source of truth and all authorised parties have real-time access to the same information, this transparency lowers the likelihood of disagreements. When handling sensitive health data, security is of utmost importance. Blockchain uses sophisticated encryption algorithms to address this issue. Claims information and patient data are kept in encrypted blocks, and consensus processes make sure that any modifications to the data need network approval (Marano, 2019). The possibility of illegal access and data breaches is greatly decreased with this degree of protection.

Smart contracts are essential to blockchain-based claims management because they are self-executing contracts with explicit terms encoded into the code. Smart contracts have the potential to automate several claims process steps in the health insurance industry, including fund disbursement, eligibility verification, and claims validation. This automation lowers the possibility of errors and fraud while also speeding up the claims processing timeframe. Blockchain provides a strong answer to the enduring problem of fraud detection in the insurance sector. The blockchain ledger's transparency and immutability facilitate the process of tracking down the source of a claim, spotting anomalies, and spotting possible fraudulent activity. Insurance companies are better equipped to detect and stop fraudulent claims because of this increased visibility. Increased operational efficiency results from blockchain's decentralised structure, which lessens reliance on a central authority. The claims management process can be made more efficient by minimising the need for intermediaries and third-party administrators. This will also lead to faster decision-making and lower administrative expenses. Although the use of blockchain in health insurance is uplifting, issues including regulatory compliance, industry standards, and interoperability with current systems need to be resolved. Blockchain has the potential to completely transform health insurance claims management, offering not only a more secure and efficient system but also one that is more transparent and accountable as stakeholders work together to overcome these obstacles and the technology advances.

- **Telemedicine platforms:**

By revolutionising the way healthcare is delivered and enhancing policyholder accessible, telemedicine platforms have emerged as essential parts of health insurance. With a number of advantages that improve healthcare as a whole, these platforms use technology to enable remote medical consultations. The wider accessibility of healthcare services is one of the main benefits of telemedicine platforms when it comes to health insurance. Through the use of these platforms, policyholders can communicate virtually with medical experts, removing geographical limitations and facilitating prompt medical advice without requiring in-person visits to healthcare institutions. This is especially helpful for policyholders who may have trouble getting to healthcare professionals since they live in rural or underserved locations.

Platforms for telemedicine reduce costs for policyholders as well as insurers. Enabling virtual consultations can save healthcare costs by preventing needless ER visits and urgent care sessions. Policyholders save money by paying less out-of-pocket for in-person visits, and insurers profit from decreased claims costs. One major aspect propelling telemedicine systems' adoption in health insurance is the ease they provide. Policyholders can receive medical consultations without having to travel or wait in queue by visiting the convenience of their homes or places of employment. For minor health conditions, routine check-ups, or follow-up visits, this convenience is especially helpful as it enables people to receive care on time without interfering with their everyday life.

Early intervention and preventive care are greatly aided by telemedicine. Healthcare providers can regularly interact with policyholders via virtual consultations and remote monitoring to monitor chronic conditions, evaluate the policyholders' state of health, and provide timely interventions. Better health outcomes and lower long-term healthcare expenditures for policyholders and insurers can result from this proactive strategy. Telemedicine systems are beneficial for health insurance since they increase client satisfaction. Insurers who incorporate telemedicine into their products frequently discover that it improves their overall value proposition, and policyholders like the flexibility and accessibility of virtual healthcare services. Increased client retention and loyalty can result from positive telemedicine encounters. It's crucial to remember that, in order to secure sensitive health information, privacy and security precautions must be taken into account when integrating telemedicine into health insurance. In virtual healthcare exchanges, maintaining the confidentiality and integrity of patient data requires adherence to standards such as the Health Insurance Portability and Accountability Act (HIPAA).

- **Wearables and health apps for policyholders:**

In the world of health insurance, wearables and health apps have grown to be indispensable tools that give policyholders greater control over their health and give insurers useful information for individualised treatment plans. Health apps on smartphones and wearable technology like smartwatches and fitness trackers offer a host of advantages for insurance companies as well as customers. For policyholders, the ability to track and monitor multiple aspects of their health in real-time is a major benefit of wearables and health applications. These gadgets have the ability to record information on heart rate, sleep patterns, physical activity, and other health parameters (Nayak et al., 2019). Policyholders can use this information to better understand their lifestyle and make changes that will enhance their general health and well-being.

Insurers can gain a more precise and up-to-date picture of policyholders' health thanks to the data produced by wearables and health applications. With the use of this data, insurers can use personalised risk assessment to customise coverage and rates according to the health habits and results of each policyholder. The move to customised insurance plans encourages a more fair sharing of risk and could encourage subscribers to lead healthier lives. Wearables and health applications greatly aid preventive care. These gadgets can offer timely alerts or warnings for possible health problems by constantly tracking health parameters. With this information, insurers may better serve their policyholders' long-term health by lowering the likelihood of costly medical procedures and by providing proactive health interventions like wellness programmes and specialised health coaching. Policyholders' participation and account-ability are increased when wearables and health apps are incorporated into health insurance policies. As a result, insurers gain from a healthier and possibly lower-risk client base, while policyholders are encouraged to adopt healthy habits. The usage of wearables and health applications in the context of health insurance requires careful consideration of privacy and data security. Insurers must guarantee that stringent protocols are implemented to safeguard the privacy and accuracy of health information gathered from policyholders. Establishing and preserving trust with policyholders requires adherence to pertinent legislation, such as the General Data Protection Regulation (GDPR), as well as regulations unique to the healthcare industry, such as the Health Insurance Portability and Accountability Act (HIPAA). By enabling policyholders to take an active role in their health management and enabling insurers to transition to more individualised and preventive healthcare models, wearables and health apps have completely changed the landscape of health insurance. These technologies are expected to become more deeply integrated into health insurance policies as they develop, opening up new avenues for better health outcomes and a more customer-focused and sustainable insurance sector.

- **Automated processes for customer onboarding:**

The health insurance sector has evolved to rely heavily on automated customer onboarding procedures, which expedite the accurate and efficient enrollment of new subscribers. Using cutting-edge systems and technology, automated onboarding procedures provide several benefits regarding efficiency, precision, and general client satisfaction. Enrollment process acceleration is one of the main advantages of auto-mated customer onboarding in health insurance (Malika Shuxratovna & Nuriddin Rustam Ugli, 2021). By using electronic signatures, digital forms, and automated document verification, new policyholders can expedite the onboarding process and eliminate the need for copious paperwork. This not only short-ens the enrollment process but also improves the client experience by offering a smooth and intuitive onboarding process. Accuracy and consistency in the data gathered from policyholders are guaranteed via automation in customer onboarding. The possibility of errors resulting from manual data entry is reduced when data inputs are validated in real-time by automated systems. This precision is crucial when it comes to health insurance, as it is required for the construction of policies, the computation of premiums, and the precise assessment of coverage.

Automated onboarding processes aid compliance with regulatory regulations. Adherence to data protection standards, such as the Health Insurance Portability and Accountability Act (HIPAA), is crucial since health insurance entails the acquisition of sensitive personal and medical information. In order to lower the risk of regulatory problems and guarantee the security and confidentiality of client data, automated systems can be built with the ability to enforce and audit compliance procedures. Automated workflows can guide new policyholders through the process, giving them the appropriate documentation and clear instructions. This enhances the onboarding process and lessens the possibility of incomplete or inaccurate submissions, which lowers the need for additional follow-ups and adjustments. Health insurance companies' scalability is improved via automated onboarding procedures. Automated sys-tems can handle higher enrollment numbers as the client base expands without causing a corresponding rise in administrative workload. For insurance companies looking to effectively handle a sizable and varied customer, this scalability is essential. A human-centric approach and automation must coexist in harmony. Although common activities can be handled by automated procedures, complicated inquiries, individualised support, and making sure that clients feel supported throughout the onboarding process still requires human intervention.

- **Automating KYC/AML Compliance:**

In the health insurance industry, automating Know Your Customer (KYC) and Anti-Money Laundering (AML) compliance procedures has become a crucial endeavour, as it improves customer onboarding speed and conforms to regulatory standards. Automated KYC/AML compliance in health insurance enables a comprehensive and standardised approach to customer identity verification and potential financial crime detection by utilising technology and sophisticated algorithms. The speed and accuracy of customer identity verification is one of the main benefits of automating KYC/AML compliance in health insurance. Automated solutions could evaluate and cross-reference vast amounts of client data quickly across many databases, which guarantees an accurate and timely identification assessment. This reduces the possibility of human error connected with conventional verification techniques while simultaneously speeding up the onboarding process. Overall fraud detection efficacy is improved by automation in KYC/AML compliance. A more advanced and proactive method of spotting possible money laundering or fraudulent activity is to use machine learning algorithms to examine trends, abnormalities, and warning signs in client data. In industries like healthcare and finance where preventing financial crimes and adhering to regulations are critical, this degree of monitoring is crucial.

Health insurance companies can reduce costs by implementing automated KYC/AML compliance procedures. Insurers can minimise the operating costs related to compliance by decreasing the amount of documentation required and the need on manual labour. Because of its affordability, insurers can spend resources more effectively while maintaining constant compliance with regulatory standards. Automation guarantees that KYC/AML compliance is handled uniformly and consistently for all of the clientele. Insurers can lower the risk of errors or overlook by establishing a consistent standard of due diligence by doing the same thorough checks on every customer. This strengthens the compliance process's overall integrity and assists in meeting regulatory requirements. Since health insurance data is sensitive and strong privacy protections are required, the industry needs to integrate automation into KYC/AML compliance. To guarantee that client data is handled securely and privately, automated systems can be made to abide by healthcare laws. Even though automation makes routine compliance operations more efficient, human oversight is still necessary. Human knowledge should be added to automated systems, particularly when managing difficult cases, dealing with unusual situations, and reaching well-informed choices that could call for delicate judgment. A complete and comprehensive compliance framework is ensured by a balanced approach that blends automation and human intuition. To comply with regulations, improve operational effectiveness, and enhance fraud prevention strategies, health insurance companies must automate KYC/AML compliance. The landscape of health insurance will become safer and more compliant as technology develops and intelligent automation in compliance processes becomes more sophisticatedly integrated.

- **Tools for Data Security and Privacy:**

In the health insurance sector, where sensitive personal and medical data is handled, maintaining strong data security and privacy is crucial. To protect information, adhere to legal requirements, and foster confidence with policyholders, a range of instruments and technologies are used. One essential tool for safeguarding data while it's in transit and at rest is encryption. Information including patient records, policy details, and financial transactions can be safely encoded using sophisticated encryption methods, limiting illegal access even if the data is intercepted. The management and restriction of user access to sensitive health data requires the use of access controls and authentication procedures. The use of multi-factor authentication, biometric verification, and role-based access restrictions can effectively mitigate the risk of data breaches by limiting access to specific information to only authorised persons. These instruments are essential for preserving patient record integrity and confidentiality in health insurance systems.

The prevention of sensitive data from being transmitted without authorization is greatly aided by data loss prevention (DLP) solutions (Shevchuk et al., 2020). These instruments keep an eye on and regulate information flow, preventing unintentional or deliberate data leaks. DLP tools reduce risks associated with human mistake or malicious intent by preventing the unintentional disclosure of private information, which is crucial in the health insurance industry where patient privacy is of utmost importance. In the health insurance industry, privacy-enhancing technologies (PETs) like homomorphic encryption and differential privacy are becoming more and more popular. These technologies enable the study of encrypted data without the need to decrypt it, protecting personal information while still yielding insightful results. This is especially important when exchanging data is required for analysis or study without jeopardising the privacy of the individual. Programmes for employee awareness and training are essential for encouraging a data security and privacy-conscious culture in health insurance companies. The first line of defence against possible security threats is knowledgeable people, and training initiatives make sure that workers are prepared to identify and address security issues (Gorchakova, 2019). Strong data security and privacy in the health insurance sector require a multipronged strategy that includes encryption, access controls, DLP, blockchain, privacy-enhancing technology, compliance management, and employee training. To keep ahead of potential dangers and safeguard the private data entrusted to health insurance carriers, it is imperative to continuously integrate cutting-edge tools and technology.

- **Mobile Apps and Portals:**

Mobile applications and portals, which enable policyholders to manage their healthcare needs simply and effectively, have become vital components of the health insurance landscape. These digital platforms offer several features that increase overall customer happiness, speed up administrative processes, and give customers the ability to take control of their health and insurance coverage. The convenience that mobile apps and portals provide to policyholders is one of the main benefits of health insurance. From the palm of their hands, users may access these platforms' insurance information, policy data, and pertinent health resources. Mobile apps offer real-time information for verifying coverage, monitoring claims status, and accessing digital insurance cards. This eliminates the need for policyholders to negotiate convoluted phone systems or wait for help. Mobile apps for health insurance often provide features that make processing claims easier. Through the app, policyholders can easily file claims, add supporting documents, and monitor the progress of their claims. This improves transparency by updating users on the status of their submissions and speeds up the claims process.

To improve communication between insurers and policyholders, mobile apps and portals are essential. Users are alerted about impending renewals, critical updates, and payment reminders using push notifications and alerts. Furthermore, by giving insurers a direct line of communication for pertinent health and wellness information, these platforms encourage policyholders to lead healthy lifestyles and receive preventive treatment. Policyholders can obtain virtual healthcare consultations thanks to the growing integration of telemedicine technologies into health insurance smartphone apps. This feature offers policyholders a prompt and simple substitute for in-person visits in the event of non-emergency medical difficulties. This helps policyholders and insurers save money while also improving accessibility to healthcare services. Mobile apps and portals greatly aid the promotion of health and wellness programmes. Features that measure exercise, track fitness objectives and offer individualised health advice are available from many health insurance companies. These resources motivate policyholders to pursue healthier lifestyles, which may have long-term advantages including lower medical expenses and enhanced general health. The way that policyholders interact with their health insurance plans has evolved through the advent of mobile apps and portals. These online resources provide an intuitive user interface for managing tasks linked to insurance, accessing healthcare services, and learning about health and wellness (Lin & Chen, 2020). As technology advances, it is projected that adding new features and functionality to health insurance apps would encourage a more proactive approach to healthcare management and enhance the user experience in general.

The Role of Autonomous Systems in Operational Excellence and Customer-Centric Services of the Health Insurance Industry

The use of autonomous systems in the health insurance sector is a paradigm-shifting development that will fundamentally alter how healthcare is handled, delivered, and experienced. These autonomous systems, which use a variety of technologies including automation, machine learning, and artificial intelligence (AI), have played a crucial role in tackling persistent issues and advancing the sector's focus on operational excellence and customer-centric services.

- Claims Processing Streamlining:

The integration of diverse technologies, such as automation, machine learning, and artificial intelligence, is causing a disruptive shift in the health insurance sector by streamlining many parts of operations. Claims processing is one area where these technologies have had a big influence. Specifically, automation has sped up the appraisal and settlement of claims by decreasing manual intervention and streamlining the claims procedure. As a result, compared to previous, manual processing methods, there has been a decrease in errors and an increase in operational efficiency. An innovative factor in the healthcare sector is the ability of autonomous systems to expedite the processing of health insurance claims (Kumar, 2017). These solutions bring in a new era of efficacy and openness by utilising artificial intelligence to deliver previously unheard-of speed, precision, and efficiency. A more responsive and user-friendly ecosystem is anticipated for the health insurance market in the future thanks to the convergence of human expertise and autonomous capabilities brought about by technological advancements.

The conventional method of processing health insurance claims has long been linked to complications, hold-ups, and the possibility of mistakes (Mueller, n.d.). Due to the increased volume of healthcare data and the complex nature of medical records, manual processing frequently results in inefficiencies, which aggravate stakeholders and cause reimbursements to be delayed. Acknowledging these difficulties, the sector has resorted to self-governing platforms to transform the complete claims-handling process.

The Insurtech startup Lemonade, situated in New York, put autonomous technologies in place to improve customer satisfaction and expedite the processing of claims. Their AI-powered technology automates certain parts of managing claims by utilising machine learning algorithms and natural language processing. For example, in a matter of seconds, the AI system evaluates a policyholder's claim submitted via Lemonade's app, confirms the policy's coverage, and determines the payout amounts. Lemonade dramatically speeds up the claims process by removing the need for human interaction in common chores; many claims are handled quickly. Lemonade has received recognition for this novel strategy's effectiveness and openness, which has raised the bar for the sector.

One of the biggest insurers in China, Ping An Insurance Group, uses autonomous systems to reduce insurance fraud and improve operational effectiveness. To find suspicious trends and anomalies suggestive of fraud, Ping An's AI-driven fraud detection system examines enormous volumes of data, including claim histories, medical records, and social media activity. Ping An has been able to save billions of dollars a year by drastically reducing the amount of money paid out for false claims by automating the detection process. Furthermore, Ping An can keep ahead of new fraud schemes and successfully defend the interests of its policyholders since the AI system is always learning from fresh data.

These case studies show how autonomous systems are revolutionising the health insurance market by increasing consumer satisfaction, speeding up the processing of claims, and boosting accuracy. The insurance business has enormous room for innovation and disruption as long as insurers keep investing in AI and machine learning technology. This bodes well for a day when insurance services will be more streamlined, easily accessed, and individually tailored than ever before.

- **Fraud Detection and Prevention:**

Artificial intelligence and machine learning have been incorporated into health insurance, resulting in more advanced fraud detection and prevention. In order to spot trends, abnormalities, and warning signs that can point to possible fraud, these systems examine enormous datasets. Insurance companies can protect the integrity of the insurance market and safeguard their financial interests by using predictive analytics to proactively identify and stop fraudulent claims (Prakhar Harit, 2021). Machine learning models are able to adjust to changing fraud strategies due to their continual learning capabilities, which makes fraud detection methods more effective overall.

The health insurance sector has seen a major transformation in fraud detection because to artificial intelligence (AI), which has significantly increased efficiency and accuracy. AI-powered fraud detection systems can analyse enormous volumes of data with unmatched speed and precision by utilising cutting-edge algorithms and machine learning techniques. This allows insurers to identify and stop fraudulent activity more successfully than in the past. These real-time systems can adjust and learn from fresh data over time to increase their accuracy. They also continuously monitor incoming claims and transactions for suspicious activity.

- **Enhancing Customer Experience:**

One of the top priorities for health insurance companies is improving the client experience, and technology is essential to reaching this objective. The relationships between insurers and policyholders are streamlined via chatbots, automated communication systems, and self-service portals driven by artificial intelligence (Joshi et al., 2020). In addition to facilitating quicker inquiry resolution and instantaneous information access, these technologies also improve customer responsiveness and personalisation. Policyholders gain from this increased sense of participation and satisfaction with their insurance companies.

With their ability to provide policyholders with individualised services, expedited response times, and innovative features, autonomous systems are essential to improving the customer experience in the health insurance sector. These systems provide customised healthcare plans or wellness programmes based on the medical histories and lifestyle characteristics of individual policyholders, via the use of artificial intelligence and powerful data analytics. Additionally, policyholder concerns can be instantly answered by AI-powered chatbots and virtual assistants, which speeds up response times and simplifies the claims procedure. Cutting-edge elements that enhance the policyholder experience further include personalised health insights and incentives for continuing healthy behaviours, such as wearable technology and health-tracking apps coupled with autonomous systems. All things considered, policyholders benefit from a smooth and frictionless experience provided by autonomous systems, which strengthens their bonds with insurers and eventually raises customer satisfaction and loyalty.

- **Data-Driven Decision Making:**

In the health insurance sector, data-driven decision-making is becoming essential to efficient management practices. This paradigm is supported by automation, machine learning, and artificial intelligence, which offer useful insights from enormous datasets. With the use of these technologies, insurers may better understand individual and population health data, evaluate risk, adjust pricing, and customise insurance plans (Cappiello, 2018). Making well-informed decisions helps to improve risk management, allocate resources more effectively, and provide insurance products that are focused on the needs of the consumer.

Data-driven decision-making in the health insurance industry has significantly evolved with the integration of autonomous systems, allowing insurers to use data in previously unheard-of ways. These cutting-edge technologies examine enormous volumes of organised and unstructured data, from claim histories and medical records to demographic data and socioeconomic determinants of health, by utilising artificial intelligence, machine learning, and data analytics.

- Autonomous systems give insurers important insights into trends, patterns, and risk factors by processing and interpreting this data in real-time. This allows insurers to make well-informed decisions that spur strategic growth and innovation. Predictive analytics, for instance, can be used by insurers to anticipate patterns in healthcare utilisation, allocate resources optimally, and provide focused treatments that enhance health outcomes and reduce risks. Additionally, based on the unique needs and preferences of each policyholder, autonomous systems allow insurers to improve customer experience, customise offerings, and personalise services. The health insurance industry has seen a revolution in data-driven decision-making due to the integration of autonomous systems. This has allowed insurers to stay ahead of the curve, adjust to shifting market dynamics, and provide better value to stakeholders and policyholders alike.

Compliance and Regulation

In the health insurance business, adherence to laws like the Health Insurance Portability and Accountability Act (HIPAA) is a requirement that cannot be compromised. By automating regulatory inspections, keeping an eye on compliance with data protection regulations, and enabling audit trails, automation and artificial intelligence help to ensure compliance. By informing policyholders that their sensitive health data is managed in compliance with strict regulatory criteria, this not only helps insurers avoid legal ramifications but also builds trust.

Several facets of the health insurance sector are undergoing radical change as a result of the industry's adoption of automation, machine learning, and artificial intelligence. These technologies, which range from claims processing to fraud detection, customer experience enhancement, data-driven decision-making, and compliance management, all help to make the health insurance market more effective, safe, and focused on the needs of the consumer. Future developments in these fields are probably going to influence how health insurance is run as technology progresses.

Regulatory Framework for Autonomous Systems in Health Insurance Industry

The regulation of autonomous systems that are redefining health insurance is essential to ensuring that these innovations uphold moral and legal obligations, safeguard patient privacy and security, and keep policyholders' trust. Providing customer-centric services and achieving operational excellence must take place within a clear regulatory framework. Here are some key regulations and considerations for autonomous systems in health insurance:

- **Data Privacy and Security Regulations:**

Health insurance autonomous systems need to abide by data privacy laws, like the Health Insurance Portability and Accountability Act (HIPAA) in the US. Strict requirements are established by HIPAA to secure sensitive health information. These criteria require the use of security measures, risk assessments, and safeguards to guarantee the confidentiality, availability, and integrity of patient data.

- **Consent Mechanisms:**

Before setting up autonomous systems that process personal health data, obtaining informed consent from policyholders is imperative. Consent procedures that are transparent and unambiguous must be in place, outlining how self-governing systems will handle and interpret patient data. Adherence to laws such as the General Data Protection Regulation (GDPR) in the European Union is very important in this context.

- **Healthcare Provider Compliance:**

Autonomous systems must comply with rules regulating communications with healthcare providers. To guarantee a smooth integration with the current healthcare infrastructure, these regulations cover data sharing, interoperability, and adherence to Electronic Health Record (EHR) standards.

- **Standards and Best Practices:**

The deployment of autonomous systems ethically and efficiently depends on adherence to industry standards and best practices. A standardised and responsible approach is ensured by adhering to recommendations from organisations such as the International Organisation for Standardisation (ISO) and industry-specific agencies.

- **Monitoring Regulatory Compliance:**

It's critical to keep an eye on any updates or modifications to regulations. Regulations change over time, and autonomous systems need to be flexible enough to modify accordingly. Compliance monitoring makes sure that changes are done on time to keep adherence to the law.

- **Regulatory Reporting:**

Reporting protocols need to be in place to adhere to the transparency requirements outlined by regulations. This includes reporting any incidents, like as data breaches and system failures, that might have an impact on the security or privacy of policyholders' health information.

- **Anti-Fraud Regulations:**

Autonomous systems ought to abide by anti-fraud guidelines in the context of health insurance. To identify and stop fraudulent activity, these systems should use machine learning and advanced analytics, in accordance with industry-specific anti-fraud regulations.

- **International Regulations:**

When operating internationally, health insurers have to pay attention to international legislation. Comprehending and adhering to the diverse nations' health data protection regulations is imperative to guarantee the legitimate handling and international transfer of medical records.

- **Fraud Detection and Reporting:**

Autonomous systems should adhere to anti-fraud legislation as well as have procedures in place for identifying and reporting possible fraudulent activity. This involves collaborating with industry networks to exchange information about emerging fraud patterns, real-time surveillance, and pattern recognition.

- **Ethical Considerations:**

Ethical considerations, beyond legal requirements, are paramount. The utilisation of autonomous systems requires accountability, justice, and transparency. Establishing and upholding ethical standards requires cooperation between policymakers, insurers, and technologists.

- **Consumer Protection:**

A primary concern is making sure that customers are protected. Policyholders' well-being should be improved by autonomous systems, not jeopardized. The provision of channels for dispute resolution and decision-making transparency are essential elements of consumer protection.

- **Transparency and Explainability:**

AI systems for health insurance must be transparent and understandable. The right to know how decisions made by autonomous systems affect policyholders' coverage or care is guaranteed. People should be able to understand the reasoning behind algorithmic judgments through the integration of comprehension methods.

- **Access Control and Encryption:**

Strong encryption techniques and access control systems are essential for protecting health information. Strong access controls guarantee that sensitive information can only be accessed by those who are permitted, and encryption protects data both during communication and storage.

The implementation of autonomous systems in the health insurance industry necessitates a thorough comprehension of and adherence to a wide range of rules and factors. This entails abiding by the law as well as adhering to moral standards, openness, and the defence of consumer rights. Continued attention to detail and flexibility are crucial to the responsible application of autonomous systems in the health insurance industry as the regulatory environment changes. Insurance companies are obligated to make sure that their autonomous systems not only increase efficiency but also comply with the intricate web of healthcare and insurance rules to achieve operational excellence and deliver customer-centric services. Respecting these rules promotes trust, safeguards policyholders' rights, and upholds the integrity of the health insurance sector.

Key Challenges of Increased Automation in the Health Insurance Sector

The increase in automation in the health insurance industry offers both great opportunities and serious moral conundrums. The most significant of these difficulties is the possibility of biassed decision-making in automated systems, which could result in unequal access to healthcare services and coverage. Existing biases in healthcare data, such as inequities based on race, ethnicity, or socioeconomic position, run the risk of being perpetuated as algorithms analyse massive volumes of data to decide insurance rates, coverage eligibility, and claims processing. It is critical to maintain social justice ideals and prevent escalating already-existing healthcare disparities by ensuring fairness and equity in automated decision-making systems.

Concerns regarding data security and privacy are also raised by the automation of health insurance procedures. The growing digitization of medical records and personal health data makes it morally important to protect sensitive information against abuse, breaches, and unauthorised access. Patients need to have confidence that automated systems respect strict privacy standards and laws, like the Health Insurance Portability and Accountability Act (HIPAA) in the US, and that their private health information is handled safely. Retaining confidence in the healthcare system and assuring ethical behaviour in the health insurance industry requires striking a balance between the advantages of automation in expediting administrative procedures and enhancing productivity and the requirement to safeguard patient privacy and data security.

Findings of the Study

After extensive research, several important results come to light regarding how autonomous systems affect the health insurance industry. First of all, the claims processing sector has seen a radical transformation thanks to the quick response times and streamlined operations provided by these state-of-the-art technologies. Routine chores like data input and document processing can be handled by automated systems with previously unheard-of speed and accuracy, which benefits policyholder happiness and speeds up payments for healthcare providers. Second, by using AI algorithms to analyse enormous volumes of data and find patterns suggestive of fraudulent conduct, autonomous systems have revolutionised the field of fraud detection. By taking a proactive stance, insurers can protect the integrity of the insurance market and lessen the financial losses caused by fraud. Insurance companies are now able to improve client experience by offering personalised services, faster response times, and cutting-edge features thanks to the integration of autonomous systems. Using AI-driven insights, insurers can better make decisions, customise products to meet the demands of specific clients, and build closer bonds with policyholders.

Autonomous systems have a wide-ranging and significant effect on health insurance overall. These technologies have enabled insurers to provide policyholders with a more individualised and responsive level of service, in addition to increasing efficiency and accuracy in claims processing and fraud detection. Insurance companies are now able to maintain their competitiveness in a market that is changing quickly thanks to the industry's increased use of autonomous systems, which has also encouraged innovation and distinction. Therefore, autonomous systems have a transformative overall effect on health insurance, resulting in improvements to consumer experience, operational efficiency, and, eventually, healthcare service-delivery.

FUTURE RESEARCH DIRECTIONS

Future research will have a wide range of areas to explore, including applications of autonomous systems in the health insurance industry. Promising research areas include the investigation of robotic process automation (RPA) in claims processing to improve efficiency and accuracy, AI-driven disease prediction and prevention based on health data of policyholders, and the adoption of blockchain for safe and transparent health data sharing. Further, the integration of IoT devices for real-time health monitoring and the effect of telemedicine adoption on healthcare access and policyholder satisfaction present exciting research directions. The notion of investigating standardised data interoperability protocols, utilising AI for fraud investigation, and creating predictive models for pandemic preparedness is quite promising. Finally, insurers using autonomous systems can monitor and improve customer happiness and loyalty by developing service measures that are centred on the needs of the consumer. Together, these study areas help to advance the application of autonomous systems in health insurance by promoting improved effectiveness, client-centeredness, and data-driven services.

CONCLUSION

In essence, the use of autonomous systems in the health insurance industry represents a major change. It is a journey towards improved operational effectiveness, client-focused services, and a reaffirmed commitment to serving policyholder demands. In order to support a new era of healthcare coverage that puts the patient at its centre, the health insurance sector is poised to become more effective, responsive, and technologically sophisticated as autonomous systems continue to develop and broaden their capabilities. The study reveals the vital role of autonomous systems in expediting fraud detection, optimising claims processing, improving customer satisfaction, enabling data-driven decision-making, and assuring compliance with the complex web of healthcare regulations. We will shed light on the revolutionary power that autonomous systems represent by investigating these aspects, not just as instruments for automation but also as the designers of a paradigm shift in the health insurance ecosystem.

REFERENCES

Akter, S., Michael, K., Uddin, M. R., McCarthy, G., & Rahman, M. (2022). Transforming business using digital innovations: The application of AI, blockchain, cloud and data analytics. *Annals of Operations Research*, *308*(1–2), 7–39. doi:10.1007/s10479-020-03620-w

Cappiello, A. (2018). Digital Disruption and InsurTech Start-ups: Risks and Challenges. In Technology and the Insurance Industry (pp. 29–50). Springer International Publishing. doi:10.1007/978-3-319-74712-5_3

Eckert, C., Neunsinger, C., & Osterrieder, K. (2022). (Repeat J)Managing customer satisfaction: Digital applications for insurance companies. *The Geneva Papers on Risk and Insurance. Issues and Practice*, *47*(3), 569–602. doi:10.1057/s41288-021-00257-z

Eling, M., Nuessle, D., & Staubli, J. (2022). The impact of artificial intelligence along the insurance value chain and on the insurability of risks. *The Geneva Papers on Risk and Insurance. Issues and Practice*, *47*(2), 205–241. doi:10.1057/s41288-020-00201-7

Flückiger, I., & Duygun, M. (2022). (LR 111)New technologies and data in insurance. In Geneva Papers on Risk and Insurance: Issues and Practice, 47(3). Palgrave Macmillan. doi:10.1057/s41288-022-00274-6

Gellweiler, C., & Krishnamurthi, L. (2020). Editorial: How digital innovators achieve customer value. In Journal of Theoretical and Applied Electronic Commerce Research, 15(1). Universidad de Talca. doi:10.4067/S0718-18762020000100101

Gorchakova, E. R. (2019). *The impact of digitalization on the health insurance system.* doi:10.18411/lj-03-2019-48

Guzmán-Ortiz, C. V., Navarro-Acosta, N. G., Florez-Garcia, W., & Vicente-Ramos, W. (2020). (LR 122)Impact of digital transformation on the individual job performance of insurance companies in peru. *International Journal of Data and Network Science*, *4*(4), 337–346. doi:10.5267/j.ijdns.2020.9.005

Harit, P. (2021). (LR 83)The Rise of Insurtech: The Ups and Downs of New Trend. SSRN *Electronic Journal*. doi:10.2139/ssrn.3799576

Joshi, V., Joshi, V. V., Pawar, N., & Acharya, S. (2020). *Digitalisation of Health Care in India: Initiatives and Challenges. 40.* https://www.researchgate.net/publication/354586176

Kumar, A. (2017). (LR 117) Impact of Digitalisation on Service Sector in India. *Reviewed Refereed Research Journal*, 8(15). https://www.researchgate.net/publication/360782465

Lin, L., & Chen, C. (2020). (LR 82)The promise and perils of insurtech. *SSRN, 2020*, 115–142. doi:10.2139/ssrn.3463533

Malika Shuxratovna, U., & Nuriddin Rustam Ugli, A. (2021). (LR 114)DIGITALIZATION OF THE INSURANCE MARKET. In Multidisciplinary Peer Reviewed Journal ISSN, 7(2).

Marano, P. (2019). (LR 112)Navigating insurtech: The digital intermediaries of insurance products and customer protection in the EU. *Maastricht Journal of European and Comparative Law*, 26(2), 294–315. doi:10.1177/1023263X19830345

Mueller, J. (n.d.). *InsurTech Rising: A Profile of the InsurTech Landscape DECEMBER 2018.*

Nayak, B., Bhattacharyya, S. S., & Krishnamoorthy, B. (2019). LR 77: Integrating wearable technology products and big data analytics in business strategy: A study of health insurance firms. *Journal of Systems and Information Technology*, 21(2), 255–275. doi:10.1108/JSIT-08-2018-0109

Ostrowska, M. (2021). (LR 110)Does new technology put an end to policyholder risk declaration? The impact of digitalisation on insurance relationships. *The Geneva Papers on Risk and Insurance. Issues and Practice*, 46(4), 573–592. doi:10.1057/s41288-020-00191-6

Sarkar, S. (2021). LR 81: The Evolving Role of Insurtech in India: Trends, Challenges and The Road Ahead. *The Management Accountant Journal*, 56(12), 30–37. doi:10.33516/maj.v56i12.30-37p

Shah, A., Mehrotra, P., Sinha, S., & Sha, J. (2021). Bcg Insurtech Report India Insurtech Landscape And Trends. In Boston Consulting Group.

Shevchuk, O., Kondrat, I., & Stanienda, J. (2020). (LR 115)Pandemic as an accelerator of digital transformation in the insurance industry: Evidence from Ukraine. *Insurance Markets and Companies*, 11(1), 30–41. doi:10.21511/ins.11(1).2020.04

Stoeckli, E., Dremel, C., & Uebernickel, F. (2018). LR 63; Exploring characteristics and transformational capabilities of InsurTech innovations to understand insurance value creation in a digital world. *Electronic Markets*, 28(3), 287–305. Advance online publication. doi:10.1007/s12525-018-0304-7

Yaneva, T. (n.d.). *Digital Transformation of Insurance Sector.*

Chapter 11
Artificial Intelligence in Robotics

Preethiya T.
https://orcid.org/0000-0003-3504-1884
SRM Institute of Science and Technology, India

Priyanga Subbiah
https://orcid.org/0000-0002-2395-7492
SRM Institute of Science and Technology, India

Pandiarajan T.
https://orcid.org/0009-0007-7808-8961
Rajalakshmi Institute of Technology, India

Stephen Ojo
College of Engineering, Anderson University, USA

Vijayalakshmi S.
SNS College of Engineering, India

ABSTRACT

The advent of artificial intelligence (AI) has had a profound impact on the realm of robotics, fundamentally altering the capabilities of self-governing devices. This abstract examines the significant influence of artificial intelligence (AI) on the field of robotics, emphasizing notable progress and practical implementations. Artificial intelligence (AI)-powered robots demonstrate improved capabilities in perception, decision-making, and adaptability, which allows them to thrive in a wide range of jobs across several domains such as industry, healthcare, space exploration, and autonomous vehicles. Machine learning methodologies, such as deep learning and reinforcement learning, enable robots to acquire aptitudes, enhance their performance, and engage in intelligent interactions with their surroundings. The ethical considerations, safety measures, and societal repercussions pertaining to AI-driven robots are also examined and analyzed.

DOI: 10.4018/979-8-3693-1962-8.ch011

INTRODUCTION

The incorporation of AI has resulted in significant shifts in the ways in which we interact with and make use of robotic systems as a result of its profound impact on the area of robotics. Robotics, which examines and advances intelligent systems that are capable of mimicking human activities, is currently in a leading position in the field of AI research and practical application (Nehal, 2023). This is due to the fact that robotics comprises the examination and improvement of such systems. The field of robotics, which is well-known for having qualities that are both dynamic and transdisciplinary, has been witness to considerable breakthroughs in recent years, which has led to the production of increasingly sophisticated robots with expanded capabilities. A new era that is characterised by the adoption of intelligent automation has begun with the introduction of AI into the field of robotics. This new age will be known as the Fourth Industrial Revolution. Robotic creatures have experienced a major transformation since their original purpose as simply mechanical tools. They have transitioned into cognitive beings capable of sensing, learning knowledge, and modifying their behaviour in reaction to the environment in which they find themselves. The shift that was described earlier has had a significant influence on a variety of spheres of activity, including manufacturing, healthcare, the exploration of space, and everyday life.

The purpose of this statement is to offer a framework for investigating the intricate and multidimensional nature of the connection that exists between robotics and artificial intelligence (Gurjeet, 2022). The purpose of this research is to analyse the fundamental components and technological progressions that are driving the incorporation of artificial intelligence inside the domain of robotics. In addition to this, the objective is to investigate the real-world uses of this technology in a variety of contexts and to kick off a conversation about the potential benefits and difficulties that are associated with this rapidly developing area of research. The combination of AI and Robotics is more than simply a technological convergence; it is a profound and revolutionary shift that is redefining a wide range of industries as well as significantly altering our way of life and the professional techniques that we use.

THE ROLE OF NLP IN HUMAN-ROBOT COMMUNICATION

The field of human-robot interaction has witnessed the emergence of Natural Language Processing (NLP) as a crucial technology. NLP facilitates the ability of computers to understand, produce, and react to human language in a manner that is more intuitive and akin to human behaviour. The advent of this transformative invention has inaugurated a novel epoch of communication between human beings and robots, which exhibits considerable potential for many applications across several industries and in our everyday existence.

This investigation examines the significance of natural language processing (NLP) in facilitating communication between people and robots, highlighting its tremendous influence on bridging this gap (Jonathan, 2023). This study aims to investigate the fundamental technologies, strategies, and algorithms that enable robots to comprehend and produce human language. Natural Language Processing (NLP) is of utmost importance in facilitating smooth communication between humans and various machines, including chatbots, virtual assistants, service robots, and autonomous cars.

Moreover, this discourse underscores the practical implementations of Natural Language Processing (NLP) within the field of robotics, placing particular emphasis on its ability to augment human-robot cooperation, improve customer service, better healthcare practises, and facilitate educational endeavours, among various other domains. This study also addresses the emerging difficulties and ethical implications related to natural language processing (NLP) in the context of human-robot communication, as we explore the dynamic intersection of technology and human contact.

The incorporation of natural language processing (NLP) into the realm of human-robot communication is fundamentally transforming the manner in which we engage with and derive advantages from robotic systems. AI has the capacity to enhance our interactions with machines by making them more intuitive, efficient, and engaging (Nam et al., 2021). This has the potential to create a future in which robots possess a genuine understanding of human behaviour and can respond to us in a manner that is both natural and reminiscent of human-to-human communication.

CONTROL OF THE ROBOT AND DETAILED ROUTE PLANNING

The optimisation of robotic control and the meticulous design of routes are fundamental components of robotics that have a direct influence on their operational efficiency and practicality. Within the domain of robotics, the term "control" pertains to the assortment of techniques and algorithms employed for the purpose of regulating a robot's locomotion, behaviours, and engagements with its surrounding milieu (Nagadevi, 2021). In contrast, route planning is the meticulous determination of pathways and trajectories that a robotic system must adhere to in order to accomplish its designated goals. These elements play a crucial role in a wide range of applications, including as industrial automation, autonomous cars, and even space exploration.

The Management of the Robot

The process of robot control entails the integration of both hardware and software elements. The hardware generally encompasses sensory components for perception and actuation mechanisms for motion. In addition, the software component contains control algorithms, feedback systems, and decision-making processes. These various components collaborate to facilitate the locomotion, execution of tasks, and responsiveness of the robot to its environment. Control tactics encompass a spectrum of approaches, spanning from rudimentary teleoperation facilitated by a human operator to comprehensive autonomy, wherein the robot independently makes decisions.

Control systems can be classified into two main categories: open-loop systems and closed-loop systems. Open-loop control refers to a control system in which predetermined actions are conducted without receiving feedback from the surrounding environment. In contrast, closed-loop control refers to the utilisation of ongoing feedback from sensors to dynamically modify the robot's operations, hence augmenting precision and flexibility.

In-Depth Route Planning

Thorough route planning plays a pivotal role in facilitating the navigation of robots in intricate situations. The task encompasses the process of ascertaining the most appropriate routes, circumventing hindrances, and optimising for variables such as velocity, energy conservation, and security. The significance of route planning is particularly pronounced in the context of autonomous vehicles, unmanned aerial vehicles (UAVs), and industrial robotic systems.

The process of planning routes for robots frequently utilises sophisticated algorithms and methodologies derived from the fields of computational geometry, artificial intelligence, and machine learning. Prominent methodologies encompass the utilisation of A* and Dijkstra algorithms in the context of graph-based pathfinding, the employment of rapidly exploring random trees (RRT) in scenarios involving dynamic surroundings, and the application of artificial neural networks to acquire knowledge regarding ideal paths. In addition, the process of route planning involves the incorporation of the robot's environmental perception, which is facilitated by sensors like as cameras, lidar, or radar (Gaur et al., 2021). The aforementioned information is included into the decision-making process in order to effectively adjust to real-world circumstances.

The management of robotic systems and the meticulous design of navigation paths play a crucial role in the domain of robotics. Several factors influence the ability of robots to efficiently carry out tasks, successfully navigate complex situations, and effectively interact with their surroundings. The ongoing development of control systems and route planning algorithms has been crucial in the advancement of robots, leading to their enhanced versatility and increased capabilities across many applications.

THE PERCEPTION OF ROBOTS

The presence of robots, which was formerly restricted to the realm of fantastic fiction and entertainment, has now become profoundly interwoven in our day-to-day lives. A discernible shift is taking place in our understanding and interpretation of robots as a result of the growing prevalence of intelligent devices across all spheres of society. The current shifts in how robots are perceived, how they are involved in society, and what roles they play hold a tremendous amount of importance (Yinong, 2021). The shift in perspective that has been described above gives rise to questions and complications that are intellectually stimulating and are related to technology, ethics, and the dynamics of social interaction.

During the modern era, robots were most commonly associated with operations that took place within controlled environments, such as assembly lines located within manufacturing facilities. These entities were typically seen as rigid, impersonal constructions that possessed limited capabilities. The fields of artificial intelligence, machine learning, and robotics have made major strides in recent years, which has resulted in considerable advancements in the capabilities and possible uses of robotic systems. One such improvement is the ability to learn on their own. At this time, people are actively participating in a wide variety of fields, including healthcare, service industries, autonomous transportation, and taking on duties as carers for individuals of all ages, including the elderly and the young. The way in which people of different age groups and cultural backgrounds think about robots differs significantly from one another. There are some people who view robots as a way to improve ease of use and productivity, which would, in turn, optimise day-to-day activities and raise the overall level of living. Individuals are finding themselves confronted with ethical and existential questions as a result of concerns regarding the displacement of employment, issues linked to privacy, and the prospect of robots surpassing humans in certain fields. These anxieties and challenges have led to the emergence of these questions.

In this study, a variety of sociological perspectives on robots are investigated from different angles. The major purpose of this research is to analyse the impacts of human-robot contact, the psychological phenomena known as anthropomorphism, and the role that the media and popular culture play in the process of influencing our perspectives (Shaukat et al., 2020). In the modern setting of robotics, it is absolutely necessary to have an understanding of how robots are perceived. This is because the perception of robots is not only significant as an academic endeavour, but also as a crucial determinant in the development and application of these intelligent machines. The acquisition of a complete grasp of this idea is essential if one wants to be certain that the use of robots will result in positive outcomes rather than in outcomes that will have a negative impact on our society and the activities we engage in on a daily basis.

LEARNING AND ADAPTATION CAPABILITIES OF ROBOTS

The learning and adaption skills exhibited by robots signify a significant breakthrough within the realm of robotics. Historically, robots have been linked to pre-programmed and repetitive duties. However, the incorporation of AI has enabled them to acquire knowledge from their interactions and adjust their behaviour accordingly in novel circumstances. This significant advancement presents a multitude of potentialities and practical implementations. Robotic systems that are equipped with AI utilise machine learning methodologies in order to augment their functionalities (Mir et al., 2020). This encompasses computational methods such as deep learning and reinforcement learning. Deep learning enables robots to efficiently analyse large volumes of data, identify recurring patterns, and subsequently make informed decisions using this acquired knowledge. Reinforcement learning facilitates the acquisition of knowledge by robots through iterative experimentation, leading to progressive enhancement of their operational capabilities.

Robotic systems are endowed with the capability to detect their surroundings through the utilisation of sophisticated sensors, including cameras, lidar, and touch sensors. These entities possess the capability to discern and recognise various entities, including items, individuals, and barriers, hence facilitating their ability to traverse intricate environments and engage with objects in a cognitively advanced manner. Robots possessing the capacity to learn are capable of modifying their behaviour in accordance with dynamic circumstances. An instance of a robot developed for the purpose of environmental monitoring possesses the capability to adapt its data collecting methodologies in accordance with the distinct attributes of the environment within which it is functioning. Learning robots have the ability to partake in interactions with people that are more natural and intuitive in nature. These entities possess the ability to perceive and react to human movements, verbal communication, and even emotional cues. This is particularly advantageous in domains like as healthcare, wherein robots may offer aid to patients and offer companionship. Learning robots has the ability to autonomously make real-time decisions. Autonomous vehicles employ AI algorithms to effectively manoeuvre through intricate traffic scenarios and promptly execute judgements in order to uphold safety standards. Robotic systems have the capacity to acquire novel abilities and enhance their overall performance through iterative learning processes. This capability holds significant value in industrial contexts such as manufacturing, as it enables robots to effectively adjust to novel production procedures and engage in cooperative endeavours alongside human operators (Bartneck et al., 2021). Learning robots has the capability to identify anomalies or malfunctions within their operational frameworks and subsequently adjust their behaviour in order to address and minimise these concerns. Individuals have the capability to engage in self-diagnosis and deploy backup procedures, so augmenting their overall reliability. Learning robots continuously strive for improvement. Through repeated interactions and experiences, individuals enhance their abilities, gradually improving their proficiency in the tasks allocated to them.

Learning robots possess the capability to be tailored to certain activities and surroundings. The inherent adaptability of these entities enables them to thrive in a wide range of contexts, spanning from the exploration of outer space to the realm of agriculture. The potential of robots' learning and adaptability skills is vast, however, it is accompanied by various challenges. In order to enable responsible and safe deployment of learning robots, it is imperative to address ethical aspects, including decision-making openness, accountability, and safety precautions. The learning and adaptability skills exhibited by robots are significantly influencing the trajectory of automation, hence enhancing their versatility, responsiveness, and intelligence. With the continuous advancement of AI, the proficiency of robots in acquiring knowledge from their experiences is expected to increase, leading to a greater convergence of human and machine skills.

COLLABORATIVE EFFORTS BETWEEN HUMANS AND ROBOTS

The cutting edge of technological progress is currently experiencing a substantial concentration on joint undertakings between humans and robots, with particular attention placed on the fields of manufacturing, healthcare, and autonomous systems. This coordinated effort will involve the integration of human workers and robots in the workplace, with the goal of capitalising on each group's unique capabilities and advantages to improve operational efficacy, worker safety, and output.

The industrial industry has undergone a profound sea change as a direct result of the widespread adoption of collaborative efforts between humans and robots. Robots and human workers are able to work together in modern industrial settings thanks to the integration of complex sensors and artificial intelligence (Belk, 2021). This allows for the efficient completion of tasks that are both repetitive and taxing on the body. The use of automation not only reduces the amount of physical labour that workers are required to perform, but it also increases accuracy and uniformity, which ultimately leads to the creation of higher-quality items. In contrast, human labourers take on the responsibility of managing operations, participating in complex decision-making processes, and carrying out tasks that require innovative thinking and flexibility in order to complete successfully. The establishment of this collaboration has resulted in substantial changes to modern manufacturing practises, resulting in an increase in both the competitiveness of these practises and their flexibility in response to the ever-changing demands of the market.

Within the field of healthcare, robots are quickly becoming indispensable helpers for medical personnel, playing an increasingly significant part in the sector overall. Surgical robots, like the ones that were mentioned, make it possible to execute minimally invasive surgeries with a level of precision that has never been seen before. The use of these robots, which are operated by surgeons, enables them to do sophisticated surgical procedures, which in turn reduces patient trauma and shortens the amount of time needed for recovery. In the realm of eldercare, robots play an important role in assisting with the lifting of patients, distributing medication, and providing companionship to people who are in need. It has been demonstrated that the utilisation of collaborative efforts can improve the standard of care provided to patients while also reducing the amount of work required of healthcare professionals.

The field of autonomous systems, which includes things like self-driving automobiles and unmanned aerial aircraft, is a field in which people and robots work together on various projects. This is because autonomous systems comprise entities like these. Robots that are driven by AI do in-depth analyses on the most recent and relevant data that is acquired from sensors in order to make crucial decisions. In exceptional situations or in situations that are outside the scope of the capabilities of the robots' programming, the participation of humans is still absolutely necessary. The convergence of human and machine intelligence is propelling forward progress in a variety of industries, including transportation, agriculture, and logistics.

However, there are still challenges to overcome in this attempt involving multiple people. It is of the utmost importance that, wherever robots are present, the protection of people be given top priority. Especially in the fields of healthcare and autonomous systems, it is absolutely necessary to address ethical problems (Oksanen et al., 2020). In addition, it is projected that the ongoing development of AI and robotics will make it increasingly difficult to differentiate the skills of humans and machines, which could lead to a re-evaluation of job responsibilities and duties.

The collaboration of humans and robots is an intriguing field that holds the promise of bringing about profound changes in the ways in which we perform work, the amount of output we achieve, and the way we live our lives. These phenomena will continue to exist as a result of the continued advancement of technology, which will eventually lead to a change in our attitude towards a variety of enterprises and activities. Table1, a streamlined table that compares the amount of effort put forward by humans versus robots in a variety of contexts.

ETHICS OF ROBOTS AND THE PROTECTION OF AI

The topic of "Ethics of Robots and the Protection of AI" is strongly rooted in the significant influence that AI and robotics have on different elements of our society, the economy, and our day-to-day lives. This influence can be seen in the title of the course, which is "Ethics of Robots and the Protection of AI."

Table 1. Contrasting human versus robotic efforts in several domains

Aspect	Humans	Robots
Physical Strength	Variable, depending on individual strength	Consistent and can be tailored for tasks
Repetitive Tasks	Fatigue-prone over time	Efficient and consistent
Precision	Prone to errors, especially with fatigue	Extremely precise and accurate
Speed	Variable, may decrease with fatigue	Consistently fast
Learning	Learning curve, variable learning speed	Rapid learning through AI algorithms
Adaptability	Learn and adapt, but with limitations	Quick adaptation based on programming
24/7 Availability	Requires rest and sleep	Can operate continuously
Safety in Hazardous Environments	Limited without protective gear	Designed for safety in hazardous settings
Endurance in Repetitive Tasks	Fatigue sets in over time	Unaffected by repetitive tasks
Collaboration	Effective but may have interpersonal issues	Collaborate efficiently with other robots
Emotional Intelligence	Emotionally intelligent, understand context	Lacks emotional understanding
Creativity	Highly creative and innovative	Performs predefined tasks
Scalability	Limited by human workforce availability	Scalable by adding more robots

The relentless advancement of artificial intelligence technology provides us with important ethical and practical questions regarding the utilisation of AI systems, the regulation of AI systems, and the protection of AI systems. The history of and current circumstances surrounding this topic are summarised in the following paragraphs for your convenience.

AI Advancements: The fast advancements made in the fields of AI and robotics have led to the creation of systems that are both extremely advanced and completely autonomous. The application of AI in a wide variety of fields, including healthcare, finance, transportation, and others, calls for a thorough investigation into the ethical issues that are raised by this progress.

Autonomous Decision-Making: Robotics, self-driving cars, and unmanned aerial vehicles (UAVs) that are powered by AI have the potential to independently form opinions and make decisions. The aforementioned conditions give rise to ethical questions regarding the probable outcomes of these decisions and the people or organisations who are responsible for them.

Safety and Security: The provision of assurances on the safety and security of AI systems is of the utmost significance. Failures in the decision-making processes of AI have the potential to lead to a variety of undesirable consequences, such as accidents, data breaches, or unforeseen effects. It is of the utmost significance to protect AI systems from being compromised by cyberattacks.

Bias and Fairness: It is possible for AI algorithms to pick up biases from the data that they are trained on, which could lead to results that are unfair or discriminatory. In order to fulfil our ethical commitment, we need to address these shortcomings and ensure that the decision-making process that artificial intelligence uses is fair.

Human-AI Collaboration: The integration of human and artificial intelligence in working together is becoming increasingly common in today's society. Ethical questions are raised both by the assignment of responsibilities to AI and by the dynamics of the relationships that exist between humans and AI.

Long-Term Impact: When thinking about the future, it is essential to give serious consideration to the long-term effects that AI will have on the job market, the workings of society, and the possibility of a peaceful cohabitation between humans and AI.

Research and Development: The field of artificial intelligence research and development falls under the purview of ethical considerations as well. It is of the utmost importance to place a high priority on responsible innovation and to take preventative measures against the development of artificial intelligence systems that could be harmful.

Education and Awareness: In order to support informed decision-making, it is necessary for developers, users, and policymakers to create a complete grasp of AI ethics. This understanding will facilitate informed decision-making.

THE ROLE OF ROBOTS IN MEDICAL CARE

The utilisation of robots in the sphere of medical care has seen significant development over the course of time. This change has been spurred by advances in technology, an increasing demand for healthcare services, and the urge to improve patient outcomes. It is becoming increasingly common practise to employ robots in a variety of aspects of patient care, including diagnosis, treatment, surgery, rehabilitation, and support for patients. These robots are playing an increasingly important role in these areas. Throughout the course of their history, the majority of robots used in the medical field have been put to work in specific fields such as robot-assisted surgery. In spite of this, recent developments have resulted in a major expansion of the potential applications of artificial intelligence (AI), machine learning, and robotics in the field of healthcare. An in-depth analysis of the various environmental considerations that are relevant to the application of robots in the field of medical care is presented in the following paragraphs.

Surgical Robotics: One of the most well-known applications of robotics in the field of health is the utilisation of surgical robots, which are utilised to carry out minimally invasive procedures with a high degree of precision and accuracy. This application of robotics is one of the most commonly recognised applications of robotics in the field of medicine. Surgeons utilise these robotic devices in order to improve the quality of their work, reduce the amount of invasiveness involved in procedures, and shorten the amount of time it takes for patients to recuperate.

Telemedicine and Remote Monitoring: The practise of telemedicine, in which medical professionals are able to examine patients without physically being present at their bedsides, is made possible by the utilisation of robots that are equipped with cameras and sensors. In addition to this, they provide a hand in the continuous monitoring of patients by collecting important physiological indicators and communicating this data to medical professionals.

Rehabilitation: There has been a discernible uptick in the number of programmes that include robotic assistance for physical therapy and rehabilitation. Physical therapists play an essential position in the process of helping patients regain their mobility and strength, which is especially important in the aftermath of traumatic events such as injuries, strokes, or surgical procedures. These robotic systems are able to provide exercise regimens that are not only consistent but also tailored to the specific requirements of each unique user.

Medication Management: The distribution of medication and its subsequent administration are both significantly aided by the utilisation of robotic devices. Professionals in the healthcare industry have the ability to assure that patients will receive the correct dosages of their medications at the proper intervals, hence reducing the likelihood that mistakes will be made.

Mental Health and Social Support: Robots have the potential to act as companions and provide therapeutic support to people who are in need of it in the field of mental health. Healthcare providers are expected to take an active part in conversations, offer folks help with empathy, and push patients to adhere to the therapeutic regimens they have been prescribed.

Laboratory and Diagnostic Robots: It has been demonstrated that automating testing procedures in laboratories can both improve the testing process's overall efficiency while simultaneously lowering the number of opportunities for human error. Sample processing, test analysis, and data management are only some of the activities that can be successfully carried out by robotic systems, which also have the capacity to carry out a broad variety of other jobs.

Patient Transport and Logistics: Robotic systems are used in hospitals and other healthcare institutions to ensure the safe and efficient movement of patients, supplies, and equipment. Robotic systems can also be used to diagnose and treat patients. The application of this strategy both lessens the possibility of contamination from one source to another and increases the effectiveness of business operations.

Emergency Response: Robots can be used in situations such as crisis management and first response to get access to areas that are difficult to reach, analyse the situation, and provide emergency teams with up-to-date information. This can be accomplished through the utilisation of robots.

Patient Education: Patients can benefit from the interactive capabilities of robots by learning more about their medical conditions, the various treatment options that are accessible, and the choices they can make regarding their lifestyle. The ability to react to questions and provide pertinent information in a way that is both simple to understand and patient-friendly is a skill that is essential for individuals working in the healthcare industry.

The inclusion of robots into the field of medical care is driven by the aim to improve healthcare outcomes, enhance the experience of patients, and maximise the efficiency of healthcare operations. Nevertheless, there are also substantial obstacles that arise as a result of this issue. These challenges include the necessity for sufficient training, the maintenance of the human element in healthcare, and the consequences of regulatory and ethical questions. It is projected that, as technology continues to advance, there will be a marked uptick in the use of robots in the field of medical care, which will have a revolutionary effect.

SIMULATIONS OF ROBOTIC SYSTEMS IN VIRTUAL ENVIRONMENTS

The utilisation of virtual environments for the purpose of simulating robotic systems is of the utmost importance in the research and development activities being carried out in the field of robotics in the modern day. These facilities provide a controlled environment that is also secure for the purpose of testing, improving, and evaluating robotic systems and the software that goes with them. Engineers, researchers, and developers can examine various aspects of robotics more easily with the use of virtual environments, which serve as digital representations of the physical world and are used in the simulations. This eliminates the need for expensive physical prototypes and makes it possible to investigate both individual components and complex systems. Individuals have the capacity to build and manipulate a diverse range of scenarios within these virtual settings, including a variety of landscapes, items that are constantly changing, and labor-intensive jobs. This makes comprehensive testing and training possibilities much easier to access. The following domains benefit greatly from the utilisation of simulations: Engineers and developers make use of virtual environments for the purpose of designing, prototyping, and iterating robotic system designs. In order to improve the functionality of robots, researchers are able to conduct experiments using a variety of robot configurations, sensor arrangements, and algorithmic approaches.

Virtual environments offer a way to train and assess autonomous robots without having to expose the robots to the risks that are present in the real world. For instance, self-driving cars can be put through rigorous testing in simulated urban environments before being used on actual roads. This can happen before the cars are put into use. Researchers are able to efficiently validate complex algorithms such as those linked to computer vision, path planning, and machine learning within regulated and repeatable settings. This technique helps to ensure that robots are capable of successfully comprehending sensory information and making decisions based on that knowledge. When it comes to the preliminary assessment and risk assessment of deploying robots in high-stakes environments, such as nuclear facilities or disaster zones, simulations are an extremely important part of the process. The protection of human lives and the preservation of valuable resources can be significantly aided by the analysis of potential threats in virtual environments and the implementation of appropriate countermeasures. Building and maintaining actual prototypes can be an expensive and time-consuming procedure that can also entail major costs. It has been discovered that substituting digital simulations for physical testing in virtual settings can result in significant cost savings. This can be accomplished by using virtual environments. The ability to scale is one of the benefits that virtual environments offer.

Researchers are able to examine a wide variety of applications for robotics because of their capacity to simulate a wide variety of scenarios. These scenarios range from small-scale robotic swarms to large-scale smart cities. The study of human-robot interaction also makes use of simulations in a number of different ways. Researchers are able to optimise robot behaviour and usability across a wide variety of settings by simulating human-robot interactions and using the data from such simulations. It is essential for robots to demonstrate predictable conduct in order for them to be deployed in real-world environments. The smooth adaptation of robots to unforeseen conditions in the actual world can be greatly aided by the use of virtual simulations, which play an important part in this process. In light of the aforementioned circumstances, it is clear that simulations are of critical significance to the development of the robotics discipline. Researchers and engineers have the ability, with the help of virtual environments, to speed up the development of cutting-edge robotic systems, reduce the risk of potential hazards, and ultimately improve the capabilities, efficiency, and safety of robots used in a wide variety of applications.

AUTOMATION OF ROBOTIC PROCESSES

The phenomena of automating robotic processes, also known as Robotic Process Automation (RPA), is a rapidly increasing technology-oriented paradigm within the modern sphere of business. RPA is an abbreviation for the acronym "Robotic Process Automation." The activity of utilising software robots, sometimes known as "bots," to mechanise recurrent responsibilities and procedures in an organisational environment is known as "bot farming." Input of data, processing of invoices, communications with customers, and analysis of data are some of the many tasks included in the range of responsibilities. Understanding the setting in which the automation of robotic processes occurs can be enhanced by taking into consideration the following three crucial points: In the modern business climate, which is marked by fierce rivalry, businesses are constantly working to improve their efficiency, limit their operational expenses, and maximise their production. The automation of robotic processes is a solution that satisfies the demand that was indicated above. This solution provides a way to optimise operations and dedicate human resources to occupations that require strategic thinking and creativity.

Rise of Digital Transformation: As a consequence of the introduction of digital transformation across a variety of sectors, businesses have found themselves confronted with a substantial influx of data and an increased incidence of processes that are repetitive. Robotic Process Automation, also known as RPA, is an essential component in efficiently capitalising on the potential of data and integrating a wide variety of digital systems without a hitch. This is of utmost importance in light of the movement of businesses towards utilising cloud-based services, the Internet of Things (IoT), and big data analytics. Robotic process automation, often known as RPA, gives businesses the ability to improve the overall quality and effectiveness of the client services they provide by facilitating the delivery of services in a more timely and efficient manner. Robotic process automation (RPA), when used to the financial services sector, has the ability to hasten the procedures for the approval of loans and increase the effectiveness of dispute resolution. As a direct consequence of this, increased levels of customer satisfaction and brand loyalty are generated.

Accuracy and Compliance: Errors caused by humans can have major effects on finances and can lead to a violation of regulations if they are not caught in time. Robotic Process Automation, abbreviated to RPA, ensures a greater level of precision and uniformity in work by virtue of the fact that automated bots carry out identical tasks with very few variations. Additionally, it is feasible to train these bots in a way that ensures strict adherence to certain compliance and regulatory criteria. This can be accomplished through the use of specific programming. Functionalities related to AI and machine learning are regularly incorporated into robotic process automation (RPA) systems in order to improve their performance. This functionality provides the artificial intelligence agents with the ability to learn knowledge from datasets, modify their behaviour in response to changing situations, and carry out activities that require the processing of unorganised information or the making of judgements. The term "Intelligent Process Automation" (IPA) is also used to refer to this occurrence on occasion.

Employee Empowerment: Employees are able to allocate their time and efforts to work that provides greater value, needing creativity, decision-making, and human connection, thanks to the implementation of automation for occupations that are of a repetitive nature and have the potential to be done again. This phenomenon not only improves the level of happiness enjoyed by workers, but it also enables businesses to maximise the potential of their human capital.

Industry Applications: Robotic process automation, often known as RPA, can be utilised in virtually any sector of the economy. This technology is useful in many different fields, including banking, healthcare, manufacturing, customer service, supply chain management, and a great many more. Robotic process automation (RPA) has been put to use in a wide variety of industries, which is a testament to its inherent versatility. The field of robotic process automation, also known as RPA, is always undergoing new developments and expanding its capabilities. The development of new technologies paves the way for the introduction of automation capabilities that are progressively more intricate and varied. Companies that want to keep their advantage in the marketplace absolutely need to make it a priority to remain current on the most recent developments in robotic process automation (RPA).

Robotic process automation (RPA) presents a number of challenges in addition to offering a variety of benefits. These include worries about the security of data, the loss of employment opportunities, and the requirement for appropriate governance. The application of automation across a variety of industries calls for thoughtful deliberation and investigation due to the ethical considerations that are raised by this trend. The imperative to boost efficiency, precision, and productivity as a response to the process of digital transformation is the driving force behind the rationale behind the automation of robotic processes. This change is being driven by digital technology. The implementation of this technology offers businesses operating in a wide variety of markets a plethora of benefits that can help them compete more effectively. Nevertheless, it also raises a number of issues, including ethical concerns, which demand careful management on the part of the responsible party.

CONCLUSION

The emergence of AI has initiated a paradigm shift in the field of robotics. This abstract elucidates the significant influence of AI on the domain of robotics, emphasising the noteworthy advancements and practical implementations that have arisen. AI-driven robots currently demonstrate improved abilities in perception, decision-making, and adaptability, hence enabling them to thrive in a wide range of jobs across various industries such as manufacturing, healthcare, space exploration, and autonomous vehicles. By utilising machine learning techniques, such as deep learning and reinforcement learning, these robotic systems are capable of acquiring novel abilities, consistently enhancing their efficiency, and intelligently interacting with their environment. Nevertheless, it is important to note that this abstract also emphasises the presence of ethical considerations, safety precautions, and societal repercussions associated with this evolution. The utilisation of artificially intelligent robots in many industries gives rise to inquiries regarding their implications on labour, privacy, and security. It is of utmost importance to address these problems and prioritise responsible development of AI and robotics, given the ongoing intersection of these fields. Looking towards the future, the continuous progress of AI presents significant possibilities for the merging of AI and robotics, which has the potential to revolutionise automation and reshape the dynamics of collaboration between humans and machines. The symbiotic association between AI and robots is anticipated to profoundly transform several industries, enhance operational effectiveness, and facilitate the emergence of novel prospects for innovation. As we find ourselves on the verge of this promising frontier, it is imperative to effectively address the obstacles and capitalise on the potential advantages presented by this integration. This will ultimately contribute to a future characterised by a symbiotic and efficient collaboration between humans and machines. As AI and robotics continue to merge, it will be crucial to conduct interdisciplinary research, collaborate, and prioritise ethical concerns if we want to create a future where AI-powered robots positively impact society.

REFERENCES

Bartneck, C., Lütge, C., Wagner, A., & Welsh, S. (2021). *An introduction to ethics in robotics and AI.* Springer Nature. doi:10.1007/978-3-030-51110-4

Belk, R. (2021). Ethical issues in service robotics and artificial intelligence. *Service Industries Journal, 41*(13-14), 860–876. doi:10.1080/02642069.2020.1727892

Gaur, L., Afaq, A., Singh, G., & Dwivedi, Y. K. (2021). Role of artificial intelligence and robotics to foster the touchless travel during a pandemic: A review and research agenda. *International Journal of Contemporary Hospitality Management, 33*(11), 4079–4098. doi:10.1108/IJCHM-11-2020-1246

Gurjeet, S. (2022). *Vijay, Kumar, Banga., Thaweesak, Yingthawornsuk.* Artificial Intelligence and Industrial Robot., doi:10.1109/SITIS57111.2022.00098

Jonathan, A. (2023). *Development of an AI-Robotics 3D Printed Circle of Command for Enhancing Accessibility and Mobility in Individuals with Mobility Issues.* IEEE. doi:10.5121/csit.2023.130910

Mir, U. B., Sharma, S., Kar, A. K., & Gupta, M. P. (2020). Critical success factors for integrating artificial intelligence and robotics. *Digital Policy. Regulation & Governance, 22*(4), 307–331. doi:10.1108/DPRG-03-2020-0032

Nagadevi, D. (2021). *A Comprehensive Study on Artificial Intelligence and Robotics for Machine Intelligence.* Springer. doi:10.4018/978-1-7998-7701-1.ch011

Nam, K., Dutt, C. S., Chathoth, P., Daghfous, A., & Khan, M. S. (2021). The adoption of artificial intelligence and robotics in the hotel industry: Prospects and challenges. *Electronic Markets, 31*(3), 553–574. doi:10.1007/s12525-020-00442-3

Nehal, R. (2023). AI in Robotics: Advancements, Applications and Challenges. *Journal of Information Technology and Digital World.* doi:10.36548/jitdw.2023.2.009

Oksanen, A., Savela, N., Latikka, R., & Koivula, A. (2020). Trust toward robots and artificial intelligence: An experimental approach to human–technology interactions online. *Frontiers in Psychology*, *11*, 568256. doi:10.3389/fpsyg.2020.568256 PMID:33343447

Shaukat, K., Iqbal, F., Alam, T. M., Aujla, G. K., Devnath, L., Khan, A. G., & Rubab, A. (2020). The impact of artificial intelligence and robotics on the future employment opportunities. *Trends in Computer Science and Information Technology, 5*(1), 50-54.

Yinong, C. (2021). Technologies Supporting Artificial Intelligence and Robotics Application Development. doi:10.37965/jait.2020.0065

Chapter 10
Synergistic Swarm:
Multi–Robot Systems in Healthcare

Jaspreet Kaur
Chandigarh University, India

ABSTRACT

The "synergistic swarm" investigates the incorporation of multi-robot systems in healthcare, introducing a fundamental change in patient care and medical operations. This abstract emphasises the collaborative synergy achieved by intelligently coordinating several robotic entities, resulting in improved efficiency, precision, and adaptability in healthcare environments. By utilising cutting-edge technology like artificial intelligence, robotics, and sensor networks, the system seeks to enhance many functions, including diagnostics and patient support, to their maximum efficiency. This chapter highlights the significant potential of combining different approaches to healthcare in order to improve the delivery of medical services. This could lead to more effective, patient-focused, and adaptable healthcare robotics in the changing healthcare industry.

INTRODUCTION

Automating daily operations by understanding the existing routines and practices, generally, it refers to software that imitates an online workforce and carries out repetitive tasks and responsibilities, reducing the requirement for social interaction. In today's competitive world of work, everyone strives to outperform their rivals in order to acquire a competitive advantage. Automating repetitive tasks with Multi-Robots/ Synergistic swarm (RPA) technology significantly enhances the profitability and efficiency of commercial organizations. Automation allows workers to focus on higher-level tasks, unleash their creativity, and devote themselves to advancing their knowledge and skills in the sector. Every Multi-Robots / Synergistic swarm project consists of three main stages: design, execution, and assessment and tracking (Alsamhi & Lee, 2020).

Multi-Robots / Synergistic swarm is considered a significant technological advancement that is capable, resilient, flexible, and reliable enough to make it feasible for use in major corporations. Experts predict that once Multi-Robots / Synergistic swarm (RPA) becomes stable and reliable in the next decade or

DOI: 10.4018/979-8-3693-1962-8.ch010

two, it will lead to significant improvements in efficiency and effectiveness among the working people in terms of emergence of concept of synergistic swarm or Multi-robotic systems. Multi-Robotic system is an emerging technology, aims to provide a sustainable alternative that reduces costs and shipping times while improving the quality of firm operations It is an innovative technology that is increasingly being adopted in businesses that include monotonous activities. Businesses that employ Multi-Robots / Synergistic swarm experience decreased expenses and enhanced operational efficiency (Cao et al., 2022). Introducing Multi-robots to the medical field is an example of such an endeavor as presented in figure 1 below:

The purpose of this study is to shed light on Multi-robotics' significance in healthcare and to lay the groundwork for integrating various strategies to boost productivity and contentment in the workplace . The healthcare sector's operational efficiency has been greatly improved by the application of technology breakthroughs. By streamlining the processing of massive amounts of data, algorithms for machine learning have benefited the healthcare industry (Kaur, 2024).

As compared to the human mind, Multi-Robots / Synergistic swarm can acquire and recall a lot more quickly. This goes against what the human brain is capable of doing cognitively. Systematic optimization of the distribution of healthcare professionals, hospital beds, and resources is possible with the use of AI. Better operational efficiency and lower costs are the outcomes of this optimization (Cao et al., 2022).

The use of cutting-edge robotic technology has made distant surgical procedures a reality, expanding patients' access to highly specialized medical care. By collecting data on a massive scale, Multi-Robots / Synergistic swarm make it possible to study populations for trends and patterns. Multi-Robots / Synergistic swarm is utilized to do this. The management of healthcare for the general public might stand to benefit greatly from this. According to Troccaz et al., (2019), patients and medical professionals can receive continuous and immediate feedback about the patient's status thanks to robotic technology integrated into rehabilitation and prosthetic devices. Accordingly, it becomes easier to tailor rehabilitation programs to each patient's unique requirements, track their progress, and make adjustments as needed (Das et al., 2015).

According to Kaur (2024), as shown in figure 2 & figure 3 below, Synergistic swarm in multi-robot system is a novel concept in healthcare and has numerous advantages:

According to the aforementioned evaluation, Multi-Robots / Synergistic swarm has the potential to be used in virtually every business in a manner that is both exact and does not involve a change to the existing framework. Control will be accomplished by the utilization of intelligent robotics. In addition to this, it has the ability to optimize data analytic for the numerous companies that provide online resources. Automated processes are expected to have a rapid and consistent rise in popularity in the coming years as an increasing number of businesses become aware of the benefits that Multi-Robots / Synergistic swarm can provide through its implementation (Duggal et al., 2022).

The fields of artificial intelligence and robotics are distinct from one another, despite the fact that both may continue to be utilized independently. Over the course of the next few years, Multi-Robots / Synergistic swarm is anticipated to develop into artificial intelligence. This implies that the technology will encompass all aspects of artificial intelligence. By integrating machine learning with the support of staff and instruments, businesses, particularly those in the healthcare industry, are quickly realizing that this combination will lead to full and advanced personnel by boosting the efficacy and effectiveness of the business as a whole, which will eventually serve its stakeholders. The online evolution that involves artificial intelligence analysis is anticipated to be a further significant transformation.

Figure 1. Present state of healthcare and the requirement of multi- robotics

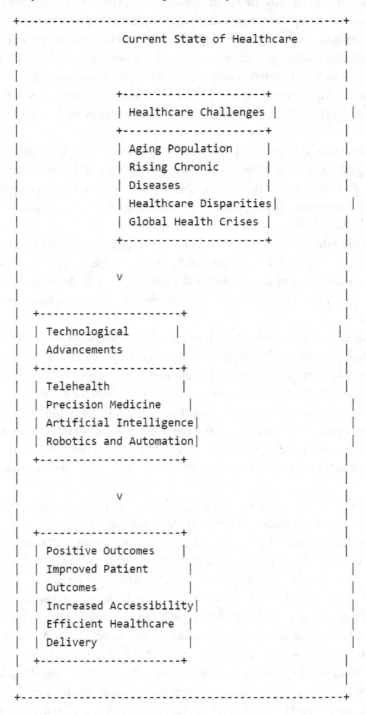

This is because employees who are equipped with automated tools will be able to construct a virtual healthcare staff that encompasses all aspects of monitoring and increases profitability across key domains (Fisher et al., 2017).

Figure 2. Synergistic swarm in multi-robot systems in healthcare

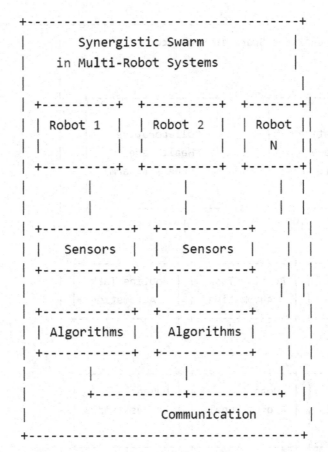

In the not too distant future, Multi-Robots / Synergistic swarm is going to be utilized extensively in a wide range of healthcare-related fields, such as the manufacturing of medical equipment, the analysis of medical data, and the administration of healthcare compliance. In the not too distant future, the extensive information and processing that the Administration is responsible for will be carried out automatically. To be more specific, the installation of Multi-Robots / Synergistic swarm will have a significant impact on the ensuing healthcare programs. It is the core technology that drives the expansion of drug research and development, which is universally accepted as an essential advance in healthcare. It acts as the driving force behind the growth of technology. It typically takes the form of algorithms that are designed for learning (Foroutannia et al., 2021; Kaur, 2024).

By utilizing unique functions and functionalities, health-care automation technologies have the potential to enhance the efficiency, effectiveness, precision, and safety of the delivery of medical services. This is accomplished through the utilization of novel functions and capabilities. The expanding field of artificial intelligence is likely to result in the introduction of a whole new facet to the field of machine learning. As is anticipated, the utilization of machines and artificial intelligence would not only expedite the operations but also greatly enhance the level of safety throughout the process. Furthermore, statistical analysis and developments in software and physical components are likely to have the effect of expanding the scope of applications for robotics in additional medical settings.

Figure 3. Uses of multi-robot system/synergistic swarm

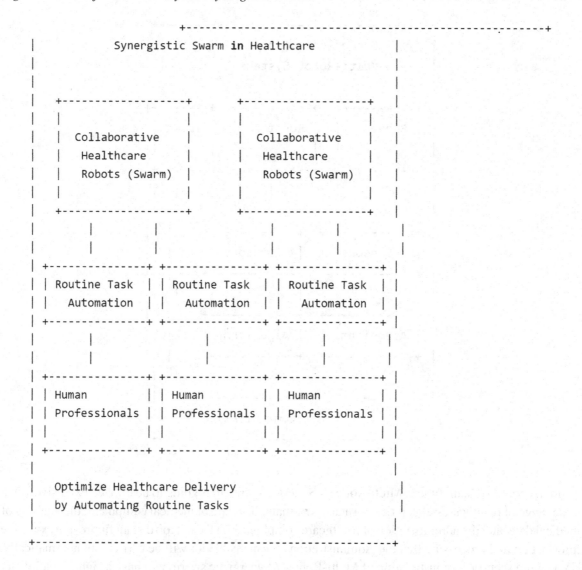

As a result of investments and collaborations between digital companies and medical specialists, the demand from customers for medical robotics is expected to increase even further (Haken & Levi, 2012; Fosch-Villaronga & Drukarch, 2021).

Despite the fact that earlier attempts to make suggestions for examination and treatment were already challenging, experts believe that the installation of Multi-Robots / Synergistic swarm will eventually become proficient in such an area as well. As a result of the rapid advancements that have been made in artificial intelligence related to computed tomography processing, it is becoming increasingly conceivable that the bulk of radio-logical and pathological imaging will soon be examined by a computer. The use of voice and optical character recognition for a variety of reasons, such as therapeutic exchanges and the transcription of diagnostic records, is going to become increasingly frequent (Holland et al., 2021).

Challenges to be Faced by Multi-Robots / Synergistic Swarm

The most significant obstacle that Multi-Robots / Synergistic swarm faces in the health care industry is merely assessing whether or not the technology advancements would be capable of being actually beneficial, rather than ensuring that they will be accepted for diagnostic reasons. In order for Multi-Robots / Synergistic swarm to be widely adopted, it is necessary for it to be endorsed by regulatory bodies, incorporated into electronic health records, sufficiently streamlined so that it is designed to imitate function similarly, the training of healthcare professionals, adequate compensation from either privately funded or publicly funded institutions, and improvement over the course of its use. It is possible that these challenges will be handled in the future; nevertheless, it will take far more time than was originally envisaged for such technology to improve under these circumstances (Humaidi et al., 2020).

As a result, experts estimate that the use of Multi-Robots / Synergistic swarm in therapeutic settings will be restricted during the next twenty years. It is important to emphasize that the introduction of Multi-Robots / Synergistic swarm will not significantly replace physicians in the treatment of patients; rather, it will merely support them in their work. It is possible that in the future, modern physicians may gravitate toward responsibilities and work arrangements that make use of special mental talents such as compassion, understanding, and motivation. It is possible that in the future, these health professionals who refuse to work together with machine learning will be the only ones who are forced to give up their own professions (Karpov & Tarassov, 2017; Kaur, 2024; Kaur & Arora, 2023).

SIGNIFICANCE OF MULTI-ROBOTICS/SYNERGISTIC SWARM

Improved patient diagnosis and remote patient monitoring are two areas where Multi-Robots / Synergistic swarm has shown to be an invaluable asset to healthcare operations. Among its many contributions to healthcare are the following: better health outcomes, more precise patient diagnoses, more effective treatment regimens, and more efficient administration of healthcare facilities (Kernbach, 2011; Lestingi et al., 2022).

By analyzing X-rays, CT images, and MRI's, diagnostic imaging—which includes Multi-Robots / Synergistic swarm systems—assists radiologists in their work. Analyzing these medical images accomplishes this. Radiologists can improve the diagnosis procedure with the help of these technologies by spotting abnormalities more easily. Robots can spot irregularities and minor patterns that a human eye might miss in the early stages of an investigation. Better early detection is made possible by this. Neurological problems like Parkinson's disease and cancer can now be detected much more quickly. Many systematic processes and procedures are followed when new medications are being created (Li et al., 2021).

Our goal in implementing these measures is to make the process of developing and testing novel pharmaceutical substances much faster. In order to find new treatments and evaluate their effectiveness, Multi-Robots / Synergistic swarm-can analyze massive amounts of data, including genetic information. The data analysis procedure does this. The time and money needed for drug trials is thus significantly reduced. When it comes to clinical studies, Multi-Robots / Synergistic swarm-also makes participant selection much easier. To do this, we look at the participants' personality qualities to see if they are a good fit for the study. According to Troccaz et al., (2019)., this means that the experiment has a better chance of succeeding. Robotic technologies help medical professionals make more educated diagnosis and treatment processes by expediting data analysis and providing decision support (Ma et al., 2015; Moura, 2012).

Individualized treatment regimens are made feasible by Robotics' utilization of personal genetic information. This enables for tailored treatment regimens and the capacity to forecast the effectiveness of specific treatments, while also decreasing the risk of unwanted responses. Customizing medications to fit with the specific demands of individual patients can considerably boost the success of treatment optimization. Previous studies (Rizk et al., 2019; Sahu et al., 2022) indicates that Multi-Robots / Synergistic swarm-can increase the quality of procedures in the medical industry-also. Despite the fact that the Synergistic Swarm model has a great deal of promise, there are ethical and regulatory difficulties associated with doing so as depicted in figure 4 below:

The Synergistic Swarm idea, which is used in multi-robot systems, is a revolutionist conceptualization that has the prospective to modify a variety of fields of study as presented in figure 5 below:

- Multi-Robots / Synergistic swarm-enables continual professional education and career growth for healthcare practitioners by leveraging telemedicine and telehealth technology. Telemedicine is the transmission of healthcare information and delivery of medical care to patients who are geographically remote. It does not belong to the realm of technology or represent a novel or revolutionary area of medicine. Telemedicine is the employment of technology to enable the interchange of data, speech, and video between patients and healthcare practitioners during their visits. It enables the supply of healthcare services to distant locations and fosters fair access to medical treatment while maintaining a peaceful interaction between urban and rural inhabitants (ŞEN et al., 2022).

- The implementation of Multi-Robots / Synergistic swarm in the healthcare industry aids in overcoming the issues arising from the geographical distance between healthcare practitioners. The recruitment and retention of healthcare workers in remote regions can offer major obstacles. However, these issues can be overcome by applying multi-robotics, as revealed by numerous research (Kaur, 2024).

- Multi-Robotic surgical aid technology can boost the professional development of healthcare personnel by facilitating the transfer of learning data to remote places and enhancing the sharing of information and knowledge in the field of surgical support. Therefore, it is crucial to determine

Figure 4. Characteristic of synergistic swarm model

Promising Aspects of Synergistic Swarm Model	Ethical and Regulatory Difficulties
• High Efficiency in Task Execution • Improved Problem Solving • Adaptability to Dynamic Environments • Increased Robustness and Resilience	• Lack of Transparent Decision-Making • Privacy and Security Concerns • Accountability in Autonomous Systems • Potential Job Displacement

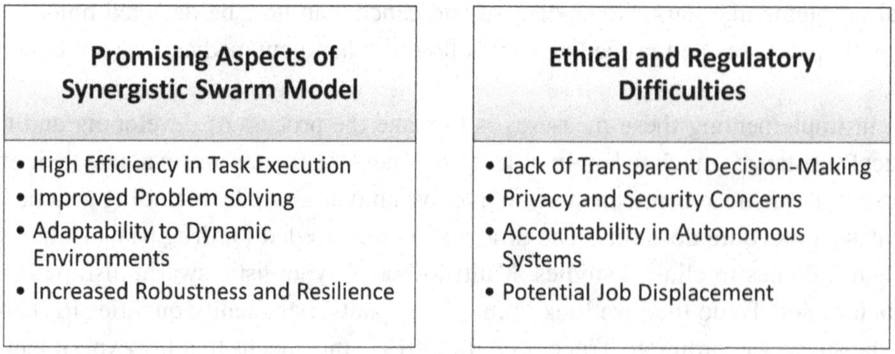

Figure 5. Potential impact across various fields

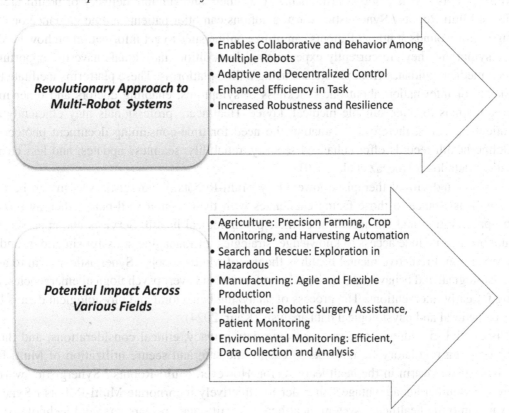

Revolutionary Approach to Multi-Robot Systems
- Enables Collaborative and Behavior Among Multiple Robots
- Adaptive and Decentralized Control
- Enhanced Efficiency in Task
- Increased Robustness and Resilience

Potential Impact Across Various Fields
- Agriculture: Precision Farming, Crop Monitoring, and Harvesting Automation
- Search and Rescue: Exploration in Hazardous
- Manufacturing: Agile and Flexible Production
- Healthcare: Robotic Surgery Assistance, Patient Monitoring
- Environmental Monitoring: Efficient, Data Collection and Analysis

the most effective use of robots to boost the knowledge and learning of healthcare professionals, so supplying them with the necessary foundation for their professional development .

- When it comes to fraud protection, algorithms driven by Multi- Robotics evaluate payment records to discover any discrepancies that may suggest fraudulent activity. Early detection of fraudulent activity is attainable due to this. Implementing Multi-Robots / Synergistic swarm boosts cyber-security measures, thereby enhancing the protecting of patient data and healthcare information systems (Shallal et al., 2020).

- The utilization of Multi-Robots / Synergistic swarm enables the use of wearable technology, such as trackers, that can continually monitor vital signs and capture real-time data. This data can be promptly communicated to the physician, alerting them to any potential difficulties that may arise. Remote monitoring has the potential to provide major benefits to those with chronic diseases. Some advantages of this technology include the ability to proactively manage symptoms and a decrease in the need for frequent hospital visits (Sugiyama et al., 2010; Kaur & Arora, 2023).

- Assistance in Medical Decision-Making: Robotics provides support to healthcare professionals in determining the best course of action for diagnosing and treating patients. It achieves this by providing them with evidence-based information. To enhance patient safety, it is advisable to utilize the alerts and notifications generated by clinical decision support systems. It is crucial for these cautions and warnings to specifically address the potential occurrence of pharmacological mistakes or interactions (Kaur, 2024).

- Multi-Robots / Synergistic swarm-enables the timely and suitable delivery of healthcare to patients. Multi-Robots / Synergistic swarm-solutions can offer patients online guidance on managing minor wounds at home. Patients can utilize online sites to get information on how to identify the symptoms they are currently experiencing. In addition, individuals have the opportunity to seek medical guidance from physicians using online platforms. These platforms facilitate the exchange of information about one's sickness or symptoms, enabling doctors and other medical professionals to offer suitable medical advice. Healthcare professionals may efficiently access patients' records, therefore eliminating the need for time-consuming document photocopying. Online health records offer enhanced security, reliability, seamless updates, and less chance of patient data loss (Troccaz et al., 2019).

- Chat-bots and virtual therapists powered by Multi-Robots / Synergistic swarm can be utilized to offer assistance to those facing challenges with their mental well-being, thereby promoting the preservation and enhancement of their psychological health. Services encompassed in this support area include access to knowledge, strategies for managing stressful situations, and crisis intervention. Predictive mental health is the use of Multi-Robots / Synergistic swarm to analyze physiological and behavioral data in order to foresee and avert psychological emergencies, allowing for early interventions. The process of analyzing behavioral and physiological data is known as behavioral and physiological data analysis (Kaur, 2024).

- It is crucial to address concerns regarding data privacy, ethical considerations, and the need for ongoing regulatory frameworks to ensure the safe and secure utilization of Multi-Robots / Synergistic swarm in the healthcare sector. However, Multi-Robots / Synergistic swarm still provides numerous advantages. In order to effectively incorporate Multi-Robots / Synergistic swarm into the healthcare system, healthcare practitioners, researchers, and technology developers must collaborate. Population health management can be achieved by employing data analytic to identify patterns and trends found among populations. To accomplish this objective, it is important to carry out a more extensive examination of the data generated by Robotics. This has the potential to significantly assist in the administration of healthcare for the overall population (Troccaz et al., 2019).

Regarding the implementation of measures to improve the health of a population, the healthcare industry can effectively manage its supply chain by utilizing Multi-Robots / Synergistic swarm-devices. These devices can monitor and regulate the storage conditions of pharmaceuticals, immunizations, and other essential supplies. The prevention of spoilage, reduction of waste, and guarantee of essential commodity supply are achieved as a consequence of this. Multi-Robots / Synergistic swarm can be employed in healthcare facilities to monitor and maintain cleanliness, as well as control infections. This utilization could be advantageous for all parties involved. Intelligent sensors possess the capability to monitor the quality of air, assess the extent to which individuals comply with hand hygiene practices, and detect upcoming epidemics. This is achieved by the examination of patterns in patient symptoms or diseases. Integrating biometric authentication methods with Multi-Robots / Synergistic swarm-technology has the potential to enhance the safety and efficiency of healthcare services. This was deliberated within the framework of authentication and security. As a result, this contributes to safeguarding patients' privacy and ensuring compliance with legislation governing the protection of sensitive information. Restricted staff members will be granted exclusive access to patients' personal information (Sugiyama et al., 2010; Kaur & Arora, 2023).

Robotic surgical equipment, powered by Multi-Robots, can swiftly and effectively support surgeons by providing them with up-to-date and valuable information during surgical procedures. The surgeons can acquire this information. These systems may include feedback mechanisms and sensors to optimize surgical outcomes, enhance precision, and minimize errors. By employing Multi Robots, it is possible to carry out the identification and surveillance of indicators of mental health. Here, we can find signs such as stress levels, sleep habits, and mood disorders. Potential exists for employing sensors, adaptations, wearable devices, and smartphone applications. All of them are potential options. Sharing data with healthcare practitioners can facilitate the adoption of personalized psychological treatments, expediting the process (Kaur, 2024). To encourage patient engagement, connected devices in Multi-Robots / Synergistic swarm-can be used to provide individualized health education, medication reminders, and lifestyle counseling opportunities.

In the field of healthcare, the implementation of Multi-Robots / Synergistic swarm (RPA) raises a variety of ethical concerns that need to be taken into consideration. Throughout the course of history, the vast majority of decisions concerning medical treatment were made decisions by individuals. Consequently, the utilization of intelligent technology to either produce treatment decisions or provide support in making them has developed as a result of this (Sugiyama et al., 2010; Kaur & Arora, 2023).

ETHICAL CONCERNS AND CONSIDERATIONS

There are concerns regarding the ethical standards and rules of communication, as well as the preservation of sensitive information, truthfulness, and agreement. Considering the rapid pace at which technological advancements are currently taking place, finding a solution to the issue of openness can be an activity that is fraught with an incredible amount of difficulty. Due to the vast complexity of certain systems, it can be quite challenging to comprehend or interpret them. This is especially true for systems that incorporate deep learning in visual analytic. In the event that patients are presented with information regarding the function that a graphic plays in the process of cancer diagnosis, it is quite probable that they will be interested in acquiring an understanding of the factors that contribute to the diagnosis of their cancer. The fact that it is difficult to articulate the context is something that may come as a surprise to medical professionals who are normally well-versed in the inner-workings of data augmentation .

When it comes to evaluating and treating patients, the utilization of Multi-Robots / Synergistic swarm is prone to errors, which can make the process of holding them accountable for carelessness more difficult. Patients can be evaluated and treated by Multi-Robots / Synergistic swarm. When it comes to providing patients with information that they would rather acquire from a compassionate physician, there will be situations in the not too distant future in which Multi-Robots / Synergistic swarm will fulfill the job of presenting patients with that information. Despite the fact that gender and racial origin are not the actual causes of the disease, it is conceivable for medical artificial intelligence to exhibit computational bias. This might result in larger disease probability estimates based on these factors, despite the fact that these factors are not the actual causes of the disease.

Using the information that is provided by the individual who is ill, an automated system is able to reliably diagnose illnesses using the information that is provided by the one who is ill.In addition to this, it has the potential to offer additional assistance after the completion of therapy. A number of automated algorithms have been developed for the purpose of supporting individuals in performing essential duties, such as the administration of their prescribed medications, the consumption of their nourishment, and the planning of their diet. An individual who has been discharged from the hospital can receive assistance from a caregiver in their recuperation at home after being discharged from the hospital. In light of this, any data or information

The application of an automated system has the ability to control and monitor seventeen distinct health illnesses in an effective manner. These disorders include blood pressure and cardiovascular health issues. According to Sugiyama et al., (2010)., it is feasible that this may be advantageous for the health of an individual because it would enable them to quickly get in touch with their physicians in the event that they experience changes that they had not anticipated.

A variety of advancements in the fields of ethics, medicine, professional practice, and scientific research are anticipated to be brought about as a consequence of the implementation of Multi-Robots / Synergistic swarm (RPA) in healthcare facilities. The construction of protocols for monitoring big circumstances, responding in a responsible manner, and building management systems to prevent adverse effects is an imperative necessity for health systems, as well as for politicians and organizations within the government. This is a necessity that cannot be avoided. Due to the fact that this technology will have a large and long-lasting impact on mankind, it will entail the design of regulations that are severe and will demand constant attention for several generations.

CONCLUSION

In the field of medicine, the use of robots that are independently operated is becoming increasingly common. Medical institutions are confronted with a multitude of demanding operations and stringent criteria, such as the organization of patients and the processing of reimbursements. The consequence of this is a string of discrepancies, increased operational expenses, and procedures that move at a snail's pace. Through the utilization of robotics and machine learning, medical practitioners are able to efficiently address difficulties in the healthcare industry.

Surgical procedures, the overall experience of patients, and the efficiency of medical institutions are all areas that need to be improved, and there are three primary issues that need to be addressed in order to accomplish these goals. Through the utilization of technology and the implementation of effective automated processes, such as Multi-Robots / Synergistic swarm, medical professionals and nurses are able to relieve themselves of the time-consuming and costly responsibilities associated with keeping up with technological advancements. It makes it possible for businesses to concentrate their resources on providing treatment in a more efficient manner.

By utilizing workstation automation to conduct a wide variety of routine duties, ranging from simple to complex, Multi-Robots / Synergistic swarm can be of assistance to medical institutions. This is especially prevalent in situations where enterprises are expanding and handling big customer lists. It is projected that the deployment of Multi-Robots / Synergistic swarm would assist businesses in generating income from a variety of operations that take place on the server side. Also, it is anticipated that Multi-Robots / Synergistic swarm would make it possible to manage huge numbers of patients in healthcare facilities and also supply knowledge about upgraded amenities that will be available in the future.The creation of algorithms that can be utilized for a variety of purposes is becoming an important priority for several suppliers.

Both consumers and medical facilities have made investments in the adoption of automated process solutions. These investments are being made in order to improve the efficiency and lifespan of organizational structures, as well as to increase their market share. In the field of medicine, the development of autonomous robots will be facilitated by the increasing application of cutting-edge technology such as artificial intelligence, data mining, and the internet of things. The use of Multi-Robots / Synergistic swarm is becoming increasingly prevalent in medical facilities as a means of simplifying operations and managing big datasets. Through the utilization of machine learning, organizations are able to independently improve their business procedures and practices.

REFERENCES

Alsamhi, S. H., & Lee, B. (2020). Blockchain-empowered multi-robot collaboration to fight COVID-19 and future pandemics. *IEEE Access : Practical Innovations, Open Solutions, 9*, 44173–44197. doi:10.1109/ACCESS.2020.3032450 PMID:34786312

Cao, K., Chen, Y., Dang, H., Gao, S., & Yan, K. (2022, July). Multi-robot Coverage System Based on Health Optimization Management Algorithm. In *Proceedings of 2021 5th Chinese Conference on Swarm Intelligence and Cooperative Control* (pp. 902-911). Singapore: Springer Nature Singapore.

Cao, K., Chen, Y., Gao, S., Zhang, H., & Dang, H. (2022). Multi-Robot Formation Control Based on CVT Algorithm and Health Optimization Management. *Applied Sciences (Basel, Switzerland), 12*(2), 755. doi:10.3390/app12020755

Das, G. P., McGinnity, T. M., Coleman, S. A., & Behera, L. (2015). A distributed task allocation algorithm for a multi-robot system in healthcare facilities. *Journal of Intelligent & Robotic Systems, 80*(1), 33–58. doi:10.1007/s10846-014-0154-2

Duggal, A. S., Malik, P. K., Gehlot, A., Singh, R., Gaba, G. S., Masud, M., & Al-Amri, J. F. (2022). A sequential roadmap to Industry 6.0: Exploring future manufacturing trends. *IET Communications, 16*(5), 521–531. doi:10.1049/cmu2.12284

Foroutannia, A., Shoryabi, M., Anaraki, A. A., & Rowhanimanesh, A. (2021, March). SIN: A Programmable Platform for Swarm Robotics. In *2021 26th International Computer Conference, Computer Society of Iran (CSICC)* (pp. 1-5). IEEE. 10.1109/CSICC52343.2021.9420596

Fosch-Villaronga, E., & Drukarch, H. (2021). On Healthcare Robots: Concepts, definitions, and considerations for healthcare robot governance. arXiv preprint arXiv:2106.03468.

Haken, H., & Levi, P. (2012). *Synergetic agents: From multi-robot systems to molecular robotics*. John Wiley & Sons. doi:10.1002/9783527659524

Holland, J., Kingston, L., McCarthy, C., Armstrong, E., O'Dwyer, P., Merz, F., & McConnell, M. (2021). Service robots in the healthcare sector. *Robotics (Basel, Switzerland), 10*(1), 47. doi:10.3390/robotics10010047

Humaidi, A. J., Ibraheem, I. K., Azar, A. T., & Sadiq, M. E. (2020). A new adaptive synergetic control design for single link robot arm actuated by pneumatic muscles. *Entropy (Basel, Switzerland)*, *22*(7), 723. doi:10.3390/e22070723 PMID:33286496

Karpov, V. E., & Tarassov, V. B. (2017, September). Synergetic artificial intelligence and social robotics. In *International Conference on Intelligent Information Technologies for Industry* (pp. 3-15). Cham: Springer International Publishing.

Kaur, J. (2024). Green Finance 2.0: Pioneering Pathways for Sustainable Development and Health Through Future Trends and Innovations. In Sustainable Investments in Green Finance (pp. 294-319). IGI Global.

Kaur, J. (2024). Fueling Healthcare Transformation: The Nexus of Startups, Venture Capital, and Innovation. In Fostering Innovation in Venture Capital and Startup Ecosystems (pp. 327-351). IGI Global.

Kaur, J. (2024). Towards a Sustainable Triad: Uniting Energy Management Systems, Smart Cities, and Green Healthcare for a Greener Future. In Emerging Materials, Technologies, and Solutions for Energy Harvesting (pp. 258-285). IGI Global.

Kaur, J., & Arora, R. (2023, June). Exploring the dimensionality of employee silence in healthcare sector. In AIP conference proceedings (Vol. 2782, No. 1). AIP Publishing. doi:10.1063/5.0154178

Kaur, J., & Arora, R. (2023, June). Exploring the impact of employee silence in private hospitals-a structural equation modeling approach. In AIP Conference Proceedings (Vol. 2782, No. 1). AIP Publishing. doi:10.1063/5.0154173

Kernbach, S. (2011). Robot companions: Technology for humans. arXiv preprint arXiv:1111.5207.

Lestingi, L., Sbrolli, C., Scarmozzino, P., Romeo, G., Bersani, M. M., & Rossi, M. (2022, May). Formal modeling and verification of multi-robot interactive scenarios in service settings. In *Proceedings of the IEEE/ACM 10th International Conference on Formal Methods in Software Engineering* (pp. 80-90). IEEE. 10.1145/3524482.3527653

Li, Y., Jiao, X. Y., Sun, B. Q., Zhang, Q. H., & Yang, J. Y. (2021, March). Multi-welfare-robot cooperation framework for multi-task assignment in healthcare facilities based on multi-agent system. In *2021 IEEE International Conference on Intelligence and Safety for Robotics (ISR)* (pp. 413-416). IEEE. 10.1109/ISR50024.2021.9419496

Ma, Y., Zhang, Y., Wan, J., Zhang, D., & Pan, N. (2015). Robot and cloud-assisted multi-modal healthcare system. *Cluster Computing*, *18*(3), 1295–1306. doi:10.1007/s10586-015-0453-9

Moura, V. (2012). Magnetically Actuated Multiscale Medical Robots. In *IROS 2012 Full-day Workshop* (p. 48). IEEE.

Rizk, Y., Awad, M., & Tunstel, E. W. (2019). Cooperative heterogeneous multi-robot systems: A survey. *ACM Computing Surveys*, *52*(2), 1–31. doi:10.1145/3303848

Sahu, B., Das, P. K., Kabat, M. R., & Kumar, R. (2022). Prevention of Covid-19 affected patient using multi robot cooperation and Q-learning approach: A solution. *Quality & Quantity*, *56*(2), 793–821. doi:10.1007/s11135-021-01155-1 PMID:33972809

Şen, M. O., Okumuş, F., & Kocamaz, F.ŞEN. (2022). Application of blockchain powered mobile robots in healthcare: Use cases, research challenges and future trends. *Türk Doğa ve Fen Dergisi*, *11*(2), 27–35. doi:10.46810/tdfd.1017499

Shallal, A. H., Ucan, O. N., Humaidi, A. J., & Bayat, O. (2020). Multi-robot systems formation control with maneuvring target in system applicable in the hospitality and care-health industry of medical internet of things. *Journal of Medical Imaging and Health Informatics*, *10*(1), 268–278. doi:10.1166/jmihi.2020.2840

Sugiyama, O., Shinozawa, K., Akimoto, T., & Hagita, N. (2010). Case study of a multi-robot healthcare system: Effects of docking and metaphor on persuasion. In *Social Robotics: Second International Conference on Social Robotics*. Singapore.

Troccaz, J., Dagnino, G., & Yang, G. Z. (2019). Frontiers of medical robotics: From concept to systems to clinical translation. *Annual Review of Biomedical Engineering*, *21*(1), 193–218. doi:10.1146/annurev-bioeng-060418-052502 PMID:30822100

Chapter 11
Cogwheels of Care:
Robotic Marvels in the Hospital Landscape

Jaspreet Kaur
Chandigarh University, India

ABSTRACT

"Cogwheels of Care: Robotic Marvels in the Hospital Landscape" examines the incorporation of sophisticated robotics in contemporary healthcare. This abstract explores the profound influence of robots in hospitals, fundamentally changing patient care and enhancing medical capabilities. The chapter explores the ways in which these advanced robots enhance and simplify many jobs, ranging from surgical procedures to everyday activities, by maximising efficiency and accuracy. It emphasises the interdependent connection between technology and healthcare practitioners, focusing on the ethical considerations and societal consequences of this technological transformation. This research highlights the changing healthcare landscape, where the complex interaction between human expertise and robotic innovation is transforming the principles of compassionate and effective patient-centered care.

INTRODUCTION

Currently, healthcare organizations are facing significant pressure to excel in the market due to intense competition. Healthcare professionals experience the burden of meeting expectations in order to preserve and safeguard their status within the organization. Organizations, in response to intense competition, must implement cost reduction measures, which may include downsizing their workforce and increasing the task of the remaining employees. An excessive workload results in an escalation of work-related stress, job discontent, and demotivate. Furthermore, these employees struggle to achieve a harmonious equilibrium between their professional and personal lives (Etukudoh et al., 2024). Hospitals in India face the dual challenge of coping with a scarcity of healthcare personnel while also managing a surge in patient numbers. Healthcare personnel, including nurses, resident physicians, and specialists, are responsible for attending to patients. Due to a scarcity of staff, they are required to work in unconventional shifts and extended hours. It is observed that

DOI: 10.4018/979-8-3693-1962-8.ch011

these staff experience significant pressure to manage the heightened patient workload, resulting in workplace stress and discontent. Additionally, as a result of irregular and excessive working hours, these employees struggle to achieve a harmonious equilibrium between their professional and home lives. Investing additional time in their professional responsibilities and experiencing work-related exhaustion can disrupt their personal lives. This can diminish the productivity of people in their work. Employees may resign from their employment in severe circumstances of overwhelming strain. This issue is prevalent throughout numerous healthcare organizations. Content and satisfied personnel contribute to a positive and prosperous organization.Employees are crucial to the functioning of any organization. Therefore, it is imperative to take proactive measures to address this issue in order to remain competitive in today's market (Ala'a, 2023).

One example of such an endeavour is the implementation of robotics in the healthcare industry. This can be accomplished by acknowledging and valuing an employee's right to a satisfying existence both within and outside of their job, resulting in advantages for the individual, the organization, and society as a whole. Work-family balance refers to a situation when the demands and expectations of one's work and family roles are in conflict and cannot be reconciled in some way.The integration of robotics in healthcare has a crucial role in enhancing overall pleasure in all aspects of life, including personal well-being, professional success, and family dynamics. It aids in mitigating stress and lowering staff turnover and job-related stress. This study illuminates the significance of Robotics for healthcare and aims to establish a foundation for implementing various methods to enhance employee job happiness and productivity. These kind of activities will assist employees in achieving a harmonious work-life balance and attaining personal contentment, fulfillment, and overall well-being both in their personal lives and within the organization. The use of advances in technology initiatives has led to a substantial improvement in the operational effectiveness of the healthcare industry. The utilization of algorithms for machine learning has been advantageous to the healthcare industry as it has streamlined the task of analyzing vast quantities of data.

Robotics is capable of retaining and acquiring knowledge at a significantly faster rate than the human brain does. This is in comparison to the performance of the human brain. The distribution of medical experts, hospital beds, and resources can be optimized with the use of solutions that are powered by artificial intelligence. This optimization leads to enhanced operational efficiency and decreased expenses. In order to shed light on the benefits that may be acquired by using Artificial Intelligence, Robotics, Robotic Process Automation, and Machine Learning algorithms in the healthcare industry, the objective of this study is to shine light on those benefits. This opens the door for the development of less invasive operations that require shorter recovery times as depicted in figure 1 below.

Through the utilization of cutting-edge robotic equipment, it is now feasible to perform surgical procedures remotely, which in turn expands the availability of specialized medical care. The Robotics generates data that has the potential to be researched on a more extensive scale in order to identify patterns and trends among populations. This is accomplished through the use of the Robotics. There is a possibility that this will prove to be of considerable aid in the management of health care for the general population. When it comes to prosthetics and rehabilitation equipment, the implementation of Robotics technology makes it feasible to provide patients and medical professionals with quick and continuous feedback regarding the patient's status (Aggarwal et al., 2019). Because of this, both the personification of rehabilitation programme and the tracking of changes, as well as the tweaking of these programme to match the specific requirements of each individual patient, are less difficult to do (AlShamsi et al., 2022). Furthermore, the implementation of robots in the sphere of eldercare

Figure 1. Flowchart depicting the utilization of robotics in the healthcare industry

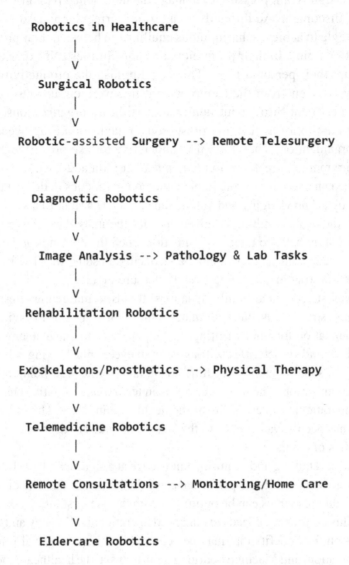

```
                Robotics in Healthcare
                        |
                        V
                  Surgical Robotics
                        |
                        V
        Robotic-assisted Surgery --> Remote Telesurgery
                        |
                        V
                 Diagnostic Robotics
                        |
                        V
          Image Analysis --> Pathology & Lab Tasks
                        |
                        V
               Rehabilitation Robotics
                        |
                        V
        Exoskeletons/Prosthetics --> Physical Therapy
                        |
                        V
                Telemedicine Robotics
                        |
                        V
       Remote Consultations --> Monitoring/Home Care
                        |
                        V
                  Eldercare Robotics
```

guarantees enhanced mobility and safety for the senior population (AlShamsi et al., 2022) as depicted in figure 2 below:

The purpose of this study is to provide an overview of the research approaches that were utilized in order to find, locate, and analyse papers that were relevant. The research questions that were utilized to investigate the content of the study are summarized in this paragraph, which provides an overview of those questions. Both the criteria that were used to include or exclude content, as well as the method that was used to gather data, will be discussed in this text. In order to complete the evaluation of the pertinent literature, four independent research inquiries were devised. The objective of this evaluation is to provide aid in the process of data extraction by assessing whether or not the papers that were selected address any of the study subjects. This evaluation will be carried out in order to accomplish this purpose. The

Figure 2. Application of robots in the domain of eldercare

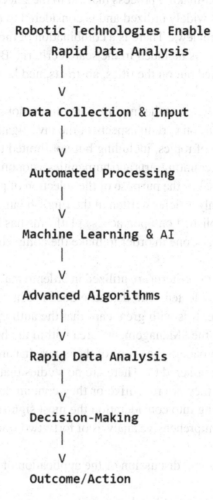

```
Robotic Technologies Enable
   Rapid Data Analysis
            |
            V
   Data Collection & Input
            |
            V
   Automated Processing
            |
            V
   Machine Learning & AI
            |
            V
   Advanced Algorithms
            |
            V
   Rapid Data Analysis
            |
            V
   Decision-Making
            |
            V
   Outcome/Action
```

following questions, which together make up the guiding principles, served as the basis for the research that was carried out for this project.

1. To what extent does the implementation of Robotics in the field of healthcare allow for the provision of a wide range of advantageous advantages?
2. What are the many advantages that the Robotics delivers to the field of healthcare as a whole, and to what extent does it bring these advantages?
3. What are the numerous advantages that the implementation of robotic process automation provides to the field of healthcare, and how may these advantages be utilized successfully?
4. When it comes to the healthcare industry, what are the numerous advantages that machine learning algorithms offer? This is the fourth research subject that needs investigating.

It is necessary to make use of the published literature that is accessible through the Scopus database in order to carry out the research. An inquiry is conducted into the Scopus database in order to discover publications that are pertinent to the study that is currently being conducted. There were two distinct elements that had a role in the decision-making process that led to the selection of this particular database. In addition, the Scopus database is widely utilized and is considered to be one of the most comprehensive databases for doing literature reviews. There is a combination of the terms "Artificial Intelligence" or "Robotics" and "Healthcare" that is included in the search criteria. By making use of the string that was specified, the search was carried out on the titles, abstracts, and keywords of the articles that were being considered.

For the aim of establishing the scope of the inquiry, some limitations were placed, meaning that the investigators were obligated to focus on certain aspects of the investigation.

This study covers a wide range of topics, including but not limited to the following: the social sciences, business management and accounting, arts and humanities, economics, econometrics, and finance, as well as multidisciplinary studies. For the purpose of the selection of publications, an extra constraint was imposed; more specifically, only articles written in the English language were taken into consideration. The study that has been published on open access platforms has been chosen with great care in order to extract the results. This was done in order to make the complete document more accessible to the general public.

Additional inclusion and exclusion criteria are utilized in order to make a decision regarding the final collection of research that will be selected. The database does not include any research that has been repeated as a result of its existence. It is with great care that the authors choose the study that will be reviewed, with a specific focus on the "Management" area within the healthcare industry. In addition, the incorporation of research that broadens the scope of the issues that are being investigated is the most important concept that needs to be adhered to. There are no studies that are included because they fall into one of two categories: either they are repetitive or they contain conclusions that are limited to a particular aspect of the issue. Taking into consideration the most significant findings from each of the studies, the authors conducted a comprehensive analysis of forty-two study investigations. This analysis was carried out by the authors.

This study presents the findings and discussion of the application of Robotics(AI) in the healthcare industry.

Robotics(AI) has the potential to be utilized in a wide range of various ways within the field of medical care (Cao & Rogers, 2007). Significant advancements have been made in the areas of diagnosis and therapy over the course of the past few years (Lloyd et al., 2024). Although it is anticipated that Robotics(AI) will serve as a supplement to human work, it is not anticipated that AI will totally replace human employment. Using Robotics(AI) assists with the monitoring of patients and provides individualized support through the analysis of images and the automation of medical equipment (Bogue, 2011).This is accomplished through the use of AI. Further, Robotics(AI) is a factor that contributes to the development of a wide range of industries, such as robotic-assisted surgery, data analysis, research in the pharmaceutical business, and many others. Tasks are completed more quickly and with greater efficiency thanks to artificial intelligence. The process of making decisions regarding patient diagnoses and the process of remotely monitoring patients are both areas in which the utilization of Robotics facilitates both of these processes (Butter et al., 2008).

Robotics makes a contribution to the improvement of healthcare operations in a variety of domains, including the optimization of health facility administration, the correct diagnosis of patients, the development of treatment plans, and the improvement of health outcomes. Furthermore, robotic equipment contribute to the diagnostic procedure by offering support, as depicted in figure 3:

The diagnostic imaging, which includes:

Figure 3. Effect of robotic surgical platforms on both diagnosis and operation

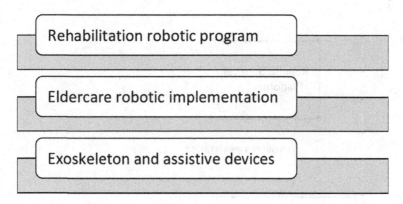

Robotics systems offer support to radiologists working in the field of radiology by analyzing X-rays, CT scans, and MRIs. This is accomplished through the study of these medical images. The use of these systems assists radiologists in identifying abnormalities and contributes to the process of diagnosis.

Early Detection: Robotics has the ability to recognize anomalies and minute patterns that human vision can overlook. This facilitates more accurate early detection. The quick diagnosis of diseases such as cancer and neurological disorders such as Parkinson's disease is made possible as a result of this (Kim et al., 2024). In the process of developing new medications, there are a variety of processes and procedures that are carried out in a methodical manner. These processes and actions are designed to facilitate the development of novel pharmaceutical substances and their subsequent testing.

Robotics has the capability to study enormous amounts of data, including genetic information, in order to discover potential new treatments and to estimate how effective they might be. This is accomplished through the process of data analysis. This consequently results in a significant reduction in the amount of time and money that is required for the study of medications (Khang et al., 2024).

When it comes to clinical trials, Robotics makes the process of selecting trial participants more efficient. This is accomplished by analyzing the characteristics of the individuals to evaluate whether or not they are suitable for the research being conducted. As a consequence of this, the probability that the experiment would be successful is increased (Gonzalo et al., 2024). In addition, robotic technologies facilitate swift data analysis and decision support, aiding medical personnel in making educated diagnosis and treatment processes, as depicted in figure 4 below:

Plans of treatment that are individualized:

The utilization of personal genetic information by Robotics makes it possible to personalize treatment regimens, which in turn makes it possible to forecast the efficacy of specific medications and reduce the possibility of adverse reactions caused by those medications. It is possible to considerably improve the efficacy of treatment optimization through the process of customizing medications to match the specific requirements of each individual patient (Etukudoh et al., 2024). Existing literature suggests that robotics has the ability to enhance the quality of processes in medical field, as depicted in figure 5 below.

Figure 4. Flowchart depicting the process by which robotic technologies facilitate swift data processing and decision-making

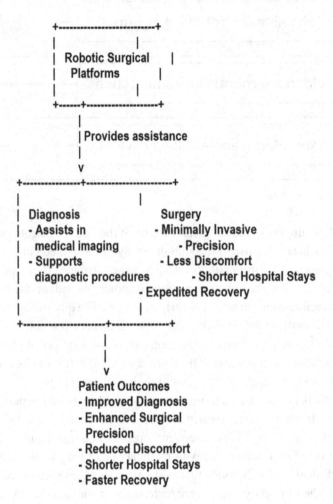

Advanced Analytic

Robotics enables ongoing professional education and advancement of healthcare practitioners through the use of telemedicine and telehealth. Telemedicine is the process of exchanging healthcare data and providing medical treatment to patients who are located far away. It does not fall within the category of technology or constitute a distinct or novel field of medicine. Telemedicine refers to the use of technology to facilitate the interchange of data, voice, and video between patients and healthcare professionals during their interactions. It facilitates the provision of healthcare services to remote regions and promotes equal access to medical care while preserving a balance between urban and rural communities.

The utilization of robotics in the healthcare sector helps to mitigate the challenges caused by the geographical separation of healthcare workers. In rural regions, the task of recruiting and retaining healthcare personnel is frequently challenging. This difficulty can be tackled by employing robot-

Figure 5. Ability of robotics in medical field

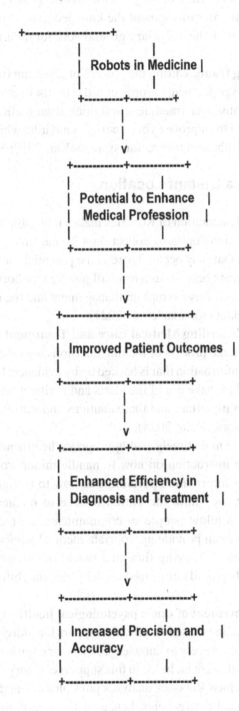

```
                    +--------------------+
                    |                    |
                    |  Robots in Medicine|
                    |                    |
                    +---------+----------+
                              |
                              |
                              v
                    +--------------------+
                    |                    |
                    |  Potential to Enhance  |
                    |  Medical Profession    |
                    |                    |
                    +---------+----------+
                              |
                              v
                    +--------------------+
                    |                    |
                    |  Improved Patient Outcomes  |
                    |                    |
                    +---------+----------+
                              |
                              v
                    +--------------------+
                    |                    |
                    |  Enhanced Efficiency in  |
                    |  Diagnosis and Treatment |
                    |                    |
                    +---------+----------+
                              |
                              v
                    +--------------------+
                    |                    |
                    |  Increased Precision and  |
                    |  Accuracy               |
                    |                    |
                    +--------------------+
```

ics (Aggarwal et al., 2019; Cresswell et al., 2018; Elendu et al., 2023; Javaid et al., 2022; Guntur et al., 2019).

Robotic surgical assistance technology has the potential to enhance the professional development of healthcare staff by facilitating the exchange of learning data to rural areas and improving the sharing of information and knowledge in the field of surgical assistance. Hence, it is crucial to ascertain the optimal utilization of robotics in order to augment the knowledge and learning of healthcare professionals, thereby providing them with the necessary groundwork for their professional growth (Joseph et al., 2018).

When it comes to preventing fraud: During the process of detecting fraudulent activity, algorithms powered by Robotics(AI) look over payment records in order to discover any inconsistencies that may have occurred. It is possible to discover fraudulent activities at an earlier stage because to this. The application of Robotics(AI) helps to improve cybersecurity standards, which in turn helps to boost the protection of patient data and healthcare information systems(Kar, 2019; Katevas, 2001).

Observing Patients From a Distant Location

Wearable technology: The implementation of Robotics makes it feasible to wear trackers that not only continuously monitor your vital signs but also collect data in real time and immediately notify your physician of any potential issues that may occur. There is the potential for individuals who suffer from chronic conditions to have significant benefits as a result of remote monitoring. A few examples of these advantages are the facilitation of proactive symptom management and the reduction in the necessity of making frequent trips to the hospital (Kavidha et al., 2021).

Help in Making Decisions Regarding Medical Care and Treatment Provision: Robotics(AI) offers aid to medical practitioners in the process of making decisions regarding how to diagnose and treat patients by supplying them with information that is backed up by evidence. For the purpose of enhancing patient safety, it is recommended to make use of the alerts and notifications that are produced by clinical decision support systems. It is important that these cautions and warnings address the possibility of pharmaceutical errors or interactions (Kaur, 2024).

Robotics facilitates the provision of timely and appropriate healthcare to patients.Robotics tools can provide patients with online instruction on how to handle minor wounds at home. Patients can utilise online resources to access information pertaining to how to recognise the symptoms they are now experiencing. Additionally, they have the option to receive medical advice from doctors via online platforms.These platforms allow people to communicate their illness or symptoms, while doctors and other medical experts can provide appropriate medical advice. The healthcare personnel can easily get the patients' records, so saving time that would otherwise be spent on photocopying documents. Online health records provide improved security, dependability, easy upgrading, and less risk of patient data loss.

The preservation and improvement of one's psychological health: Chat-bots and virtual therapists that are driven by Robotics can be used to provide support for individuals who are experiencing difficulties with their mental health. Access to knowledge, ways for coping with stressful situations, and crisis intervention are all services that are included in this support category. The term "predictive mental health" refers to the process by which Robotics analyses physiological and behavioral data in order to anticipate and prevent psychological emergencies, hence enabling early interventions. This process is referred to as behavioral and physiological data analysis (Kaur, 2024).

It is vital to address issues such as data privacy, ethical considerations, and the demand for continual regulatory frameworks in order to guarantee the safe and secure use of Robotics(AI) in the healthcare industry. This is the case despite the fact that Robotics(AI) offers a variety of benefits. For the purpose of achieving the objective of successfully integrating Robotics(AI) into the ecosystem of healthcare, it will be required for healthcare practitioners, researchers, and technology developers to collaborate with one another. The management of population health can be accomplished through the utilization of data analytic in order to find patterns and trends observed among populations. In order to achieve this goal, it is necessary to conduct a more comprehensive analysis of the data that is produced by Robotics. There is a possibility that this will prove to be of considerable aid in the management of health care for the general population. Specifically with reference to the deployment of preventative measures with the intention of improving the health of a populations (Kaur, 2024).

The supply chain in the healthcare industry can be managed through the implementation of Robotics devices that are able to monitor and regulate the conditions under which pharmaceuticals, immunizations, and other important supplies are stored. It is as a result of this that the prevention of spoilage, the reduction of waste, and the guarantee of the supply of essential commodities are all accomplished (Maalouf et al., 2018).

Robotics have the potential to be utilized in healthcare facilities for the goal of monitoring and maintaining cleanliness as well as infection control. This usage could be beneficial for all parties involved. Intelligent sensors have the ability to monitor air quality, evaluate the degree to which persons adhere to hand hygiene measures, and identify future epidemics. This is accomplished by the analysis of patterns of patient symptoms or diseases. The introduction of biometric authentication methods into Robotics technology has the potential to increase the efficiency of healthcare systems in terms of safety. This was discussed in the context of authentication and security. The result of this is that it contributes to the protection of patients' privacy and assures compliance with the regulations that regulate the protection of sensitive information. Staff members who are restricted in their access will be provided exclusive access to the personal information of patients (Kolpashchikov et al., 2022; Kim et al., 2016).

Current information: During surgical procedures, robotic surgical equipment that is enabled by the Robotics has the ability to provide surgeons with quick and valuable assistance by giving them with information that is current. This information can be obtained by the surgeons. It is possible that these systems will incorporate feedback mechanisms and sensors in order to enhance the outcomes of surgical procedures, as well as to improve precision and cut down on the amount of errors that take place.

Through the utilization of Robotics, it is feasible to perform detection and monitoring of markers of mental health. Stress levels, sleep patterns, and mood problems are some of the indicators that can be found here. There is the potential for the utilization of sensors, modifications, wearable devices, and applications for smartphones. These are all possibilities. It is possible to share the data with healthcare practitioners in order to expedite the process of adopting psychological treatments that are specifically suited to the individual (Kaur, 2024).

Patient Engagement and Education: As a means of encouraging patients to take an active role in their own healthcare, devices that are connected to the Robotics can be utilized to provide patients with individualized health education, medication prompts, and lifestyle counselling opportunities. Patients are motivated to take an active role in the management of their own health as a result of the implementation of this method, which in turn enhances the likelihood that they will adhere to the treatment regimens that have been prescribed to them (Kyrarini et al., 2021; Kaur, 2024).

Robotics is a technology that enables Real-time position Services (RTLS) to monitor the precise location of patients, medical staff, and medical equipment within a healthcare institution or clinic in real time. This is made possible by the Robotics. Consequently, this not only enhances the entire patient experience but also boosts the efficiency of the procedure, which in turn reduces the length of time that patients are required to wait. The integration of block-chain technology with Robotics technology has the potential to increase the dependability and security of health data management. Smart prostheses and rehabilitation equipment are now able to provide fast feedback to both patients and healthcare practitioners thanks to Robotics, which makes this capability possible. Robotics technology is responsible for making this capability a reality. The customization of rehabilitation programme, the monitoring of these programme progress, and the modification of these programme to match the specific requirements of each individual patient are all made simpler as a result of this reason. When it comes to the healthcare industry, it is required to solve issues such as data security, interoperability, and ethical considerations in order to make use of Robotics in a manner that is both suitable and successful.

Challenges

There are a number of challenges that the healthcare business must contend with, some of which include the complexity of procedures, the integration of data from a wide variety of sources, the management of information systems, and laboratory information systems. The software robotics that are currently accessible allow for the extraction of data from a wide number of sources and its subsequent utilization within businesses. Through the use of robotic process automation, there has been a notable reduction in the number of processes that are repetitive. It is possible to relate this to the fact that robots are more efficient than humans in terms of their operational capabilities. There is the opportunity for individuals to commit their time to tasks that require them to engage in direct interaction with other consumers (Morgan et al., 2022; Pee et al., 2019; Narula et al., 2014; Kaur, 2024).When it comes to aspects such as speed, efficiency, quality, and intellect, there is no comparison that can be made between humans and robots. The utilization of robotic process automation will result in a reduction of the expenses that are associated with human resources.

There will be a huge rise in productivity as a consequence of job automation processes. As a consequence of the implementation of automation, the total efficiency of the organization will experience an improved state.

Through the implementation of a digital workplace, the organization will be able to enhance its capacity to optimize and supervise data management, which will result in enhanced efficiency. There will be an increase in the organization's overall efficiency as a consequence of the introduction of robotic process automation as well as other technical advancements. It is currently being worked on to automate the procedures for requesting information regarding the status of claims. The fact that claim requests are handled automatically is one factor that contributes to the overall satisfaction of the target audience. Robotics techniques that enable computers to learn and generate predictions without being explicitly programmed and without the need for human interaction are referred to as "machine learning" techniques.

Predictive analytic is a term that refers to the process of applying machine learning algorithms to the analysis of data that is obtained from a range of health records. This analytic is being conducted with the intention of identifying patterns and trends that can be utilized in the process of formulating policies pertaining to public health. There is not a single piece of technology that does not make a major contribution to the enhancement of organizational efficiency and the facilitation of predictive analytic. By doing so, the organization is able to acquire a more comprehensive understanding of its patients and to make decisions concerning the health of those individuals. It becomes abundantly evident, as a result of the process of analyzing the data, which clients require particular types of treatment. In order to expedite the patient's recovery even further, individualized medication may also be supplied to the person. The implementation of robotic process automation has led to a major improvement in both the speed and quality of surgical treatments. Additionally, it has been responsible for a large reduction in the number of errors that occur during surgical procedures.

CONCLUSION

The application of robotic technology exemplifies the unwavering commitment to improving patient care through innovative advancements in the ever-changing and developing field of healthcare. The adoption of robotics in healthcare facilities has complex repercussions. These technological marvels have demonstrated their capacity to significantly enhance healthcare standards in various domains, such as providing logistical assistance and performing surgical procedures with utmost accuracy. An examination of the relevant facts has revealed the chronological progression of robotics, starting from the initial prototypes and ending with the most advanced systems currently in operation (Ragno et al., 2023; Kaur, 2024; (Sarker et al., 2021). Nevertheless, the research emphasizes that the proper implementation of these technologies, together with their flexibility and training, are crucial factors that could enhance the efficiency of these technologies. This is a finding underlined by the research (Kaur, 2024).

This comprehensive analysis leads to the conclusion that robotic technology is poised to play a significant role in the future of healthcare. Based on the investigation's results, this conclusion was reached. Several proposals have been put forward for future research endeavour focused on enhancing existing systems, tackling identified limitations, and managing ethical issues arising from the increasing automation in healthcare settings. These recommendations have been put up in the last few years. In order to ensure the ethical and safe integration of robots into healthcare services, it is crucial for technologists, healthcare practitioners, ethicists, and policymakers to collaborate and set comprehensive guidelines. This will enable the assurance of proper implementation of robots in healthcare services (Soriano et al., 2022; Stahl & Coeckelbergh, 2016).

The future of healthcare will be shaped by the integration of human skill with the advancement of technical innovation. This will be the case as the future of healthcare necessitates the combination of both. The combination of a visually realistic medical environment, along with the seamless integration of human empathy and precise robotic capabilities, has the potential to bring about a new era of patient-centered healthcare. This would represent a substantial advancement in the realm of healthcare. As healthcare becomes more complex, it is crucial to handle the issue with caution to ensure that compassion remains a vital aspect of technological advancements in the healthcare profession. The rationale behind this is that compassion plays a crucial role in the progress of technology innovations in the healthcare sector. In summary, the integration of robotics into healthcare facilities leads to numerous impressive achievements, as well as the potential for confronting challenges. To ensure that healthcare evolves into a future where human creativity and technology proficiency seamlessly merge, it is crucial for the various individuals involved to collaborate and contribute their diverse areas of knowledge. This will enable the path to be directed in order to accomplish the intended result (Vallès-Peris & Domènech, 2023; Vallès-Peris et al., 2021; Yoon & Lee, 2018).

This conclusion provides a succinct evaluation of the significant findings, viewpoints, and suggestions. Additionally, it introduces a thought-provoking topic of the harmonious existence of individuals and technology within the healthcare domain. Robotics is progressively becoming a significant component of the daily tasks performed by healthcare professionals. The significance of technology, particularly Robotics, in the healthcare industry has been widely acknowledged. Health-care professionals must possess computer abilities to efficiently navigate the ever expanding environment.Healthcare workers will dedicate time utilising Robotics tools.This technology would also facilitate the professional development of healthcare personnel in terms of knowledge and lifelong learning by enabling the sharing of educational data to rural areas and enhancing the transfer of data and expertise among faculty, students, and colleagues. Hence, it is crucial to ascertain the utilisation of Robotics in augmenting the comprehension and education of healthcare professionals, thereby providing them with the necessary groundwork for their professional advancement.

REFERENCES

Aggarwal, S., Gupta, D., & Saini, S. (2019, November). A literature survey on robotics in healthcare. In *2019 4th International Conference on Information Systems and Computer Networks (ISCON)* (pp. 55-58). IEEE. 10.1109/ISCON47742.2019.9036253

Ala'a, A. M. (2023). Adoption of Roboticsand Robotics in Healthcare: A Systematic Literature Review. [IJCMIT]. *International Journal of Contemporary Management and Information Technology*, *3*(6), 1–16.

AlShamsi, S., AlSuwaidi, L., & Shaalan, K. (2022). Robotics and AI in Healthcare: A Systematic Review. *Recent Innovations in Roboticsand Smart Applications*, 319-343.

Antony, V. N., Li, M., Lin, S. H., Li, J., & Huang, C. M. (2024). *Social Robots for Sleep Health: A Scoping Review*. arXiv preprint arXiv:2403.04169.

Bakshi, G., Kumar, A., & Puranik, A. N. (2021). Adoption of robotics technology in healthcare sector. In Advances in Communication, Devices and Networking [Singapore: Springer Singapore.]. *Proceedings of ICCDN*, *2020*, 405–414.

Bogue, R. (2011). Robots in healthcare. Industrial Robot. *International Journal (Toronto, Ont.)*, *38*(3), 218–223.

Butter, M., Rensma, A., Kalisingh, S., Schoone, M., Leis, M., Gelderblom, G. J., & Korhonen, I. (2008). *Robotics for healthcare*.

Cao, C. G., & Rogers, G. (2007). *Robotics in health care: HF issues in surgery. Handbook of Human Factors and Ergonomics in Health Care and Patient Safety*. Lawrence Earlbaum & Associates.

Cresswell, K., Cunningham-Burley, S., & Sheikh, A. (2018). Health care robotics: Qualitative exploration of key challenges and future directions. *Journal of Medical Internet Research*, *20*(7), e10410. doi:10.2196/10410 PMID:29973336

Elendu, C., Amaechi, D. C., Elendu, T. C., Jingwa, K. A., Okoye, O. K., Okah, M. J., & Alimi, H. A. (2023). Ethical implications of AI and robotics in healthcare. *Revista de Medicina (São Paulo)*, *102*(50), e36671. PMID:38115340

Etukudoh, N. S., Esame, N. V., Obeta, U. M., Ejinaka, O. R., & Khang, A. (2024). Automations and Robotics Improves Quality Healthcare in the Era of Digital Medical Laboratory. In Computer Vision and AI-Integrated IoT Technologies in the Medical Ecosystem (pp. 419-434). CRC Press. doi:10.1201/9781003429609-24

Gonzalo de Diego, B., González Aguña, A., Fernández Batalla, M., Herrero Jaén, S., Sierra Ortega, A., Barchino Plata, R., & Santamaría García, J. M. (2024, March). Competencies in the Robotics of Care for Nursing Robotics: A Scoping Review. In Healthcare (Vol. 12, No. 6, p. 617). MDPI. doi:10.3390/healthcare12060617

Guntur, S. R., Gorrepati, R. R., & Dirisala, V. R. (2019). Robotics in healthcare: an internet of medical robotic things (IoMRT) perspective. In *Machine learning in bio-signal analysis and diagnostic imaging* (pp. 293–318). Academic Press. doi:10.1016/B978-0-12-816086-2.00012-6

Javaid, M., Haleem, A., Singh, R. P., Rab, S., Suman, R., & Kumar, L. (2022). Utilization of Robotics for Healthcare: A Scoping Review. *Journal of Industrial Integration and Management, 2250015.*

Joseph, A., Christian, B., Abiodun, A. A., & Oyawale, F. (2018). A review on humanoid robotics in healthcare. In *MATEC Web of Conferences* (Vol. 153, p. 02004). EDP Sciences. 10.1051/matecconf/201815302004

Kar, S. (2019, October). Robotics in HealthCare. In *2019 2nd International Conference on Power Energy, Environment and Intelligent Control (PEEIC)* (pp. 78-83). IEEE. 10.1109/PEEIC47157.2019.8976668

Katevas, N. (Ed.). (2001). *Mobile robotics in healthcare* (Vol. 7). IOS Press.

Kaur, J. (2024). Green Finance 2.0: Pioneering Pathways for Sustainable Development and Health Through Future Trends and Innovations. In Sustainable Investments in Green Finance (pp. 294-319). IGI Global.

Kaur, J. (2024). Fueling Healthcare Transformation: The Nexus of Startups, Venture Capital, and Innovation. In Fostering Innovation in Venture Capital and Startup Ecosystems (pp. 327-351). IGI Global.

Kaur, J. (2024). Towards a Sustainable Triad: Uniting Energy Management Systems, Smart Cities, and Green Healthcare for a Greener Future. In Emerging Materials, Technologies, and Solutions for Energy Harvesting (pp. 258-285). IGI Global.

Kaur, J., & Arora, R. (2023, June). Exploring the dimensionality of employee silence in healthcare sector. In AIP conference proceedings (Vol. 2782, No. 1). AIP Publishing. doi:10.1063/5.0154178

Kaur, J., & Arora, R. (2023, June). Exploring the impact of employee silence in private hospitals-a structural equation modeling approach. In AIP Conference Proceedings (Vol. 2782, No. 1). AIP Publishing. doi:10.1063/5.0154173

Kavidha, V., Gayathri, N., & Kumar, S. R. (2021). AI, IoT and robotics in the medical and healthcare field. *AI and IoT-Based Intelligent Automation in Robotics*, 165-187.

Khang, A., Rath, K. C., Anh, P. T. N., Rath, S. K., & Bhattacharya, S. (2024). Quantum-Based Robotics in the High-Tech Healthcare Industry: Innovations and Applications. In Medical Robotics and AI-Assisted Diagnostics for a High-Tech Healthcare Industry (pp. 1-27). IGI Global.

Kim, H., Kwon, D., Son, J., & Choi, J. (2024). A Novel Robotic Healthcare Device for Treating Chronic Venous Insufficiency in People Who Sit for Prolonged Periods. *IEEE Transactions on Medical Robotics and Bionics*, 6(2), 618–631. doi:10.1109/TMRB.2024.3373909

Kim, J., Gu, G. M., & Heo, P. (2016). Robotics for healthcare. *Biomedical Engineering: Frontier Research and Converging Technologies*, 489-509.

Kolpashchikov, D., Gerget, O., & Meshcheryakov, R. (2022). *Robotics in healthcare. Handbook of Roboticsin Healthcare* (Vol. 2). Practicalities and Prospects.

Kyrarini, M., Lygerakis, F., Rajavenkatanarayanan, A., Sevastopoulos, C., Nambiappan, H. R., Chaitanya, K. K., Babu, A. R., Mathew, J., & Makedon, F. (2021). A survey of robots in healthcare. *Technologies*, 9(1), 8. doi:10.3390/technologies9010008

Lloyd, P., Dall'Armellina, E., Schneider, J. E., & Valdastri, P. (2024). *Future cardiovascular healthcare via magnetic resonance imaging-driven robotics*.

Maalouf, N., Sidaoui, A., Elhajj, I. H., & Asmar, D. (2018). Robotics in nursing: A scoping review. *Journal of Nursing Scholarship*, 50(6), 590–600. doi:10.1111/jnu.12424 PMID:30260093

Mois, G., & Beer, J. M. (2020). The role of healthcare robotics in providing support to older adults: A socio-ecological perspective. *Current Geriatrics Reports*, 9(2), 82–89. doi:10.1007/s13670-020-00314-w PMID:32435576

Morgan, A. A., Abdi, J., Syed, M. A., Kohen, G. E., Barlow, P., & Vizcaychipi, M. P. (2022). Robots in healthcare: A scoping review. *Current Robotics Reports*, 3(4), 271–280. doi:10.1007/s43154-022-00095-4 PMID:36311256

Narula, A., Narula, N. K., Khanna, S., Narula, R., Narula, J., & Narula, A. (2014). Future prospects of Roboticsin robotics software, a healthcare perspective. *International Journal of Applied Engineering Research: IJAER*, 9(22), 10271–10280.

Oña, E. D., Garcia-Haro, J. M., Jardón, A., & Balaguer, C. (2019). Robotics in health care: Perspectives of robot-aided interventions in clinical practice for rehabilitation of upper limbs. *Applied Sciences (Basel, Switzerland)*, 9(13), 2586. doi:10.3390/app9132586

Patel, A. R., Patel, R. S., Singh, N. M., & Kazi, F. S. (2017). Vitality of robotics in healthcare industry: Robotics perspective. *Robotics and big data technologies for next generation healthcare*, 91-109.

Pee, L. G., Pan, S. L., & Cui, L. (2019). Roboticsin healthcare robots: A social informatics study of knowledge embodiment. *Journal of the Association for Information Science and Technology*, 70(4), 351–369. doi:10.1002/asi.24145

Ragno, L., Borboni, A., Vannetti, F., Amici, C., & Cusano, N. (2023). Application of Social Robots in Healthcare: Review on Characteristics, Requirements, Technical Solutions. *Sensors (Basel)*, 23(15), 6820. doi:10.3390/s23156820 PMID:37571603

Sarker, S., Jamal, L., Ahmed, S. F., & Irtisam, N. (2021). Robotics and Roboticsin healthcare during CO-VID-19 pandemic: A systematic review. *Robotics and Autonomous Systems*, *146*, 103902. doi:10.1016/j.robot.2021.103902 PMID:34629751

Silvera-Tawil, D. (2024). Robotics in Healthcare: A Survey. *SN Computer Science*, *5*(1), 189. doi:10.1007/s42979-023-02551-0

Soriano, G. P., Yasuhara, Y., Ito, H., Matsumoto, K., Osaka, K., Kai, Y., & Tanioka, T. (2022, August). Robots and robotics in nursing. In Healthcare (Vol. 10, No. 8, p. 1571). MDPI. doi:10.3390/healthcare10081571

Stahl, B. C., & Coeckelbergh, M. (2016). Ethics of healthcare robotics: Towards responsible research and innovation. *Robotics and Autonomous Systems*, *86*, 152–161. doi:10.1016/j.robot.2016.08.018

Vallès-Peris, N., Barat-Auleda, O., & Domènech, M. (2021). Robots in healthcare? What patients say. *International Journal of Environmental Research and Public Health*, *18*(18), 9933. doi:10.3390/ijerph18189933 PMID:34574861

Vallès-Peris, N., & Domènech, M. (2023). Caring in the in-between: A proposal to introduce responsible AI and robotics to healthcare. *AI & Society*, *38*(4), 1685–1695. doi:10.1007/s00146-021-01330-w

Yoon, S. N., & Lee, D. (2018). Roboticsand robots in healthcare: What are the success factors for technology-based service encounters? *International Journal of Healthcare Management*.

Chapter 12
Bio–Inspired Nanorobots for Cancer Diagnosis and Therapy

Anshit Mukherjee
(iD) https://orcid.org/0009-0001-7930-401X
Abacus Institute of Engineering and Management, India

Gunjan Mukherjee
(iD) https://orcid.org/0000-0002-3959-3718
Brainware University, India

ABSTRACT

Cancer is one of the most serious threats to human health and life. Despite the advances in conventional therapies, such as surgery, chemotherapy, radiotherapy, and immunotherapy, there are still many challenges and limitations in achieving effective and precise cancer treatment. Nanorobots, inspired by natural biological nanomachines, offer a promising alternative for cancer diagnosis and therapy. Nanorobots are nanoscale devices that can perform various tasks under the guidance of external stimuli, such as magnetic fields, light, ultrasound, or chemical gradients. Nanorobots can be designed to target specific cancer cells or tissues, deliver drugs or genes, sense tumor biomarkers, perform minimally invasive surgery, or combine multiple functions for comprehensive treatment. In this chapter, the authors review the recent progress and applications of bio-inspired nanorobots for cancer diagnosis and therapy, with a focus on magnetic field-driven nanorobots. They also discuss the challenges and future perspectives of nanorobots in clinical translation.

INTRODUCTION

Bio-inspired nanorobots are a type of nanomedicine that mimics the natural, physical, and chemical properties of biological systems or processes. They have great potential for cancer diagnosis and therapy, as they can access remote and hard-to-reach body regions, perform various medical tasks, and improve the efficiency and effectiveness of treatment with reduced toxicity and side effects. Bio-inspired nanorobots can be designed and constructed using different materials, such as metals,

DOI: 10.4018/979-8-3693-1962-8.ch012

polymers, lipids, proteins, DNA, or cells. Depending on the material (Jun-Bing Fan,2022), they can have different shapes, sizes, functions, and biocompatibility. Some examples of bio-inspired nanorobots are magnetic nanorobots, DNA nanorobots, cell-based nanorobots, etc. Bio-inspired nanorobots can be driven by various methods, such as magnetic fields, light, ultrasound, chemical reactions, or biological motors. These methods(Xiangyi Kong,2023) can provide different levels of control, speed, and power for the nanorobots. Some examples of driving methods are water propulsion, enzyme catalysis, bacterial flagella, etc. Bio-inspired nanorobots can be applied for various purposes in cancer diagnosis and therapy, such as drug delivery, tumor sensing and diagnosis, targeted therapy, minimally invasive surgery, and immunotherapy. These applications can enhance the accuracy, sensitivity, specificity, and efficacy of cancer treatment. Some examples of applications are tumor targeting, tumor imaging, tumor ablation, tumor surgery, etc. Bio-inspired nanorobots are a promising and emerging field of research that could revolutionize cancer treatment in the near future. However, there are still many challenges and opportunities for further development, such as improving the biostability, biodegradability, biosafety, and bioethics of nanorobots; optimizing the design, fabrication, and integration of nanorobots; exploring new materials, driving methods, and functions of nanorobots; and validating the clinical feasibility and effectiveness of nanorobots(Lianging Liu, 2022). They have emerged as a promising platform for cancer diagnosis and therapy, owing to their advantages of high specificity, low toxicity, and self-assembly. In this book chapter, we will review the recent advances in the design, fabrication, and application of bio-inspired nanorobots for cancer detection and treatment. We also discuss the challenges and opportunities for the future development of bio-inspired nanorobots in the field of nanomedicine. Some of the possible key points we are going to discuss this chapter are:

- The advantages and disadvantages of different materials, shapes, sizes, and biocompatibility of bio-inspired nanorobots.
- Framework of bio-inspired nanorobots that can mimic the natural functions of biological entities, such as bacteria, viruses, cells, and enzymes, for cancer detection and therapy.
- How can bio-inspired nanorobots be driven by different methods, such as magnetic fields, light, ultrasound, chemical reactions, or biological motors? What are the trade-offs between control, speed, and power of these methods?
- How can bio-inspired nanorobots be applied for various purposes in cancer diagnosis and therapy, such as drug delivery, tumor sensing and diagnosis, targeted therapy, minimally invasive surgery, and immunotherapy? What are the benefits and limitations of these applications?
- How can bio-inspired nanorobots improve the accuracy, sensitivity, specificity, and efficacy of cancer treatment with reduced toxicity and side effects?

REVIEW

Bio-inspired nanorobots are nanoscale devices that mimic the functions and behaviors of natural biological systems, such as bacteria, viruses, enzymes, and cells. They can perform various tasks, such as sensing, targeting, delivery, diagnosis, and therapy, in complex biological environments. Bio-inspired nanorobots have great potential for cancer diagnosis and therapy, as they can overcome some of the limitations of conventional methods, such as low specificity, high toxicity, and drug resistance.

One of the main challenges in designing bio-inspired nanorobots is to achieve autonomous and controllable motion in biological fluids. Various propulsion mechanisms have been explored, such as chemical, magnetic, acoustic, optical, and electrical. Chemical propulsion is based on the catalytic decomposition of fuel molecules by nanomotors, which generates thrust from the reaction products. Magnetic propulsion relies on the application of external magnetic fields to manipulate the orientation and movement of magnetic nanomotors. Acoustic propulsion utilizes ultrasound waves to induce acoustic streaming around nanomotors, which results in fluid flow and propulsion. Optical propulsion exploits light energy to generate thermal gradients or optical forces that drive the motion of nanomotors. Electrical propulsion employs electric fields to induce electrokinetic effects, such as electrophoresis and electro-osmosis, that propel nanomotors.

Another challenge in designing bio-inspired nanorobots is to achieve specific and efficient targeting of cancer cells or tissues. Various targeting strategies have been developed, such as passive targeting, active targeting, and stimuli-responsive targeting. Passive targeting exploits the enhanced permeability and retention (EPR) effect of tumors, which allows nanomotors to accumulate in tumor sites due to their leaky vasculature and impaired lymphatic drainage. Active targeting involves the functionalization of nanomotors with ligands that can bind to receptors or antigens overexpressed on cancer cells or tissues. Stimuli-responsive targeting utilizes external or internal stimuli, such as pH, temperature, enzymes, or redox potential, to trigger the release or activation of nanomotors at tumor sites.

Bio-inspired nanorobots can perform various functions for cancer diagnosis and therapy, such as drug delivery, tumor sensing and diagnosis, targeted therapy, minimally invasive surgery, and other comprehensive treatments. Drug delivery is one of the most common applications of bio-inspired nanorobots, which can transport drugs or other therapeutic agents to tumor sites with high efficiency and specificity. Tumor sensing and diagnosis is another important application of bio-inspired nanorobots, which can detect tumor biomarkers or microenvironmental changes with high sensitivity and selectivity. Targeted therapy is a promising application of bio-inspired nanorobots, which can destroy cancer cells or tissues by physical or chemical means, such as mechanical drilling, photothermal ablation, or gene silencing. Minimally invasive surgery is an emerging application of bio-inspired nanorobots, which can perform surgical tasks at the microscale or nanoscale level with minimal damage to healthy tissues. Other comprehensive treatments are also possible with bio-inspired nanorobots, which can integrate multiple functions into one platform for synergistic effects.

The Table -1 summarizes some of the recent research work on bio-inspired nanorobots for cancer diagnosis and therapy:

FRAMEWORK OF BIO-INSPIRED NANOROBOTS THAT CAN MIMIC THE NATURAL FUNCTIONS OF BIOLOGICAL ENTITIES, SUCH AS BACTERIA, VIRUSES, CELLS, AND ENZYMES, FOR CANCER DETECTION AND THERAPY

The nanorobot based testing process has taken place in numberof steps. Figure 1 presents the detailed steps testing starting from the Material selection process.

One possible way is as follows (Calvalcanti, 2008):

Table 1. Review works of recent research works

Researcher's Name	Methodologies Used	Accuracy in Result
(Kong et al.,2023)	Nanosubmarines powered by chemical fuels for cancer treatment	Achieved autonomous navigation in blood vessels and selective destruction of cancer cells with high speed and precision
(Wang et al.,2020)	AuNPs-based micro/nanomotors for cancer-targeted delivery, diagnosis and imaging-guided therapy	Achieved efficient delivery of drugs or imaging agents to tumor sites with enhanced therapeutic efficacy or imaging contrast
(Li et al.,2020)	DNA origami-based photothermal motors for tumor ablation	Achieved light-driven motion in biological fluids and effective ablation of tumor cells with low laser power
(Li et al.,2019)	DNA origami-based gene motors for RNA interference therapy	Achieved electric field-driven motion in biological fluids and efficient delivery of siRNA to tumor cells with high gene silencing efficiency
(Wang et al.,2019)	Enzyme-powered micromotors for tumor microenvironment modulation	Achieved urease-driven motion in biological fluids and effective modulation of tumor acidity with enhanced drug efficacy
(Liu et al.,2018)	Magnetic helical microrobots for minimally invasive surgery	Achieved magnetic field-driven motion in biological fluids and precise manipulation of microscale objects with high dexterity
(Gao et al.,2017)	Ultrasound-powered nanorobots for tumor penetration and therapy	Achieved ultrasound-driven motion in biological fluids and deep penetration into tumor tissues with improved drug delivery
(Medina-Sánchez et al.,2017)	Magnetically actuated sperm-hybrid micromotors for drug delivery	Achieved magnetic field-driven motion in biological fluids and targeted delivery of drugs to tumor sites with high biocompatibility
(Esteban-Fernández de Ávila et al.,2017)	Bacteria-powered microrobots for tumor targeting and therapy	Achieved bacteria-driven motion in biological fluids and selective accumulation at tumor sites with enhanced drug efficacy
(Li et al.,2016)	Catalytic nanomotors for tumor sensing and diagnosis	Achieved catalytic motion in biological fluids and rapid detection of tumor biomarkers with high sensitivity and specificity

Figure 1. The steps n nanorobot testing from the material selection process

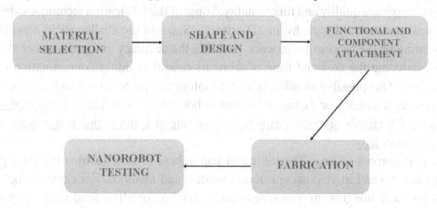

- First step is material selection. The material for the nanorobot body should be
- biocompatible, stable, and functionalizable. Biocompatibility means that the material should not cause adverse reactions or toxicity in the biological environment. Stability means that the material should not degrade or lose its properties over time. Functionalizability means that the material should allow the attachment of functional components, such as sensors, actuators, or drugs. Some of the challenges in material selection are finding materials that meet all these criteria, ensuring the quality and purity of the materials, and controlling the size and shape of the materials. One possible solution is to use natural biomolecules, such as DNA,

proteins, or lipids, as building blocks for the nanorobot body. <u>These biomolecules are inherently biocompatible, stable under certain conditions, and functionalizable through molecular interactions</u> .

- Second step is shape and size design. The shape and size of the nanorobot should be designed according to the desired function and target. For example, spherical nanorobots can be used for drug delivery, rod-shaped nanorobots can be used for cell penetration, or helical nanorobots can be used for propulsion. Some of the challenges in shape and size design are optimizing the geometry and dimensions of the nanorobot for maximum performance, minimizing the drag and friction forces on the nanorobot, and avoiding aggregation or clearance of the nanorobot by the immune system. <u>One possible solution is to use computer-aided design (CAD) tools to model and simulate the nanorobot shape and size under different conditions and scenarios</u> .

- Third step is functional component attachment.The functional components are the parts of the nanorobot that enable sensing, actuation, communication, or drug release. These components can be derived from natural biomolecules, such as antibodies, enzymes, DNA, or peptides, or from synthetic materials, such as magnetic nanoparticles, quantum dots, or organic molecules. Some of the challenges in functional component attachment are selecting the appropriate components for the specific function and target, ensuring the compatibility and functionality of the components with the nanorobot body and the biological environment, and controlling the number and location of the components on the nanorobot surface. <u>One possible solution is to use self-assembly methods to attach the functional components to the nanorobot body through specific molecular interactions, such as DNA hybridization, antigen-antibody binding, or enzyme-substrate recognition</u> .

- Fourth step is fabrication. The fabrication of nanorobots involves creating large quantities of nanorobots with consistent quality and functionality. Some of the fabrication techniques are self-assembly, chemical synthesis,lithography, or 3D printing. Some of the challenges in nanorobot fabrication are scaling up the production process, ensuring the accuracy and precision of the fabrication technique, reducing the cost and time of fabrication, and avoiding contamination or defects in the nanorobots. One possible solution is to use biological systems, such as bacteria,viruses,cells, or enzymes, as templates or factories for nanorobot fabrication. <u>These biological systems can provide natural scaffolds or mechanisms for assembling or synthesizing nanorobots with high efficiency and specificity</u> .

- Fifth test is nanorobot testing. The testing of nanorobots involves evaluating their performance and safety in vitro and in vivo using relevant models and methods. For example, optical microscopy, fluorescence imaging, magnetic resonance imaging, or ultrasound imaging can be used to monitor the location and movement of the nanorobots. Cell culture, animal models, or human trials can be used to evaluate the efficacy and toxicity of the nanorobots. <u>Some of the challenges in nanorobot testing are measuring and analyzing the behavior and interactions of nanorobots at different scales and levels, ensuring the validity and reliability of the testing models and methods, addressing ethical issues related to animal or human experiments, and complying with regulatory standards and guidelines for clinical applications.</u>

HOW BIO-INSPIRED NANOROBOTS CAN BE USED FOR CANCER DETECTION?

They can be used for cancer detection by performing tasks such as(Wang,2019):

- Navigating through the blood vessels and tissues to reach the tumor site.
- Recognizing and binding to specific cancer cells or markers using molecular recognition or targeting strategies.
- Transmitting signals or data to external devices or receivers using optical, magnetic, electrical, or acoustic methods.
- Delivering contrast agents or tracers to enhance the visibility of cancer cells under various imaging modalities, such as MRI, PET, CT, or ultrasound.
- Collecting samples or biopsies from the tumor tissue for further analysis or diagnosis.

However, using bio-inspired nanorobots for cancer detection is not easy. There are many challenges and limitations that need to be solved, such as:

- Biocompatibility: How to make sure that the nanorobots do not harm the healthy cells or tissues in the body?
- Safety: How to prevent the nanorobots from causing unwanted side effects, such as inflammation, infection, or immune response?
- Specificity: How to ensure that the nanorobots only target the cancer cells or markers and not the normal ones?
- Stability: How to protect the nanorobots from degradation or damage by the body's enzymes or fluids?
- Scalability: How to produce and deliver enough nanorobots for effective cancer detection?

One possible solution to overcome these challenges is to use living cells or biological materials as building blocks for nanorobots. This way, the nanorobots can mimic natural functions and behaviors and avoid being rejected by the body. For example, some researchers have used bacteria as nanorobots that can sense and respond to oxygen levels in the tumor microenvironment. Other researchers have used DNA as nanorobots that can self-assemble into various shapes and perform logic operations. These are some of the examples of how bio-inspired nanorobots can be improved by using living cells or biological materials. However, ethical, social, and regulatory issues also need to be considered before nanorobots can be widely used in clinical settings.

HOW CAN BIO-INSPIRED NANOROBOTS BE DRIVEN BY DIFFERENT METHODS, SUCH AS MAGNETIC FIELDS, LIGHT, ULTRASOUND, CHEMICAL REACTIONS, OR BIOLOGICAL MOTORS? WHAT ARE THE TRADE-OFFS BETWEEN CONTROL, SPEED, AND POWER OF THESE METHODS? WHAT ARE THE BENEFITS AND LIMITATIONS OF THESE APPLICATIONS?

Bio-inspired nanorobots can be driven by different methods depending on their design, size, and function. Some of the common methods are:

Figure 2. Replica of nanorobot

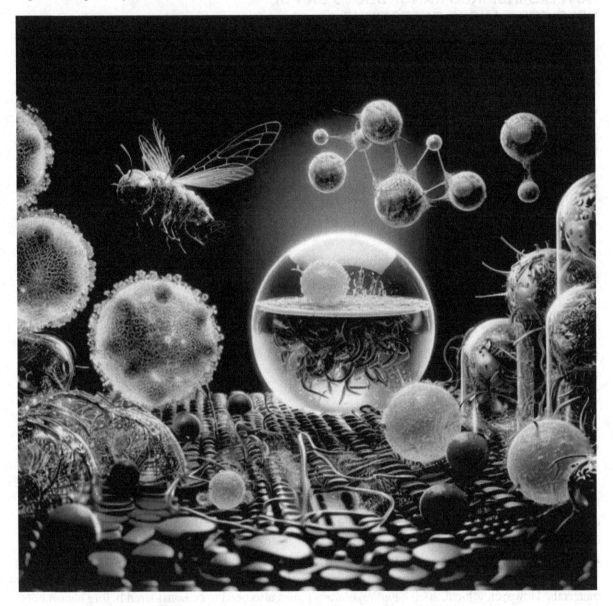

- Magnetic fields: This method uses an external magnetic field to generate torque and force on the nanorobots that have magnetic materials or components(Yan, 2019). The advantages of this method are that it is non-invasive, wireless, and can be controlled remotely and precisely. The disadvantages are that it requires a strong and uniform magnetic field, which may interfere with other devices or biological tissues, and that it may cause heating or damage to the nanorobots or the surrounding environment .
- Light: This method uses light to activate or power the nanorobots that have light-sensitive materials or components, such as photochromic molecules, photovoltaic cells, or optical fibers. The advantages of this method are that it is wireless, biocompatible, and can be modulated by changing

the wavelength, intensity, or direction of the light(Martel,2009). The disadvantages are that it may have limited penetration depth in biological tissues, which may reduce the range and efficiency of the nanorobots, and that it may cause photodamage or photobleaching to the nanorobots or the surrounding environment .

- Ultrasound: This method uses ultrasound waves to generate acoustic radiation force or streaming on the nanorobots that have acoustic materials or components, such as piezoelectric crystals, microbubbles, or microcapsules. The advantages of this method are that it is wireless, biocompatible, and can be focused and steered by changing the frequency, amplitude, or phase of the ultrasound waves. The disadvantages are that it may have limited resolution and accuracy in controlling the nanorobots, and that it may cause cavitation or heating to the nanorobots or the surrounding environment .

- Chemical reactions: This method uses chemical reactions to generate propulsion or power for the nanorobots that have catalytic materials or components, such as metal nanoparticles, enzymes, or fuel molecules. The advantages of this method are that it is self-powered, autonomous, and can be triggered by specific stimuli, such as pH, temperature, or biomolecules. The disadvantages are that it may have limited control and directionality of the nanorobots, and that it may cause toxicity or depletion of the nanorobots or the surrounding environment .

- Biological motors: This method uses biological motors to drive the nanorobots that have biological materials or components, such as flagella, cilia, or muscle cells. The advantages of this method are that it is biocompatible, bio functional, and can be integrated with natural systems. The disadvantages are that it may have limited stability and durability of the nanorobots, and that it may cause immune response or infection to the nanorobots or the surrounding environment .

The trade-offs between control, speed, and power of these methods depend on various factors, such as the design parameters of the nanorobots, the properties of the external fields or stimuli, and the characteristics of the operating environment. Generally speaking, magnetic fields and light offer high control and speed but low power; ultrasound and chemical reactions offer moderate control and speed but high power; biological motors offer low control and speed but moderate power . However, these trade-offs are not fixed and can be optimized by combining different methods or improving the performance of the nanorobots.

HOW CAN BIO-INSPIRED NANOROBOTS BE APPLIED FOR VARIOUS PURPOSES IN CANCER DIAGNOSIS AND THERAPY, SUCH AS DRUG DELIVERY, TUMOR SENSING AND DIAGNOSIS, TARGETED THERAPY, MINIMALLY INVASIVE SURGERY, AND IMMUNOTHERAPY?

Bio-inspired nanorobots are nanoscale devices that mimic the behavior and functions of natural biological systems, such as bacteria, viruses, enzymes, and cells. They can be applied for various purposes in cancer diagnosis and therapy, such as drug delivery, tumor sensing and diagnosis, targeted therapy, minimally invasive surgery, and immunotherapy. Here are some examples of how bio-inspired nanorobots can work in each of these applications:

Figure 3. Application of nanorobot in the cancer diagnosis

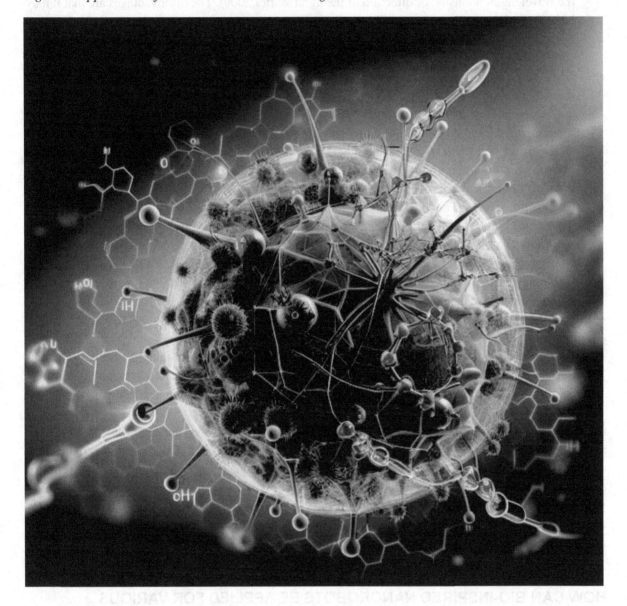

- Drug delivery: Bio-inspired nanorobots can carry anticancer drugs and deliver them to the tumor cells with high precision and efficiency. For example, researchers have invented self-propelling nanorobots that can precisely target and deliver an anticancer drug to human colon cancer cells. The nanorobots are made of magnesium nanoparticles coated with a biocompatible polymer and a layer of red blood cell membranes. The magnesium nanoparticles react with water to produce hydrogen bubbles, which propel the nanorobots toward the tumor cells (Banerjee, 2020). The red blood cell membranes help the nanorobots evade the immune system and recognize the tumor cells by binding to their surface receptors. The nanorobots release the drug slowly at the target cancer cells, enabling the drug to kill cancer cells at a low dose, sparing healthy cells.

The benefit of using bio-inspired nanorobots for drug delivery is that they can enhance the specificity, efficiency, and safety of anticancer drugs. They can target tumor cells with high accuracy, deliver drugs at a controlled rate and dose, and avoid harming healthy cells or causing systemic toxicity. The limitation of this process is that it may face challenges such as immune clearance, biofouling, biodegradation, and drug resistance. The nanorobots may be recognized and eliminated by the immune system, or they may lose their functionality due to the accumulation of biological molecules or the degradation of their materials. The tumor cells may also develop resistance to the drugs delivered by the nanorobots, reducing their effectiveness.

- Tumor sensing and diagnosis: Bio-inspired nanorobots can sense and detect tumor cells in the blood or tissue samples of cancer patients. For example, researchers have designed efficient, light-emitting magnetic nanorobots that can capture circulating tumor cells (CTCs) in the blood samples of cancer patients. The nanorobots are made of iron oxide nanoparticles coated with a fluorescent polymer and antibodies that recognize CTCs. The iron oxide nanoparticles allow the nanorobots to be controlled by a magnetic field and to be separated from the blood sample. The fluorescent polymer emits light when excited by a laser, making the nanorobots visible under a microscope. The antibodies help the nanorobots capture CTCs by binding to their surface antigens. The captured CTCs can be used for further analysis and diagnosis.

The benefit of using bio-inspired nanorobots for tumor sensing and diagnosis is that they can improve the sensitivity, specificity, and speed of cancer detection. They can capture and identify tumor cells or biomarkers in blood or tissue samples with high affinity and selectivity. They can also provide real-time and non-invasive imaging of tumor location and progression. The limitation of this process is that it may encounter difficulties such as low signal-to-noise ratio, interference from background substances, and false-positive or false-negative results. The nanorobots may not be able to generate enough signal or contrast to distinguish tumor cells or biomarkers from normal cells or molecules. They may also be affected by other substances in the biological environment that may interfere with their sensing or imaging functions. They may also fail to capture or detect some tumor cells or biomarkers due to their heterogeneity or variability.

- Targeted therapy: Bio-inspired nanorobots can deliver therapeutic agents or signals to specific tumor cells or tissues, enhancing the efficacy and reducing the side effects of cancer treatment. For example, researchers have developed DNA-based nanorobots that can deliver thrombin molecules to tumor-associated blood vessels, inducing blood clotting and cutting off the blood supply to the tumor (Wavhale,2021). The nanorobots are made of DNA origami structures that fold into hollow tubes with two open ends. One end is closed by a DNA aptamer that binds to nucleolin, a protein overexpressed on the surface of tumor-associated endothelial cells. The other end is loaded with thrombin molecules that are released when the aptamer binds to nucleolin. The thrombin molecules trigger coagulation cascade in the blood vessels, leading to tumor necrosis.

The benefit of using bio-inspired nanorobots for targeted therapy is that they can induce tumor cell death or inhibit tumor growth by delivering therapeutic agents or signals to specific tumor cells or tissues. They can overcome the limitations of conventional therapies such as low efficacy, high toxicity, and adverse effects. They can also achieve synergistic effects by combining different therapeutic modalities such as chemotherapy, radiotherapy, gene therapy, immunotherapy, and phototherapy. The limitation of this process is that it may face challenges such as poor penetration, low retention, and undesired side effects. The nanorobots may not be able to reach deep-seated tumors or diffuse tumors due to the physical barriers or physiological factors in the body. They may also be quickly cleared from the circulation or the tumor site due to their size, shape, charge, or surface properties. They may also cause unwanted side effects such as inflammation, infection, or immunogenicity due to their interaction with the biological system..

- Minimally invasive surgery: Bio-inspired nanorobots can perform surgical tasks in hard-to-reach or delicate body regions, reducing the trauma and risk of infection associated with conventional surgery. For example, researchers have created magnetic helical nanorobots that can drill through biological barriers and remove unwanted tissue or foreign objects. The nanorobots are made of nickel–gold–iron hybrid nanoparticles that form helical shapes under a magnetic field. The magnetic field also controls the rotation and direction of the nanorobots, enabling them to drill through mucus layers or cell membranes. The nanorobots can also carry functional molecules or nanoparticles that can degrade or detach unwanted tissue or foreign objects.

The benefit of using bio-inspired nanorobots for minimally invasive surgery is that they can perform surgical tasks in hard-to-reach or delicate body regions, reducing the trauma and risk of infection associated with conventional surgery. They can drill through biological barriers, remove unwanted tissue or foreign objects, repair damaged tissue or organs, and deliver drugs or biomaterials to the surgical site. They can also provide feedback and guidance for the surgeon during the operation. The limitation of this process is that it may encounter difficulties such as navigation, control, communication, and coordination. The nanorobots may not be able to navigate through complex and dynamic environments in the body due to the lack of reliable sensors or actuators. That may also be difficult to control remotely due to the interference from electromagnetic fields or biological signals. They may also have problems with communication and coordination with other nanorobots or external devices due to the limited bandwidth or power.

- Immunotherapy: Bio-inspired nanorobots can modulate the immune system to fight against cancer cells or prevent tumor recurrence. For example, researchers have fabricated biomimetic nanorobots that can activate dendritic cells (DCs), which are key players in initiating adaptive immune responses. The nanorobots are made of mesoporous silica nanoparticles coated with red blood cell membranes and loaded with antigen peptides and adjuvants. The red blood cell membranes help the nanorobots evade the immune system and target DCs by binding to their surface receptors. The antigen peptides and adjuvants stimulate DCs to mature and present antigens to T cells, which then recognize and kill tumor cells.

The benefit of using bio-inspired nanorobots for immunotherapy is that they can modulate the immune system to fight against cancer cells or prevent tumor recurrence. They can activate or suppress immune cells, enhance or inhibit immune responses, and deliver antigens or adjuvants to elicit specific immune reactions. They can also evade or overcome immune evasion mechanisms of tumor cells such as antigen loss, immunosuppression, or tolerance. The limitation of this process is that it may face challenges such as immunogenicity, immunotoxicity, and autoimmunity. The nanorobots may be recognized and attacked by the immune system, reducing their functionality or causing inflammation. They may also trigger excessive or inappropriate immune responses that may damage normal tissues or organs. They may also induce autoimmune diseases by stimulating self-reactive immune cells.

DEVELOP AND EVALUATE NOVEL BIOSENSING CHIPS THAT CAN CAPTURE AND ISOLATE CIRCULATING TUMOR CELLS FROM BLOOD SAMPLES USING NANOROBOTS

One possible way to develop biosensing chips that can capture and isolate CTCs from blood samples using nanorobots is to use magnetic nanowires as the building blocks of the nanorobots. Magnetic nanowires are thin rods of magnetic materials that can be manipulated by external magnetic fields. They can also be functionalized with antibodies or other molecules that can specifically bind to CTCs. By applying a rotating magnetic field, the magnetic nanowires can form helical structures that can propel themselves in fluid and capture CTCs on their surface (Yan, 2019). The captured CTCs can then be isolated from the blood sample by applying a gradient magnetic field that pulls the nanowires out of the fluid.

To evaluate the performance of the biosensing chips, one could measure the capture efficiency, purity, and viability of the CTCs. Capture efficiency is the ratio of the number of captured CTCs to the number of CTCs in the blood sample. Purity is the ratio of the number of captured CTCs to the number of total cells on the chip. Viability is the percentage of captured CTCs that are alive and functional. These metrics can be assessed by using various techniques, such as fluorescence microscopy, flow cytometry, or polymerase chain reaction (PCR).

How can bio-inspired nanorobots improve the accuracy, sensitivity, specificity, and efficacy of cancer treatment with reduced toxicity and side effects?

Bio-inspired nanorobots are nanoscale devices that mimic the structure and function of natural biological systems, such as bacteria, viruses, or cells. They can improve the accuracy, sensitivity, specificity, and efficacy of cancer treatment with reduced toxicity and side effects by performing the following tasks:

- **Drug delivery**: Bio-inspired nanorobots can carry and deliver large amounts of anti-cancer drugs into cancerous cells without harming healthy cells, reducing the side effects related to current therapies such as chemotherapy damage. For example, researchers have designed nanorobots that can self-assemble into helical structures that can propel themselves in fluid and capture circulating tumor cells (CTCs) on their surface. The captured CTCs can then be isolated from the blood sample by applying a gradient magnetic field that pulls the nanorobots out of the fluid.

- **Tumor sensing and diagnosis**: Bio-inspired nanorobots can detect and measure biological signals, such as DNA, proteins, or cells, that are associated with cancer. They can also provide real-time feedback and imaging of the tumor microenvironment. For example, researchers have developed nanorobots that can use DNA origami to fold into tubular structures that can recognize and bind to specific nucleic acid sequences on the surface of cancer cells. The binding triggers a conformational change in the nanorobots that exposes a fluorescent dye for optical detection.

- **Targeted therapy**: Bio-inspired nanorobots can selectively destroy cancer cells by using various mechanisms, such as mechanical drilling, thermal ablation, or gene editing. For example, researchers have used nanorobots to drill into cancer cells, killing them in just 60 seconds. They are now experimenting on micro-organisms and small fish, before moving on to rodents (Martel,

2009). <u>Clinical trials in humans are expected to follow and it is hoped that the results may have the potential to save millions of lives.</u>

- **Minimally invasive surgery**: <u>Bio-inspired nanorobots can perform surgical tasks at the nanoscale, such as cutting, suturing, or removing tissue, with minimal damage to the surrounding healthy tissue. For example, researchers have proposed nanorobots that can use carbon nanotubes as surgical blades to cut through tissue with high precision and low friction.</u>

THE ADVANTAGES AND DISADVANTAGES OF DIFFERENT MATERIALS, SHAPES, SIZES, AND BIOCOMPATIBILITY OF BIO-INSPIRED NANOROBOTS FOR THE TOPIC BIO-INSPIRED NANOROBOTS FOR CANCER DIAGNOSIS AND THERAPY

Some of the advantages and disadvantages of different materials, shapes, sizes, and biocompatibility of bio-inspired nanorobots for cancer diagnosis and therapy (Datta, 2022):

- **Materials**: Different materials can be used to make bio-inspired nanorobots, depending on what they are supposed to do and where they are going to be used. For instance, nanorobots made of metals can be good for optical or thermal applications, such as finding or destroying cancer cells with light or heat. But metal nanorobots may not be very friendly to the body and may cause harm by releasing metal ions or causing oxidative stress. So, metal nanorobots need to be covered with biocompatible materials or made by green methods to make them safer. Another example is nanorobots made of polymers, which can be good for drug delivery applications, as they can hold and release drugs in a controlled way. Polymer nanorobots can also change their behavior according to different stimuli, such as pH, temperature, light, or magnetic fields. But polymer nanorobots may not last long and degrade in biological environments. So polymer nanorobots need to be adjusted for their physical and chemical properties and biodegradability. A third example is nanorobots made of DNA, which can be good for tumor sensing and targeted therapy applications. DNA nanorobots can form various shapes and structures that can recognize and bind to specific DNA sequences on the surface of cancer cells. When the nanorobots bind to their targets, they change their shape and show a bright dye for optical detection or a gene-editing tool for therapeutic delivery. But DNA nanorobots may not be stable and specific in complex biological fluids due to nuclease degradation or off-target binding. So, DNA nanorobots need to be protected by chemical modifications or encapsulation.
- **Shapes**: The shape of the nanorobots can vary, such as round, stick-like, tube-like, spiral, or complex shapes. The shape influences how they move and interact in fluid environments and with biological components, such as cells, proteins, or receptors. For instance, round nanorobots move easily and quickly in fluids because they have low drag force and high diffusion coefficient. But round nanorobots may not enter cells well because they have low aspect ratio and surface area. So round nanorobots may need to have targeting ligands or stimuli-responsive moieties on their surface to improve their cellular uptake. Another example is stick-like or tube-like nanorobots that have high aspect ratio and surface area that can help them enter cells better. But stick-like or tube-like nanorobots move slowly and hard in fluids because they have high drag force and low diffusion coefficient. So, stick-like or tube-like nanorobots may need to be controlled by external forces

or self-propelling mechanisms to overcome the hydrodynamic resistance. A third example is spiral nanorobots that can copy the structure and function of natural spiral microorganisms. Spiral nanorobots can move themselves in fluids by spinning under external magnetic fields. Spiral nanorobots can also catch circulating tumor cells on their surface by applying a gradient magnetic field that pulls them out of the fluid. But spiral nanorobots may have complex fabrication process and low biocompatibility because of their metallic components. So spiral nanorobots need to be covered with biocompatible materials or made by green methods to make them safer.

- **Sizes**: The nanorobots can be different sizes from a few nanometers to a few micrometers. The size influences how they spread, move, and leave in the body. The size also influences how they interact with biological obstacles, such as blood vessels, tumor environment, and immune system. For instance, tiny nanorobots (smaller than 10 nm) move easily and quickly in fluids because they have low drag force and high diffusion coefficient. But tiny nanorobots may not last long and stay in the body because they are quickly removed by kidney filtration or phagocytosis. So tiny nanorobots may need to have stealth agents or targeting ligands on their surface to increase their circulation time and tumor accumulation. Another example is big nanorobots (bigger than 100 nm) move slowly and hard in fluids because they have high drag force and low diffusion coefficient. But big nanorobots may last long and stay in the body because they are less removed by kidney filtration or phagocytosis. So big nanorobots may need to be made to overcome the biological obstacles such as the endothelial gaps, the extracellular matrix, and the interstitial pressure that prevent their tumor penetration and delivery. A third example is medium-sized nanorobots (between 10 and 100 nm) that can balance the trade-off between lasting long and being removed in the body. Medium-sized nanorobots can also use the enhanced permeability and retention (EPR) effect that lets them passively accumulate in tumor tissues due to the leaky blood vessels and impaired lymphatic drainage. But medium-sized nanorobots may have different and unpredictable EPR effect depending on the tumor type, location, and stage. So medium-sized nanorobots may need to be combined with active targeting strategies or stimuli-responsive mechanisms to improve their tumor specificity and efficacy.

- **Biocompatibility:** The nanorobots need to be highly biocompatible to avoid causing harm such as toxicity, inflammation, immunogenicity, or thrombogenicity in the body. Biocompatibility depends on how the nanorobots look and behave, such as their material, shape, size, and surface functionalization. For instance, nanorobots made of materials that can break down or are friendly to the body, such as polymers, lipids, proteins, or DNA, can reduce their toxicity and immunogenicity. But these nanorobots may not last long and work well in the body because they can be degraded or denatured by biological factors. So, these nanorobots need to be adjusted for their physical and chemical properties and biodegradability. Another example is nanorobots made of materials that do not break down or are not friendly to the body, such as metals or synthetic polymers, can last long and work well in the body. But these nanorobots may cause high toxicity and immunogenicity because they can accumulate or be recognized by biological components. So these nanorobots need to be covered with biocompatible materials or made by green methods to make them safer. A third example is nanorobots with different shapes and sizes that can affect their biocompatibility. Nanorobots that are round and tiny can reduce their inflammation and thrombogenicity because they have low interaction with blood components. But these nanorobots may not enter cells well and reach tumor tissues because they have low aspect ratio and surface area. So these nanorobots may need to have targeting ligands or stimuli-responsive moieties on their surface to improve their cellular uptake and tumor accumulation. On the other hand, nanorobots that are stick-like, tube-like, spiral, or complex shapes and big sizes can enter cells well and reach tumor tissues because they have high aspect ratio and surface area. But these nanorobots may cause high inflammation and thrombogenicity because they have high interaction with blood components. So, these nanorobots may need to have stealth agents or anti-coagulants on their surface to reduce their inflammation and thrombogenicity.

BIONANO ROBOTS FOR CANCER THERAPY: A FOE OR A FRIEND?

Cancer is one of the leading causes of death worldwide, and despite the advances in diagnosis and treatment, it remains a major challenge for medicine (Mavroidis, 2013). Nanotechnology, the manipulation of matter at the nanoscale, offers new possibilities for improving cancer therapy. Among the various nanomaterials, bionano robots, or biohybrid nanomachines, are emerging as a promising and innovative approach. Bionano robots are composed of biological components, such as cells, proteins, or DNA, integrated with synthetic materials, such as metals, polymers, or carbon nanotubes. These hybrid structures can perform specific functions, such as sensing, targeting, drug delivery, or imaging, in response to external stimuli or environmental cues (Webster, 2012). Bionano robots have the potential to overcome some of the limitations of conventional cancer therapies, such as low specificity, systemic toxicity, drug resistance, or poor penetration. However, bionano robots also pose significant challenges and risks for their clinical application. The safety, biocompatibility, stability, and ethical implications of bionano robots need to be carefully evaluated before they can be used in humans. Moreover, the regulation and standardization of bionano robots are still lacking and require further development. Therefore, bionano robots for cancer therapy can be seen as both a foe and a friend, depending on how they are designed, used, and controlled (Elsevier, 2012).

FUTURE DIRECTIONS

Bio-inspired nanorobots are a promising field of research that aims to create nanoscale devices that can perform various tasks in the human body (Fan, 2020), such as cancer diagnosis and treatment. Some of the future directions of bio-inspired nanorobots for cancer diagnosis are:

- Developing nanorobots that can harvest energy from the body or external sources, such as light, magnetic fields, or ultrasound, to power their functions and movements.
- Designing nanorobots that can sense and respond to specific stimuli in the tumor microenvironment (Kong,2023), such as pH, temperature, enzymes, or biomarkers, to activate their diagnostic or therapeutic actions.
- Integrating nanorobots with biosensors, imaging agents, or drug delivery systems to enable simultaneous detection and treatment of cancer cells.
- Creating nanorobots that can self-assemble, self-repair, or self-destruct after completing their tasks to avoid accumulation or toxicity in the body.
- Exploring the use of living cells or biological materials as building blocks for nanorobots that can mimic natural functions and behaviors.

These are some of the possible ways that bio-inspired nanorobots can advance the field of cancer diagnosis and treatment in the future. However, there are also many challenges and limitations that need to be overcome, such as ensuring biocompatibility, safety, specificity, stability, and scalability of nanorobots. Moreover, ethical, social, and regulatory issues also need to be addressed before nanorobots can be widely applied in clinical settings.

CONCLUSION

Bio-inspired nanorobots are a promising approach for cancer diagnosis and therapy, as they can mimic the natural functions of biological systems and interact with the tumor microenvironment. In this paper, we reviewed the recent advances in the design, fabrication, and evaluation of bio-inspired nanorobots for cancer applications(Grumezescu, 2016). We discussed the advantages and challenges of different types of bio-inspired nanorobots, such as DNA origami, bacterial, enzymatic, and cell-based nanorobots. We also highlighted the potential clinical implications and future directions of bio-inspired nanorobotics for cancer management (Jiang, 2010). We concluded that bio-inspired nanorobots have great potential to revolutionize cancer diagnosis and therapy, but they also face significant technical and ethical hurdles that need to be overcome before they can be translated into clinical practice.

REFERENCES

Banerjee, S. S., Andhari, S. S., Wavhale, R. D., Dhobale, K. D., Tawade, B. V., Chate, G. P., & Khandare, J. J. (2020). Self-propelling targeted magneto-nanobots for deep tumor penetration and pH-responsive intracellular drug delivery. *Scientific Reports*, *10*(1), 1–14. PMID:31913322

Cavalcanti, A., Shirinzadeh, B., Freitas, R. A. Jr, & Hogg, T. (2008). Nanorobot architecture for medical target identification. *Nanomedicine; Nanotechnology, Biology, and Medicine*, *4*(2), 134–152. PMID:18455965

Cavalcanti, A., Shirinzadeh, B., Freitas, R. A. Jr, & Hogg, T. (2008). Nanorobot architecture for medical target identification. *Nanomedicine; Nanotechnology, Biology, and Medicine*, *4*(2), 134–152. PMID:18455965

Datta Burton, S. (2022). Not Anytime Soon: The Clinical Translation of Nanorobots and Its Biocompat-ibility Constraints. In *Interactive Robotics: Legal, Ethical, Social and Economic Aspects* (pp. 123–136). Springer. doi:10.1007/978-3-031-04305-5_35

Jiang, L., & Feng, L. (Eds.). (2010). *Bioinspired Intelligent Nanostructured Interfacial Materials*. Springer. doi:10.1142/7380

Martel, S., Mohammadi, M., Felfoul, O., Lu, Z., & Pouponneau, P. (2009). Flagellated magnetotactic bacteria as controlled MRI-trackable propulsion and steering systems for medical nanorobots operating in the human microvasculature. *The International Journal of Robotics Research*, *28*(4), 571–582. doi:10.1177/0278364908100924 PMID:19890435

Martel, S., Mohammadi, M., Felfoul, O., Lu, Z., & Pouponneau, P. (2009). Flagellated magnetotactic bacteria as controlled MRI-trackable propulsion and steering systems for medical nanorobots operating in the human microvasculature. *The International Journal of Robotics Research*, 28(4), 571–582. doi:10.1177/0278364908100924 PMID:19890435

Nanobiomaterials in Drug Delivery. (2016). *Applications of Nanobiomaterials* (A. M. Grumezescu, Ed.). Vol. 9). Elsevier.

Wang, J., & Lee, J. (2019). Bioinspired Nanorobots for Cancer Detection and Therapy. In *Bioinspired Nanomaterials and Nanostructures from Nanobiology to Nanomedicine* (pp. 1–31). Springer.

Wavhale, R. D., Andhari, S. S., Dhobale, K. D., Tawade, B. V., Chate, G. P., Patil, Y. N., ... Banerjee, S. S. (2021). Self-propelling magnetic nanorobots for capturing circulating tumor cells in blood samples of cancer patients. *Communications Chemistry*, 4(1), 1–12. PMID:36697560

Yan, H., & Fan, C. (2019). DNA nanotechnology and its biological applications. In D. N. A. Nanotechnology (Ed.), (pp. 1–22). Springer.

Yan, H., & Fan, C. (2019). DNA nanotechnology and its biological applications. In D. N. A. Nanotechnology (Ed.), (pp. 1–22). Springer.

Chapter 13
Advanced Biomimetic Compound Continuum Robot for Minimally Invasive Surgical Applications

Ranjit Barua

(iD) https://orcid.org/0000-0003-2236-3876

Omdayal Group of Institutions, India

ABSTRACT

the bio-inspired compound continuum robot represents a groundbreaking innovation in the realm of minimally invasive surgery (MIS). Drawing inspiration from the flexibility and adaptability observed in nature, this robotic system employs a novel approach to navigating complex anatomical structures with enhanced precision. Mimicking the serpentine motion of snakes, the robot utilizes a compound continuum structure composed of interconnected segments. This design allows for unparalleled maneuverability, enabling the robot to navigate through confined spaces and intricate pathways within the human body. By emulating the biomechanics of natural organisms, the robot can reach anatomical locations that traditional rigid instruments might struggle to access. In this chapter, the authors will discuss the advanced biomimetic compound continuum robot for minimally invasive surgical applications.

INTRODUCTION

The Biomimetic Compound Continuum Robot represents a groundbreaking fusion of robotics and biomimicry, revolutionizing the landscape of minimally invasive surgery (MIS) (Zhang et al., 2022). Drawing inspiration from nature's adaptability, this innovative robotic system is designed to navigate complex anatomical structures with unparalleled precision and flexibility (Barua et al., 2022) (Li et al., 2013). The Advanced Biomimetic Compound Continuum Robot (ABCCR) has emerged as a transformative force in modern minimally invasive surgery, revolutionizing the way surgeons approach and perform intricate procedures. With its soft and flexible structure, inspired by the biomechanics of natural organ-

DOI: 10.4018/979-8-3693-1962-8.ch013

isms, ABCCR addresses key challenges associated with traditional rigid surgical instruments, offering significant advantages in terms of precision, maneuverability, and patient outcomes. One of the primary contributions of ABCCR to minimally invasive surgery lies in its ability to navigate through confined and delicate anatomical structures with unparalleled flexibility (Zhang et al., 2022). Unlike conventional rigid tools, ABCCR's snake-like motion enables it to access hard-to-reach areas, reducing the need for large incisions. This minimizes trauma to surrounding tissues, decreases postoperative pain, and accelerates patient recovery. The biomimetic design of ABCCR is particularly advantageous in procedures where intricate movements are required. In tasks such as suturing, tissue manipulation, and dissection, the robot's adaptability allows surgeons to replicate the nuanced dexterity of their hands with greater precision (Li et al., 2013). This is crucial in surgeries involving complex anatomical structures or procedures requiring meticulous attention to detail. The integration of advanced control systems and machine learning further enhances ABCCR's performance in the surgical arena. Surgeons can manipulate the robot with a high degree of accuracy, aided by real-time feedback from sensors and cameras embedded in the robot (Barua et al., 2022). Additionally, machine learning algorithms enable the robot to learn from each procedure, optimizing its movements and responses over time, ultimately contributing to improved surgical outcomes (Zhang et al., 2022). The impact of ABCCR in modern minimally invasive surgery extends beyond traditional procedures to include novel applications (Barua et al., 2022). For instance, in interventions requiring access to challenging locations, such as brain surgeries or procedures involving intricate vascular structures, ABCCR proves to be an invaluable asset. Its ability to navigate tight spaces and adapt to the contours of the human body makes it a versatile tool for a wide range of surgical specialties. As ABCCR continues to evolve, ongoing research and development promise even greater advancements in its capabilities. The seamless integration of this biomimetic robot into the surgical workflow underscores its potential to redefine the standard of care in minimally invasive surgery, offering patients safer procedures, faster recovery times, and improved overall outcomes. In the modern era of surgical innovation, ABCCR stands as a testament to the successful fusion of nature-inspired design and cutting-edge technology in the service of advancing medical practice.

REVIEWS OF THE LITERATURE

The advanced biomimetic compound continuum robot (ABCCR) represents a revolutionary leap in the field of robotics, drawing inspiration from nature to create a versatile and adaptive robotic system. Its development has been marked by a series of breakthroughs and innovations, transforming the landscape of robotics and opening up new possibilities for applications in various fields (Barua et al., 2022). The roots of ABCCR can be traced back to the early 21st century when researchers began exploring the concept of soft robotics. Traditional rigid robots faced limitations in terms of flexibility, adaptability, and safety. Soft robotics, inspired by the flexibility and resilience of biological organisms, aimed to overcome these challenges (Zhang et al., 2022). This laid the foundation for the development of continuum robots, which emulate the structure and motion of natural organisms. In the early stages of ABCCR development, researchers drew inspiration from the biomechanics of animals like octopuses and snakes. These creatures exhibit exceptional flexibility and dexterity, allowing them to navigate complex environments with ease. The idea was to create a robot that could mimic the continuous, snake-like motion while maintaining the ability to deform and adapt to its surroundings (Li et al., 2013) (Datta et al., 2023). The breakthrough came with the integration of biomimetic materials and advanced control systems. Researchers focused on developing flexible materials that could withstand various environmental conditions and deform without losing structural integrity (Barua et al., 2023) (Anderson et al., 1970). The incorporation of smart materials, such as shape-memory alloys and soft polymers, allowed the robot to bend and twist in ways that were previously unattainable with traditional rigid structures.

The control system of ABCCR was equally crucial to its success. Advanced algorithms enabled precise control of the robot's movements, allowing it to navigate tight spaces and execute complex tasks (Anderson et al., 1970). Machine learning played a significant role, as the robot could adapt and learn from its interactions with the environment, continuously improving its performance over time. As the technology matured, ABCCR found applications in a wide range of fields. In the medical industry, the robot's ability to navigate through delicate and confined spaces made it invaluable for minimally invasive surgeries. Its soft and flexible structure reduced the risk of tissue damage and improved patient recovery times. Surgeons could now perform intricate procedures with unprecedented precision. In search and rescue missions, ABCCR's flexibility allowed it to navigate through rubble and debris, reaching areas inaccessible to traditional robots. Equipped with sensors and cameras, the robot became an essential tool for locating and assisting survivors in disaster-stricken environments. Its adaptability to unpredictable terrains made it a game-changer in emergency response scenarios. The industrial sector also embraced ABCCR for tasks that required precision and flexibility (Zhang et al., 2022). The robot's dexterity made it suitable for intricate assembly processes, and its ability to reach confined spaces increased efficiency in manufacturing. With advancements in automation, ABCCR became an integral part of smart factories, contributing to increased productivity and safety. In the field of exploration, ABCCR demonstrated its capabilities in space missions and underwater exploration. Its adaptability allowed it to traverse uneven surfaces and navigate complex environments, making it an ideal candidate for missions where traditional rigid robots faced limitations. The evolution of ABCCR has been marked by continuous innovation and collaboration across various scientific disciplines. Researchers and engineers worked hand in hand to refine the robot's design, enhance its capabilities, and explore new avenues of application. The synergy of biology, materials science, robotics, and artificial intelligence has propelled ABCCR to the forefront of technological advancements (Li et al., 2013). Looking ahead, the future of ABCCR holds even greater promise. As research continues, the robot is likely to become more sophisticated, with improved sensory capabilities, faster response times, and enhanced adaptability (Barua et al., 2023). The impact of ABCCR on industries, healthcare, and exploration is expected to grow, solidifying its place as a groundbreaking technology that has reshaped the landscape of robotics. Top of Form Biomimicry involves emulating biological systems and processes to inspire technological innovations. In the case of the Biomimetic Compound Continuum Robot, nature serves as the blueprint for its design (Datta et al., 2023) (Barua et al., 2023). The flexible and snake-like movements (Figure 1) observed in various organisms become the basis for creating a robotic system capable of navigating intricate pathways within the human body (Zhang et al., 2022). However, robot manipulators don't always need to be made of rigid linkages. In this study, we address an alternate design possibility: building a robot with a continuous form, or backbone. When compared to the "vertebrate" design of traditional rigid-link robots, these robots, also known as continuum robots, can be thought of as "invertebrate" robots. Continuum robots are able to bend at any point along its structure, as well as frequently stretch or contract and twist (Barua et al., 2023). Their capabilities surpass those of their counterparts with stiff links as a result. In the past, there has been interest in continuous backbone robots since the 1960s. Regarding the initial continuum robot, it seems that the Tensor Arm (Anderson et al., 1970) by Anderson and Horn was the first model documented in the literature. The early version was meant for undersea uses, but it never made it out of the lab.

Initial designs could produce a wide range of shapes, but it soon became apparent that the relationship between the shapes and inputs was extremely complex, considerably more so than for rigid-link robots, and certainly difficult to construct using the computing systems available at the time. Complementary to the aforementioned advancements in hardware, continuum robot modeling, especially with regard to kinematics, saw growth and innovation in the 1990s. "Bottom-up" continuum robot kinematics models were created in a set of papers (Jones et al., 2006) (Gravagne et al., 2000) (Hannan et al., 2003). These works developed backbone kinematics starting from the limitations of physical continuum robot backbones. The first published "top-down" theory of (Chirikjian et al., 1994) can be used to build the models emerging from these "bottom-up" techniques, as is evident. The new models allowed for model-based implementations and consequently real-time computer control of continuum robot shapes because they matched closely to hardware restrictions.

At the heart of the Biomimetic Compound Continuum Robot is its unique compound continuum structure (Russo et al., 2023). Unlike traditional rigid robotic systems, this design mimics the segmented flexibility found in organisms like snakes or invertebrates (Garfjeld Roberts et al., 2023). The robot consists of interconnected segments, allowing it to move with a serpentine motion. This inherent flexibility enables the robot to navigate through confined spaces and complex anatomical structures, providing surgeons with a tool capable of reaching locations that were once challenging with conventional surgical instruments (Barua et al., 2023).Minimally invasive surgery (MIS) has become a preferred approach due to its potential for reduced postoperative pain, shorter recovery times, and smaller incisions (Zhu et al., 2023) (Barua et al., 2023). The Biomimetic Compound Continuum Robot takes these advantages a step further by minimizing tissue trauma during surgery (Das et al., 2023) (Datta et al., 2023). The segmented structure allows the robot to adapt to the contours of the body, reducing the risk of damage to surrounding tissues (Wei et al., 2023). This feature is particularly crucial in delicate procedures where precision is paramount (Waidi et al., 2023). The applications of the Biomimetic Compound Continuum Robot are diverse, spanning various surgical specialties (Zhang et al., 2022) (Dupont et al., 2022). This innovative robotic system, inspired by the flexibility and adaptability of natural organisms, introduces new possibilities for surgical interventions across various medical specialties (Barua et al., 2022). One of the key features of the Biomimetic Compound Continuum Robot (Figure 2) is its ability to achieve

Figure 1. The robotic system attains unparalleled dexterity by leveraging the biological framework inspired by bionic snakes
(Zhang et al., 2022).

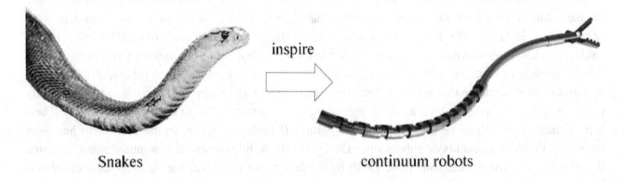

Snakes   continuum robots

precise navigation within the human body (Wei et al., 2022). Surgeons can remotely control the robot, guiding it with a high degree of accuracy to the targeted surgical site (Morton et al., 2022). The biomimetic design enables the robot to traverse challenging anatomical pathways, making it suitable for a wide range of surgical applications (Barua et al., 2023).

MINIMALLY INVASIVE SURGERY (MIS)

Minimally Invasive Surgery (MIS) has emerged as a transformative approach to medical interventions, revolutionizing the field of surgery over the past few decades (Chen et al., 2022). This essay explores the evolution, techniques, benefits, challenges, and future prospects of minimally invasive procedures, shedding light on the profound impact they have had on patient outcomes and the practice of surgery (Barua et al., 2020) (Li et al., 2021).

Figure 2. The configuration of the compound continuum robot is depicted as follows: (a) The overarching structure, (b) The cable-driven mode and radial dimensions of the robot, and (c) The axial dimensions of the robot joints
(Wei et al., 2022)

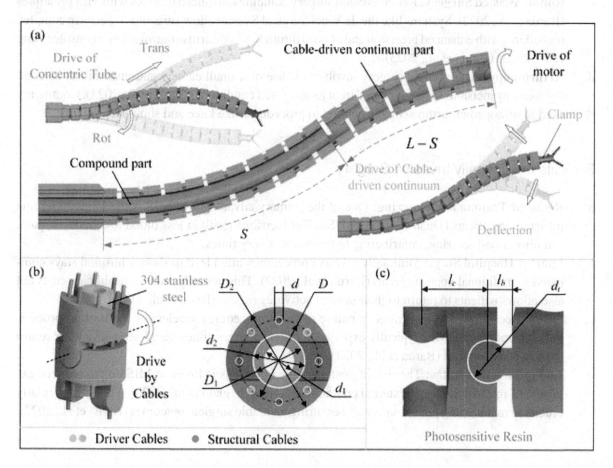

Evolution of Minimally Invasive Surgery

The roots of minimally invasive techniques can be traced back to the early 20th century with the advent of laparoscopy (Morizane et al., 2023) (Shimizu et al., 2022). However, it wasn't until the latter half of the century that technological advancements allowed for the widespread adoption of minimally invasive procedures (Barua et al., 2023) (Azizi et al., 2018). The development of fiber-optic technology, video cameras, and improved instrumentation paved the way for more sophisticated and less invasive surgical approaches.

Techniques in Minimally Invasive Surgery

a. **Laparoscopy:** Laparoscopy, also known as keyhole surgery, involves making small incisions through which a laparoscope and specialized instruments are inserted (Shimizu et al., 2022). It is commonly used in abdominal and pelvic surgeries, such as cholecystectomy, appendectomy, and hysterectomy (Barua et al., 2021).
b. **Endoscopy:** Endoscopic procedures involve the use of a flexible tube with a light and camera (endoscope) to visualize and operate within the body (Siau et al., 2019). Gastrointestinal endoscopy, bronchoscopy, and cystoscopy are examples of endoscopic techniques widely employed in diagnostic and therapeutic interventions.
c. **Robot-Assisted Surgery:** Robot-assisted surgery combines advanced robotics with MIS principles (Barua et al., 2022). Systems like the da Vinci Surgical System allow surgeons to perform complex procedures with enhanced precision and control through robotic arms controlled by a console (Yang et al., 2023) (Barua et al., 2023).
d. **Arthroscopy:** Arthroscopic surgery involves the use of a small camera and instruments inserted through tiny incisions to diagnose and treat joint-related conditions (Barua et al., 2023). Commonly used in orthopedics, arthroscopy is applied to procedures like knee and shoulder surgeries.

Benefits of Minimally Invasive Surgery

a. **Reduced Trauma and Scarring:** One of the primary advantages of MIS is the minimal trauma inflicted on patients (Duan et al., 2023). Smaller incisions result in less blood loss, reduced pain, and diminished scarring, contributing to quicker recovery times.
b. **Shorter Hospital Stays:** Minimally invasive procedures often lead to shorter hospital stays compared to traditional open surgeries (Barua et al., 2022). This not only reduces healthcare costs but also allows patients to return to their normal activities sooner [Datta et al., 2018].
c. **Faster Recovery:** The less invasive nature of these procedures accelerates the healing process. Patients undergoing MIS typically experience faster recovery times, facilitating a quicker return to their daily routines (Barua et al., 2023).
d. **Lower Infection Rates:** The risk of postoperative infections is lower in MIS due to reduced exposure of internal tissues to external contaminants [Marchegiani et al., 2023]. This is particularly crucial in maintaining patient safety and ensuring favorable surgical outcomes (Barua et al., 2022).

Figure 3. Minimally invasive surgery
(Azizi et al., 2018)

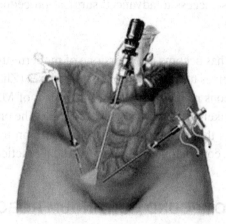

Challenges and Limitations

While minimally invasive surgery has transformed the field of surgery, it is not without challenges:

a. **Learning Curve:** Adopting MIS techniques requires specialized training and a steep learning curve for surgeons. Proficiency in manipulating instruments through small incisions or using robotic interfaces demands dedicated practice (Datta et al., 2023).

b. **Costs and Equipment:** The initial costs associated with acquiring and maintaining advanced equipment for MIS, such as robotic surgical systems, can be substantial. However, the long-term benefits in terms of patient outcomes and reduced postoperative care may offset these costs.

c. **Limited Application in Complex Cases:** In some complex surgeries or cases with anatomical challenges, traditional open procedures may still be preferred (Duan et al., 2023). The adaptability of MIS to all surgical scenarios is an ongoing area of research and development.

Future Prospects of MIS

The future of minimally invasive surgery holds exciting possibilities:

a. **Technological Advancements:** Continued technological innovations, including improved imaging, enhanced robotics, and smarter instrumentation, will further refine MIS techniques, making them more accessible and efficient.

b. **Integration of Artificial Intelligence (AI):** The integration of AI in MIS can contribute to real-time decision-making, automated assistance during surgery, and personalized treatment plans, enhancing the precision and effectiveness of these procedures (Barua et al., 2023).

c. **Expanding Surgical Specialties:** As technology evolves, the application of MIS is expected to expand into various surgical specialties (Yang et al., 2023). Ongoing research explores its feasibility in areas such as cardiac surgery, neurosurgery, and vascular surgery.

d.   **Global Access to Advanced Surgery:** The development of cost-effective and portable MIS technologies could increase access to advanced surgical procedures in resource-limited settings, benefiting patients worldwide.

Minimally Invasive Surgery has become a cornerstone of modern surgical practice, offering patients safer and more efficient alternatives to traditional open procedures (Zhang et al., 2022). As technology continues to advance and surgeons refine their skills, the impact of MIS on patient outcomes and the overall healthcare landscape is likely to grow (Yang et al., 2023). The ongoing commitment to research, training, and innovation ensures that the future holds even more promising developments, cementing minimally invasive surgery as a cornerstone of modern medical practice.

WHAT IS BIOMIMETIC COMPOUND CONTINUUM ROBOT?

The term "Biomimetic Compound Continuum Robot" refers to a type of robotic system designed for various applications, particularly in the field of minimally invasive surgery (MIS) (Zhang et al., 2022). Let's break down the key components of this term to understand its meaning:

Biomimetic

"Biomimetic" means imitating or inspired by biological systems and processes found in nature. In the context of robotics, biomimicry involves designing machines that replicate or mimic the form, function, or behavior of living organisms (Zhang et al., 2022).

Compound Continuum

"Compound continuum" refers to a flexible and segmented structure that allows for continuous, snake-like motion (Russo et al., 2023). Unlike traditional rigid robots, a continuum robot is characterized by

Figure 4. Surgical instrumentation criteria for surgical procedures
(Zhang et al., 2022)

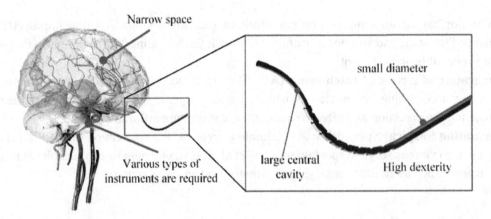

its ability to move in a more flexible and adaptable manner, much like the way some animals, such as snakes or worms, can navigate through confined spaces.

Robot

A "robot" in this context refers to a machine capable of carrying out tasks autonomously or under remote human control (Barua et al., 2023). In the case of the Biomimetic Compound Continuum Robot, the design is inspired by the flexibility and adaptability observed in natural organisms (Datta et al., 2023).

Combining these elements, the Biomimetic Compound Continuum Robot is a robotic system that mimics the flexible and segmented motion seen in certain living organisms [Yang et al., 2023] (Barua et al., 2023). This design is particularly advantageous in applications like minimally invasive surgery, where the robot can navigate through intricate anatomical structures with reduced impact on surrounding tissues (Duan et al., 2023). The term emphasizes the robot's biomimetic inspiration and its compound continuum structure, allowing for more versatile and less invasive movements in various medical and technological scenarios (Li et al., 2021). Here are a few examples of of research prototypes and projects that embody the principles of biomimicry and compound continuum robotics in the context of minimally invasive surgery.

a. **i-Snake:**
   ◦ *Description:* Developed by the European Union-funded project RAS (Robotic Assisted Surgery), i-Snake is a research initiative that explores the use of a flexible robotic system for minimally invasive surgery (Wu et al., 2013). It aims to mimic the dexterity and flexibility of a snake to navigate through complex anatomical structures.

b. **CardioArm:**
   ◦ *Description:* The CardioArm is a robotic catheter system designed for navigating through the cardiovascular system (Wang et al., 2017). Inspired by the agility of snakes, this system allows for precise movements within blood vessels during minimally invasive cardiac procedures.

c. **RoboSnake:**
   ◦ *Description:* RoboSnake is a biomimetic robotic system designed to replicate the undulating motion of snakes (Cuperman et al., 2019). While not exclusively developed for surgery, its bio-inspired design has potential applications in minimally invasive procedures, particularly in navigating confined spaces.

d. **Flex System:**
   ◦ *Description:* The Flex System, developed by FlexDex Surgical, incorporates principles of continuum robotics (Remacle et al., 2015). Although not explicitly biomimetic in its design, it utilizes a flexible robotic arm to enable minimally invasive surgery with enhanced dexterity, providing surgeons with intuitive control.

e. **STIFF-FLOP:**
   ◦ *Description:* STIFF-FLOP (STIFFness controllable Flexible and Learnable manipulator for surgical OPerations) is a research project that focuses on developing a robotic system with a flexible structure inspired by octopus tentacles (Dawood et al., 2021). The aim is to provide surgeons with a tool that can adapt to various surgical scenarios.

Figure 5. Continuum robots: a. Octopus leg); and b. tentacle-inspired
(a), (McMahan et al., 2009); (b), (Sanan et al., 2011)

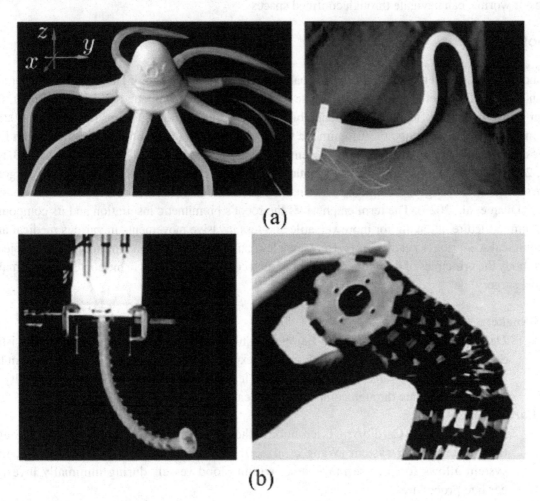

(a)

(b)

APPLICATIONS IN SURGICAL PROCEDURES

The applications of the Biomimetic Compound Continuum Robot span a wide range of surgical procedures (Figure 5), offering transformative capabilities in the field of minimally invasive surgery (MIS) (Zhang et al., 2022). In neurosurgery, where precision and access to intricate structures are critical, the robot's ability to navigate through tight spaces becomes invaluable. Similarly, in abdominal surgeries, the robot's flexibility allows it to reach and manipulate organs with reduced invasiveness.

Neurosurgery

In neurosurgery, where precision and access to delicate structures are paramount, the Biomimetic Compound Continuum Robot demonstrates significant advantages (Burgner-Kahrs et al., 2015). The snake-like motion of the robot allows it to navigate through intricate pathways in the brain with reduced trauma to surrounding tissues. Surgeons can remotely guide the robot to reach specific regions that may be challenging to access using traditional surgical instruments (Zhang et al., 2022). This capability enhances the accuracy of procedures such as tumor removal, biopsies, and the placement of therapeutic devices.

Abdominal Surgery

The flexibility of the compound continuum structure makes the robot well-suited for abdominal surgeries. It can navigate through the confined spaces of the abdominal cavity, providing surgeons with enhanced dexterity in manipulating organs and tissues (Burgner-Kahrs et al., 2015). The reduced invasiveness of the robot contributes to faster recovery times and minimizes postoperative pain. Applications in abdominal surgery include procedures such as laparoscopic cholecystectomy, gastrointestinal surgeries, and organ resections.

Cardiovascular Interventions

In the realm of cardiovascular surgery, the Biomimetic Compound Continuum Robot holds promise for a range of interventions. The robot's ability to navigate through intricate blood vessels with precision is particularly beneficial for procedures such as angioplasty, stent placement, and the treatment of vascular abnormalities (Zhang et al., 2022). The minimally invasive nature of these procedures, facilitated by the robot, reduces the risk of complications and shortens recovery times for patients undergoing cardiovascular interventions.

Gynecological Procedures

Gynecological surgeries, including hysterectomies and ovarian procedures, can benefit from the Biomimetic Compound Continuum Robot. The robot's flexible structure allows it to navigate through the pelvic region with greater ease, providing surgeons with improved access to target areas (Russo et al., 2023). The minimally invasive approach reduces scarring and enhances patient recovery, making it an attractive option for various gynecological interventions (Barua et al., 2023).

Urological Interventions

In urology, the robot's adaptability is valuable for procedures such as prostate surgeries and kidney interventions. Its snake-like motion enables precise navigation through complex anatomical structures, reducing the risk of damage to adjacent tissues (Zhang et al., 2022). The minimally invasive approach enhances patient outcomes by decreasing postoperative pain and shortening hospital stays (Yang et al., 2023). The robot's remote surgical capabilities also contribute to the surgeon's ability to perform intricate procedures with increased precision.

Orthopedic Surgery

The Biomimetic Compound Continuum Robot holds potential in orthopedic surgery, particularly in procedures involving joints and soft tissues. The robot's flexibility allows for precise navigation around bones and articulations, making it suitable for arthroscopic surgeries (Russo et al., 2023). Surgeons can use the robot to access joint spaces and perform repairs with reduced invasiveness, contributing to quicker recovery and improved functional outcomes for patients undergoing orthopedic interventions (Li et al., 2021).

Head and Neck Surgery

In head and neck surgeries, the Biomimetic Compound Continuum Robot offers advantages in accessing challenging anatomical structures (Zhang et al., 2022). Its flexible design allows for maneuverability in confined spaces, making it suitable for procedures such as throat surgeries, tongue base surgeries, and minimally invasive approaches to tumors in the head and neck region. The robot's ability to navigate through complex anatomies enhances the precision of these interventions (Yang et al., 2023).

Ophthalmic Procedures

The robot's adaptability extends to ophthalmic surgeries, where delicate and precise maneuvers are essential (Li et al., 2021). In procedures such as retinal surgeries and cataract removal, the Biomimetic Compound Continuum Robot's snake-like motion provides surgeons with enhanced control and access to intricate ocular structures (Zhang et al., 2022). The minimally invasive nature of the robot contributes to reduced postoperative complications and faster visual recovery for patients undergoing ophthalmic interventions (Chen et al., 2022).

FUTURE IMPLICATIONS AND ETHICAL AND REGULATORY CONSIDERATIONS

As technology continues to advance, the Biomimetic Compound Continuum Robot holds promise for further developments (Barua et al., 2023). The biomimetic compound continuum robot, inspired by nature's adaptability, revolutionizes minimally invasive surgery (Li et al., 2021). This robotic system emulates the flexible and snake-like movements found in biological organisms. Comprising interconnected segments, it navigates complex anatomical structures with precision, reaching confined spaces traditional tools cannot (Yang et al., 2023). Its biomimicry enhances surgical capabilities, reducing tissue trauma and allowing for intricate procedures. Surgeons remotely guide the robot, offering unparalleled dexterity and access (Datta et al., 2023). This innovative technology holds promise for diverse surgical applications, marking a significant advancement in improving patient outcomes through less invasive and more precise interventions.

Continued research and innovation may lead to even more refined and specialized versions of the robot, catering to specific surgical procedures and anatomical challenges (Li et al., 2021). Integration with advanced imaging technologies could enhance the robot's ability to navigate with even greater precision (Yang et al., 2023). The biomimetic approach of the robot contributes to a reduction in patient trauma. The flexibility of its continuum structure minimizes the impact on surrounding tissues, leading to less postoperative pain and faster recovery times. Patients undergoing surgeries assisted by this robotic system may experience shorter hospital stays and quicker returns to daily activities (Li et al., 2021). The Biomimetic Compound Continuum Robot offers the advantage of remote surgical capabilities. Surgeons can operate the robot from a console, providing them with a more ergonomic and comfortable environment (Zhang et al., 2022). This not only enhances the precision of movements but also allows for improved focus during lengthy procedures. The remote control feature is particularly beneficial in situations where the surgical site may be challenging to access directly (Zhang et al., 2022). The introduction of advanced robotic systems in surgery raises ethical and regulatory considerations. Ensuring patient safety, ethical use of technology, and comprehensive training for surgeons are crucial aspects that need careful attention (Yang et al., 2023). Regulatory bodies play a vital role in establishing guidelines and standards to govern the integration of such innovative technologies into clinical practice.

CONCLUSION

The Biomimetic Compound Continuum Robot presents a transformative paradigm in minimally invasive surgery, with diverse applications across multiple medical specialties. Its biomimetic design, inspired by nature's flexibility, provides surgeons with a tool that enhances precision, reduces tissue trauma, and expands the scope of minimally invasive interventions. As technology continues to advance, the robot's applications are likely to grow, offering new possibilities for improving patient outcomes and redefining the future of surgical care. The application of this bio-inspired technology in MIS holds immense promise. Surgeons can remotely control the robot, guiding it with precision to perform targeted medical interventions. The inherent flexibility of the compound continuum structure reduces the risk of tissue damage and trauma during the surgical procedure, contributing to faster recovery times and improved patient outcomes. While the applications of the Biomimetic Compound Continuum Robot are promising, challenges remain in terms of technological refinement, training, and regulatory considerations. Continued research is necessary to optimize the robot's capabilities, ensuring its safety and efficacy in a variety of surgical scenarios. Training programs for surgeons need to be developed to familiarize them with the unique features and operational aspects of the robot. Additionally, regulatory bodies play a crucial role in establishing guidelines and standards for the integration of such advanced robotic systems into clinical practice. Ethical considerations surrounding patient safety, consent, and the responsible use of technology must be addressed to ensure that the benefits of the robot are maximized while minimizing potential risks. Moreover, the robot's adaptability makes it well-suited for a variety of surgical procedures, ranging from delicate neurosurgery to intricate abdominal surgeries. Its ability to access challenging anatomical sites with minimal invasiveness marks a paradigm shift in surgical techniques, paving the way for more effective and patient-friendly procedures. In brief, the Bio-Inspired Compound Continuum Robot represents a remarkable fusion of engineering and biology, revolutionizing the landscape of minimally invasive surgery by providing surgeons with an advanced tool that combines precision, flexibility, and adaptability for improved patient care.

Conflicts of Interest

The authors declare that there are no conflicts of interest regarding the publication of this chapter.

Funding

No funding has been provided for this work.

Ethical approval

Not required.

ACKNOWLEDGEMENTS

The authors would like to thank IIEST Shibpur, and IISc Bengalore, and thanks to Mrs. Nibedita Bardhan for language proof reading.

REFERENCES

Anderson, V. C., & Horn, R. C. (1970). *U.S. Patent No. 3,497,083*. Washington, DC: U.S. Patent and Trademark Office.

Azizi, A., Hortamani, R., & Zabihollah, A. (2018). Sensing the material by minimally invasive surgery grasper. *International Robotics & Automation Journal*, 4(3). doi:10.15406/iratj.2018.04.00117

Barua, R., Bhowmik, S., Dey, A., Das, S., & Datta, S. (2022, September). Analysis of Robotically Controlled Percutaneous Needle Insertion into Ex Vivo Kidney Tissue for Minimally Invasive Percutaneous Nephrolithotomy (PCNL) Surgery. *In International Conference on Emergent Converging Technologies and Biomedical Systems* (pp. 249-257). Singapore: Springer Nature Singapore.

Barua, R., Bhowmik, S., Dey, A., & Mondal, J. (2023). Advances of the Robotics Technology in Modern Minimally Invasive Surgery. In M. Mellal (Ed.), *Design and Control Advances in Robotics* (pp. 91–104). IGI Global.

Barua, R., Das, S., Datta, P., & Chowdhury, A. (2022). Computational FEM Application on Percutaneous Nephrolithotomy (PCNL) Minimum Invasive Surgery Through Needle Insertion Process. In P. Pain, S. Banerjee, & G. Bose (Eds.), *Advances in Computational Approaches in Biomechanics* (pp. 210-222). IGI Global. doi:10.4018/978-1-7998-9078-2.ch013

Barua, R., Das, S., Datta, S., Datta, P., & Roy Chowdhury, A. (2021). Analysis of surgical needle insertion modeling and viscoelastic tissue material interaction for minimally invasive surgery (MIS). *Materials Today: Proceedings*, 57, 259–264. doi:10.1016/j.matpr.2022.02.498

Barua, R., Das, S., Datta, S., Datta, P., & Roy Chowdhury, A. (2023). Study and experimental investigation of insertion force modeling and tissue deformation phenomenon during surgical needle-soft tissue interaction. *Proceedings of the Institution of Mechanical Engineers. Part C, Journal of Mechanical Engineering Science*, 237(5), 1007–1014. doi:10.1177/09544062221126628

Barua, R., Das, S., Datta, S., Roy Chowdhury, A., & Datta, P. (2022). Experimental study of the robotically controlled surgical needle insertion for analysis of the minimum invasive process. In *Emergent Converging Technologies and Biomedical Systems: Select Proceedings of ETBS 2021* (pp. 473-482). Singapore: Springer Singapore. 10.1007/978-981-16-8774-7_38

Barua, R., Das, S., & Mondal, J. (2023). Emerging Applications of Artificial Intelligence (AI) and Machine Learning (ML) in Modern Urology. In R. Queirós, B. Cunha, & X. Fonseca (Eds.), *Exploring the Convergence of Computer and Medical Science Through Cloud Healthcare* (pp. 117–133). IGI Global. doi:10.4018/978-1-6684-5260-8.ch006

Barua, R., Das, S., Roy Chowdhury, A., & Datta, P. (2023). Experimental and simulation investigation of surgical needle insertion into soft tissue mimic biomaterial for minimally invasive surgery (MIS). *Proceedings of the Institution of Mechanical Engineers. Part H, Journal of Engineering in Medicine*, 237(2), 254–264. doi:10.1177/09544119221143860 PMID:36527297

Barua, R., Das, S., RoyChowdhury, A., & Datta, P. (2023). Simulation and experimental investigation of the surgical needle deflection model during the rotational and steady insertion process. *The International Journal of Artificial Organs*, 46(1), 40–51. doi:10.1177/03913988221136154 PMID:36397288

Barua, R., Datta, P., Chowdhury, A. R., & Das, S. (2022). Computational Study of In-Vitro Ureter Urine Flow in DJ Stent. In P. Pain, S. Banerjee, & G. Bose (Eds.), *Advances in Computational Approaches in Biomechanics* (pp. 198–209). IGI Global. doi:10.4018/978-1-7998-9078-2.ch012

Barua, R., & Datta, S. (2022). Study of the surgical needle and biological soft tissue interaction phenomenon during insertion process for medical application: A Survey. *Proceedings of the Institution of Mechanical Engineers, Part H: Journal of Engineering in Medicine, 236*(10), 1465-1477.

Barua, R., & Datta, S. (2023). Emerging Surgical Robotic Applications for Modern Minimally Invasive Surgery (MIS). In M. Habib (Ed.), *Global Perspectives on Robotics and Autonomous Systems: Development and Applications* (pp. 314–332). IGI Global. doi:10.4018/978-1-6684-7791-5.ch014

Barua, R., & Datta, S. (2023). Artificial Intelligence in Modern Medical Science: A Promising Practice. In S. Rajest, B. Singh, A. J. Obaid, R. Regin, & K. Chinnusamy (Eds.), *Recent Developments in Machine and Human Intelligence* (pp. 1–12). IGI Global. doi:10.4018/978-1-6684-9189-8.ch001

Barua, R., Datta, S., & Sarkar, A. (2023). Artificial Intelligence and Robotics-Based Minimally Invasive Surgery: Innovations and Future Perceptions. In G. Karthick & S. Karupusamy (Eds.), *Contemporary Applications of Data Fusion for Advanced Healthcare Informatics* (pp. 350–368). IGI Global. doi:10.4018/978-1-6684-8913-0.ch015

Barua, R., Giria, H., Datta, S., Roy Chowdhury, A., & Datta, P. (2020). Force modeling to develop a novel method for fabrication of hollow channels inside a gel structure. *Proceedings of the Institution of Mechanical Engineers. Part H, Journal of Engineering in Medicine, 234*(2), 223–231. doi:10.1177/0954411919891654 PMID:31774361

Barua, R., & Mondal, J. (2023). Study of the Current Trends of CAD (Computer-Aided Detection) in Modern Medical Imaging. In L. Panigrahi, S. Biswal, A. Bhoi, A. Kalam, & P. Barsocchi (Eds.), *Machine Learning and AI Techniques in Interactive Medical Image Analysis* (pp. 35–50). IGI Global., doi:10.4018/978-1-6684-4671-3.ch002

Barua, R., Sarkar, A., & Datta, S. (2023). Modern Lab-on-Chip Biosensors Application on Infectious COVID-19 Detection. In R. Singh, R. Phanden, B. Sikarwar, & J. Davim (Eds.), *Advances in MEMS and Microfluidic Systems* (pp. 258–270). IGI Global. doi:10.4018/978-1-6684-6952-1.ch013

Burgner-Kahrs, J., Rucker, D. C., & Choset, H. (2015). Continuum robots for medical applications: A survey. *IEEE Transactions on Robotics*, *31*(6), 1261–1280. doi:10.1109/TRO.2015.2489500

Chen, K., Zhang, J., Beeraka, N. M., Sinelnikov, M. Y., Zhang, X., Cao, Y., & Lu, P. (2022). Robot-Assisted Minimally Invasive Breast Surgery: Recent Evidence with Comparative Clinical Outcomes. *Journal of Clinical Medicine*, *11*(7), 1827. doi:10.3390/jcm11071827 PMID:35407434

Chirikjian, G. S. (1994). Hyper-redundant manipulator dynamics: A continuum approximation. *Advanced Robotics*, *9*(3), 217–243. doi:10.1163/156855395X00175

Cuperman, D., & Verner, I. M. (2019). Fostering analogical reasoning through creating robotic models of biological systems. *Journal of Science Education and Technology*, *28*(2), 90–103. doi:10.1007/s10956-018-9750-4

Das, S., Datta, S., Barman, A., & Barua, R. (2023). Smart Biodegradable and Bio-Based Polymeric Biomaterials for Biomedical Applications. In A. Kumar, P. Kumar, A. Srivastava, & V. Goyat (Eds.), *Modeling, Characterization, and Processing of Smart Materials* (pp. 56–82). IGI Global. doi:10.4018/978-1-6684-9224-6.ch003

Datta, S., & Barua, R. (2023). Fluorescent Nanomaterials and Its Application in Biomedical Engineering. In A. Rakha, A. Munawar, V. Khanna, & S. Bansal (Eds.), *Modeling and Simulation of Functional Nanomaterials for Forensic Investigation* (pp. 164–186). IGI Global. doi:10.4018/978-1-6684-8325-1.ch009

Datta, S., & Barua, R. (2023). Advanced Materials for Surgical Tools and Biomedical Implants. *Advanced Materials and Manufacturing Techniques for Biomedical Applications*, 25-35.

Datta, S., Barua, R., & Das, J. (2020). *A review on electro-rheological fluid (er) and its various technological applications*. Extremophilic Microbes and Metabolites-Diversity, Bioprospecting and Biotechnological Applications.

Datta, S., Barua, R., & Das, S. (2023). Role and Challenges of Bioprinting in Bone Tissue Engineering. In R. Ranjith & J. Davim (Eds.), *Handbook of Research on Advanced Functional Materials for Orthopedic Applications* (pp. 205–218). IGI Global. doi:10.4018/978-1-6684-7412-9.ch012

Datta, S., Barua, R., & Prasad, A. (2023). Additive Manufacturing for the Development of Artificial Organs. *Advanced Materials and Manufacturing Techniques for Biomedical Applications*, 411-427.

Datta, S., Barua, R., Sarkar, R., Barui, A., Chowdhury, A. R., & Datta, P. (2018, September). Design and development of alginate: Poly-l-lysine scaffolds by 3D bio printing and studying their mechanical, structural and cell viability properties. []. IOP Publishing.]. *IOP Conference Series. Materials Science and Engineering, 402,* 012113. doi:10.1088/1757-899X/402/1/012113

Datta, S., Das, S., & Barua, R. (2023). Self-Sustained Nanobiomaterials: Innovative Materials for Biomedical Applications. *Advanced Materials and Manufacturing Techniques for Biomedical Applications,* 303-323.

Dawood, A. B., Fras, J., Aljaber, F., Mintz, Y., Arezzo, A., Godaba, H., & Althoefer, K. (2021). Fusing dexterity and perception for soft robot-assisted minimally invasive surgery: What we learnt from STIFF-FLOP. *Applied Sciences (Basel, Switzerland), 11*(14), 6586. doi:10.3390/app11146586

Duan, W., Akinyemi, T., Du, W., Ma, J., Chen, X., Wang, F., Omisore, O., Luo, J., Wang, H., & Wang, L. (2023). Technical and Clinical Progress on Robot-Assisted Endovascular Interventions: A Review. *Micromachines, 14*(1), 197. doi:10.3390/mi14010197 PMID:36677258

Dupont, P. E., Simaan, N., Choset, H., & Rucker, C. (2022). Continuum Robots for Medical Interventions. *Proceedings of the IEEE*. Institute of Electrical and Electronics Engineers.

Garfjeld Roberts, P., Glasbey, J. C., Abram, S., Osei-Bordom, D., Bach, S. P., & Beard, D. J. (2020). Research quality and transparency, outcome measurement and evidence for safety and effectiveness in robot-assisted surgery: Systematic review. *BJS Open, 4*(6), 1084–1099. doi:10.1002/bjs5.50352 PMID:33052029

Gravagne, I., & Walker, I. D. (2000). Kinematics for constrained continuum robots using wavelet decomposition. *Robotics, 2000,* 292–298.

Hannan, M. W., & Walker, I. D. (2003). Kinematics and the implementation of an elephant's trunk manipulator and other continuum style robots. *Journal of Robotic Systems, 20*(2), 45–63. doi:10.1002/rob.10070 PMID:14983840

Jones, B. A., & Walker, I. D. (2006). Kinematics for multisection continuum robots. *IEEE Transactions on Robotics, 22*(1), 43–55. doi:10.1109/TRO.2005.861458

Li, W., Kong, K., Li, P., Wang, G., Cui, B., Zhu, L., & Zhu, S. (2021). Robot-assisted sleeve gastrectomy in patients with obesity with a novel Chinese domestic MicroHand SII surgical system. *BMC Surgery, 21*(1), 260. doi:10.1186/s12893-021-01259-3 PMID:34034737

Li, Z., & Du, R. (2013). Design and analysis of a bio-inspired wire-driven multi-section flexible robot. *International Journal of Advanced Robotic Systems, 10*(4), 209. doi:10.5772/56025

Marchegiani, F., Siragusa, L., Zadoroznyj, A., Laterza, V., Mangana, O., Schena, C. A., Ammendola, M., Memeo, R., Bianchi, P. P., Spinoglio, G., Gavriilidis, P., & de'Angelis, N. (2023). New Robotic Platforms in General Surgery: What's the Current Clinical Scenario? *Medicina (Kaunas, Lithuania), 59*(7), 1264. doi:10.3390/medicina59071264 PMID:37512075

McMahan, W., & Walker, I. D. (2009, February). Octopus-inspired grasp-synergies for continuum manipulators. In *2008 IEEE International Conference on Robotics and Biomimetics* (pp. 945-950). IEEE. 10.1109/ROBIO.2009.4913126

Morizane, S., Stein, H., Komiya, T., Kaneta, H., & Takenaka, A. (2023). Retroperitoneal robot-assisted laparoscopic nephroureterectomy using the da Vinci Xi and SP systems: Initial experiences in cadaveric models. *Investigative and Clinical Urology*, *64*(4), 380–387. doi:10.4111/icu.20230021 PMID:37417563

Morton, J., Hardwick, R. H., Tilney, H. S., Gudgeon, A. M., Jah, A., Stevens, L., Marecik, S., & Slack, M. (2021). Preclinical evaluation of the versius surgical system, a new robot-assisted surgical device for use in minimal access general and colorectal procedures. *Surgical Endoscopy*, *35*(5), 2169–2177. doi:10.1007/s00464-020-07622-4 PMID:32405893

Remacle, M. M. N., Prasad, V., Lawson, G., Plisson, L., Bachy, V., & Van der Vorst, S. (2015). Transoral robotic surgery (TORS) with the Medrobotics Flex™ System: First surgical application on humans. *European Archives of Oto-Rhino-Laryngology*, *272*, 1451–1455. doi:10.1007/s00405-015-3532-x PMID:25663191

Russo, M., Gautreau, E., Bonnet, X., & Laribi, M. A. (2023). Continuum Robots: From Conventional to Customized Performance Indicators. *Biomimetics*, *8*(2), 147. doi:10.3390/biomimetics8020147 PMID:37092399

Sanan, S., Moidel, J., & Atkeson, C. G. (2011, June). A continuum approach to safe robots for physical human interaction. In *International Symposium on Quality of Life Technology*. IEEE.

Schranz, M., Umlauft, M., Sende, M., & Elmenreich, W. (2020). Swarm Robotic Behaviors and Current Applications. *Frontiers in Robotics and AI*, *7*, 36. doi:10.3389/frobt.2020.00036 PMID:33501204

Shimizu, A., Ito, M., & Lefor, A. K. (2022). Laparoscopic and Robot-Assisted Hepatic Surgery: An Historical Review. *Journal of Clinical Medicine*, *11*(12), 3254. doi:10.3390/jcm11123254 PMID:35743324

Siau, K., Hodson, J., Ingram, R., Baxter, A., Widlak, M. M., Sharratt, C., Baker, G. M., Troth, T., Hicken, B., Tahir, F., Magrabi, M., Yousaf, N., Grant, C., Poon, D., Khalil, H., Lee, H. L., White, J. R., Tan, H., Samani, S., & Major, G. (2019). Time to endoscopy for acute upper gastrointestinal bleeding: Results from a prospective multicentre trainee-led audit. *United European Gastroenterology Journal*, *7*(2), 199–209. doi:10.1177/2050640618811491 PMID:31080604

Waidi, Y. O., Barua, R., & Datta, S. (2023). Metals, Polymers, Ceramics, Composites Biomaterials Used in Additive Manufacturing for Biomedical Applications. In A. Kumar, P. Kumar, A. Srivastava, & V. Goyat (Eds.), *Modeling, Characterization, and Processing of Smart Materials* (pp. 165–184). IGI Global. doi:10.4018/978-1-6684-9224-6.ch008

Wang, H., Zhang, R., Chen, W., Wang, X., & Pfeifer, R. (2017). A cable-driven soft robot surgical system for cardiothoracic endoscopic surgery: Preclinical tests in animals. *Surgical Endoscopy*, *31*(8), 3152–3158. doi:10.1007/s00464-016-5340-9 PMID:27858208

Wei, H., Zhang, G., Wang, S., Zhang, P., Su, J., & Du, F. (2023). Coupling Analysis of Compound Continuum Robots for Surgery: Another Line of Thought. *Sensors (Basel)*, *23*(14), 6407. doi:10.3390/s23146407 PMID:37514701

Wu, X., & Ma, S. (2013). Neurally controlled steering for collision-free behavior of a snake robot. *IEEE Transactions on Control Systems Technology*, *21*(6), 2443–2449. doi:10.1109/TCST.2012.2237519

Yang, Y., Li, D., Sun, Y., Wu, M., Su, J., Li, Y., Yu, X., Li, L., & Yu, J. (2023). Muscle-inspired soft robots based on bilateral dielectric elastomer actuators. *Microsystems & Nanoengineering*, *9*(1), 124. doi:10.1038/s41378-023-00592-2 PMID:37814608

Zhang, G., Du, F., Xue, S., Cheng, H., Zhang, X., Song, R., & Li, Y. (2022). Design and Modeling of a Bio-Inspired Compound Continuum Robot for Minimally Invasive Surgery. *Machines*, *10*(6), 468. doi:10.3390/machines10060468

Zhu, J., Lyu, L., Xu, Y., Liang, H., Zhang, X., Ding, H., & Wu, Z. (2021). Intelligent Soft Surgical Robots for Next-Generation Minimally Invasive Surgery. *Advanced Intelligent Systems*, *3*(5), 2100011. doi:10.1002/aisy.202100011

KEY TERMS AND DEFINITIONS

Laparoscope: A laparoscope is a minimally invasive surgical instrument equipped with a thin, flexible tube and a tiny camera that allows surgeons to visualize the inside of the abdominal or pelvic cavity. It is inserted through small incisions, enabling procedures like gallbladder removal, appendectomy, and exploratory surgery with reduced scarring and shorter recovery times compared to traditional open surgery. The camera transmits real-time images to a monitor, guiding surgeons during the procedure, and offering a detailed view of the organs and tissues.

MIS: A medical technique that uses small incisions and specialized tools to perform procedures within the body, reducing the need for large surgical openings. It offers advantages such as faster recovery, less scarring, and reduced risk of complications compared to traditional open surgery.

Robotics: Basically a interdisciplinary field of designing, building, and operating robots. These autonomous or remote-controlled machines perform tasks, often in manufacturing, healthcare, exploration, and more. Utilizing sensors, actuators, and artificial intelligence, robotics aims to enhance efficiency and safety while advancing automation and technology across various industries.

Soft Tissue: Soft tissue refers to a group of connective tissues in the body that includes muscles, tendons, ligaments, fat, and blood vessels. It provides support and flexibility, enabling bodily movements, and plays a crucial role in various bodily functions. Injuries to soft tissues can lead to pain and mobility issues.

Surgical robot: A sophisticated medical device designed to assist surgeons in performing complex procedures with precision. Controlled by a surgeon from a console, these robots use advanced technology, such as robotic arms and cameras, to provide enhanced dexterity, visualization, and minimally invasive capabilities, improving surgical outcomes and patient recovery.

Chapter 14
An Intelligent Robotic Fogger System for Predicting Dengue Outbreaks

D. Raveena Judie Dolly

(iD) https://orcid.org/0000-0001-9837-2213

Karunya Institute of Technology and Sciences, India

D. J Jagannath

Karunya Institute of Technology and Sciences, India

J. Dinesh Peter

(iD) https://orcid.org/0000-0002-4357-7163

Karunya Institute of Technology and Sciences, India

ABSTRACT

Humans may encounter an arboviral illness through viruses transmitted by mosquitoes, commonly result-ing in a fever known as breakbone fever. This term reflects the severity of muscle spasms and joint pains associated with the illness. While some cases are asymptomatic, others can be fatal. Dengue awareness often arises during seasonal changes. The integration of AI in dengue prediction becomes crucial for early diagnosis and treatment. Utilizing appropriate deep learning classifiers can aid in categorizing cases based on their severity. This article advocates for the implementation of an intelligent robotic fogger system in predicted areas. This approach employs interprofessional strategies to safeguard health workers and residents in regions prone to dengue outbreaks.

INTRODUCTION

Dengue, a viral infection transmitted by mosquitoes, is particularly common during seasonal and monsoonal shifts. The causative agents, Dengue types 1 to 4, and the Chikungunya virus fall under the Flavivirus genus. Without proper diagnosis and treatment, Dengue can lead to severe consequences. The

DOI: 10.4018/979-8-3693-1962-8.ch014

southern regions of India are at increased risk due to climatic variations, with 28,578 cases reported in 2021 and a total of 1.93 lakh cases nationwide during the same year. This emphasizes the urgent need for heightened awareness and proactive measures to address potential outbreaks.

While predicting Dengue outbreaks remains challenging, artificial intelligence emerges as a promising solution. Integrating AI holds the potential for accurate outbreak predictions, potentially saving lives through timely warnings. After identifying an outbreak period, deploying a smart Fogger Robot becomes a valuable strategy to control the virus's spread, ensuring the safety of both the general public and healthcare workers.

DISCUSSION

Two cases of around 14 years of age were reported in southern parts of Tamilnadu where severe fever was observed in both the cases. The first case had high temperature, which didn't ease even after several medications. The patient had several pills before proper diagnosis. The third day of fever instigated the doctors that it could be dengue and the blood test revealed the same. By then the patient felt so weak and was admitted where, the platelet count went on decreasing from 2.55 Lakh to 32,000 and found that the liver was also affected.

Clinical tests were advised for the patient. As per the direction, it was observed that on the onset day of fever, the patient had a test report with 48.0 mg/L of CRP – Turbidometry but the reference range is <6 mg/L. The CBC showed incremental increase in Neutrophils which was about 93%, where the reference range was about 40-75% and the Lymphocytes was 04% where the reference range was around 15-45%. The platelet count was found to be 2.55 Lakhs/cumm. The first day, the platelet count seemed to be normal. As per the literature survey, CRP helps in distinguishing the bacterial and viral infection. The test was repeated on the third day and the CRP – Turbidometry was found to be 46.1 mg/L. The total WBC count was reduced to 2000 cells/cumm from 6800 cells/cumm. The platelet count had a decremental phase of 1.57 Lakhs/cumm. Hence Dengue NS1 Antigen was found to be positive. Dengue IgM Antibody and Dengue IgG Antibody was tested negative. Counselling was provided which boosted the patient mentally. The test was repeated on the fourth day where again the WBC count was noticed to be 1700 cells/cumm. Lymphocytes was observed as 49%. The platelet count was observed to be 1.25 Lakhs/cumm. The next day, the patient was tested with SGOT, Liver function test and was observed to have 201 U/L where, the reference range need to be up to 40U/L. SGPT was observed as 103 U/L where, the reference range need to be up to 41 U/L. Medications started immediately to improve the liver functioning of the patient. The next day, platelet count was 32000 / cumm. IV fluids was suggested and was initiated immediately on the third day. Proper medication was then provided by the doctors for recovering. Again the platelet count was checked on the next day and was found that it was 60000 / cumm. As per the advice, the next day, platelet count was checked and found to be 145000/cumm. The medications for liver continued and the patient was discharged on the next day.

The other case had severe fever but the platelet count was observed to be lingering around 2 Lakh. It was also observed that after the fifth day of the fever, the platelet count started to decrease and on the seventh day the patient could recover. Rashes appeared after the 6th day of the fever.

It is recommended that, A prediction (Brasier et al., 2012; Gomes et al., 2010; Guzman et al., 2010) in this case could warn the mosquito borne areas during the outbreak. Diverse Machine learning algorithms (Chen et al., 2015; Lee et al., 2012; Mushtaque et al., 2020; National Vector Borne Disease

Control Programme (NVBDCP), 2015; Potts et al., 2010; Ranjit & Kissoon, 2011; Rao & Kumar, 2012; Side et al., 2020) have been adopted to predict the outbreak. In many literatures, RNA-Seq data have been widely deployed for evolving predictive model of the different categories of dengue. Several classifiers are also adopted to classify the various types of dengue. Tropical areas are more prone to mosquitoes; hence the outbreak can be suggested by predictive modelling methods as indicated in Husin (2012). The southern Parts of India encounter more dengue cases. As observed in Figure 1, the total reported cases in India has been decreased in 2022 (National Vector Borne Disease Control Programme (NVBDCP), 2015). But when compared to 2017, there is a significant increase in the number of cases. Appropriate prediction and prevention techniques need to be enforced to prevent diseases that spread through mosquitoes.

The number of Dengue cases in India was observed to be 1,88,401 in the year 2017. A decline of 87,209 in the number of cases was observed in the year 2018. Again a substantial increase of around 1,57,315 was observed in the year 2019. But, again a decline of 44,585 was observed in the year 2020. There is a rapid increase in the number of cases around 1,93,245 in the year 2021. Till 30th Sep, 2022, the number of cases was around 63,280. As observed in Fig.2, there is a significant decrease in the states like Andhra Pradesh, Karnataka, Kerala and Tamilnadu. But, comparatively Telangana seems to have a hike in the number of reported cases in the year 2022.

It seems to be a real concern in reducing the number of cases. Artificial intelligence has played a vital role in predicting the dengue outbreak. Learning points are highlighted where, investigation report claims that the Dengue fever has to be treated immediately with greater concern.

Dengue Viral Prediction Using Artificial Neural Networks

Aburas (2010) suggested a neural network model for predicting the Dengue confirmed-cases. The authors have contributed an article to predict dengue using Artificial Neural Networks (ANNs).

Figure 1. Dengue cases in India from 2017 to 2022 (National Vector Borne Disease Control Programme (NVBDCP), 2015)

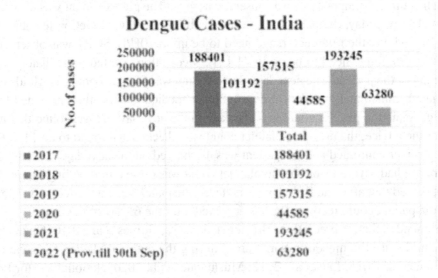

Figure 2. Dengue cases in South India from 2017 to 2022 (National Vector Borne Disease Control Programme (NVBDCP), 2015)

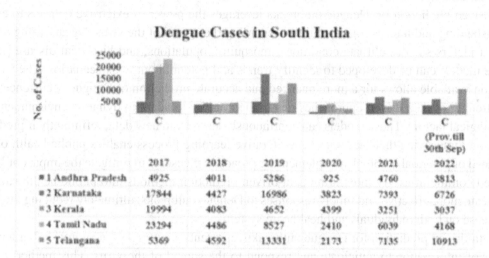

	2017	2018	2019	2020	2021	2022 (Prov.till 30th Sep)
▪ 1 Andhra Pradesh	4925	4011	5286	925	4760	3813
▪ 2 Karnataka	17844	4427	16986	3823	7393	6726
▪ 3 Kerala	19994	4083	4652	4399	3251	3037
▪ 4 Tamil Nadu	23294	4486	8527	2410	6039	4168
▪ 5 Telangana	5369	4592	13331	2173	7135	10913

Based on the real data provided by Singaporean National Environment Agency (NEA) the behavior of dengue cases were predicted based on the physical parameters of mean temperature, mean relative humidity and total rainfall. Around 14,209 dengue reported confirmed-cases have been analyzed by using the ANNs.

Forecasting Dengue virus outbreaks poses a considerable challenge, yet Artificial Neural Networks (ANNs) emerge as a promising tool to improve the precision and effectiveness of predictions. Taking inspiration from the neural structure of the human brain, ANNs have the capacity to analyze extensive datasets, uncovering intricate patterns that conventional methods might overlook. In the Dengue context, these networks can process diverse variables, including climate data, mosquito population dynamics, and historical infection rates, to generate forecasts. ANNs' adaptability and capacity to learn from a variety of inputs make them especially well-suited for addressing the dynamic and multifaceted nature of Dengue prediction.

The application of ANNs in predicting Dengue viral activity holds substantial potential for early detection, enabling prompt and targeted public health interventions. Through training on historical data and continuous updates with real-time information, these networks can discern subtle trends preceding outbreaks. This proactive approach empowers authorities to implement preventive measures, allocate resources efficiently, and heighten public awareness during periods of elevated Dengue transmission risk. The integration of Artificial Neural Networks into Dengue prediction thus signifies a pivotal advancement in mitigating the impact of the virus on public health.

Data Driven Prediction for Dengue Outbreak

Buczak (2012) has suggested a epidemiological prediction method for dengue outbreaks using local and remote sensing data. Althouse (2011) suggested prediction using search query. A prediction method employing Fuzzy Association Rule Mining was adopted to extract relationships between clinical, meteorological, climatic, and socio-political data from Peru. The relationships are rule based. The best set of rules are automatically chosen and forms a classifier. HIGH (outbreak) or LOW (no outbreak) is predicted based on the novel methodology

Data-driven prediction for Dengue outbreaks leverages the power of extensive datasets to enhance our understanding and forecasting capabilities regarding the spread of the virus. By analyzing a variety of relevant factors such as climate conditions, mosquito populations, and historical disease patterns, predictive models can be developed to identify trends and potential outbreak scenarios. The wealth of information available allows for a more nuanced and accurate prediction of Dengue occurrences.

The strength of data-driven approaches lies in their ability to adapt to dynamic environmental and epidemiological factors. These models can continuously learn from new data, refining their predictions over time and improving their accuracy. This iterative learning process enables public health officials to stay ahead of potential outbreaks, implementing proactive measures to mitigate the impact of Dengue on affected communities. By integrating data-driven prediction methods into public health strategies, we can create more effective and timely responses to Dengue outbreaks, ultimately reducing the burden of the disease on both individuals and healthcare systems.

The data-driven prediction for Dengue outbreaks represents a cutting-edge approach that harnesses the power of information to anticipate and respond to the spread of the virus. This method not only enhances our ability to forecast potential outbreaks but also empowers public health initiatives to take targeted actions in a timely manner, contributing to the overall control and prevention of Dengue.

Dengue Prediction Based on Linear Regression

Karim (2012), Model for dengue prediction in Dhaka city based on the Climatic factors influencing dengue cases. Githeko (2012) developed a climate-based dengue outbreak model in Dhaka, Bangladesh. Linear regression method is adopted for predicting the outbreak. To normalize data for linear regression, Log transformation is adopted. Average monthly humidity, rainfall, minimum and maximum temperature were used as independent variables and number of dengue cases reported monthly was used as dependent variable. Accuracy of the model for predicting outbreak was assessed through receiver operative characteristics (ROC) curve.

Dengue prediction employing linear regression involves utilizing statistical techniques to model the relationship between various factors and the likelihood of Dengue outbreaks. Linear regression identifies and quantifies the linear associations between independent variables, such as climate parameters, mosquito populations, and historical Dengue incidence, to predict the dependent variable, which is the likelihood of a Dengue outbreak. This method enables a systematic analysis of the impact of different factors on Dengue occurrences, providing a quantitative basis for predictions.

The strength of linear regression lies in its simplicity and interpretability, making it a valuable tool for understanding the potential risk factors contributing to Dengue outbreaks. By establishing a linear relationship between input variables and Dengue incidence, this method facilitates the identification of key drivers and allows for straightforward predictions based on new data. However, it's essential to recognize the limitations of linear regression, particularly in capturing non-linear and complex relationships within the Dengue ecosystem. Despite its simplicity, linear regression can serve as a foundational step in Dengue prediction, offering valuable insights into the factors influencing the likelihood of outbreaks.

Dengue prediction based on linear regression provides a systematic and interpretable approach to forecasting outbreaks by analyzing the relationships between various contributing factors. While it may not capture the full complexity of Dengue dynamics, it serves as a valuable initial step in understanding and predicting the incidence of Dengue, providing a basis for further exploration and refinement of predictive models.

SIRI Model for Dengue

Syafruddin (2020), Analysis and Simulation of SIRI Model for Dengue Fever Transmission was suggested in the article. The re-infection of dengue fever is predicted based on SIRI model. It is mentioned that the dengue cases always occur at a certain time in a region.

The SIRI (Susceptible-Infectious-Recovered-Immune) model offers a structured framework for understanding and predicting the dynamics of Dengue outbreaks. In this model, the population is divided into four compartments: Susceptible, Infectious, Recovered, and Immune. The Susceptible population represents individuals who are at risk of contracting Dengue, the Infectious population includes those currently infected and capable of transmitting the virus, the Recovered group consists of individuals who have overcome the infection, and the Immune group comprises those who have developed immunity. Through a system of differential equations, the SIRI model simulates the flow of individuals between these compartments, allowing for the exploration of how Dengue spreads through a population over time.

The SIRI model for Dengue is particularly valuable for understanding the impact of various intervention strategies and vaccination programs. By adjusting parameters related to the transmission rate and recovery rate, researchers can simulate different scenarios to assess the effectiveness of control measures. This modeling approach aids in optimizing public health strategies, as it provides insights into the potential outcomes of interventions and helps guide decision-making processes. The SIRI model thus serves as a valuable tool in the broader effort to mitigate the impact of Dengue on public health.

The SIRI model offers a comprehensive and dynamic framework for studying Dengue outbreaks. Its compartmental structure and differential equations provide a systematic way to explore the transmission dynamics and assess the effectiveness of interventions, contributing to the development of informed strategies for Dengue prevention and control.

Dengue Forecast Model Using Machine Learning

Guo (2017) suggested a forecast model using machine learning. A case study in China was reported where, it demonstrated the SVR model to track the dynamics of dengue outbreaks in China. The ML technique adopted in the article has provided a superior performance compared to the existing methods.

Creating a Dengue forecast model using machine learning involves leveraging advanced algorithms to analyze historical data and identify patterns that contribute to the spread of the virus. Machine learning models, such as decision trees, random forests, or support vector machines, can process vast datasets containing variables like climate conditions, mosquito populations, and past Dengue incidences. By training the model on this data, it learns to recognize complex relationships and make predictions about future Dengue outbreaks. The predictive power of these models lies in their ability to adapt and improve as more data becomes available, allowing for dynamic and accurate forecasts.

One significant advantage of machine learning in Dengue forecasting is its capability to handle diverse and non-linear relationships within the data. Unlike traditional statistical models, machine learning algorithms can capture intricate patterns and dependencies, providing a more nuanced understanding of the factors influencing Dengue outbreaks. This adaptability is particularly crucial in the context of a dynamic and evolving disease environment. The integration of machine learning into Dengue forecasting not only enhances prediction accuracy but also empowers public health officials to implement timely interventions and allocate resources effectively, ultimately mitigating the impact of Dengue on communities.

Employing machine learning for Dengue forecasting represents a cutting-edge approach that harnesses the power of advanced algorithms to predict outbreaks more accurately. By extracting insights from diverse datasets, machine learning models contribute to a more comprehensive understanding of the complex dynamics of Dengue transmission, enabling proactive measures to be taken for the prevention and control of this infectious disease.

Artificial Intelligence as a Dengue Surveillance and Prediction Tool

Sundram (2019) has proposed the Bayesian network system Using Artificial Intelligence for Dengue Surveillance and Prediction. The authors claim that the proposed system has the ability to predict the next dengue outbreaks in real-time. Data entry and other functionalities are user friendly and the system is able to report advance outbreak predictions.

Artificial Intelligence (AI) is rapidly becoming a pivotal tool in Dengue surveillance and prediction, revolutionizing our approach to understanding and managing the disease. AI applications, such as machine learning algorithms and predictive modeling, can analyze vast and diverse datasets, including climate data, demographic information, and historical Dengue cases, to identify intricate patterns and correlations. These algorithms can then generate accurate predictions and assist in early detection of potential outbreaks, allowing public health officials to implement timely interventions.

The strength of AI in Dengue surveillance lies in its ability to adapt and learn from new data continuously. As it processes real-time information, AI algorithms can dynamically adjust predictions, improving their accuracy over time. This adaptability is crucial in addressing the dynamic nature of Dengue, where factors influencing the spread of the virus can change rapidly. Additionally, AI can provide valuable insights into the risk factors and variables contributing to Dengue outbreaks, aiding in the development of targeted prevention and control strategies.

By harnessing the power of AI, Dengue surveillance and prediction can move beyond traditional methods, offering a more proactive and efficient approach to managing the disease. The integration of AI technologies not only enhances our ability to forecast Dengue outbreaks accurately but also empowers public health systems to take preemptive actions, ultimately contributing to the effective control and reduction of Dengue's impact on communities.

Predictive Models for Dengue using ANN and SVM

Jorge (2019) has proposed that SVM polynomial and ANN-MLP have proved their superiority in objective analysis in terms of Accuracy, Sensitivity and Specificity for prediction of Dengue. ANN and SVM classifiers can be incorporated to forewarn the outbreak of Dengue. The ANN-MLP shows 96% of accuracy.

Predictive models for Dengue utilizing Artificial Neural Networks (ANN) and Support Vector Machines (SVM) represent advanced applications of machine learning in disease forecasting. Artificial Neural Networks, inspired by the human brain's neural structure, can handle complex relationships within Dengue-related data, such as climate variables, mosquito populations, and historical Dengue incidences. ANN excels in recognizing intricate patterns, enabling accurate predictions by learning from diverse inputs. On the other hand, Support Vector Machines, a powerful classification algorithm, are adept at identifying patterns and creating decision boundaries in multidimensional data spaces. SVMs excel in separating different classes within the data, making them effective tools for predicting Dengue outbreaks based on various factors.

The combination of ANN and SVM in Dengue prediction allows for a comprehensive and complementary approach. ANN can capture nonlinear relationships and complex dependencies in the data, while SVM can effectively classify instances and delineate distinct patterns. Integrating these models enhances the overall accuracy and robustness of Dengue predictions. The adaptability of both ANN and SVM to changing conditions, along with their ability to learn from new data, positions them as valuable tools in creating dynamic and responsive predictive models for Dengue. This sophisticated fusion of machine learning methodologies holds great promise for improving our understanding of Dengue dynamics and enhancing our capacity to implement proactive public health measures.

Dengue Predictive Models Using ANN and Discriminant Analysis

Silitonga (2021) has compared Dengue Predictive Models using ANN and Discriminant Analysis. The model developed would aid in predicting the severity level before entering into the critical phase. ANN models based on logistic and hyperbolic tangent activation function with 70% training data yielded the highest accuracy (90.91%), sensitivity (91.11%), and specificity (95.51%). These predictive models can aid in monitoring the severity level based on laboratory test results.

Dengue predictive models, employing Artificial Neural Networks (ANN) and Discriminant Analysis, showcase a synergistic blend of advanced machine learning techniques for accurate disease forecasting. Artificial Neural Networks, inspired by the human brain's neural architecture, excel in capturing intricate patterns and relationships within Dengue-related datasets. They are particularly adept at handling nonlinear and complex dependencies, making them invaluable for discerning the multifaceted factors influencing Dengue outbreaks. In parallel, Discriminant Analysis, a statistical technique, focuses on classifying and distinguishing between different groups within the data. Applied to Dengue prediction, Discriminant Analysis helps identify key variables that contribute significantly to outbreak occurrences.

The combination of ANN and Discriminant Analysis in Dengue predictive modeling brings complementary strengths to the forefront. While ANN excels in recognizing subtle patterns and nonlinear relationships, Discriminant Analysis enhances the interpretability of the model by identifying the most discriminative features for classifying Dengue outbreaks. This integrated approach improves the overall robustness of Dengue predictions, providing a more comprehensive understanding of the complex interplay of variables. The adaptability and learning capabilities of both techniques ensure that the predictive models stay dynamic and responsive to changing conditions, ultimately contributing to more effective and timely public health interventions for Dengue prevention and control.

Deep Learning Classifiers

Employing deep learning classifiers proves instrumental in precisely categorizing the severity of Dengue cases. Specifically, convolutional neural networks (CNNs) excel in image-based analysis, while recurrent neural networks (RNNs) effectively capture temporal dependencies in patient data. These classifiers, leveraging advanced techniques like long short-term memory (LSTM) networks, play a crucial role in distinguishing between Dengue Fever (DF) and the more severe Dengue Hemorrhagic Fever (DHF) by evaluating clinical indicators such as C-reactive protein (CRP). Furthermore, LSTM networks contribute to forecasting the disease's progression, facilitating timely intervention strategies.

In the envisioned robotic fogger system, the success of deployment relies on interprofessional strategies. Collaboration among healthcare professionals, data scientists, and robotics experts proves indispensable for the effective implementation of this technology. Healthcare providers bring crucial domain expertise in comprehending Dengue epidemiology, while data scientists contribute insights into refining predictive models and classifiers. Robotics experts are vital in ensuring the Smart Fogger Robot's efficient operation and navigation. Consistent communication and collaboration among these professionals are paramount to customizing the technology to the specific requirements of Dengue-prone areas.

Despite the immense potential of integrating AI and a Smart Fogger Robot, certain challenges and limitations necessitate careful consideration. Concerns related to data privacy, model interpretability, and the robot's adaptability to changing environmental conditions require focused attention. Additionally, successful implementation requires addressing potential resistance or skepticism within communities and ensuring equitable access to healthcare resources. Tackling these challenges is essential for the sustainable and ethical deployment of advanced technologies in Dengue prevention and control.

Smart Fogger Robot During Dengue Outbreak

Once the prediction is performed using Machine learning or Deep learning based on the varied climatic conditions and the available data, a Mosquito fogger robot can be designed to automatically spray the disinfectant. The engagement of the public health workers need not be physically required thereby ensuring no health hazards among them. The fogger Robot can alarm the surrounding before spraying the disinfectant and based on a threshold level of time, it can move into various places of a home, mall, industry etc. and end spraying. This could help the health workers to stay safe.

The deployment of a Smart Fogger Robot during a Dengue outbreak presents a compelling and forward-thinking approach to disease control. Dengue, transmitted by mosquitoes, poses a significant public health threat, especially in regions susceptible to outbreaks. The Smart Fogger Robot, equipped with intelligent technologies, can play a crucial role in mitigating the spread of the virus. By autonomously navigating through affected areas and dispersing targeted insecticides, the robot can efficiently reduce mosquito populations, interrupting the transmission cycle and minimizing the risk of Dengue infection.

Implementing a Smart Fogger Robot not only enhances the effectiveness of vector control but also addresses challenges faced by human workers in accessing high-risk environments. The robot's precision in delivering interventions can lead to more targeted and resource-efficient strategies, optimizing the impact of disease control efforts. Furthermore, the use of such technology aligns with the broader trend of leveraging automation and artificial intelligence to augment public health initiatives, offering a proactive and innovative solution to combat Dengue outbreaks. Overall, the incorporation of a Smart Fogger Robot represents a promising and scalable tool in the ongoing battle against mosquito-borne diseases.

Intelligent Robotic Fogger System

A Smart Fogger Robot for Dengue is a specialized robotic device designed to combat Dengue fever by efficiently and effectively applying fogging treatments to control and reduce mosquito populations. Dengue is a mosquito-borne viral disease, and controlling mosquito populations is crucial in preventing its spread. Here are key features and functionalities of a Smart Fogger Robot for Dengue:

Autonomous Navigation: The robot is equipped with autonomous navigation capabilities, using sensors, cameras, and mapping technology to move through designated areas, such as neighborhoods, parks, or urban areas.

Mosquito Detection: Some models may incorporate mosquito detection technology, including sensors or cameras that can identify mosquito breeding sites or mosquito activity in real-time.

Fogging Equipment: The robot is equipped with a fogging system that disperses insecticides or larvicides in the form of fine droplets. The fogging equipment should be adjustable to control the droplet size and distribution for maximum effectiveness.

Precision Targeting: The robot uses precision targeting to ensure that the fogging treatment is applied only to areas where mosquito breeding or activity is detected. This reduces the environmental impact and minimizes the exposure of non-target organisms.

Real-Time Monitoring: The robot may have sensors to monitor environmental conditions such as temperature, humidity, and wind speed, which can affect the effectiveness of the fogging treatment. Real-time data analysis allows for adjustments to the fogging process.

Remote Operation: Operators can control the robot remotely, monitoring its progress and making adjustments as needed. Remote operation allows for flexibility and adaptability in response to changing conditions.

Integrated Safety Features: Safety features are crucial to prevent accidents or unintended exposure. This includes emergency stop buttons, obstacle detection sensors, and safety protocols for human interaction.

Data Collection and Reporting: The robot collects data on fogging operations, mosquito activity, and environmental conditions. This data can be used for analysis and reporting to assess the effectiveness of mosquito control efforts.

Sustainability: To promote environmental sustainability, the robot may use environmentally friendly insecticides or larvicides and minimize chemical usage through precision targeting.

Communication: The robot can communicate with local authorities or a central control system to provide real-time updates on its operations and any issues encountered during fogging.

Community Engagement: In some cases, the robot may be equipped with communication features to engage with the local community, providing information about Dengue prevention and mosquito control efforts.

A Smart Fogger Robot for Dengue can significantly enhance mosquito control efforts in areas affected by Dengue outbreaks. By automating and optimizing fogging operations, it can help reduce the spread of the disease, protect public health, and contribute to the overall well-being of communities at risk of Dengue fever.

The illustrated Intelligent Robotic Fogger System depicted in Fig. 3 offers a viable solution for enhancing public safety. Embracing this mechanism can effectively mitigate potential risks and ensure the well-being of the public.

Figure 3. Intelligent robotic fogger system

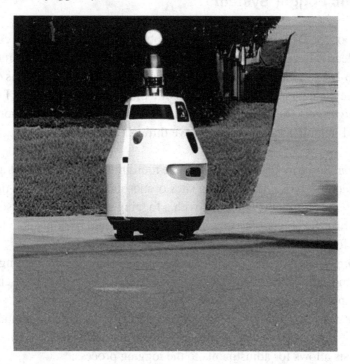

CONCLUSION

Leveraging Artificial Intelligence in Dengue prediction models proves instrumental in effectively forecasting the occurrence of Dengue fever in regions prone to the disease. By employing sophisticated classifiers, such as those distinguishing between DENV-1, DENV-2, DENV-3, and DENV-4, these models can provide a targeted approach to identify specific strains and tailor appropriate treatments accordingly. Furthermore, the severity of Dengue cases, whether classified as DF or DHF, can be accurately assessed by incorporating classifiers based on factors like CRP (C-reactive protein). Implementing a computer-aided diagnosis approach, driven by AI, offers a proactive strategy to predict Dengue outbreaks, enabling timely warnings and preemptive measures in areas susceptible to the virus.

To enhance control and prevention efforts, a Smart Fogger Robot emerges as a valuable tool deployed at regular intervals in predicted Dengue-prone areas. This autonomous device, guided by AI-driven insights, aids in curtailing the spread of Dengue by precisely dispersing targeted interventions. The integration of AI and the deployment of a smart Fogger Robot represent a comprehensive and forward-thinking approach to Dengue management, utilizing technology to predict, classify, and proactively address the complexities associated with Dengue outbreaks.

Conflict of Interest

The authors declare that the research was conducted in the absence of any commercial or financial relationships that could be construed as a potential conflict of interest.

Author Contributions

DRJD, DJJ and JDP devised the work. DRJD provided the main conceptual ideas, DJJ and JDP verified the proof outline, and worked out almost all of the technical details. DJJ and JDP worked on the manuscript. All authors contributed to the article and approved the submitted version.

ACKNOWLEDGMENT

Authors express their sincere thanks to Karunya Institute of Technology and Sciences for the research environment and infrastructure that has been extended.

REFERENCES

Brasier, A. R., Ju, H., Garcia, J., Spratt, H. M., Victor, S. S., Forshey, B. M., ... Rocha, C. (2012). A three-component biomarker panel for prediction of dengue hemorrhagic fever. *The American Journal of Tropical Medicine and Hygiene*, 86(2), 341–348. doi:10.4269/ajtmh.2012.11-0469 PMID:22302872

Chen, C. C., Lee, I.-K., Liu, J.-W., Huang, S.-Y., & Wang, L. (2015). Utility of C-Reactive Protein Levels for Early Prediction of Dengue Severity in Adults. *BioMed Research International*, 2015, 1–6. doi:10.1155/2015/936062 PMID:26247033

Gomes, A. L. V., Wee, L. J., Khan, A. M., Gil, L. H., Marques, E. T. Jr, Calzavara-Silva, C. E., & Tan, T. W. (2010). Classification of dengue fever patients based on gene expression data using support vector machines. *PLoS One*, 5(6), 11267. doi:10.1371/journal.pone.0011267 PMID:20585645

Guzman, M. G., Halstead, S. B., Artsob, H., Buchy, P., Farrar, J., Gubler, D. J., & Nathan, M. B. (2010). Dengue: A continuing global threat. *Nature Reviews. Microbiology*, 8(S12), S7–S16. doi:10.1038/nrmicro2460 PMID:21079655

Lee, V. J., Chow, A., Zheng, X., Carrasco, L. R., Cook, A. R., Lye, D. C., Ng, L.-C., & Leo, Y. S. (2012). Simple clinical and laboratory predictors of Chikungunya versus dengue infections in adults. *PLoS Neglected Tropical Diseases*, 6(9), 1786. doi:10.1371/journal.pntd.0001786 PMID:23029573

Mushtaque, R. S., Ahmad, S. M., Mushtaque, R., & Baloch, S. (2020). Case Report, A Curious Case of Dengue Fever: A Case Report of Unorthodox Manifestations. *Case Reports in Medicine*, 2020, 1–4. doi:10.1155/2020/1701082 PMID:32774384

National Vector Borne Disease Control Programme (NVBDCP). (2015). Retrieved from https://nvbdcp.gov.in/index4.php?lang=1&level=0&linkid=431&lid=3715

Potts, J. A., Gibbons, R. V., Rothman, A. L., Srikiatkhachorn, A., Thomas, S. J., Supradish, P. O., Lemon, S. C., Libraty, D. H., Green, S., & Kalayanarooj, S. (2010). Prediction of dengue disease severity among pediatric Thai patients using early clinical laboratory indicators. *PLoS Neglected Tropical Diseases*, 4(8), 769. doi:10.1371/journal.pntd.0000769 PMID:20689812

Ranjit, S., & Kissoon, N. (2011). Dengue hemorrhagic fever and shock syndromes. *Pediatric Critical Care Medicine*, *12*(1), 90–100. doi:10.1097/PCC.0b013e3181e911a7 PMID:20639791

Rao, V. S. H., & Kumar, M. N. (2012). A new intelligence-based approach for computer-aided diagnosis of dengue fever. *IEEE Transactions on Information Technology in Biomedicine*, *16*(1), 112–118. doi:10.1109/TITB.2011.2171978 PMID:22010159

Side, S., Pratama, M. I., Badwi, N., & Sanusi, W. (2020). Analysis and Simulation of SIRI Model for Dengue Fever Transmission. *Indian Journal of Science and Technology*, *13*(3), 340–351. doi:10.17485/ijst/2020/v13i03/147852

Compilation of References

. Ma, Y., Wang, Z., Yang, H., & Yang, L. (2020). Artificial intelligence applications in the development of autonomous vehicles: A survey. *IEEE/CAA Journal of AutomaticaSinica, 7*(2), 315-329.

. Milledge, J. (2020). Hypobaria: high altitude, aviation physiology, and medicine. *Cotes' lung function*, 615-637.

Aggarwal, S., Gupta, D., & Saini, S. (2019, November). A literature survey on robotics in healthcare. In *2019 4th International Conference on Information Systems and Computer Networks (ISCON)* (pp. 55-58). IEEE. 10.1109/IS-CON47742.2019.9036253

Agrawal, S., Kumar, V., Anand, N., Agarwal, V. K., & Islam, A. (2016). *Development of Data Acquisition System and Data Analysis Technique for Automotive Applications. 50*(Ic), 3–6.

Aguirre, S., & Rodriguez, A. (2017). *Automation of a Business Process Using Robotic Process Automation (RPA): A Case Study.* Springer. . doi:10.1007/978-3-319-66963-2_7

Akter, S., Michael, K., Uddin, M. R., McCarthy, G., & Rahman, M. (2022). Transforming business using digital innovations: The application of AI, blockchain, cloud and data analytics. *Annals of Operations Research, 308*(1–2), 7–39. doi:10.1007/s10479-020-03620-w

Ala'a, A. M. (2023). Adoption of Roboticsand Robotics in Healthcare: A Systematic Literature Review. [IJCMIT]. *International Journal of Contemporary Management and Information Technology, 3*(6), 1–16.

Al-Ani, R., Zhou, B., Shi, Q., & Sagheer, A. (2018). A survey on secure safety applications in vanet. In *2018 IEEE 20th International Conference on High Performance Computing and Communications; IEEE 16th International Conference on Smart City; IEEE 4th International Conference on Data Science and Systems (HPCC/SmartCity/DSS)* (pp. 1485-1490). IEEE. 10.1109/HPCC/SmartCity/DSS.2018.00245

Alsamhi, S. H., & Lee, B. (2020). Blockchain-empowered multi-robot collaboration to fight COVID-19 and future pandemics. *IEEE Access : Practical Innovations, Open Solutions, 9*, 44173–44197. doi:10.1109/ACCESS.2020.3032450 PMID:34786312

AlShamsi, S., AlSuwaidi, L., & Shaalan, K. (2022). Robotics and AI in Healthcare: A Systematic Review. *Recent Innovations in Roboticsand Smart Applications*, 319-343.

Amestica, O. E., Melin, P. E., Duran-Faundez, C. R., & Lagos, G. R. (2019). An Experimental Comparison of Arduino IDE Compatible Platforms for Digital Control and Data Acquisition Applications. *IEEE CHILEAN Conference on Electrical, Electronics Engineering, Information and Communication Technologies, CHILECON 2019*, (pp. 1–6). IEEE. 10.1109/CHILECON47746.2019.8986865

Amrutkar, C., Satav, A., Sonawwanay, P. D., & Pawar, A. H. (2024). Overview of Autonomous Vehicle and Its Challenges. Techno-Societal 2022. *ICATSA, 2022*, 243–251. doi:10.1007/978-3-031-34648-4_25

Anderson, V. C., & Horn, R. C. (1970). *U.S. Patent No. 3,497,083*. Washington, DC: U.S. Patent and Trademark Office.

Antoniadi, A. M., Du, Y., Guendouz, Y., Wei, L., Mazo, C., Becker, B. A., & Mooney, C. (2021). Current challenges and future opportunities for XAI in machine learning-based clinical decision support systems: A systematic review. *Applied Sciences (Basel, Switzerland)*, *11*(11), 5088. doi:10.3390/app11115088

Antony, V. N., Li, M., Lin, S. H., Li, J., & Huang, C. M. (2024). *Social Robots for Sleep Health: A Scoping Review*. arXiv preprint arXiv:2403.04169.

Aouf, A., Boussaid, L., & Sakly, A. (2019). Same fuzzy logic controller for two-wheeled mobile robot navigation in strange environments. *Journal of Robotics*, *2019*, 2465219. doi:10.1155/2019/2465219

Arrieta, A. B., Díaz-Rodríguez, N., Del Ser, J., Bennetot, A., Tabik, S., Barbado, A., & Herrera, F. (2020). Explainable Artificial Intelligence (XAI): Concepts, taxonomies, opportunities and challenges toward responsible AI. *Information Fusion*, *58*, 82–115. doi:10.1016/j.inffus.2019.12.012

Atakishiyev, S., Salameh, M., Yao, H., & Goebel, R. (2021). Explainable artificial intelligence for autonomous driving: A comprehensive overview and field guide for future research directions. *arXiv preprint arXiv:2112.11561*.

Azizi, A., Hortamani, R., & Zabihollah, A. (2018). Sensing the material by minimally invasive surgery grasper. *International Robotics & Automation Journal*, *4*(3). doi:10.15406/iratj.2018.04.00117

Aziz, L., Salam, M. S. B. H., Sheikh, U. U., & Ayub, S. (2020). Exploring deep learning-based architecture, strategies, applications and current trends in generic object detection: A comprehensive review. *IEEE Access : Practical Innovations, Open Solutions*, *8*, 170461–170495. doi:10.1109/ACCESS.2020.3021508

Bae, I., Moon, J., & Seo, J. (2019). Toward a comfortable driving experience for a self-driving shuttle bus. *Electronics (Basel)*, *8*(9), 943. doi:10.3390/electronics8090943

Bajwa, J., Munir, U., Nori, A., & Williams, B. (2021, July). Artificial intelligence in healthcare: Transforming the practice of medicine. *Future Healthcare Journal*, *8*(2), e188–e194. doi:10.7861/fhj.2021-0095 PMID:34286183

Bakdi, A., Bounoua, W., Guichi, A., & Mekhilef, S. (2021). Real-time fault detection in PV systems under MPPT using PMU and high-frequency multi-sensor data through online PCA-KDE-based multivariate KL divergence. *International Journal of Electrical Power & Energy Systems*, *125*, 106457. doi:10.1016/j.ijepes.2020.106457

Bakshi, G., Kumar, A., & Puranik, A. N. (2021). Adoption of robotics technology in healthcare sector. In Advances in Communication, Devices and Networking [Singapore: Springer Singapore.]. *Proceedings of ICCDN*, *2020*, 405–414.

Banerjee, S. S., Andhari, S. S., Wavhale, R. D., Dhobale, K. D., Tawade, B. V., Chate, G. P., & Khandare, J. J. (2020). Self-propelling targeted magneto-nanobots for deep tumor penetration and pH-responsive intracellular drug delivery. *Scientific Reports*, *10*(1), 1–14. PMID:31913322

Bangotra, D. K., Singh, Y., & Selwal, A. (2018). Machine learning in wireless sensor networks: Challenges and opportunities. In *2018 Fifth International Conference on Parallel, Distributed and Grid Computing (PDGC)* (pp. 534-539). IEEE. 10.1109/PDGC.2018.8745845

Bao, J., Li, D., & Qiao, X. (2020). Integrated navigation for autonomous underwater vehicles in aquaculture: A review. *Information Processing in Agriculture, 7*(1).

Baoquan, G. (2011). *Time-domain Analysis and Research on blasting vibration signals Based on Fourier I°*. Research Gate.

Bartneck, C., Lütge, C., Wagner, A., & Welsh, S. (2021). *An introduction to ethics in robotics and AI*. Springer Nature. doi:10.1007/978-3-030-51110-4

Barua, R., & Datta, S. (2022). Study of the surgical needle and biological soft tissue interaction phenomenon during insertion process for medical application: A Survey. *Proceedings of the Institution of Mechanical Engineers, Part H: Journal of Engineering in Medicine, 236*(10), 1465-1477.

Barua, R., Bhowmik, S., Dey, A., Das, S., & Datta, S. (2022, September). Analysis of Robotically Controlled Percutaneous Needle Insertion into Ex Vivo Kidney Tissue for Minimally Invasive Percutaneous Nephrolithotomy (PCNL) Surgery. *In International Conference on Emergent Converging Technologies and Biomedical Systems* (pp. 249-257). Singapore: Springer Nature Singapore.

Barua, R., Das, S., Datta, P., & Chowdhury, A. (2022). Computational FEM Application on Percutaneous Nephrolithotomy (PCNL) Minimum Invasive Surgery Through Needle Insertion Process. In P. Pain, S. Banerjee, & G. Bose (Eds.), *Advances in Computational Approaches in Biomechanics* (pp. 210-222). IGI Global. doi:10.4018/978-1-7998-9078-2.ch013

Barua, R., Das, S., Datta, S., Roy Chowdhury, A., & Datta, P. (2022). Experimental study of the robotically controlled surgical needle insertion for analysis of the minimum invasive process. In *Emergent Converging Technologies and Biomedical Systems: Select Proceedings of ETBS 2021* (pp. 473-482). Singapore: Springer Singapore. 10.1007/978-981-16-8774-7_38

Barua, R., Bhowmik, S., Dey, A., & Mondal, J. (2023). Advances of the Robotics Technology in Modern Minimally Invasive Surgery. In M. Mellal (Ed.), *Design and Control Advances in Robotics* (pp. 91–104). IGI Global.

Barua, R., Das, S., Datta, S., Datta, P., & Roy Chowdhury, A. (2021). Analysis of surgical needle insertion modeling and viscoelastic tissue material interaction for minimally invasive surgery (MIS). *Materials Today: Proceedings, 57*, 259–264. doi:10.1016/j.matpr.2022.02.498

Barua, R., Das, S., Datta, S., Datta, P., & Roy Chowdhury, A. (2023). Study and experimental investigation of insertion force modeling and tissue deformation phenomenon during surgical needle-soft tissue interaction. *Proceedings of the Institution of Mechanical Engineers. Part C, Journal of Mechanical Engineering Science, 237*(5), 1007–1014. doi:10.1177/09544062221126628

Barua, R., Das, S., & Mondal, J. (2023). Emerging Applications of Artificial Intelligence (AI) and Machine Learning (ML) in Modern Urology. In R. Queirós, B. Cunha, & X. Fonseca (Eds.), *Exploring the Convergence of Computer and Medical Science Through Cloud Healthcare* (pp. 117–133). IGI Global. doi:10.4018/978-1-6684-5260-8.ch006

Barua, R., Das, S., Roy Chowdhury, A., & Datta, P. (2023). Experimental and simulation investigation of surgical needle insertion into soft tissue mimic biomaterial for minimally invasive surgery (MIS). *Proceedings of the Institution of Mechanical Engineers. Part H, Journal of Engineering in Medicine, 237*(2), 254–264. doi:10.1177/09544119221143860 PMID:36527297

Barua, R., Das, S., RoyChowdhury, A., & Datta, P. (2023). Simulation and experimental investigation of the surgical needle deflection model during the rotational and steady insertion process. *The International Journal of Artificial Organs, 46*(1), 40–51. doi:10.1177/03913988221136154 PMID:36397288

Barua, R., Datta, P., Chowdhury, A. R., & Das, S. (2022). Computational Study of In-Vitro Ureter Urine Flow in DJ Stent. In P. Pain, S. Banerjee, & G. Bose (Eds.), *Advances in Computational Approaches in Biomechanics* (pp. 198–209). IGI Global. doi:10.4018/978-1-7998-9078-2.ch012

Barua, R., & Datta, S. (2023). Artificial Intelligence in Modern Medical Science: A Promising Practice. In S. Rajest, B. Singh, A. J. Obaid, R. Regin, & K. Chinnusamy (Eds.), *Recent Developments in Machine and Human Intelligence* (pp. 1–12). IGI Global. doi:10.4018/978-1-6684-9189-8.ch001

Barua, R., & Datta, S. (2023). Emerging Surgical Robotic Applications for Modern Minimally Invasive Surgery (MIS). In M. Habib (Ed.), *Global Perspectives on Robotics and Autonomous Systems: Development and Applications* (pp. 314–332). IGI Global. doi:10.4018/978-1-6684-7791-5.ch014

Barua, R., Datta, S., & Sarkar, A. (2023). Artificial Intelligence and Robotics-Based Minimally Invasive Surgery: Innovations and Future Perceptions. In G. Karthick & S. Karupusamy (Eds.), *Contemporary Applications of Data Fusion for Advanced Healthcare Informatics* (pp. 350–368). IGI Global. doi:10.4018/978-1-6684-8913-0.ch015

Barua, R., Giria, H., Datta, S., Roy Chowdhury, A., & Datta, P. (2020). Force modeling to develop a novel method for fabrication of hollow channels inside a gel structure. *Proceedings of the Institution of Mechanical Engineers. Part H, Journal of Engineering in Medicine, 234*(2), 223–231. doi:10.1177/0954411919891654 PMID:31774361

Barua, R., & Mondal, J. (2023). Study of the Current Trends of CAD (Computer-Aided Detection) in Modern Medical Imaging. In L. Panigrahi, S. Biswal, A. Bhoi, A. Kalam, & P. Barsocchi (Eds.), *Machine Learning and AI Techniques in Interactive Medical Image Analysis* (pp. 35–50). IGI Global., doi:10.4018/978-1-6684-4671-3.ch002

Barua, R., Sarkar, A., & Datta, S. (2023). Modern Lab-on-Chip Biosensors Application on Infectious COVID-19 Detection. In R. Singh, R. Phanden, B. Sikarwar, & J. Davim (Eds.), *Advances in MEMS and Microfluidic Systems* (pp. 258–270). IGI Global. doi:10.4018/978-1-6684-6952-1.ch013

Belk, R. (2021). Ethical issues in service robotics and artificial intelligence. *Service Industries Journal, 41*(13-14), 860–876. doi:10.1080/02642069.2020.1727892

Bhoi, S. K., & Khilar, P. M. (2013). A secure routing protocol for Vehicular Ad Hoc Network to provide ITS services. In *2013 International Conference on Communication and Signal Processing* (pp. 1170-1174). IEEE. 10.1109/iccsp.2013.6577240

Biswas, A. K., & Dasgupta, M. (2020). A secure hybrid routing protocol for mobile ad-hoc networks (MANETs). In *2020 11th International Conference on Computing, Communication and Networking Technologies (ICCCNT)* (pp. 1-7). IEEE.

Bogue, R. (2011). Robots in healthcare. Industrial Robot. *International Journal (Toronto, Ont.), 38*(3), 218–223.

Bourdon, P., Ahmed, O. B., Urruty, T., Djemal, K., & Fernandez-Maloigne, C. (2021). Explainable ai for medical imaging: Knowledge matters. *Multi-faceted Deep Learning: Models and Data.*

Brasier, A. R., Ju, H., Garcia, J., Spratt, H. M., Victor, S. S., Forshey, B. M., ... Rocha, C. (2012). A three-component biomarker panel for prediction of dengue hemorrhagic fever. *The American Journal of Tropical Medicine and Hygiene, 86*(2), 341–348. doi:10.4269/ajtmh.2012.11-0469 PMID:22302872

Brown, B. (2016). The social life of autonomous cars. *MIT Technology Review, 50*(2).

Burgner-Kahrs, J., Rucker, D. C., & Choset, H. (2015). Continuum robots for medical applications: A survey. *IEEE Transactions on Robotics, 31*(6), 1261–1280. doi:10.1109/TRO.2015.2489500

Butter, M., Rensma, A., Kalisingh, S., Schoone, M., Leis, M., Gelderblom, G. J., & Korhonen, I. (2008). *Robotics for healthcare.*

Cai, Y., Luan, T., Gao, H., Wang, H., Chen, L., Li, Y., Sotelo, M. A., & Li, Z. (2021). YOLOv4-5D: An effective and efficient object detector for autonomous driving. *IEEE Transactions on Instrumentation and Measurement, 70*, 1–13. doi:10.1109/TIM.2021.3065438

Cao, K., Chen, Y., Dang, H., Gao, S., & Yan, K. (2022, July). Multi-robot Coverage System Based on Health Optimization Management Algorithm. In *Proceedings of 2021 5th Chinese Conference on Swarm Intelligence and Cooperative Control* (pp. 902-911). Singapore: Springer Nature Singapore.

Cao, C. G., & Rogers, G. (2007). *Robotics in health care: HF issues in surgery. Handbook of Human Factors and Ergonomics in Health Care and Patient Safety.* Lawrence Earlbaum & Associates.

Cao, K., Chen, Y., Gao, S., Zhang, H., & Dang, H. (2022). Multi-Robot Formation Control Based on CVT Algorithm and Health Optimization Management. *Applied Sciences (Basel, Switzerland), 12*(2), 755. doi:10.3390/app12020755

Cappiello, A. (2018). Digital Disruption and InsurTech Start-ups: Risks and Challenges. In Technology and the Insurance Industry (pp. 29–50). Springer International Publishing. doi:10.1007/978-3-319-74712-5_3

Carranza-García, M., Torres-Mateo, J., Lara-Benítez, P., & García-Gutiérrez, J. (2021). On the performance of one-stage and two-stage object detectors in autonomous vehicles using camera data. *Remote Sensing (Basel), 13*(1), 89. doi:10.3390/rs13010089

Cavalcanti, A., Shirinzadeh, B., Freitas, R. A. Jr, & Hogg, T. (2008). Nanorobot architecture for medical target identification. *Nanomedicine; Nanotechnology, Biology, and Medicine, 4*(2), 134–152. PMID:18455965

Chaurasia, A., Parashar, B., & Kautish, S. (2024). Artificial Intelligence and Automation for Industry 4.0. In S. Kautish, P. Chatterjee, D. Pamucar, N. Pradeep, & D. Singh (Eds.), *Computational Intelligence for Modern Business Systems. Disruptive Technologies and Digital Transformations for Society 5.0.* doi:10.1007/978-981-99-5354-7_18

Chellaswamy, C., Famitha, H., Anusuya, T., & Amirthavarshini, S. B. (2018). *IoT Based Humps and Pothole Detection on Roads and Information Sharing.* Research Gate.

Chen, E. N. (2009). Remote analysis of mechanical vibration based on client/server architecture. *ICEMI 2009 - Proceedings of 9th International Conference on Electronic Measurement and Instruments*, (pp. 10–13). IEEE. 10.1109/ICEMI.2009.5274399

Chen, S., & Xu, H. (2023). A pneumatic–hydraulic hybrid actuator for underwater soft robot swimming and crawling. *Sensors and Actuators A: Physical, 356.* doi:10.1016/j.sna.2023.114284

Chen, Z., Liu, Q., & Lian, C. (2019, June). Pointlanenet: Efficient end-to-end cnns for accurate real-time lane detection. In 2019 IEEE intelligent vehicles symposium (IV) (pp. 2563-2568). IEEE.

Chen, C. C., Lee, I.-K., Liu, J.-W., Huang, S.-Y., & Wang, L. (2015). Utility of C-Reactive Protein Levels for Early Prediction of Dengue Severity in Adults. *BioMed Research International, 2015*, 1–6. doi:10.1155/2015/936062 PMID:26247033

Chen, K., Zhang, J., Beeraka, N. M., Sinelnikov, M. Y., Zhang, X., Cao, Y., & Lu, P. (2022). Robot-Assisted Minimally Invasive Breast Surgery: Recent Evidence with Comparative Clinical Outcomes. *Journal of Clinical Medicine, 11*(7), 1827. doi:10.3390/jcm11071827 PMID:35407434

Chirikjian, G. S. (1994). Hyper-redundant manipulator dynamics: A continuum approximation. *Advanced Robotics, 9*(3), 217–243. doi:10.1163/156855395X00175

Chiu, Y. C., Tsai, C. Y., Ruan, M. D., Shen, G. Y., & Lee, T. T. (2020, August). Mobilenet-SSDv2: An improved object detection model for embedded systems. In *2020 International conference on system science and engineering (ICSSE)* (pp. 1-5). IEEE. 10.1109/ICSSE50014.2020.9219319

Chopra, H., Baig, A. A., Cavalu, S., Singh, I., & Emran, T. B. (2022, August 17). Robotics in surgery: Current trends. *Annals of Medicine and Surgery (London), 81*, 104375. doi:10.1016/j.amsu.2022.104375 PMID:36051814

Cresswell, K., Cunningham-Burley, S., & Sheikh, A. (2018). Health care robotics: Qualitative exploration of key challenges and future directions. *Journal of Medical Internet Research, 20*(7), e10410. doi:10.2196/10410 PMID:29973336

Cui, Q., Wang, Y., Chen, K.-C., Ni, W., Lin, I.-C., Tao, X., & Zhang, P. (2019). Big data analytics and network calculus enabling intelligent management of autonomous vehicles in a smart city. *IEEE Internet of Things Journal*, *6*(2), 2021–2034. doi:10.1109/JIOT.2018.2872442

Cuperman, D., & Verner, I. M. (2019). Fostering analogical reasoning through creating robotic models of biological systems. *Journal of Science Education and Technology*, *28*(2), 90–103. doi:10.1007/s10956-018-9750-4

Da Silva Assis, L., da Silva Soares, A., Coelho, C. J., & Van Baalen, J. (2016). An evolutionary algorithm for autonomous robot navigation. *Procedia Computer Science*, *80*, 2261–2265. doi:10.1016/j.procs.2016.05.404

Daniel, T. (2023). Autonomous AI Systems in Conflict: Emergent Behavior and Its Impact on Predictability and Reliability. *Journal of Military Ethics*, *22*(1), 2–17. doi:10.1080/15027570.2023.2213985

Das, G. P., McGinnity, T. M., Coleman, S. A., & Behera, L. (2015). A distributed task allocation algorithm for a multi-robot system in healthcare facilities. *Journal of Intelligent & Robotic Systems*, *80*(1), 33–58. doi:10.1007/s10846-014-0154-2

Das, S., Datta, S., Barman, A., & Barua, R. (2023). Smart Biodegradable and Bio-Based Polymeric Biomaterials for Biomedical Applications. In A. Kumar, P. Kumar, A. Srivastava, & V. Goyat (Eds.), *Modeling, Characterization, and Processing of Smart Materials* (pp. 56–82). IGI Global. doi:10.4018/978-1-6684-9224-6.ch003

Datta Burton, S. (2022). Not Anytime Soon: The Clinical Translation of Nanorobots and Its Biocompatibility Constraints. In *Interactive Robotics: Legal, Ethical, Social and Economic Aspects* (pp. 123–136). Springer. doi:10.1007/978-3-031-04305-5_35

Datta, S., & Barua, R. (2023). Advanced Materials for Surgical Tools and Biomedical Implants. *Advanced Materials and Manufacturing Techniques for Biomedical Applications*, 25-35.

Datta, S., Barua, R., & Prasad, A. (2023). Additive Manufacturing for the Development of Artificial Organs. *Advanced Materials and Manufacturing Techniques for Biomedical Applications*, 411-427.

Datta, S., Das, S., & Barua, R. (2023). Self-Sustained Nanobiomaterials: Innovative Materials for Biomedical Applications. *Advanced Materials and Manufacturing Techniques for Biomedical Applications*, 303-323.

Datta, S., & Barua, R. (2023). Fluorescent Nanomaterials and Its Application in Biomedical Engineering. In A. Rakha, A. Munawar, V. Khanna, & S. Bansal (Eds.), *Modeling and Simulation of Functional Nanomaterials for Forensic Investigation* (pp. 164–186). IGI Global. doi:10.4018/978-1-6684-8325-1.ch009

Datta, S., Barua, R., & Das, J. (2020). *A review on electro-rheological fluid (er) and its various technological applications*. Extremophilic Microbes and Metabolites-Diversity, Bioprospecting and Biotechnological Applications.

Datta, S., Barua, R., & Das, S. (2023). Role and Challenges of Bioprinting in Bone Tissue Engineering. In R. Ranjith & J. Davim (Eds.), *Handbook of Research on Advanced Functional Materials for Orthopedic Applications* (pp. 205–218). IGI Global. doi:10.4018/978-1-6684-7412-9.ch012

Datta, S., Barua, R., Sarkar, R., Barui, A., Chowdhury, A. R., & Datta, P. (2018, September). Design and development of alginate: Poly-l-lysine scaffolds by 3D bio printing and studying their mechanical, structural and cell viability properties. []. IOP Publishing.]. *IOP Conference Series. Materials Science and Engineering*, *402*, 012113. doi:10.1088/1757-899X/402/1/012113

Dawood, A. B., Fras, J., Aljaber, F., Mintz, Y., Arezzo, A., Godaba, H., & Althoefer, K. (2021). Fusing dexterity and perception for soft robot-assisted minimally invasive surgery: What we learnt from STIFF-FLOP. *Applied Sciences (Basel, Switzerland)*, *11*(14), 6586. doi:10.3390/app11146586

Deng, W., & Wu, R. (2019). Real-time driver-drowsiness detection system using facial features. *IEEE Access : Practical Innovations, Open Solutions*, *7*, 118727–118738. doi:10.1109/ACCESS.2019.2936663

Dixit, P., & Silakari, S. (2021). Deep learning algorithms for cybersecurity applications: A technological and status review. *Computer Science Review*, *39*, 100317. doi:10.1016/j.cosrev.2020.100317

Dong, J., Chen, S., Miralinaghi, M., Chen, T., Li, P., & Labi, S. (2023). Why did the AI make that decision? Towards an explainable artificial intelligence (XAI) for autonomous driving systems. *Transportation Research Part C, Emerging Technologies*, *156*, 104358. doi:10.1016/j.trc.2023.104358

Dongpo, L., & Xuhui, M. (2011). *Virtual Proving Ground.*

Duan, W., Akinyemi, T., Du, W., Ma, J., Chen, X., Wang, F., Omisore, O., Luo, J., Wang, H., & Wang, L. (2023). Technical and Clinical Progress on Robot-Assisted Endovascular Interventions: A Review. *Micromachines*, *14*(1), 197. doi:10.3390/mi14010197 PMID:36677258

Duggal, A. S., Malik, P. K., Gehlot, A., Singh, R., Gaba, G. S., Masud, M., & Al-Amri, J. F. (2022). A sequential roadmap to Industry 6.0: Exploring future manufacturing trends. *IET Communications*, *16*(5), 521–531. doi:10.1049/cmu2.12284

Dupont, P. E., Simaan, N., Choset, H., & Rucker, C. (2022). Continuum Robots for Medical Interventions. *Proceedings of the IEEE*. Institute of Electrical and Electronics Engineers.

Du, Y., Liu, C., Wu, D., & Li, S. (2016). Application of Vehicle Mounted Accelerometers to Measure Pavement Roughness. *International Journal of Distributed Sensor Networks*, *2016*(6), 8413146. doi:10.1155/2016/8413146

Eckert, C., Neunsinger, C., & Osterrieder, K. (2022). (Repeat J)Managing customer satisfaction: Digital applications for insurance companies. *The Geneva Papers on Risk and Insurance. Issues and Practice*, *47*(3), 569–602. doi:10.1057/s41288-021-00257-z

Elendu, C., Amaechi, D. C., Elendu, T. C., Jingwa, K. A., Okoye, O. K., Okah, M. J., & Alimi, H. A. (2023). Ethical implications of AI and robotics in healthcare. *Revista de Medicina (São Paulo)*, *102*(50), e36671. PMID:38115340

Eling, M., Nuessle, D., & Staubli, J. (2022). The impact of artificial intelligence along the insurance value chain and on the insurability of risks. *The Geneva Papers on Risk and Insurance. Issues and Practice*, *47*(2), 205–241. doi:10.1057/s41288-020-00201-7

Etukudoh, N. S., Esame, N. V., Obeta, U. M., Ejinaka, O. R., & Khang, A. (2024). Automations and Robotics Improves Quality Healthcare in the Era of Digital Medical Laboratory. In Computer Vision and AI-Integrated IoT Technologies in the Medical Ecosystem (pp. 419-434). CRC Press. doi:10.1201/9781003429609-24

Faniadis, E., & Amanatiadis, A. (2020, November). Deep learning inference at the edge for mobile and aerial robotics. In *2020 IEEE International Symposium on Safety, Security, and Rescue Robotics (SSRR)* (pp. 334-340). IEEE. 10.1109/SSRR50563.2020.9292575

Fischell, E., Stanton, T. K., Kukulya, A., & Andone, C. (1806). Lavery, Monitoring of macroalgae (kelp) farms with autonomous underwater vehicle-based split-beam sonar, September 2018. *The Journal of the Acoustical Society of America*, *144*(3).

Flückiger, I., & Duygun, M. (2022). (LR 111)New technologies and data in insurance. In Geneva Papers on Risk and Insurance: Issues and Practice, 47(3). Palgrave Macmillan. doi:10.1057/s41288-022-00274-6

Foroutannia, A., Shoryabi, M., Anaraki, A. A., & Rowhanimanesh, A. (2021, March). SIN: A Programmable Platform for Swarm Robotics. In *2021 26th International Computer Conference, Computer Society of Iran (CSICC)* (pp. 1-5). IEEE. 10.1109/CSICC52343.2021.9420596

Fosch-Villaronga, E., & Drukarch, H. (2021). On Healthcare Robots: Concepts, definitions, and considerations for healthcare robot governance. arXiv preprint arXiv:2106.03468.

Fujiyoshi, H., Hirakawa, T., & Yamashita, T. (2019). Deep learning-based image recognition for autonomous driving. *IATSS Research*, *43*(4), 244–252. doi:10.1016/j.iatssr.2019.11.008

Gadkari, M. Y., & Sambre, N. B. (2012). VANET: Routing protocols, security issues and simulation tools. *IOSR Journal of Computer Engineering*, *3*(3), 28–38. doi:10.9790/0661-0332838

Garfjeld Roberts, P., Glasbey, J. C., Abram, S., Osei-Bordom, D., Bach, S. P., & Beard, D. J. (2020). Research quality and transparency, outcome measurement and evidence for safety and effectiveness in robot-assisted surgery: Systematic review. *BJS Open*, *4*(6), 1084–1099. doi:10.1002/bjs5.50352 PMID:33052029

Gaur, L., Afaq, A., Singh, G., & Dwivedi, Y. K. (2021). Role of artificial intelligence and robotics to foster the touchless travel during a pandemic: A review and research agenda. *International Journal of Contemporary Hospitality Management*, *33*(11), 4079–4098. doi:10.1108/IJCHM-11-2020-1246

Gellweiler, C., & Krishnamurthi, L. (2020). Editorial: How digital innovators achieve customer value. In Journal of Theoretical and Applied Electronic Commerce Research, 15(1). Universidad de Talca. doi:10.4067/S0718-18762020000100101

Ghosh, U., & Datta, R. (2014). SDRP: Secure and dynamic routing protocol for mobile ad-hoc networks. *IET Networks*, *3*(3), 235–243. doi:10.1049/iet-net.2013.0056

Gomes, A. L. V., Wee, L. J., Khan, A. M., Gil, L. H., Marques, E. T. Jr, Calzavara-Silva, C. E., & Tan, T. W. (2010). Classification of dengue fever patients based on gene expression data using support vector machines. *PLoS One*, *5*(6), 11267. doi:10.1371/journal.pone.0011267 PMID:20585645

González, A., Olazagoitia, J. L., & Vinolas, J. (2018). A low-cost data acquisition system for automobile dynamics applications. *Sensors (Basel)*, *18*(2), 366. doi:10.3390/s18020366 PMID:29382039

Gonzalez, L. C., Moreno, R., Escalante, H. J., Martinez, F., & Carlos, M. R. (2017). Learning Roadway Surface Disruption Patterns Using the Bag of Words Representation. *IEEE Transactions on Intelligent Transportation Systems*, *18*(11), 2916–2928. doi:10.1109/TITS.2017.2662483

Gonzalo de Diego, B., González Aguña, A., Fernández Batalla, M., Herrero Jaén, S., Sierra Ortega, A., Barchino Plata, R., & Santamaría García, J. M. (2024, March). Competencies in the Robotics of Care for Nursing Robotics: A Scoping Review. In Healthcare (Vol. 12, No. 6, p. 617). MDPI. doi:10.3390/healthcare12060617

Gorchakova, E. R. (2019). *The impact of digitalization on the health insurance system.* doi:10.18411/lj-03-2019-48

Gravagne, I., & Walker, I. D. (2000). Kinematics for constrained continuum robots using wavelet decomposition. *Robotics*, *2000*, 292–298.

Greener, J. G., Kandathil, S. M., Moffat, L., & Jones, D. T. (2022). A guide to machine learning for biologists. *Nature Reviews. Molecular Cell Biology*, *23*(1), 40–55. doi:10.1038/s41580-021-00407-0 PMID:34518686

Guntur, S. R., Gorrepati, R. R., & Dirisala, V. R. (2019). Robotics in healthcare: an internet of medical robotic things (IoMRT) perspective. In *Machine learning in bio-signal analysis and diagnostic imaging* (pp. 293–318). Academic Press. doi:10.1016/B978-0-12-816086-2.00012-6

Guo, N., Lenzo, B., Zhang, X., Zou, Y., Zhai, R., & Zhang, T. (2020). A real-time nonlinear model predictive controller for yaw motion optimization of distributed drive electric vehicles. *IEEE Transactions on Vehicular Technology*, *69*(5), 4935–4946. doi:10.1109/TVT.2020.2980169

Gupta, A., Anpalagan, A., Guan, L., & Khwaja, A. S. (2021). Deep learning for object detection and scene perception in self-driving cars: Survey, challenges, and open issues. *Array (New York, N.Y.)*, *10*, 100057. doi:10.1016/j.array.2021.100057

Gupta, S., Upadhyay, D., & Dubey, A. K. (2019). Self-Driving Car Using Artificial Intelligence. In M. Kumar, R. Pandey, & V. Kumar (Eds.), *Advances in Interdisciplinary Engineering. Lecture Notes in Mechanical Engineering.* Springer. doi:10.1007/978-981-13-6577-5_49

Gurjeet, S. (2022). *Vijay, Kumar, Banga., Thaweesak, Yingthawornsuk.* Artificial Intelligence and Industrial Robot., doi:10.1109/SITIS57111.2022.00098

Guzman, M. G., Halstead, S. B., Artsob, H., Buchy, P., Farrar, J., Gubler, D. J., & Nathan, M. B. (2010). Dengue: A continuing global threat. *Nature Reviews. Microbiology*, *8*(S12), S7–S16. doi:10.1038/nrmicro2460 PMID:21079655

Guzmán-Ortiz, C. V., Navarro-Acosta, N. G., Florez-Garcia, W., & Vicente-Ramos, W. (2020). (LR 122)Impact of digital transformation on the individual job performance of insurance companies in peru. *International Journal of Data and Network Science*, *4*(4), 337–346. doi:10.5267/j.ijdns.2020.9.005

Haken, H., & Levi, P. (2012). *Synergetic agents: From multi-robot systems to molecular robotics.* John Wiley & Sons. doi:10.1002/9783527659524

Hamdi, M. M., Audah, L., Rashid, S. A., & Alani, S. (2021). VANET-based traffic monitoring and incident detection system: A review. *International Journal of Electrical & Computer Engineering (2088-8708)*, *11*(4).

Hamdi, M. M., Audah, L., Rashid, S. A., Mohammed, A. H., Alani, S., & Mustafa, A. S. (2020). A review of applications, characteristics and challenges in vehicular ad hoc networks (VANETs). In 2020 international congress on human-computer interaction, optimization and robotic applications (HORA) (pp. 1-7). IEEE.

Hannan, M. W., & Walker, I. D. (2003). Kinematics and the implementation of an elephant's trunk manipulator and other continuum style robots. *Journal of Robotic Systems*, *20*(2), 45–63. doi:10.1002/rob.10070 PMID:14983840

Harit, P. (2021). (LR 83)The Rise of Insurtech: The Ups and Downs of New Trend. SSRN *Electronic Journal*. doi:10.2139/ssrn.3799576

Hodge, V. J., Hawkins, R., & Alexander, R. (2021). Deep reinforcement learning for drone navigation using sensor data. *Neural Computing & Applications*, *33*(6), 2015–2033. doi:10.1007/s00521-020-05097-x

Holland, J., Kingston, L., McCarthy, C., Armstrong, E., O'Dwyer, P., Merz, F., & McConnell, M. (2021). Service robots in the healthcare sector. *Robotics (Basel, Switzerland)*, *10*(1), 47. doi:10.3390/robotics10010047

Hong, Y., Pan, H., Sun, W., & Jia, Y. (2021). Deep dual-resolution networks for real-time and accurate semantic segmentation of road scenes. *arXiv preprint arXiv:2101.06085*.

Hu, F., Chen, B., Shi, D., Zhang, X., & Pan, H. Z. (2020). Secure Routing Protocol in Wireless Ad Hoc Networks via Deep Learning. In 2020 IEEE Wireless Communications and Networking Conference (WCNC) (pp. 1-6). IEEE. doi:10.1109/WCNC45663.2020.9120545

Huang, W. (2021). Modeling soft swimming robots using discrete elastic rod method. *Proc. Bioinspired Sensing, Actuation, Control Underwater Soft Robotic Syst.*

Hu, F., He, Q., & Kong, F. (2011)... *Time-Frequency Vibration Representation for Steel Mill Condition Monitoring.*, *1*, 1–5.

Hughes, J., Culha, U., Giardina, F., Guenther, F., Rosendo, A., & Iida, F. (2016). Soft manipulators and grippers: A review. *Frontiers in Robotics and AI*, *3*, 1–12. doi:10.3389/frobt.2016.00069

Humaidi, A. J., Ibraheem, I. K., Azar, A. T., & Sadiq, M. E. (2020). A new adaptive synergetic control design for single link robot arm actuated by pneumatic muscles. *Entropy (Basel, Switzerland)*, 22(7), 723. doi:10.3390/e22070723 PMID:33286496

Hussain, F., Hussain, R., & Hossain, E. (2021). Explainable artificial intelligence (XAI): An engineering perspective. *arXiv preprint arXiv:2101.03613*.

Ilic, S., Katupitiya, J., & Tordon, M. (n.d.). *In-vehicle data logging system for fatigue analysis of drive shaft.*

Inam, M., Li, Z., Ali, A., & Zahoor, A. (2019). A novel protocol for vehicle cluster formation and vehicle head selection in vehicular ad-hoc networks. *International Journal of Electronics and Information Engineering*, 10(2), 103–119.

Jabbar, R., Shinoy, M., Kharbeche, M., Al-Khalifa, K., Krichen, M., & Barkaoui, K. (2020, February). Driver drowsiness detection model using convolutional neural networks techniques for android application. In *2020 IEEE International Conference on Informatics, IoT, and Enabling Technologies (ICIoT)* (pp. 237-242). IEEE. 10.1109/ICIoT48696.2020.9089484

Jamaludin, W. A. W. (2021). *Photovoltaic-Thermoelectric Generator Monitoring System using Arduino Based Data Acquisition system Technique.*

Javaid, M., Haleem, A., Singh, R. P., Rab, S., Suman, R., & Kumar, L. (2022). Utilization of Robotics for Healthcare: A Scoping Review. *Journal of Industrial Integration and Management, 2250015.*

Jiang, L., & Feng, L. (Eds.). (2010). *Bioinspired Intelligent Nanostructured Interfacial Materials*. Springer. doi:10.1142/7380

Jonathan, A. (2023). *Development of an AI-Robotics 3D Printed Circle of Command for Enhancing Accessibility and Mobility in Individuals with Mobility Issues*. IEEE. doi:10.5121/csit.2023.130910

Jones, B. A., & Walker, I. D. (2006). Kinematics for multisection continuum robots. *IEEE Transactions on Robotics*, 22(1), 43–55. doi:10.1109/TRO.2005.861458

Joseph, A., Christian, B., Abiodun, A. A., & Oyawale, F. (2018). A review on humanoid robotics in healthcare. In *MATEC Web of Conferences* (Vol. 153, p. 02004). EDP Sciences. 10.1051/matecconf/201815302004

Joshi, V., Joshi, V. V., Pawar, N., & Acharya, S. (2020). *Digitalisation of Health Care in India: Initiatives and Challenges. 40.* https://www.researchgate.net/publication/354586176

Junnila, S., & Niittylahti, J. (2003). Wireless technologies for data acquisition systems. *Proceedings of the 1st International Symposium on Information and Communication Technologies*, (pp. 132–137). IEEE.

Kamboj, S., & Chawla, S. (2014). Geocast routing in vehicular Ad Hoc networks: A survey. [IJCSIT]. *International Journal of Computer Science and Information Technologies*, 5(4), 5365.

Kang, Y., Yin, H., & Berger, C. (2019). Test Your Self-Driving Algorithm: An Overview of Publicly Available Driving Datasets and Virtual Testing Environments. [Google Scholar] [CrossRef]. *IEEE Transactions on Intelligent Vehicles*, 4(2), 171–185. doi:10.1109/TIV.2018.2886678

Kar, S. (2019, October). Robotics in HealthCare. In *2019 2nd International Conference on Power Energy, Environment and Intelligent Control (PEEIC)* (pp. 78-83). IEEE. 10.1109/PEEIC47157.2019.8976668

Karpov, V. E., & Tarassov, V. B. (2017, September). Synergetic artificial intelligence and social robotics. In *International Conference on Intelligent Information Technologies for Industry* (pp. 3-15). Cham: Springer International Publishing.

Katevas, N. (Ed.). (2001). *Mobile robotics in healthcare* (Vol. 7). IOS Press.

Katrolia, J. S., Mirbach, B., El-Sherif, A., Feld, H., Rambach, J., & Stricker, D. (2021). Ticam: A time-of-flight in-car cabin monitoring dataset. *arXiv preprint arXiv:2103.11719.*

Kaur, J. (2024). Fueling Healthcare Transformation: The Nexus of Startups, Venture Capital, and Innovation. In Fostering Innovation in Venture Capital and Startup Ecosystems (pp. 327-351). IGI Global.

Kaur, J. (2024). Green Finance 2.0: Pioneering Pathways for Sustainable Development and Health Through Future Trends and Innovations. In Sustainable Investments in Green Finance (pp. 294-319). IGI Global.

Kaur, J. (2024). Towards a Sustainable Triad: Uniting Energy Management Systems, Smart Cities, and Green Healthcare for a Greener Future. In Emerging Materials, Technologies, and Solutions for Energy Harvesting (pp. 258-285). IGI Global.

Kaur, J., & Arora, R. (2023, June). Exploring the dimensionality of employee silence in healthcare sector. In AIP conference proceedings (Vol. 2782, No. 1). AIP Publishing. doi:10.1063/5.0154178

Kaur, J., & Arora, R. (2023, June). Exploring the impact of employee silence in private hospitals-a structural equation modeling approach. In AIP Conference Proceedings (Vol. 2782, No. 1). AIP Publishing. doi:10.1063/5.0154173

Kavidha, V., Gayathri, N., & Kumar, S. R. (2021). AI, IoT and robotics in the medical and healthcare field. *AI and IoT-Based Intelligent Automation in Robotics*, 165-187.

Kernbach, S. (2011). Robot companions: Technology for humans. arXiv preprint arXiv:1111.5207.

Khamis, A., Patel, D., & Elgazzar, K. (2021). Deep Learning for Unmanned Autonomous Vehicles: A Comprehensive Review. In A. Koubaa & A. T. Azar (Eds.), *Deep Learning for Unmanned Systems. Studies in Computational Intelligence* (Vol. 984). Springer. doi:10.1007/978-3-030-77939-9_1

Khang, A., Rath, K. C., Anh, P. T. N., Rath, S. K., & Bhattacharya, S. (2024). Quantum-Based Robotics in the High-Tech Healthcare Industry: Innovations and Applications. In Medical Robotics and AI-Assisted Diagnostics for a High-Tech Healthcare Industry (pp. 1-27). IGI Global.

Kim, J., Gu, G. M., & Heo, P. (2016). Robotics for healthcare. *Biomedical Engineering: Frontier Research and Converging Technologies*, 489-509.

Kim, H., Kwon, D., Son, J., & Choi, J. (2024). A Novel Robotic Healthcare Device for Treating Chronic Venous Insufficiency in People Who Sit for Prolonged Periods. *IEEE Transactions on Medical Robotics and Bionics*, 6(2), 618–631. doi:10.1109/TMRB.2024.3373909

Kolpashchikov, D., Gerget, O., & Meshcheryakov, R. (2022). *Robotics in healthcare. Handbook of Robotics in Healthcare* (Vol. 2). Practicalities and Prospects.

Kumar, V., Mishra, S., & Chand, N. (2013). Applications of VANETs: present & future. *communications and network,* 5(01), 12-15.

Kumar, A. (2017). (LR 117) Impact of Digitalisation on Service Sector in India. *Reviewed Refereed Research Journal,* 8(15). https://www.researchgate.net/publication/360782465

Kumar, A., Kaur, A., & Kumar, M. (2019). Face detection techniques: A review. *Artificial Intelligence Review*, 52(2), 927–948. doi:10.1007/s10462-018-9650-2

Kumar, K. R. (2010). VANET parameters and applications: A review. *Global Journal of Computer Science and Technology*, 10(7), 72–77.

Kyrarini, M., Lygerakis, F., Rajavenkatanarayanan, A., Sevastopoulos, C., Nambiappan, H. R., Chaitanya, K. K., Babu, A. R., Mathew, J., & Makedon, F. (2021). A survey of robots in healthcare. *Technologies*, *9*(1), 8. doi:10.3390/technologies9010008

Lai, W. K., Lin, M. T., & Yang, Y. H. (2015). A machine learning system for routing decision-making in urban vehicular ad hoc networks. *International Journal of Distributed Sensor Networks*, *11*(3), 374391. doi:10.1155/2015/374391

Langarica, S., Rüffelmacher, C., & Núñez, F. (2019). An industrial internet application for real-time fault diagnosis in industrial motors. *IEEE Transactions on Automation Science and Engineering*, *17*(1), 284–295. doi:10.1109/TASE.2019.2913628

Lan, H., Hartonen, K., & Riekkola, M. L. (2020). Miniaturised air sampling techniques for analysis of volatile organic compounds in air. *Trends in Analytical Chemistry*, *126*, 115873. doi:10.1016/j.trac.2020.115873

LastMinuteEngineers.com. (2022). *Interfacing Micro SD Card Module with Arduino*. Last Minute Engineers.

Lazrag, H., Chaibi, H., Saadane, R., & Rahmani, M. D. (2018). An optimal and secure routing protocol for wireless sensor networks. In *2018 6th International Conference on Multimedia Computing and Systems (ICMCS)* (pp. 1-5). IEEE. 10.1109/ICMCS.2018.8525911

Lee, V. J., Chow, A., Zheng, X., Carrasco, L. R., Cook, A. R., Lye, D. C., Ng, L.-C., & Leo, Y. S. (2012). Simple clinical and laboratory predictors of Chikungunya versus dengue infections in adults. *PLoS Neglected Tropical Diseases*, *6*(9), 1786. doi:10.1371/journal.pntd.0001786 PMID:23029573

Lestingi, L., Sbrolli, C., Scarmozzino, P., Romeo, G., Bersani, M. M., & Rossi, M. (2022, May). Formal modeling and verification of multi-robot interactive scenarios in service settings. In *Proceedings of the IEEE/ACM 10th International Conference on Formal Methods in Software Engineering* (pp. 80-90). IEEE. 10.1145/3524482.3527653

Liang, W., Li, Z., Zhang, H., Wang, S., & Bie, R. (2015). Vehicular ad hoc networks: Architectures, research issues, methodologies, challenges, and trends. *International Journal of Distributed Sensor Networks*, *11*(8), 745303. doi:10.1155/2015/745303

Li, D., Zhang, Z., Liu, P., Wang, Z., & Zhang, L. (2020). Battery fault diagnosis for electric vehicles based on voltage abnormality by combining the long short-term memory neural network and the equivalent circuit model. *IEEE Transactions on Power Electronics*, *36*(2), 1303–1315. doi:10.1109/TPEL.2020.3008194

Lin, L., & Chen, C. (2020). (LR 82)The promise and perils of insurtech. *SSRN*, *2020*, 115–142. doi:10.2139/ssrn.3463533

Liu, L., Lu, S., Zhong, R., Wu, B., Yao, Y., Zhang, Q., & Shi, W. (2020). Computing systems for autonomous driving: State of the art and challenges. *IEEE Internet of Things Journal*, *8*(8), 6469–6486. doi:10.1109/JIOT.2020.3043716

Liu, Z., Cai, Y., Wang, H., Chen, L., Gao, H., Jia, Y., & Li, Y. (2021). Robust target recognition and tracking of self-driving cars with radar and camera information fusion under severe weather conditions. *IEEE Transactions on Intelligent Transportation Systems*, *23*(7), 6640–6653. doi:10.1109/TITS.2021.3059674

Li, W., Kong, K., Li, P., Wang, G., Cui, B., Zhu, L., & Zhu, S. (2021). Robot-assisted sleeve gastrectomy in patients with obesity with a novel Chinese domestic MicroHand SII surgical system. *BMC Surgery*, *21*(1), 260. doi:10.1186/s12893-021-01259-3 PMID:34034737

Li, Y., Jiao, X. Y., Sun, B. Q., Zhang, Q. H., & Yang, J. Y. (2021, March). Multi-welfare-robot cooperation framework for multi-task assignment in healthcare facilities based on multi-agent system. In *2021 IEEE International Conference on Intelligence and Safety for Robotics (ISR)* (pp. 413-416). IEEE. 10.1109/ISR50024.2021.9419496

Li, Z., & Du, R. (2013). Design and analysis of a bio-inspired wire-driven multi-section flexible robot. *International Journal of Advanced Robotic Systems*, *10*(4), 209. doi:10.5772/56025

Lloyd, P., Dall'Armellina, E., Schneider, J. E., & Valdastri, P. (2024). *Future cardiovascular healthcare via magnetic resonance imaging-driven robotics.*

Maalouf, N., Sidaoui, A., Elhajj, I. H., & Asmar, D. (2018). Robotics in nursing: A scoping review. *Journal of Nursing Scholarship*, *50*(6), 590–600. doi:10.1111/jnu.12424 PMID:30260093

Malika Shuxratovna, U., & Nuriddin Rustam Ugli, A. (2021). (LR 114)DIGITALIZATION OF THE INSURANCE MARKET. In Multidisciplinary Peer Reviewed Journal ISSN, 7(2).

Mallaboyev, N. M., Sharifjanovna, Q. M., Muxammadjon, Q., & Shukurullo, C. (2022, May). INFORMATION SECURITY ISSUES. In Conference Zone (pp. 241-245). IEEE.

Mankodiya, H., Jadav, D., Gupta, R., Tanwar, S., Hong, W. C., & Sharma, R. (2022). Od-xai: Explainable ai-based semantic object detection for autonomous vehicles. *Applied Sciences (Basel, Switzerland)*, *12*(11), 5310. doi:10.3390/app12115310

Manoharan, D. S. (2019). An improved safety algorithm for artificial intelligence enabled processors in self driving cars. *Journal of Artificial Intelligence and Capsule Networks*, *1*(2), 95–104. doi:10.36548/jaicn.2019.2.005

Marano, P. (2019). (LR 112)Navigating insurtech: The digital intermediaries of insurance products and customer protection in the EU. *Maastricht Journal of European and Comparative Law*, *26*(2), 294–315. doi:10.1177/1023263X19830345

Marchegiani, F., Siragusa, L., Zadoroznyj, A., Laterza, V., Mangana, O., Schena, C. A., Ammendola, M., Memeo, R., Bianchi, P. P., Spinoglio, G., Gavriilidis, P., & de'Angelis, N. (2023). New Robotic Platforms in General Surgery: What's the Current Clinical Scenario? *Medicina (Kaunas, Lithuania)*, *59*(7), 1264. doi:10.3390/medicina59071264 PMID:37512075

Martel, S., Mohammadi, M., Felfoul, O., Lu, Z., & Pouponneau, P. (2009). Flagellated magnetotactic bacteria as controlled MRI-trackable propulsion and steering systems for medical nanorobots operating in the human microvasculature. *The International Journal of Robotics Research*, *28*(4), 571–582. doi:10.1177/0278364908100924 PMID:19890435

Ma, Y., Zhang, Y., Wan, J., Zhang, D., & Pan, N. (2015). Robot and cloud-assisted multi-modal healthcare system. *Cluster Computing*, *18*(3), 1295–1306. doi:10.1007/s10586-015-0453-9

McMahan, W., & Walker, I. D. (2009, February). Octopus-inspired grasp-synergies for continuum manipulators. In *2008 IEEE International Conference on Robotics and Biomimetics* (pp. 945-950). IEEE. 10.1109/ROBIO.2009.4913126

Mehta, P. L., Kalra, R., & Prasad, R. (2021). A Backdrop Case Study of AI-Drones in Indian Demographic Characteristics Emphasizing the Role of AI in Global Cities Digitalization. *Wireless Personal Communications*, *118*(1), 301–321. doi:10.1007/s11277-020-08014-6 PMID:33424130

Mejri, M. N., & Ben-Othman, J. (2016). GDVAN: A new greedy behavior attack detection algorithm for VANETs. *IEEE Transactions on Mobile Computing*, *16*(3), 759–771. doi:10.1109/TMC.2016.2577035

Men, X., Liu, H., Chen, N., & Li, F. (2018). *A new time domain filtering method for calculating the RMS value of vibration signals. 51605191*, 2016–2019.

Mir, U. B., Sharma, S., Kar, A. K., & Gupta, M. P. (2020). Critical success factors for integrating artificial intelligence and robotics. *Digital Policy. Regulation & Governance*, *22*(4), 307–331. doi:10.1108/DPRG-03-2020-0032

Mishra, A., Cha, J., & Kim, S. (2022). Privacy-preserved in-cabin monitoring system for autonomous vehicles. *Computational Intelligence and Neuroscience*, *2022*, 2022. doi:10.1155/2022/5389359 PMID:35498178

Mohamed, A., Fouad, M. M. M., & Elhariri, E. (2014). *RoadMonitor: An Intelligent Road Surface Condition Monitoring System RoadMonitor: An Intelligent Road Surface Condition Monitoring System.* Springer. doi:10.1007/978-3-319-11310-4

Mohan, P., Sabarwal, T., & Preethiya, T. (2023). Indian Sign Language Character Recognition System. *2023 4th International Conference on Electronics and Sustainable Communication Systems (ICESC).* IEEE. 10.1109/ICESC57686.2023.10193309

Mois, G., & Beer, J. M. (2020). The role of healthcare robotics in providing support to older adults: A socio-ecological perspective. *Current Geriatrics Reports, 9*(2), 82–89. doi:10.1007/s13670-020-00314-w PMID:32435576

Mo, K., Suh, K., & Hong, S. (2000). New Approach in Vehicle Durability Evaluation, Virtual Proving Ground. *Test*, (March), 1–5.

Monterrey, C. (2018). *Road Load Data Acquisition system with SAE-J1939 Communications Network: Integration and Laboratory Test.* [Thesis, Instituto Tecnológico y de Estudios Superiores de Monterrey].

Moradi, M., Yan, K., Colwell, D., Samwald, M., & Asgari, R. (2023). Model-agnostic explainable artificial intelligence for object detection in image data. *arXiv preprint arXiv:2303.17249.* doi:10.2139/ssrn.4429462

Moreno, C., González, A., Olazagoitia, J. L., & Vinolas, J. (2020). The acquisition rate and soundness of a low-cost data acquisition system (LC-DAQ) for high frequency applications. *Sensors (Basel), 20*(2), 524. doi:10.3390/s20020524 PMID:31963552

Morgan, A. A., Abdi, J., Syed, M. A., Kohen, G. E., Barlow, P., & Vizcaychipi, M. P. (2022). Robots in healthcare: A scoping review. *Current Robotics Reports, 3*(4), 271–280. doi:10.1007/s43154-022-00095-4 PMID:36311256

Morizane, S., Stein, H., Komiya, T., Kaneta, H., & Takenaka, A. (2023). Retroperitoneal robot-assisted laparoscopic nephroureterectomy using the da Vinci Xi and SP systems: Initial experiences in cadaveric models. *Investigative and Clinical Urology, 64*(4), 380–387. doi:10.4111/icu.20230021 PMID:37417563

Morton, J., Hardwick, R. H., Tilney, H. S., Gudgeon, A. M., Jah, A., Stevens, L., Marecik, S., & Slack, M. (2021). Pre-clinical evaluation of the versius surgical system, a new robot-assisted surgical device for use in minimal access general and colorectal procedures. *Surgical Endoscopy, 35*(5), 2169–2177. doi:10.1007/s00464-020-07622-4 PMID:32405893

Moura, V. (2012). Magnetically Actuated Multiscale Medical Robots. In *IROS 2012 Full-day Workshop* (p. 48). IEEE.

Mueller, J. (n.d.). *InsurTech Rising: A Profile of the InsurTech Landscape DECEMBER 2018.*

Muhammad, K., Hussain, T., Ullah, H., Del Ser, J., Rezaei, M., Kumar, N., & de Albuquerque, V. H. C. (2022). Vision-based semantic segmentation in scene understanding for autonomous driving: Recent achievements, challenges, and outlooks. *IEEE Transactions on Intelligent Transportation Systems, 23*(12), 22694–22715. doi:10.1109/TITS.2022.3207665

Muhammad, K., Ullah, A., Lloret, J., Del Ser, J., & de Albuquerque, V. H. C. (2020). Deep learning for safe autonomous driving: Current challenges and future directions. *IEEE Transactions on Intelligent Transportation Systems, 22*(7), 4316–4336. doi:10.1109/TITS.2020.3032227

Mushtaque, R. S., Ahmad, S. M., Mushtaque, R., & Baloch, S. (2020). Case Report, A Curious Case of Dengue Fever: A Case Report of Unorthodox Manifestations. *Case Reports in Medicine, 2020*, 1–4. doi:10.1155/2020/1701082 PMID:32774384

Nagadevi, D. (2021). *A Comprehensive Study on Artificial Intelligence and Robotics for Machine Intelligence.* Springer. doi:10.4018/978-1-7998-7701-1.ch011

Nam, K., Dutt, C. S., Chathoth, P., Daghfous, A., & Khan, M. S. (2021). The adoption of artificial intelligence and robotics in the hotel industry: Prospects and challenges. *Electronic Markets, 31*(3), 553–574. doi:10.1007/s12525-020-00442-3

Nanobiomaterials in Drug Delivery. (2016). *Applications of Nanobiomaterials* (A. M. Grumezescu, Ed.). Vol. 9). Elsevier.

Narula, A., Narula, N. K., Khanna, S., Narula, R., Narula, J., & Narula, A. (2014). Future prospects of Robotics in robotics software, a healthcare perspective. *International Journal of Applied Engineering Research: IJAER, 9*(22), 10271–10280.

National Vector Borne Disease Control Programme (NVBDCP). (2015). Retrieved from https://nvbdcp.gov.in/index4.php?lang=1&level=0&linkid=431&lid=3715

Nayak, B., Bhattacharyya, S. S., & Krishnamoorthy, B. (2019). LR 77: Integrating wearable technology products and big data analytics in business strategy: A study of health insurance firms. *Journal of Systems and Information Technology, 21*(2), 255–275. doi:10.1108/JSIT-08-2018-0109

Nehal, R. (2023). AI in Robotics: Advancements, Applications and Challenges. *Journal of Information Technology and Digital World.* doi:10.36548/jitdw.2023.2.009

Nordin, I. N. A. M., Razif, M. R. M., & Natarajan, E. (2013). 3-D finite-element analysis of fiber-reinforced soft bending actuator for finger flexion. IEEE/ASME international conference on advanced intelligent mechatronic, Wollongong, Australia.

Of, A., & Signal, V. (2013). *A LabVIEW BASED DATA ACQUISITION SYSTEM FOR MONITORING Sunita Mohanta Department of Electronics and Communication Engineering National Institute of Technology Rourkela, Odisha-769008 Sunita Mohanta Dr. Umesh Chandra Pati Department of Electronics and Co.*

Ogunoiki, A. O. (2015). *University of Birmingham Research Archive.* University of Birmingham.

Oksanen, A., Savela, N., Latikka, R., & Koivula, A. (2020). Trust toward robots and artificial intelligence: An experimental approach to human–technology interactions online. *Frontiers in Psychology, 11*, 568256. doi:10.3389/fpsyg.2020.568256 PMID:33343447

Olszewska, J. I. (2022, February). Snakes in Trees: An Explainable Artificial Intelligence Approach for Automatic Object Detection and Recognition. In ICAART (3) (pp. 996-1002).

Omeiza, D., Webb, H., Jirotka, M., & Kunze, L. (2021). Explanations in autonomous driving: A survey. *IEEE Transactions on Intelligent Transportation Systems, 23*(8), 10142–10162. doi:10.1109/TITS.2021.3122865

Oña, E. D., Garcia-Haro, J. M., Jardón, A., & Balaguer, C. (2019). Robotics in health care: Perspectives of robot-aided interventions in clinical practice for rehabilitation of upper limbs. *Applied Sciences (Basel, Switzerland), 9*(13), 2586. doi:10.3390/app9132586

Ostrowska, M. (2021). (LR 110)Does new technology put an end to policyholder risk declaration? The impact of digitalisation on insurance relationships. *The Geneva Papers on Risk and Insurance. Issues and Practice, 46*(4), 573–592. doi:10.1057/s41288-020-00191-6

Ouyang, Z., Niu, J., Liu, Y., & Guizani, M. (2019). Deep CNN-based real-time traffic light detector for self-driving vehicles. *IEEE Transactions on Mobile Computing, 19*(2), 300–313. doi:10.1109/TMC.2019.2892451

Pal Singh, H., & Singh, R. (2021). Low Cost Data Acquisition System for Road-Vehicle Interaction Using Arduino Board. *Journal of Physics: Conference Series, 1831*(1), 012031. doi:10.1088/1742-6596/1831/1/012031

Pandit, C. M., & Ladhe, S. A. (2014). Secure routing protocol in MANET using TAC. In *2014 First International Conference on Networks & Soft Computing (ICNSC2014)* (pp. 107-112). IEEE. 10.1109/CNSC.2014.6906693

Paramasivan, B., Prakash, M. J. V., & Kaliappan, M. (2015). Development of a secure routing protocol using game theory model in mobile ad hoc networks. *Journal of Communications and Networks (Seoul)*, *17*(1), 75–83. doi:10.1109/JCN.2015.000012

Patel, A. R., Patel, R. S., Singh, N. M., & Kazi, F. S. (2017). Vitality of robotics in healthcare industry: Robotics perspective. *Robotics and big data technologies for next generation healthcare*, 91-109.

Patil, C., & Nataraj, K. R. (2014). A Secure Routing Protocol for VANET. *International Journal of Engine Research*, *3*(5).

Pee, L. G., Pan, S. L., & Cui, L. (2019). Roboticsin healthcare robots: A social informatics study of knowledge embodiment. *Journal of the Association for Information Science and Technology*, *70*(4), 351–369. doi:10.1002/asi.24145

Perttunen, M., Mazhelis, O., Cong, F., Ristaniemi, T., & Riekki, J. (2011). Distributed Road Surface Condition Monitoring. Lecture Notes in Computer Science. Springer. doi:10.1007/978-3-642-23641-9

PiMyLife. (2022). *Arduino Accelerometer using the ADXL345.*

Polat, F. (2017). *Journal of Engineering Research and Applied Science. Dece.*

Ponn, T., Kröger, T., & Diermeyer, F. (2020). Identification and explanation of challenging conditions for camera-based object detection of automated vehicles. *Sensors (Basel)*, *20*(13), 3699. doi:10.3390/s20133699 PMID:32630350

Poon, Y. S., Lin, C. C., Liu, Y. H., & Fan, C. P. (2022, January). YOLO-based deep learning design for in-cabin monitoring system with fisheye-lens camera. In *2022 IEEE International Conference on Consumer Electronics (ICCE)* (pp. 1-4). IEEE. 10.1109/ICCE53296.2022.9730235

Potts, J. A., Gibbons, R. V., Rothman, A. L., Srikiatkhachorn, A., Thomas, S. J., Supradish, P. O., Lemon, S. C., Libraty, D. H., Green, S., & Kalayanarooj, S. (2010). Prediction of dengue disease severity among pediatric Thai patients using early clinical laboratory indicators. *PLoS Neglected Tropical Diseases*, *4*(8), 769. doi:10.1371/journal.pntd.0000769 PMID:20689812

Preethiya, T., Muthukumar, A., & Durairaj, S. (2018) Providing Secured Data Aggregation in Mobile Wireless Sensor Network. *Proceedings of 4th IEEE International Symposium on Robotics and Manufacturing Automation.* IEEE. 10.1109/ROMA46407.2018.8986735

Preethiya, T., Muthukumar, A., & Durairaj, S. (2019a). Double Cluster Head Heterogeneous Clustering for Optimization in Hybrid Wireless Sensor Network. *Wireless Personal Communications. Wireless Personal Communications*, *110*(4), 1751–1768. doi:10.1007/s11277-019-06810-3

Preethiya, T., Muthukumar, A., & Durairaj, S. (2019b). Mobility Handling in Cluster based Mobile Wireless Sensor Network. *Proceedings of 2019 IEEE International Conference on Clean Energy and Energy Efficient Electronics Circuit for Sustainable Development (INCCES).* IEEE. 10.1109/INCCES47820.2019.9167692

Preethiya, T., Muthukumar, A., & Durairaj, S. (2020). An energy efficient clustering and multipath routing for mobile wireless sensor network using game theory. *International Journal of Communication Systems*, *33*(7), 1–18.

Priyadarshi, R., Gupta, B., & Anurag, A. (2020). Deployment techniques in wireless sensor networks: A survey, classification, challenges, and future research issues. *The Journal of Supercomputing*, *76*(9), 7333–7373. doi:10.1007/s11227-020-03166-5

RadhaKrishna Karne, D. T. (2021). Review on vanet architecture and applications. [TURCOMAT]. *Turkish Journal of Computer and Mathematics Education*, *12*(4), 1745–1749.

Ragno, L., Borboni, A., Vannetti, F., Amici, C., & Cusano, N. (2023). Application of Social Robots in Healthcare: Review on Characteristics, Requirements, Technical Solutions. *Sensors (Basel)*, *23*(15), 6820. doi:10.3390/s23156820 PMID:37571603

Rajkumar, M. N., Nithya, M., & HemaLatha, P. (2016). Overview of VANETs with its features and security attacks. *International Research Journal of Engineering and Technology, 3*(1).

Ramos-Sorroche, E., Rubio-Aparicio, J., Santa, J., Guardiola, C., & Egea-Lopez, E. (2023). In-cabin and outdoor environmental monitoring in vehicular scenarios with distributed computing. *Internet of Things : Engineering Cyber Physical Human Systems*, 101009.

Ranjit, S., & Kissoon, N. (2011). Dengue hemorrhagic fever and shock syndromes. *Pediatric Critical Care Medicine*, *12*(1), 90–100. doi:10.1097/PCC.0b013e3181e911a7 PMID:20639791

Rao, V. S. H., & Kumar, M. N. (2012). A new intelligence-based approach for computer-aided diagnosis of dengue fever. *IEEE Transactions on Information Technology in Biomedicine*, *16*(1), 112–118. doi:10.1109/TITB.2011.2171978 PMID:22010159

Rathi, B. S., Kumar, P. S., & Vo, D. V. N. (2021). Critical review on hazardous pollutants in water environment: Occurrence, monitoring, fate, removal technologies and risk assessment. *The Science of the Total Environment*, *797*, 149134. doi:10.1016/j.scitotenv.2021.149134 PMID:34346357

Rehman, S. U., Khan, M., Zia, T., & Zheng, L. (2013). Vehicular ad-hoc networks (VANETs): an overview and challenges. *Journal of Wireless Networking and communications, 3*(3), 29-38.

Remacle, M. M. N., Prasad, V., Lawson, G., Plisson, L., Bachy, V., & Van der Vorst, S. (2015). Transoral robotic surgery (TORS) with the Medrobotics Flex™ System: First surgical application on humans. *European Archives of Oto-Rhino-Laryngology*, *272*, 1451–1455. doi:10.1007/s00405-015-3532-x PMID:25663191

Rizk, Y., Awad, M., & Tunstel, E. W. (2019). Cooperative heterogeneous multi-robot systems: A survey. *ACM Computing Surveys*, *52*(2), 1–31. doi:10.1145/3303848

Rohan, A., Rabah, M., & Kim, S. H. (2019). Convolutional neural network-based real-time object detection and tracking for parrot AR drone 2. *IEEE Access : Practical Innovations, Open Solutions*, *7*, 69575–69584. doi:10.1109/ACCESS.2019.2919332

Russo, M., Gautreau, E., Bonnet, X., & Laribi, M. A. (2023). Continuum Robots: From Conventional to Customized Performance Indicators. *Biomimetics*, *8*(2), 147. doi:10.3390/biomimetics8020147 PMID:37092399

Saggi, M. K., & Sandhu, R. K. (2014). A survey of vehicular ad hoc network on attacks and security threats in VANETs. In *International Conference on Research and Innovations in Engineering and Technology (ICRIET 2014)* (pp. 19-20). IEEE.

Sahu, B., Das, P. K., Kabat, M. R., & Kumar, R. (2022). Prevention of Covid-19 affected patient using multi robot co-operation and Q-learning approach: A solution. *Quality & Quantity*, *56*(2), 793–821. doi:10.1007/s11135-021-01155-1 PMID:33972809

Saini, M., & Singh, H. (2016). VANET its characteristics attacks and routing techniques: A survey. *International Journal of Scientific Research*, *5*(5), 1595–1599.

Salokhe, N., Thakre, P., Awale, R. N., & Kambale, S. (2016). *Vibration Based Damage Detection using Overall Frequency Response and Time Domain.*

Sampoornam, K. P., Saranya, S., Vigneshwaran, S., Sofiarani, P., Sarmitha, S., & Sarumathi, N. (2020). A comparative study on reactive routing protocols in VANET. In *2020 4th International Conference on Electronics, Communication and Aerospace Technology (ICECA)* (pp. 726-731). IEEE. 10.1109/ICECA49313.2020.9297550

Sanan, S., Moidel, J., & Atkeson, C. G. (2011, June). A continuum approach to safe robots for physical human interaction. In *International Symposium on Quality of Life Technology*. IEEE.

Sarkar, S. (2021). LR 81: The Evolving Role of Insurtech in India: Trends, Challenges and The Road Ahead. *The Management Accountant Journal*, *56*(12), 30–37. doi:10.33516/maj.v56i12.30-37p

Sarker, S., Jamal, L., Ahmed, S. F., & Irtisam, N. (2021). Robotics and Roboticsin healthcare during COVID-19 pandemic: A systematic review. *Robotics and Autonomous Systems*, *146*, 103902. doi:10.1016/j.robot.2021.103902 PMID:34629751

Sarma, A. H. K. D., Kar, B. A., & Mall, C. R. (2011). Secure routing protocol for mobile wireless sensor network. In *2011 IEEE Sensors Applications Symposium* (pp. 93-99). IEEE. 10.1109/SAS.2011.5739778

Saxena, A., Khanna, A., & Gupta, D. (2020). Emotion recognition and detection methods: A comprehensive survey. *Journal of Artificial Intelligence and Systems*, *2*(1), 53–79. doi:10.33969/AIS.2020.21005

Schranz, M., Umlauft, M., Sende, M., & Elmenreich, W. (2020). Swarm Robotic Behaviors and Current Applications. *Frontiers in Robotics and AI*, *7*, 36. doi:10.3389/frobt.2020.00036 PMID:33501204

Sener, A. S. (n.d.). *Determination Of Vehicle Components Fatigue Life Based On Fea Method And Experimental Analysis Determination Of Vehicle Components Fatigue Life Based On Fea Method And.* *2*(Lcv), 133–146.

Şen, M. O., Okumuş, F., & Kocamaz, F.ŞEN. (2022). Application of blockchain powered mobile robots in healthcare: Use cases, research challenges and future trends. *Türk Doğa ve Fen Dergisi*, *11*(2), 27–35. doi:10.46810/tdfd.1017499

Shafiullah, A. K. M., & Wu, C. Q. (2013). Generation and validation of loading profiles for highly accelerated durability tests of ground vehicle components. *Engineering Failure Analysis*, *33*, 1–16. doi:10.1016/j.engfailanal.2013.04.008

Shah, A., Mehrotra, P., Sinha, S., & Sha, J. (2021). Bcg Insurtech Report India Insurtech Landscape And Trends. In Boston Consulting Group.

Shaktawat, R. S., Singh, D., & Choudhary, N. (2014). An efficient secure routing protocol in MANET Security-Enhanced AODV (SE-AODV). *International Journal of Computer Applications*, *97*(8). Advance online publication. doi:10.5120/17030-7329

Shallal, A. H., Ucan, O. N., Humaidi, A. J., & Bayat, O. (2020). Multi-robot systems formation control with maneuvring target in system applicable in the hospitality and care-health industry of medical internet of things. *Journal of Medical Imaging and Health Informatics*, *10*(1), 268–278. doi:10.1166/jmihi.2020.2840

Shaukat, K., Iqbal, F., Alam, T. M., Aujla, G. K., Devnath, L., Khan, A. G., & Rubab, A. (2020). The impact of artificial intelligence and robotics on the future employment opportunities. *Trends in Computer Science and Information Technology*, *5*(1), 50-54.

Shen, J., Wang, N., Wan, Z., Luo, Y., Sato, T., Hu, Z., & Chen, Q. A. (2022). Sok: On the semantic ai security in autonomous driving. *arXiv preprint arXiv:2203.05314*.

Shevchuk, O., Kondrat, I., & Stanienda, J. (2020). (LR 115)Pandemic as an accelerator of digital transformation in the insurance industry: Evidence from Ukraine. *Insurance Markets and Companies*, *11*(1), 30–41. doi:10.21511/ins.11(1).2020.04

Shimizu, A., Ito, M., & Lefor, A. K. (2022). Laparoscopic and Robot-Assisted Hepatic Surgery: An Historical Review. *Journal of Clinical Medicine*, *11*(12), 3254. doi:10.3390/jcm11123254 PMID:35743324

Shuai, J., Heng, S., Jing, Y., Feng, Y., Han, N., & Mengqin, Y. (2021). *Load Spectrum Acquisition, Analysis and Application of The Electric Bus in Road Simulation Test Based on*. 479–483. toptechboy.com. (n.d.). *ARDUINO LESSON 21: LOG SENSOR DATA TO AN SD CARD*.

Siau, K., Hodson, J., Ingram, R., Baxter, A., Widlak, M. M., Sharratt, C., Baker, G. M., Troth, T., Hicken, B., Tahir, F., Magrabi, M., Yousaf, N., Grant, C., Poon, D., Khalil, H., Lee, H. L., White, J. R., Tan, H., Samani, S., & Major, G. (2019). Time to endoscopy for acute upper gastrointestinal bleeding: Results from a prospective multicentre trainee-led audit. *United European Gastroenterology Journal, 7*(2), 199–209. doi:10.1177/2050640618811491 PMID:31080604

Side, S., Pratama, M. I., Badwi, N., & Sanusi, W. (2020). Analysis and Simulation of SIRI Model for Dengue Fever Transmission. *Indian Journal of Science and Technology, 13*(3), 340–351. doi:10.17485/ijst/2020/v13i03/147852

Silvera-Tawil, D. (2024). Robotics in Healthcare: A Survey. *SN Computer Science, 5*(1), 189. doi:10.1007/s42979-023-02551-0

Simon, M., Amende, K., Kraus, A., Honer, J., Samann, T., Kaulbersch, H., & Michael Gross, H. (2019). Complexer-yolo: Real-time 3d object detection and tracking on semantic point clouds. In *Proceedings of the IEEE/CVF Conference on Computer Vision and Pattern Recognition Workshops* (pp. 0-0). IEEE. 10.1109/CVPRW.2019.00158

Singh, R., Kathuria, K., & Sagar, A. K. (2018). Secure routing protocols for wireless sensor networks. In *2018 4th international conference on computing communication and automation (ICCCA)* (pp. 1-5). IEEE. 10.1109/CCAA.2018.8777557

Singh, G., Rohil, H., Rishi, R., & Ranga, V. (2019). LETSRP: A secure routing protocol for MANETs. *Int J Eng Adv Technol (IJEAT). ISSN, 9*(1), 2249–8958.

Soft Robotics Toolkit. (n.d.). Modeling and Design Tool for Soft Pneumatic Actuators. Soft Robotics Toolkit. https://softroboticstoolkit.com/book/modeling-soft-pneumatic-actuators

Sonker, A., & Gupta, R. K. (2020). A new combination of machine learning algorithms using stacking approach for misbehavior detection in VANETs. *International Journal of Computer Science and Network Security, 20*(10), 94–100.

Soriano, G. P., Yasuhara, Y., Ito, H., Matsumoto, K., Osaka, K., Kai, Y., & Tanioka, T. (2022, August). Robots and robotics in nursing. In Healthcare (Vol. 10, No. 8, p. 1571). MDPI. doi:10.3390/healthcare10081571

Stahl, B. C., & Coeckelbergh, M. (2016). Ethics of healthcare robotics: Towards responsible research and innovation. *Robotics and Autonomous Systems, 86*, 152–161. doi:10.1016/j.robot.2016.08.018

Stenius, I., Folkesson, J., Bhat, S., Sprague, C. I., Ling, L., Özkahraman, Ö., Bore, N., Cong, Z., Severholt, J., Ljung, C., Arnwald, A., Torroba, I., Gröndahl, F., & Thomas, J.-B. (2022). A System for Autonomous Seaweed Farm Inspection with an Underwater Robot. *Sensors (Basel), 22*(13), 5064. doi:10.3390/s22135064 PMID:35808560

Stoeckli, E., Dremel, C., & Uebernickel, F. (2018). LR 63; Exploring characteristics and transformational capabilities of InsurTech innovations to understand insurance value creation in a digital world. *Electronic Markets, 28*(3), 287–305. Advance online publication. doi:10.1007/s12525-018-0304-7

Sugiyama, O., Shinozawa, K., Akimoto, T., & Hagita, N. (2010). Case study of a multi-robot healthcare system: Effects of docking and metaphor on persuasion. In *Social Robotics: Second International Conference on Social Robotics*. Singapore.

Sun, L., Yang, K., Hu, X., Hu, W., & Wang, K. (2020). Real-time fusion network for RGB-D semantic segmentation incorporating unexpected obstacle detection for road-driving images. *IEEE Robotics and Automation Letters, 5*(4), 5558–5565. doi:10.1109/LRA.2020.3007457

Tarnawski, J. M., Phanishayee, A., Devanur, N., Mahajan, D., & Nina Paravecino, F. (2020). Efficient algorithms for device placement of dnn graph operators. *Advances in Neural Information Processing Systems, 33*, 15451–15463.

Thakker, D., Mishra, B. K., Abdullatif, A., Mazumdar, S., & Simpson, S. (2020). Explainable artificial intelligence for developing smart cities solutions. *Smart Cities*, *3*(4), 1353–1382. doi:10.3390/smartcities3040065

Tian, Y., Ma, S., Wen, M., Liu, Y., Cheung, S. C., & Zhang, X. (2021). To what extent do DNN-based image classification models make unreliable inferences? *Empirical Software Engineering*, *26*(5), 84. doi:10.1007/s10664-021-09985-1

Tong, W., Hussain, A., Bo, W. X., & Maharjan, S. (2019). Artificial intelligence for vehicle-to-everything: A survey. *IEEE Access : Practical Innovations, Open Solutions*, *7*, 10823–10843. doi:10.1109/ACCESS.2019.2891073

Trewartha, A., Walker, N., Huo, H., Lee, S., Cruse, K., Dagdelen, J., Dunn, A., Persson, K. A., Ceder, G., & Jain, A. (2022). Quantifying the advantage of domain-specific pre-training on named entity recognition tasks in materials science. *Patterns (New York, N.Y.)*, *3*(4), 100488. doi:10.1016/j.patter.2022.100488 PMID:35465225

Troccaz, J., Dagnino, G., & Yang, G. Z. (2019). Frontiers of medical robotics: From concept to systems to clinical translation. *Annual Review of Biomedical Engineering*, *21*(1), 193–218. doi:10.1146/annurev-bioeng-060418-052502 PMID:30822100

Tyagi, A. K., & Aswathy, S. U. (2021). Autonomous Intelligent Vehicles (AIV): Research statements, open issues, challenges and road for future. *International Journal of Intelligent Networks*, *2*, 83–102. doi:10.1016/j.ijin.2021.07.002

Ur Rehman, S., Mustafa, H., & Larik, A. R. (2021). IoT Based Substation Monitoring Control System Using Arduino with Data Logging. *Proceedings - 2021 IEEE 4th International Conference on Computing and Information Sciences, ICCIS 2021*. IEEE. 10.1109/ICCIS54243.2021.9676384

Vallès-Peris, N., Barat-Auleda, O., & Domènech, M. (2021). Robots in healthcare? What patients say. *International Journal of Environmental Research and Public Health*, *18*(18), 9933. doi:10.3390/ijerph18189933 PMID:34574861

Vallès-Peris, N., & Domènech, M. (2023). Caring in the in-between: A proposal to introduce responsible AI and robotics to healthcare. *AI & Society*, *38*(4), 1685–1695. doi:10.1007/s00146-021-01330-w

Van Wyk, F., Wang, Y., Khojandi, A., & Masoud, N. (2019). Real-time sensor anomaly detection and identification in automated vehicles. *IEEE Transactions on Intelligent Transportation Systems*, *21*(3), 1264–1276. doi:10.1109/TITS.2019.2906038

Venkat, Y., Chand, K. P., & Preethiya, T. (2023). An intrusion detection system for the Internet of Things based on machine learning. *2023 International Conference on Recent Advances in Electrical, Electronics, Ubiquitous Communication, and Computational Intelligence (RAEEUCCI)*. IEEE. 10.1109/RAEEUCCI57140.2023.10134432

Verma, A. K., Nagpal, S., Desai, A., & Sudha, R. (2021). An efficient neural-network model for real-time fault detection in industrial machine. *Neural Computing & Applications*, *33*(4), 1297–1310. doi:10.1007/s00521-020-05033-z

Vesnic-Alujevic, L., Nascimento, S., & Pólvora, A. (2020). Societal and ethical impacts of artificial intelligence: Critical notes on European policy frameworks. *Telecommunications Policy*, *44*(6), 2020. doi:10.1016/j.telpol.2020.101961

Waidi, Y. O., Barua, R., & Datta, S. (2023). Metals, Polymers, Ceramics, Composites Biomaterials Used in Additive Manufacturing for Biomedical Applications. In A. Kumar, P. Kumar, A. Srivastava, & V. Goyat (Eds.), *Modeling, Characterization, and Processing of Smart Materials* (pp. 165–184). IGI Global. doi:10.4018/978-1-6684-9224-6.ch008

Wali, S., & Areeb, M. (2018). Development of Low-Cost DAQ for Power System Signals Using Arduino. *2018 IEEE 21st International Multi-Topic Conference (INMIC)*, (pp. 1–5). IEEE. 10.1109/INMIC.2018.8595519

Wang, J., Zhao, Y., Yang, Y., & Yang, J. (2019). *Fatigue Analysis for Bogie Frame of Urban Transit Rail Vehicle under Overload Situation. Qr2mse*. Research Gate.

Wang, Q., Yan, K., & Li, H. (2009). *Motor Noise Source Identification Based on Frequency Domain Analysis*. Research Gate.

Wang, H., Zhang, R., Chen, W., Wang, X., & Pfeifer, R. (2017). A cable-driven soft robot surgical system for cardio-thoracic endoscopic surgery: Preclinical tests in animals. *Surgical Endoscopy*, *31*(8), 3152–3158. doi:10.1007/s00464-016-5340-9 PMID:27858208

Wang, J., & Lee, J. (2019). Bioinspired Nanorobots for Cancer Detection and Therapy. In *Bioinspired Nanomaterials and Nanostructures from Nanobiology to Nanomedicine* (pp. 1–31). Springer.

Wang, J., Li, Y., Zhou, Z., Wang, C., Hou, Y., Zhang, L., & Chen, S. (2022). When, where and how does it fail? A spatial-temporal visual analytics approach for interpretable object detection in autonomous driving. *IEEE Transactions on Visualization and Computer Graphics*. PMID:36040948

Wavhale, R. D., Andhari, S. S., Dhobale, K. D., Tawade, B. V., Chate, G. P., Patil, Y. N., ... Banerjee, S. S. (2021). Self-propelling magnetic nanorobots for capturing circulating tumor cells in blood samples of cancer patients. *Communications Chemistry*, *4*(1), 1–12. PMID:36697560

Wei, H., Zhang, G., Wang, S., Zhang, P., Su, J., & Du, F. (2023). Coupling Analysis of Compound Continuum Robots for Surgery: Another Line of Thought. *Sensors (Basel)*, *23*(14), 6407. doi:10.3390/s23146407 PMID:37514701

Wei, Y., Chen, Y., Ren, T., Chen, Q., Yan, C., Yang, Y., & Li, Y. (2016). A novel, variable stiffness robotic gripper based on integrated soft actuating and particle jamming. *Soft Robotics*, *3*(3), 134143. doi:10.1089/soro.2016.0027

Wu, X., & Ma, S. (2013). Neurally controlled steering for collision-free behavior of a snake robot. *IEEE Transactions on Control Systems Technology*, *21*(6), 2443–2449. doi:10.1109/TCST.2012.2237519

Xavier, M. S., Fleming, A. J., & Yong, Y. K. (2021, February). Finite element modeling of soft uidic actuators: Overview and recent developments. *Advanced Intelligent Systems*, *3*(2), 2000187. doi:10.1002/aisy.202000187

Yadav, S., Rajput, N. K., Sagar, A. K., & Maheshwari, D. (2018). Secure and reliable routing protocols for VANETs. In *2018 4th International Conference on Computing Communication and Automation (ICCCA)* (pp. 1-5). IEEE. 10.1109/CCAA.2018.8777690

Yadav, N., & Chug, U. (2019). Secure Routing in MANET: A Review. In *2019 International Conference on Machine Learning, Big Data, Cloud and Parallel Computing (COMITCon)* (pp. 375-379). IEEE.

Yaneva, T. (n.d.). *Digital Transformation of Insurance Sector*.

Yang, T., Xiangyang, X., Peng, L., Tonghui, L., & Leina, P. (2018). A secure routing of wireless sensor networks based on trust evaluation model. *Procedia Computer Science*, *131*, 1156–1163. doi:10.1016/j.procs.2018.04.289

Yang, Y., Li, D., Sun, Y., Wu, M., Su, J., Li, Y., Yu, X., Li, L., & Yu, J. (2023). Muscle-inspired soft robots based on bilateral dielectric elastomer actuators. *Microsystems & Nanoengineering*, *9*(1), 124. doi:10.1038/s41378-023-00592-2 PMID:37814608

Yan, H., & Fan, C. (2019). DNA nanotechnology and its biological applications. In D. N. A. Nanotechnology (Ed.), (pp. 1–22). Springer.

Yao, L., Fang, Z., Xiao, Y., Hou, J., & Fu, Z. (2021). An intelligent fault diagnosis method for lithium battery systems based on grid search support vector machine. *Energy*, *214*, 118866. doi:10.1016/j.energy.2020.118866

Yao, L., Xiao, Y., Gong, X., Hou, J., & Chen, X. (2020). A novel intelligent method for fault diagnosis of electric vehicle battery system based on wavelet neural network. *Journal of Power Sources*, *453*, 227870. doi:10.1016/j.jpowsour.2020.227870

Yaqoob, I., Khan, L. U., Kazmi, S. A., Imran, M., Guizani, N., & Hong, C. S. (2019). Autonomous driving cars in smart cities: Recent advances, requirements, and challenges. *IEEE Network*, *34*(1), 174–181. doi:10.1109/MNET.2019.1900120

Yinong, C. (2021). Technologies Supporting Artificial Intelligence and Robotics Application Development. doi:10.37965/jait.2020.0065

Yin, S., Rodriguez-Andina, J. J., & Jiang, Y. (2019). Real-time monitoring and control of industrial cyberphysical systems: With integrated plant-wide monitoring and control framework. *IEEE Industrial Electronics Magazine*, *13*(4), 38–47. doi:10.1109/MIE.2019.2938025

Yoon, S. N., & Lee, D. (2018). Roboticsand robots in healthcare: What are the success factors for technology-based service encounters? *International Journal of Healthcare Management*.

Zablocki, É., Ben-Younes, H., Pérez, P., & Cord, M. (2022). Explainability of deep vision-based autonomous driving systems: Review and challenges. *International Journal of Computer Vision*, *130*(10), 2425–2452. doi:10.1007/s11263-022-01657-x

Zhang, G., Du, F., Xue, S., Cheng, H., Zhang, X., Song, R., & Li, Y. (2022). Design and Modeling of a Bio-Inspired Compound Continuum Robot for Minimally Invasive Surgery. *Machines*, *10*(6), 468. doi:10.3390/machines10060468

Zhao, L., Li, Y., Meng, C., Gong, C., & Tang, X. (2016). A SVM based routing scheme in VANETs. In *2016 16th International Symposium on Communications and Information Technologies (ISCIT)* (pp. 380-383). IEEE. 10.1109/ISCIT.2016.7751655

Zhao, J., Zhao, W., Deng, B., Wang, Z., Zhang, F., Zheng, W., & Burke, A. F. (2023). Autonomous driving system: A comprehensive survey. *Expert Systems with Applications*, 122836.

Zhu, J., Lyu, L., Xu, Y., Liang, H., Zhang, X., Ding, H., & Wu, Z. (2021). Intelligent Soft Surgical Robots for Next-Generation Minimally Invasive Surgery. *Advanced Intelligent Systems*, *3*(5), 2100011. doi:10.1002/aisy.202100011

Related References

To continue our tradition of advancing academic research, we have compiled a list of recommended IGI Global readings. These references will provide additional information and guidance to further enrich your knowledge and assist you with your own research and future publications.

Abbasnejad, B., Moeinzadeh, S., Ahankoob, A., & Wong, P. S. (2021). The Role of Collaboration in the Implementation of BIM-Enabled Projects. In J. Underwood & M. Shelbourn (Eds.), *Handbook of Research on Driving Transformational Change in the Digital Built Environment* (pp. 27–62). IGI Global. https://doi.org/10.4018/978-1-7998-6600-8.ch002

Abdulrahman, K. O., Mahamood, R. M., & Akinlabi, E. T. (2022). Additive Manufacturing (AM): Processing Technique for Lightweight Alloys and Composite Material. In K. Kumar, B. Babu, & J. Davim (Ed.), *Handbook of Research on Advancements in the Processing, Characterization, and Application of Lightweight Materials* (pp. 27–48). IGI Global. https://doi.org/10.4018/978-1-7998-7864-3.ch002

Agrawal, R., Sharma, P., & Saxena, A. (2021). A Diamond Cut Leather Substrate Antenna for BAN (Body Area Network) Application. In V. Singh, V. Dubey, A. Saxena, R. Tiwari, & H. Sharma (Eds.), *Emerging Materials and Advanced Designs for Wearable Antennas* (pp. 54–59). IGI Global. https://doi.org/10.4018/978-1-7998-7611-3.ch004

Ahmad, F., Al-Ammar, E. A., & Alsaidan, I. (2022). Battery Swapping Station: A Potential Solution to Address the Limitations of EV Charging Infrastructure. In M. Alam, R. Pillai, & N. Murugesan (Eds.), *Developing Charging Infrastructure and Technologies for Electric Vehicles* (pp. 195–207). IGI Global. doi:10.4018/978-1-7998-6858-3.ch010

Aikhuele, D. (2018). A Study of Product Development Engineering and Design Reliability Concerns. *International Journal of Applied Industrial Engineering, 5*(1), 79–89. doi:10.4018/IJAIE.2018010105

Al-Khatri, H., & Al-Atrash, F. (2021). Occupants' Habits and Natural Ventilation in a Hot Arid Climate. In R. González-Lezcano (Ed.), *Advancements in Sustainable Architecture and Energy Efficiency* (pp. 146–168). IGI Global. https://doi.org/10.4018/978-1-7998-7023-4.ch007

Al-Shebeeb, O. A., Rangaswamy, S., Gopalakrishan, B., & Devaru, D. G. (2017). Evaluation and Indexing of Process Plans Based on Electrical Demand and Energy Consumption. *International Journal of Manufacturing, Materials, and Mechanical Engineering*, 7(3), 1–19. doi:10.4018/IJMMME.2017070101

Amuda, M. O., Lawal, T. F., & Akinlabi, E. T. (2017). Research Progress on Rheological Behavior of AA7075 Aluminum Alloy During Hot Deformation. *International Journal of Materials Forming and Machining Processes*, 4(1), 53–96. doi:10.4018/IJMFMP.2017010104

Amuda, M. O., Lawal, T. F., & Mridha, S. (2021). Microstructure and Mechanical Properties of Silicon Carbide-Treated Ferritic Stainless Steel Welds. In L. Burstein (Ed.), *Handbook of Research on Advancements in Manufacturing, Materials, and Mechanical Engineering* (pp. 395–411). IGI Global. https://doi.org/10.4018/978-1-7998-4939-1.ch019

Anikeev, V., Gasem, K. A., & Fan, M. (2021). Application of Supercritical Technologies in Clean Energy Production: A Review. In L. Chen (Ed.), *Handbook of Research on Advancements in Supercritical Fluids Applications for Sustainable Energy Systems* (pp. 792–821). IGI Global. https://doi.org/10.4018/978-1-7998-5796-9.ch022

Arafat, M. Y., Saleem, I., & Devi, T. P. (2022). Drivers of EV Charging Infrastructure Entrepreneurship in India. In M. Alam, R. Pillai, & N. Murugesan (Eds.), *Developing Charging Infrastructure and Technologies for Electric Vehicles* (pp. 208–219). IGI Global. https://doi.org/10.4018/978-1-7998-6858-3.ch011

Araujo, A., & Manninen, H. (2022). Contribution of Project-Based Learning on Social Skills Development: An Industrial Engineer Perspective. In A. Alves & N. van Hattum-Janssen (Eds.), *Training Engineering Students for Modern Technological Advancement* (pp. 119–145). IGI Global. https://doi.org/10.4018/978-1-7998-8816-1.ch006

Armutlu, H. (2018). Intelligent Biomedical Engineering Operations by Cloud Computing Technologies. In U. Kose, G. Guraksin, & O. Deperlioglu (Eds.), *Nature-Inspired Intelligent Techniques for Solving Biomedical Engineering Problems* (pp. 297–317). Hershey, PA: IGI Global. doi:10.4018/978-1-5225-4769-3.ch015

Atik, M., Sadek, M., & Shahrour, I. (2017). Single-Run Adaptive Pushover Procedure for Shear Wall Structures. In V. Plevris, G. Kremmyda, & Y. Fahjan (Eds.), *Performance-Based Seismic Design of Concrete Structures and Infrastructures* (pp. 59–83). Hershey, PA: IGI Global. doi:10.4018/978-1-5225-2089-4.ch003

Attia, H. (2021). Smart Power Microgrid Impact on Sustainable Building. In R. González-Lezcano (Ed.), *Advancements in Sustainable Architecture and Energy Efficiency* (pp. 169–194). IGI Global. https://doi.org/10.4018/978-1-7998-7023-4.ch008

Aydin, A., Akyol, E., Gungor, M., Kaya, A., & Tasdelen, S. (2018). Geophysical Surveys in Engineering Geology Investigations With Field Examples. In N. Ceryan (Ed.), *Handbook of Research on Trends and Digital Advances in Engineering Geology* (pp. 257–280). Hershey, PA: IGI Global. doi:10.4018/978-1-5225-2709-1.ch007

Ayoobkhan, M. U. D., Y., A., J., Easwaran, B., & R., T. (2021). Smart Connected Digital Products and IoT Platform With the Digital Twin. In P. Vasant, G. Weber, & W. Punurai (Ed.), Research Advancements in Smart Technology, Optimization, and Renewable Energy (pp. 330-350). IGI Global. https://doi.org/ doi:10.4018/978-1-7998-3970-5.ch016

Baeza Moyano, D., & González Lezcano, R. A. (2021). The Importance of Light in Our Lives: Towards New Lighting in Schools. In R. González-Lezcano (Ed.), *Advancements in Sustainable Architecture and Energy Efficiency* (pp. 239–256). IGI Global. https://doi.org/10.4018/978-1-7998-7023-4.ch011

Bagdadee, A. H. (2021). A Brief Assessment of the Energy Sector of Bangladesh. *International Journal of Energy Optimization and Engineering, 10*(1), 36–55. doi:10.4018/IJEOE.2021010103

Baklezos, A. T., & Hadjigeorgiou, N. G. (2021). Magnetic Sensors for Space Applications and Magnetic Cleanliness Considerations. In C. Nikolopoulos (Ed.), *Recent Trends on Electromagnetic Environmental Effects for Aeronautics and Space Applications* (pp. 147–185). IGI Global. https://doi.org/10.4018/978-1-7998-4879-0.ch006

Bas, T. G. (2017). Nutraceutical Industry with the Collaboration of Biotechnology and Nutrigenomics Engineering: The Significance of Intellectual Property in the Entrepreneurship and Scientific Research Ecosystems. In T. Bas & J. Zhao (Eds.), *Comparative Approaches to Biotechnology Development and Use in Developed and Emerging Nations* (pp. 1–17). Hershey, PA: IGI Global. doi:10.4018/978-1-5225-1040-6.ch001

Bazeer Ahamed, B., & Periakaruppan, S. (2021). Taxonomy of Influence Maximization Techniques in Unknown Social Networks. In P. Vasant, G. Weber, & W. Punurai (Eds.), *Research Advancements in Smart Technology, Optimization, and Renewable Energy* (pp. 351-363). IGI Global. https://doi.org/10.4018/978-1-7998-3970-5.ch017

Beale, R., & André, J. (2017). *Design Solutions and Innovations in Temporary Structures*. Hershey, PA: IGI Global. doi:10.4018/978-1-5225-2199-0

Behnam, B. (2017). Simulating Post-Earthquake Fire Loading in Conventional RC Structures. In P. Samui, S. Chakraborty, & D. Kim (Eds.), *Modeling and Simulation Techniques in Structural Engineering* (pp. 425–444). Hershey, PA: IGI Global. doi:10.4018/978-1-5225-0588-4.ch015

Ben Hamida, I., Salah, S. B., Msahli, F., & Mimouni, M. F. (2018). Distribution Network Reconfiguration Using SPEA2 for Power Loss Minimization and Reliability Improvement. *International Journal of Energy Optimization and Engineering, 7*(1), 50–65. doi:10.4018/IJEOE.2018010103

Bentarzi, H. (2021). Fault Tree-Based Root Cause Analysis Used to Study Mal-Operation of a Protective Relay in a Smart Grid. In A. Recioui & H. Bentarzi (Eds.), *Optimizing and Measuring Smart Grid Operation and Control* (pp. 289–308). IGI Global. https://doi.org/10.4018/978-1-7998-4027-5.ch012

Beysens, D. A., Garrabos, Y., & Zappoli, B. (2021). Thermal Effects in Near-Critical Fluids: Piston Effect and Related Phenomena. In L. Chen (Ed.), *Handbook of Research on Advancements in Supercritical Fluids Applications for Sustainable Energy Systems* (pp. 1–31). IGI Global. https://doi.org/10.4018/978-1-7998-5796-9.ch001

Bhaskar, S. V., & Kudal, H. N. (2017). Effect of TiCN and AlCrN Coating on Tribological Behaviour of Plasma-nitrided AISI 4140 Steel. *International Journal of Surface Engineering and Interdisciplinary Materials Science*, 5(2), 1–17. doi:10.4018/IJSEIMS.2017070101

Bhuyan, D. (2018). Designing of a Twin Tube Shock Absorber: A Study in Reverse Engineering. In K. Kumar & J. Davim (Eds.), *Design and Optimization of Mechanical Engineering Products* (pp. 83–104). Hershey, PA: IGI Global. doi:10.4018/978-1-5225-3401-3.ch005

Blumberg, G. (2021). Blockchains for Use in Construction and Engineering Projects. In J. Underwood & M. Shelbourn (Eds.), *Handbook of Research on Driving Transformational Change in the Digital Built Environment* (pp. 179–208). IGI Global. https://doi.org/10.4018/978-1-7998-6600-8.ch008

Bolboaca, A. M. (2021). Considerations Regarding the Use of Fuel Cells in Combined Heat and Power for Stationary Applications. In G. Badea, R. Felseghi, & I. Aşchilean (Eds.), *Hydrogen Fuel Cell Technology for Stationary Applications* (pp. 239–275). IGI Global. https://doi.org/10.4018/978-1-7998-4945-2.ch010

Burstein, L. (2021). Simulation Tool for Cable Design. In L. Burstein (Ed.), *Handbook of Research on Advancements in Manufacturing, Materials, and Mechanical Engineering* (pp. 54–74). IGI Global. https://doi.org/10.4018/978-1-7998-4939-1.ch003

Calderon, F. A., Giolo, E. G., Frau, C. D., Rengel, M. G., Rodriguez, H., Tornello, M., ... Gallucci, R. (2018). Seismic Microzonation and Site Effects Detection Through Microtremors Measures: A Review. In N. Ceryan (Ed.), *Handbook of Research on Trends and Digital Advances in Engineering Geology* (pp. 326–349). Hershey, PA: IGI Global. doi:10.4018/978-1-5225-2709-1.ch009

Ceryan, N., & Can, N. K. (2018). Prediction of The Uniaxial Compressive Strength of Rocks Materials. In N. Ceryan (Ed.), *Handbook of Research on Trends and Digital Advances in Engineering Geology* (pp. 31–96). Hershey, PA: IGI Global. doi:10.4018/978-1-5225-2709-1.ch002

Ceryan, S. (2018). Weathering Indices Used in Evaluation of the Weathering State of Rock Material. In N. Ceryan (Ed.), *Handbook of Research on Trends and Digital Advances in Engineering Geology* (pp. 132–186). Hershey, PA: IGI Global. doi:10.4018/978-1-5225-2709-1.ch004

Chen, H., Padilla, R. V., & Besarati, S. (2017). Supercritical Fluids and Their Applications in Power Generation. In L. Chen & Y. Iwamoto (Eds.), *Advanced Applications of Supercritical Fluids in Energy Systems* (pp. 369–402). Hershey, PA: IGI Global. doi:10.4018/978-1-5225-2047-4.ch012

Chen, H., Padilla, R. V., & Besarati, S. (2021). Supercritical Fluids and Their Applications in Power Generation. In L. Chen (Ed.), *Handbook of Research on Advancements in Supercritical Fluids Applications for Sustainable Energy Systems* (pp. 566–599). IGI Global. https://doi.org/10.4018/978-1-7998-5796-9.ch016

Chen, L. (2017). Principles, Experiments, and Numerical Studies of Supercritical Fluid Natural Circulation System. In L. Chen & Y. Iwamoto (Eds.), *Advanced Applications of Supercritical Fluids in Energy Systems* (pp. 136–187). Hershey, PA: IGI Global. doi:10.4018/978-1-5225-2047-4.ch005

Chen, L. (2021). Principles, Experiments, and Numerical Studies of Supercritical Fluid Natural Circulation System. In L. Chen (Ed.), *Handbook of Research on Advancements in Supercritical Fluids Applications for Sustainable Energy Systems* (pp. 219–269). IGI Global. https://doi.org/10.4018/978-1-7998-5796-9.ch007

Chiba, Y., Marif, Y., Henini, N., & Tlemcani, A. (2021). Modeling of Magnetic Refrigeration Device by Using Artificial Neural Networks Approach. *International Journal of Energy Optimization and Engineering*, *10*(4), 68–76. https://doi.org/10.4018/IJEOE.2021100105

Clementi, F., Di Sciascio, G., Di Sciascio, S., & Lenci, S. (2017). Influence of the Shear-Bending Interaction on the Global Capacity of Reinforced Concrete Frames: A Brief Overview of the New Perspectives. In V. Plevris, G. Kremmyda, & Y. Fahjan (Eds.), *Performance-Based Seismic Design of Concrete Structures and Infrastructures* (pp. 84–111). Hershey, PA: IGI Global. doi:10.4018/978-1-5225-2089-4.ch004

Codinhoto, R., Fialho, B. C., Pinti, L., & Fabricio, M. M. (2021). BIM and IoT for Facilities Management: Understanding Key Maintenance Issues. In J. Underwood & M. Shelbourn (Eds.), *Handbook of Research on Driving Transformational Change in the Digital Built Environment* (pp. 209–231). IGI Global. doi:10.4018/978-1-7998-6600-8.ch009

Cortés-Polo, D., Calle-Cancho, J., Carmona-Murillo, J., & González-Sánchez, J. (2017). Future Trends in Mobile-Fixed Integration for Next Generation Networks: Classification and Analysis. *International Journal of Vehicular Telematics and Infotainment Systems*, *1*(1), 33–53. doi:10.4018/IJVTIS.2017010103

Costa, H. G., Sheremetieff, F. H., & Araújo, E. A. (2022). Influence of Game-Based Methods in Developing Engineering Competences. In A. Alves & N. van Hattum-Janssen (Eds.), *Training Engineering Students for Modern Technological Advancement* (pp. 69–88). IGI Global. https://doi.org/10.4018/978-1-7998-8816-1.ch004

Cui, X., Zeng, S., Li, Z., Zheng, Q., Yu, X., & Han, B. (2018). Advanced Composites for Civil Engineering Infrastructures. In K. Kumar & J. Davim (Eds.), *Composites and Advanced Materials for Industrial Applications* (pp. 212–248). Hershey, PA: IGI Global. doi:10.4018/978-1-5225-5216-1.ch010

Dalgıç, S., & Kuşku, İ. (2018). Geological and Geotechnical Investigations in Tunneling. In N. Ceryan (Ed.), *Handbook of Research on Trends and Digital Advances in Engineering Geology* (pp. 482–529). Hershey, PA: IGI Global. doi:10.4018/978-1-5225-2709-1.ch014

Dang, C., & Hihara, E. (2021). Study on Cooling Heat Transfer of Supercritical Carbon Dioxide Applied to Transcritical Carbon Dioxide Heat Pump. In L. Chen (Ed.), *Handbook of Research on Advancements in Supercritical Fluids Applications for Sustainable Energy Systems* (pp. 451–493). IGI Global. https://doi.org/10.4018/978-1-7998-5796-9.ch013

Daus, Y., Kharchenko, V., & Yudaev, I. (2021). Research of Solar Energy Potential of Photovoltaic Installations on Enclosing Structures of Buildings. *International Journal of Energy Optimization and Engineering*, *10*(4), 18–34. https://doi.org/10.4018/IJEOE.2021100102

Daus, Y., Kharchenko, V., & Yudaev, I. (2021). Optimizing Layout of Distributed Generation Sources of Power Supply System of Agricultural Object. *International Journal of Energy Optimization and Engineering*, *10*(3), 70–84. https://doi.org/10.4018/IJEOE.2021070104

de la Varga, D., Soto, M., Arias, C. A., van Oirschot, D., Kilian, R., Pascual, A., & Álvarez, J. A. (2017). Constructed Wetlands for Industrial Wastewater Treatment and Removal of Nutrients. In Á. Val del Río, J. Campos Gómez, & A. Mosquera Corral (Eds.), *Technologies for the Treatment and Recovery of Nutrients from Industrial Wastewater* (pp. 202–230). Hershey, PA: IGI Global. doi:10.4018/978-1-5225-1037-6.ch008

Deb, S., Ammar, E. A., AlRajhi, H., Alsaidan, I., & Shariff, S. M. (2022). V2G Pilot Projects: Review and Lessons Learnt. In M. Alam, R. Pillai, & N. Murugesan (Eds.), *Developing Charging Infrastructure and Technologies for Electric Vehicles* (pp. 252–267). IGI Global. https://doi.org/10.4018/978-1-7998-6858-3.ch014

Dekhandji, F. Z., & Rais, M. C. (2021). A Comparative Study of Power Quality Monitoring Using Various Techniques. In A. Recioui & H. Bentarzi (Eds.), *Optimizing and Measuring Smart Grid Operation and Control* (pp. 259–288). IGI Global. https://doi.org/10.4018/978-1-7998-4027-5.ch011

Deperlioglu, O. (2018). Intelligent Techniques Inspired by Nature and Used in Biomedical Engineering. In U. Kose, G. Guraksin, & O. Deperlioglu (Eds.), *Nature-Inspired Intelligent Techniques for Solving Biomedical Engineering Problems* (pp. 51–77). Hershey, PA: IGI Global. doi:10.4018/978-1-5225-4769-3.ch003

Dhurpate, P. R., & Tang, H. (2021). Quantitative Analysis of the Impact of Inter-Line Conveyor Capacity for Throughput of Manufacturing Systems. *International Journal of Manufacturing, Materials, and Mechanical Engineering*, *11*(1), 1–17. https://doi.org/10.4018/IJMMME.2021010101

Dinkar, S., & Deep, K. (2021). A Survey of Recent Variants and Applications of Antlion Optimizer. *International Journal of Energy Optimization and Engineering*, *10*(2), 48–73. doi:10.4018/IJEOE.2021040103

Dixit, A. (2018). Application of Silica-Gel-Reinforced Aluminium Composite on the Piston of Internal Combustion Engine: Comparative Study of Silica-Gel-Reinforced Aluminium Composite Piston With Aluminium Alloy Piston. In K. Kumar & J. Davim (Eds.), *Composites and Advanced Materials for Industrial Applications* (pp. 63–98). Hershey, PA: IGI Global. doi:10.4018/978-1-5225-5216-1.ch004

Drabecki, M. P., & Kułak, K. B. (2021). Global Pandemics on European Electrical Energy Markets: Lessons Learned From the COVID-19 Outbreak. *International Journal of Energy Optimization and Engineering*, *10*(3), 24–46. https://doi.org/10.4018/IJEOE.2021070102

Dutta, M. M. (2021). Nanomaterials for Food and Agriculture. In M. Bhat, I. Wani, & S. Ashraf (Eds.), *Applications of Nanomaterials in Agriculture, Food Science, and Medicine* (pp. 75–97). IGI Global. doi:10.4018/978-1-7998-5563-7.ch004

Dutta, M. M., & Goswami, M. (2021). Coating Materials: Nano-Materials. In S. Roy & G. Bose (Eds.), *Advanced Surface Coating Techniques for Modern Industrial Applications* (pp. 1–30). IGI Global. doi:10.4018/978-1-7998-4870-7.ch001

Elsayed, A. M., Dakkama, H. J., Mahmoud, S., Al-Dadah, R., & Kaialy, W. (2017). Sustainable Cooling Research Using Activated Carbon Adsorbents and Their Environmental Impact. In T. Kobayashi (Ed.), *Applied Environmental Materials Science for Sustainability* (pp. 186–221). Hershey, PA: IGI Global. doi:10.4018/978-1-5225-1971-3.ch009

Ercanoglu, M., & Sonmez, H. (2018). General Trends and New Perspectives on Landslide Mapping and Assessment Methods. In N. Ceryan (Ed.), *Handbook of Research on Trends and Digital Advances in Engineering Geology* (pp. 350–379). Hershey, PA: IGI Global. doi:10.4018/978-1-5225-2709-1.ch010

Faroz, S. A., Pujari, N. N., Rastogi, R., & Ghosh, S. (2017). Risk Analysis of Structural Engineering Systems Using Bayesian Inference. In P. Samui, S. Chakraborty, & D. Kim (Eds.), *Modeling and Simulation Techniques in Structural Engineering* (pp. 390–424). Hershey, PA: IGI Global. doi:10.4018/978-1-5225-0588-4.ch014

Fekik, A., Hamida, M. L., Denoun, H., Azar, A. T., Kamal, N. A., Vaidyanathan, S., Bousbaine, A., & Benamrouche, N. (2022). Multilevel Inverter for Hybrid Fuel Cell/PV Energy Conversion System. In A. Fekik & N. Benamrouche (Eds.), *Modeling and Control of Static Converters for Hybrid Storage Systems* (pp. 233–270). IGI Global. https://doi.org/10.4018/978-1-7998-7447-8.ch009

Fekik, A., Hamida, M. L., Houassine, H., Azar, A. T., Kamal, N. A., Denoun, H., Vaidyanathan, S., & Sambas, A. (2022). Power Quality Improvement for Grid-Connected Photovoltaic Panels Using Direct Power Control. In A. Fekik & N. Benamrouche (Eds.), *Modeling and Control of Static Converters for Hybrid Storage Systems* (pp. 107–142). IGI Global. https://doi.org/10.4018/978-1-7998-7447-8.ch005

Fernando, P. R., Hamigah, T., Disne, S., Wickramasingha, G. G., & Sutharshan, A. (2018). The Evaluation of Engineering Properties of Low Cost Concrete Blocks by Partial Doping of Sand with Sawdust: Low Cost Sawdust Concrete Block. *International Journal of Strategic Engineering*, 1(2), 26–42. doi:10.4018/IJoSE.2018070103

Ferro, G., Minciardi, R., Parodi, L., & Robba, M. (2022). Optimal Charging Management of Microgrid-Integrated Electric Vehicles. In M. Alam, R. Pillai, & N. Murugesan (Eds.), *Developing Charging Infrastructure and Technologies for Electric Vehicles* (pp. 133–155). IGI Global. https://doi.org/10.4018/978-1-7998-6858-3.ch007

Flumerfelt, S., & Green, C. (2022). Graduate Lean Leadership Education: A Case Study of a Program. In A. Alves & N. van Hattum-Janssen (Eds.), *Training Engineering Students for Modern Technological Advancement* (pp. 202–224). IGI Global. https://doi.org/10.4018/978-1-7998-8816-1.ch010

Galli, B. J. (2021). Implications of Economic Decision Making to the Project Manager. *International Journal of Strategic Engineering*, 4(1), 19–32. https://doi.org/10.4018/IJoSE.2021010102

Gento, A. M., Pimentel, C., & Pascual, J. A. (2022). Teaching Circular Economy and Lean Management in a Learning Factory. In A. Alves & N. van Hattum-Janssen (Eds.), *Training Engineering Students for Modern Technological Advancement* (pp. 183–201). IGI Global. https://doi.org/10.4018/978-1-7998-8816-1.ch009

Ghosh, S., Mitra, S., Ghosh, S., & Chakraborty, S. (2017). Seismic Reliability Analysis in the Framework of Metamodelling Based Monte Carlo Simulation. In P. Samui, S. Chakraborty, & D. Kim (Eds.), *Modeling and Simulation Techniques in Structural Engineering* (pp. 192–208). Hershey, PA: IGI Global. doi:10.4018/978-1-5225-0588-4.ch006

Gil, M., & Otero, B. (2017). Learning Engineering Skills through Creativity and Collaboration: A Game-Based Proposal. In R. Alexandre Peixoto de Queirós & M. Pinto (Eds.), *Gamification-Based E-Learning Strategies for Computer Programming Education* (pp. 14–29). Hershey, PA: IGI Global. doi:10.4018/978-1-5225-1034-5.ch002

Gill, J., Ayre, M., & Mills, J. (2017). Revisioning the Engineering Profession: How to Make It Happen! In M. Gray & K. Thomas (Eds.), *Strategies for Increasing Diversity in Engineering Majors and Careers* (pp. 156–175). Hershey, PA: IGI Global. doi:10.4018/978-1-5225-2212-6.ch008

Godzhaev, Z., Senkevich, S., Kuzmin, V., & Melikov, I. (2021). Use of the Neural Network Controller of Sprung Mass to Reduce Vibrations From Road Irregularities. In P. Vasant, G. Weber, & W. Punurai (Ed.), *Research Advancements in Smart Technology, Optimization, and Renewable Energy* (pp. 69-87). IGI Global. https://doi.org/10.4018/978-1-7998-3970-5.ch005

Gomes de Gusmão, C. M. (2022). Digital Competencies and Transformation in Higher Education: Up-skilling With Extension Actions. In A. Alves & N. van Hattum-Janssen (Eds.), *Training Engineering Students for Modern Technological Advancement* (pp. 313–328). IGI Global. https://doi.org/10.4018/978-1-7998-8816-1.ch015A

Goyal, N., Ram, M., & Kumar, P. (2017). Welding Process under Fault Coverage Approach for Reliability and MTTF. In M. Ram & J. Davim (Eds.), *Mathematical Concepts and Applications in Mechanical Engineering and Mechatronics* (pp. 222–245). Hershey, PA: IGI Global. doi:10.4018/978-1-5225-1639-2.ch011

Gray, M., & Lundy, C. (2017). Engineering Study Abroad: High Impact Strategy for Increasing Access. In M. Gray & K. Thomas (Eds.), *Strategies for Increasing Diversity in Engineering Majors and Careers* (pp. 42–59). Hershey, PA: IGI Global. doi:10.4018/978-1-5225-2212-6.ch003

Güler, O., & Varol, T. (2021). Fabrication of Functionally Graded Metal and Ceramic Powders Synthesized by Electroless Deposition. In S. Roy & G. Bose (Eds.), *Advanced Surface Coating Techniques for Modern Industrial Applications* (pp. 150–187). IGI Global. https://doi.org/10.4018/978-1-7998-4870-7.ch007

Guraksin, G. E. (2018). Internet of Things and Nature-Inspired Intelligent Techniques for the Future of Biomedical Engineering. In U. Kose, G. Guraksin, & O. Deperlioglu (Eds.), *Nature-Inspired Intelligent Techniques for Solving Biomedical Engineering Problems* (pp. 263–282). Hershey, PA: IGI Global. doi:10.4018/978-1-5225-4769-3.ch013

Hamida, M. L., Fekik, A., Denoun, H., Ardjal, A., & Bokhtache, A. A. (2022). Flying Capacitor Inverter Integration in a Renewable Energy System. In A. Fekik & N. Benamrouche (Eds.), *Modeling and Control of Static Converters for Hybrid Storage Systems* (pp. 287–306). IGI Global. https://doi.org/10.4018/978-1-7998-7447-8.ch011

Hasegawa, N., & Takahashi, Y. (2021). Control of Soap Bubble Ejection Robot Using Facial Expressions. *International Journal of Manufacturing, Materials, and Mechanical Engineering, 11*(2), 1–16. https://doi.org/10.4018/IJMMME.2021040101

Hejazi, T., & Akbari, L. (2017). A Multiresponse Optimization Model for Statistical Design of Processes with Discrete Variables. In M. Ram & J. Davim (Eds.), *Mathematical Concepts and Applications in Mechanical Engineering and Mechatronics* (pp. 17–37). Hershey, PA: IGI Global. doi:10.4018/978-1-5225-1639-2.ch002

Hejazi, T., & Hejazi, A. (2017). Monte Carlo Simulation for Reliability-Based Design of Automotive Complex Subsystems. In M. Ram & J. Davim (Eds.), *Mathematical Concepts and Applications in Mechanical Engineering and Mechatronics* (pp. 177–200). Hershey, PA: IGI Global. doi:10.4018/978-1-5225-1639-2.ch009

Hejazi, T., & Poursabbagh, H. (2017). Reliability Analysis of Engineering Systems: An Accelerated Life Testing for Boiler Tubes. In M. Ram & J. Davim (Eds.), *Mathematical Concepts and Applications in Mechanical Engineering and Mechatronics* (pp. 154–176). Hershey, PA: IGI Global. doi:10.4018/978-1-5225-1639-2.ch008

Henao, J., Poblano-Salas, C. A., Vargas, F., Giraldo-Betancur, A. L., Corona-Castuera, J., & Sotelo-Mazón, O. (2021). Principles and Applications of Thermal Spray Coatings. In S. Roy & G. Bose (Eds.), *Advanced Surface Coating Techniques for Modern Industrial Applications* (pp. 31–70). IGI Global. https://doi.org/10.4018/978-1-7998-4870-7.ch002

Henao, J., & Sotelo, O. (2018). Surface Engineering at High Temperature: Thermal Cycling and Corrosion Resistance. In A. Pakseresht (Ed.), *Production, Properties, and Applications of High Temperature Coatings* (pp. 131–159). Hershey, PA: IGI Global. doi:10.4018/978-1-5225-4194-3.ch006

Hrnčič, M. K., Cör, D., & Knez, Ž. (2021). Supercritical Fluids as a Tool for Green Energy and Chemicals. In L. Chen (Ed.), *Handbook of Research on Advancements in Supercritical Fluids Applications for Sustainable Energy Systems* (pp. 761–791). IGI Global. doi:10.4018/978-1-7998-5796-9.ch021

Ibrahim, O., Erdem, S., & Gurbuz, E. (2021). Studying Physical and Chemical Properties of Graphene Oxide and Reduced Graphene Oxide and Their Applications in Sustainable Building Materials. In R. González-Lezcano (Ed.), *Advancements in Sustainable Architecture and Energy Efficiency* (pp. 221–238). IGI Global. https://doi.org/10.4018/978-1-7998-7023-4.ch010

Ihianle, I. K., Islam, S., Naeem, U., & Ebenuwa, S. H. (2021). Exploiting Patterns of Object Use for Human Activity Recognition. In A. Nwajana & I. Ihianle (Eds.), *Handbook of Research on 5G Networks and Advancements in Computing, Electronics, and Electrical Engineering* (pp. 382–401). IGI Global. https://doi.org/10.4018/978-1-7998-6992-4.ch015

Ijemaru, G. K., Ngharamike, E. T., Oleka, E. U., & Nwajana, A. O. (2021). An Energy-Efficient Model for Opportunistic Data Collection in IoV-Enabled SC Waste Management. In A. Nwajana & I. Ihianle (Eds.), *Handbook of Research on 5G Networks and Advancements in Computing, Electronics, and Electrical Engineering* (pp. 1–19). IGI Global. https://doi.org/10.4018/978-1-7998-6992-4.ch001

Ilori, O. O., Adetan, D. A., & Umoru, L. E. (2017). Effect of Cutting Parameters on the Surface Residual Stress of Face-Milled Pearlitic Ductile Iron. *International Journal of Materials Forming and Machining Processes*, 4(1), 38–52. doi:10.4018/IJMFMP.2017010103

Imam, M. H., Tasadduq, I. A., Ahmad, A., Aldosari, F., & Khan, H. (2017). Automated Generation of Course Improvement Plans Using Expert System. *International Journal of Quality Assurance in Engineering and Technology Education*, 6(1), 1–12. doi:10.4018/IJQAETE.2017010101

Injeti, S. K., & Kumar, T. V. (2018). A WDO Framework for Optimal Deployment of DGs and DSCs in a Radial Distribution System Under Daily Load Pattern to Improve Techno-Economic Benefits. *International Journal of Energy Optimization and Engineering*, 7(2), 1–38. doi:10.4018/IJEOE.2018040101

Ishii, N., Anami, K., & Knisely, C. W. (2018). *Dynamic Stability of Hydraulic Gates and Engineering for Flood Prevention*. Hershey, PA: IGI Global. doi:10.4018/978-1-5225-3079-4

Iwamoto, Y., & Yamaguchi, H. (2021). Application of Supercritical Carbon Dioxide for Solar Water Heater. In L. Chen (Ed.), *Handbook of Research on Advancements in Supercritical Fluids Applications for Sustainable Energy Systems* (pp. 370–387). IGI Global. https://doi.org/10.4018/978-1-7998-5796-9.ch010

Jayapalan, S. (2018). A Review of Chemical Treatments on Natural Fibers-Based Hybrid Composites for Engineering Applications. In K. Kumar & J. Davim (Eds.), *Composites and Advanced Materials for Industrial Applications* (pp. 16–37). Hershey, PA: IGI Global. doi:10.4018/978-1-5225-5216-1.ch002

Kapetanakis, T. N., Vardiambasis, I. O., Ioannidou, M. P., & Konstantaras, A. I. (2021). Modeling Antenna Radiation Using Artificial Intelligence Techniques: The Case of a Circular Loop Antenna. In C. Nikolopoulos (Ed.), *Recent Trends on Electromagnetic Environmental Effects for Aeronautics and Space Applications* (pp. 186–225). IGI Global. https://doi.org/10.4018/978-1-7998-4879-0.ch007

Karkalos, N. E., Markopoulos, A. P., & Dossis, M. F. (2017). Optimal Model Parameters of Inverse Kinematics Solution of a 3R Robotic Manipulator Using ANN Models. *International Journal of Manufacturing, Materials, and Mechanical Engineering*, 7(3), 20–40. doi:10.4018/IJMMME.2017070102

Kelly, M., Costello, M., Nicholson, G., & O'Connor, J. (2021). The Evolving Integration of BIM Into Built Environment Programmes in a Higher Education Institute. In J. Underwood & M. Shelbourn (Eds.), *Handbook of Research on Driving Transformational Change in the Digital Built Environment* (pp. 294–326). IGI Global. https://doi.org/10.4018/978-1-7998-6600-8.ch012

Kesimal, A., Karaman, K., Cihangir, F., & Ercikdi, B. (2018). Excavatability Assessment of Rock Masses for Geotechnical Studies. In N. Ceryan (Ed.), *Handbook of Research on Trends and Digital Advances in Engineering Geology* (pp. 231–256). Hershey, PA: IGI Global. doi:10.4018/978-1-5225-2709-1.ch006

Knoflacher, H. (2017). The Role of Engineers and Their Tools in the Transport Sector after Paradigm Change: From Assumptions and Extrapolations to Science. In H. Knoflacher & E. Ocalir-Akunal (Eds.), *Engineering Tools and Solutions for Sustainable Transportation Planning* (pp. 1–29). Hershey, PA: IGI Global. doi:10.4018/978-1-5225-2116-7.ch001

Kose, U. (2018). Towards an Intelligent Biomedical Engineering With Nature-Inspired Artificial Intelligence Techniques. In U. Kose, G. Guraksin, & O. Deperlioglu (Eds.), *Nature-Inspired Intelligent Techniques for Solving Biomedical Engineering Problems* (pp. 1–26). Hershey, PA: IGI Global. doi:10.4018/978-1-5225-4769-3.ch001

Kostić, S. (2018). A Review on Enhanced Stability Analyses of Soil Slopes Using Statistical Design. In N. Ceryan (Ed.), *Handbook of Research on Trends and Digital Advances in Engineering Geology* (pp. 446–481). Hershey, PA: IGI Global. doi:10.4018/978-1-5225-2709-1.ch013

Kumar, A., Patil, P. P., & Prajapati, Y. K. (2018). *Advanced Numerical Simulations in Mechanical Engineering*. Hershey, PA: IGI Global. doi:10.4018/978-1-5225-3722-9

Kumar, G. R., Rajyalakshmi, G., & Manupati, V. K. (2017). Surface Micro Patterning of Aluminium Reinforced Composite through Laser Peening. *International Journal of Manufacturing, Materials, and Mechanical Engineering*, 7(4), 15–27. doi:10.4018/IJMMME.2017100102

Kumar, N., Basu, D. N., & Chen, L. (2021). Effect of Flow Acceleration and Buoyancy on Thermalhydraulics of sCO2 in Mini/Micro-Channel. In L. Chen (Ed.), *Handbook of Research on Advancements in Supercritical Fluids Applications for Sustainable Energy Systems* (pp. 161–182). IGI Global. doi:10.4018/978-1-7998-5796-9.ch005

Kumari, N., & Kumar, K. (2018). Fabrication of Orthotic Calipers With Epoxy-Based Green Composite. In K. Kumar & J. Davim (Eds.), *Composites and Advanced Materials for Industrial Applications* (pp. 157–176). Hershey, PA: IGI Global. doi:10.4018/978-1-5225-5216-1.ch008

Kuppusamy, R. R. (2018). Development of Aerospace Composite Structures Through Vacuum-Enhanced Resin Transfer Moulding Technology (VERTMTy): Vacuum-Enhanced Resin Transfer Moulding. In K. Kumar & J. Davim (Eds.), *Composites and Advanced Materials for Industrial Applications* (pp. 99–111). Hershey, PA: IGI Global. doi:10.4018/978-1-5225-5216-1.ch005

Kurganov, V. A., Zeigarnik, Y. A., & Maslakova, I. V. (2021). Normal and Deteriorated Heat Transfer Under Heating Turbulent Supercritical Pressure Coolants Flows in Round Tubes. In L. Chen (Ed.), *Handbook of Research on Advancements in Supercritical Fluids Applications for Sustainable Energy Systems* (pp. 494–532). IGI Global. https://doi.org/10.4018/978-1-7998-5796-9.ch014

Li, H., & Zhang, Y. (2021). Heat Transfer and Fluid Flow Modeling for Supercritical Fluids in Advanced Energy Systems. In L. Chen (Ed.), *Handbook of Research on Advancements in Supercritical Fluids Applications for Sustainable Energy Systems* (pp. 388–422). IGI Global. https://doi.org/10.4018/978-1-7998-5796-9.ch011

Loy, J., Howell, S., & Cooper, R. (2017). Engineering Teams: Supporting Diversity in Engineering Education. In M. Gray & K. Thomas (Eds.), *Strategies for Increasing Diversity in Engineering Majors and Careers* (pp. 106–129). Hershey, PA: IGI Global. doi:10.4018/978-1-5225-2212-6.ch006

Macher, G., Armengaud, E., Kreiner, C., Brenner, E., Schmittner, C., Ma, Z., ... Krammer, M. (2018). Integration of Security in the Development Lifecycle of Dependable Automotive CPS. In N. Druml, A. Genser, A. Krieg, M. Menghin, & A. Hoeller (Eds.), *Solutions for Cyber-Physical Systems Ubiquity* (pp. 383–423). Hershey, PA: IGI Global. doi:10.4018/978-1-5225-2845-6.ch015

Madhu, M. N., Singh, J. G., Mohan, V., & Ongsakul, W. (2021). Transmission Risk Optimization in Interconnected Systems: Risk-Adjusted Available Transfer Capability. In P. Vasant, G. Weber, & W. Punurai (Ed.), *Research Advancements in Smart Technology, Optimization, and Renewable Energy* (pp. 183-199). IGI Global. https://doi.org/10.4018/978-1-7998-3970-5.ch010

Mahendramani, G., & Lakshmana Swamy, N. (2018). Effect of Weld Groove Area on Distortion of Butt Welded Joints in Submerged Arc Welding. *International Journal of Manufacturing, Materials, and Mechanical Engineering*, 8(2), 33–44. doi:10.4018/IJMMME.2018040103

Makropoulos, G., Koumaras, H., Setaki, F., Filis, K., Lutz, T., Montowtt, P., Tomaszewski, L., Dybiec, P., & Järvet, T. (2021). 5G and Unmanned Aerial Vehicles (UAVs) Use Cases: Analysis of the Ecosystem, Architecture, and Applications. In A. Nwajana & I. Ihianle (Eds.), *Handbook of Research on 5G Networks and Advancements in Computing, Electronics, and Electrical Engineering* (pp. 36–69). IGI Global. https://doi.org/10.4018/978-1-7998-6992-4.ch003

Meric, E. M., Erdem, S., & Gurbuz, E. (2021). Application of Phase Change Materials in Construction Materials for Thermal Energy Storage Systems in Buildings. In R. González-Lezcano (Ed.), *Advancements in Sustainable Architecture and Energy Efficiency* (pp. 1–20). IGI Global. https://doi.org/10.4018/978-1-7998-7023-4.ch001

Mihret, E. T., & Yitayih, K. A. (2021). Operation of VANET Communications: The Convergence of UAV System With LTE/4G and WAVE Technologies. *International Journal of Smart Vehicles and Smart Transportation*, 4(1), 29–51. https://doi.org/10.4018/IJSVST.2021010103

Mir, M. A., Bhat, B. A., Sheikh, B. A., Rather, G. A., Mehraj, S., & Mir, W. R. (2021). Nanomedicine in Human Health Therapeutics and Drug Delivery: Nanobiotechnology and Nanobiomedicine. In M. Bhat, I. Wani, & S. Ashraf (Eds.), *Applications of Nanomaterials in Agriculture, Food Science, and Medicine* (pp. 229–251). IGI Global. doi:10.4018/978-1-7998-5563-7.ch013

Mohammadzadeh, S., & Kim, Y. (2017). Nonlinear System Identification of Smart Buildings. In P. Samui, S. Chakraborty, & D. Kim (Eds.), *Modeling and Simulation Techniques in Structural Engineering* (pp. 328–347). Hershey, PA: IGI Global. doi:10.4018/978-1-5225-0588-4.ch011

Molina, G. J., Aktaruzzaman, F., Soloiu, V., & Rahman, M. (2017). Design and Testing of a Jet-Impingement Instrument to Study Surface-Modification Effects by Nanofluids. *International Journal of Surface Engineering and Interdisciplinary Materials Science*, 5(2), 43–61. doi:10.4018/IJSEIMS.2017070104

Moreno-Rangel, A., & Carrillo, G. (2021). Energy-Efficient Homes: A Heaven for Respiratory Illnesses. In R. González-Lezcano (Ed.), *Advancements in Sustainable Architecture and Energy Efficiency* (pp. 49–71). IGI Global. https://doi.org/10.4018/978-1-7998-7023-4.ch003

Msomi, V., & Jantjies, B. T. (2021). Correlative Analysis Between Tensile Properties and Tool Rotational Speeds of Friction Stir Welded Similar Aluminium Alloy Joints. *International Journal of Surface Engineering and Interdisciplinary Materials Science*, 9(2), 58–78. https://doi.org/10.4018/IJSEIMS.2021070104

Muigai, M. N., Mwema, F. M., Akinlabi, E. T., & Obiko, J. O. (2021). Surface Engineering of Materials Through Weld-Based Technologies: An Overview. In S. Roy & G. Bose (Eds.), *Advanced Surface Coating Techniques for Modern Industrial Applications* (pp. 247–260). IGI Global. doi:10.4018/978-1-7998-4870-7.ch011

Mukherjee, A., Saeed, R. A., Dutta, S., & Naskar, M. K. (2017). Fault Tracking Framework for Software-Defined Networking (SDN). In C. Singhal & S. De (Eds.), *Resource Allocation in Next-Generation Broadband Wireless Access Networks* (pp. 247–272). Hershey, PA: IGI Global. doi:10.4018/978-1-5225-2023-8.ch011

Mukhopadhyay, A., Barman, T. K., & Sahoo, P. (2018). Electroless Nickel Coatings for High Temperature Applications. In K. Kumar & J. Davim (Eds.), *Composites and Advanced Materials for Industrial Applications* (pp. 297–331). Hershey, PA: IGI Global. doi:10.4018/978-1-5225-5216-1.ch013

Mwema, F. M., & Wambua, J. M. (2022). Machining of Poly Methyl Methacrylate (PMMA) and Other Olymeric Materials: A Review. In K. Kumar, B. Babu, & J. Davim (Eds.), *Handbook of Research on Advancements in the Processing, Characterization, and Application of Lightweight Materials* (pp. 363–379). IGI Global. https://doi.org/10.4018/978-1-7998-7864-3.ch016

Mykhailyshyn, R., Savkiv, V., Boyko, I., Prada, E., & Virgala, I. (2021). Substantiation of Parameters of Friction Elements of Bernoulli Grippers With a Cylindrical Nozzle. *International Journal of Manufacturing, Materials, and Mechanical Engineering, 11*(2), 17–39. https://doi.org/10.4018/IJMMME.2021040102

Náprstek, J., & Fischer, C. (2017). Dynamic Stability and Post-Critical Processes of Slender Auto-Parametric Systems. In V. Plevris, G. Kremmyda, & Y. Fahjan (Eds.), *Performance-Based Seismic Design of Concrete Structures and Infrastructures* (pp. 128–171). Hershey, PA: IGI Global. doi:10.4018/978-1-5225-2089-4.ch006

Nautiyal, L., Shivach, P., & Ram, M. (2018). Optimal Designs by Means of Genetic Algorithms. In M. Ram & J. Davim (Eds.), *Soft Computing Techniques and Applications in Mechanical Engineering* (pp. 151–161). Hershey, PA: IGI Global. doi:10.4018/978-1-5225-3035-0.ch007

Nazir, R. (2017). Advanced Nanomaterials for Water Engineering and Treatment: Nano-Metal Oxides and Their Nanocomposites. In T. Saleh (Ed.), *Advanced Nanomaterials for Water Engineering, Treatment, and Hydraulics* (pp. 84–126). Hershey, PA: IGI Global. doi:10.4018/978-1-5225-2136-5.ch005

Nikolopoulos, C. D. (2021). Recent Advances on Measuring and Modeling ELF-Radiated Emissions for Space Applications. In C. Nikolopoulos (Ed.), *Recent Trends on Electromagnetic Environmental Effects for Aeronautics and Space Applications* (pp. 1–38). IGI Global. https://doi.org/10.4018/978-1-7998-4879-0.ch001

Nogueira, A. F., Ribeiro, J. C., Fernández de Vega, F., & Zenha-Rela, M. A. (2018). Evolutionary Approaches to Test Data Generation for Object-Oriented Software: Overview of Techniques and Tools. In M. Khosrow-Pour, D.B.A. (Ed.), Incorporating Nature-Inspired Paradigms in Computational Applications (pp. 162-194). Hershey, PA: IGI Global. https://doi.org/ doi:10.4018/978-1-5225-5020-4.ch006

Nwajana, A. O., Obi, E. R., Ijemaru, G. K., Oleka, E. U., & Anthony, D. C. (2021). Fundamentals of RF/Microwave Bandpass Filter Design. In A. Nwajana & I. Ihianle (Eds.), *Handbook of Research on 5G Networks and Advancements in Computing, Electronics, and Electrical Engineering* (pp. 149–164). IGI Global. https://doi.org/10.4018/978-1-7998-6992-4.ch005

Ogbodo, E. A. (2021). Comparative Study of Transmission Line Junction vs. Asynchronously Coupled Junction Diplexers. In A. Nwajana & I. Ihianle (Eds.), *Handbook of Research on 5G Networks and Advancements in Computing, Electronics, and Electrical Engineering* (pp. 326–336). IGI Global. https://doi.org/10.4018/978-1-7998-6992-4.ch013

Orosa, J. A., Vergara, D., Fraguela, F., & Masdías-Bonome, A. (2021). Statistical Understanding and Optimization of Building Energy Consumption and Climate Change Consequences. In R. González-Lezcano (Ed.), *Advancements in Sustainable Architecture and Energy Efficiency* (pp. 195–220). IGI Global. https://doi.org/10.4018/978-1-7998-7023-4.ch009

Osho, M. B. (2018). Industrial Enzyme Technology: Potential Applications. In S. Bharati & P. Chaurasia (Eds.), *Research Advancements in Pharmaceutical, Nutritional, and Industrial Enzymology* (pp. 375–394). Hershey, PA: IGI Global. doi:10.4018/978-1-5225-5237-6.ch017

Ouadi, A., & Zitouni, A. (2021). Phasor Measurement Improvement Using Digital Filter in a Smart Grid. In A. Recioui & H. Bentarzi (Eds.), *Optimizing and Measuring Smart Grid Operation and Control* (pp. 100–117). IGI Global. https://doi.org/10.4018/978-1-7998-4027-5.ch005

Padmaja, P., & Marutheswar, G. (2017). Certain Investigation on Secured Data Transmission in Wireless Sensor Networks. *International Journal of Mobile Computing and Multimedia Communications*, *8*(1), 48–61. doi:10.4018/IJMCMC.2017010104

Palmer, S., & Hall, W. (2017). An Evaluation of Group Work in First-Year Engineering Design Education. In R. Tucker (Ed.), *Collaboration and Student Engagement in Design Education* (pp. 145–168). Hershey, PA: IGI Global. doi:10.4018/978-1-5225-0726-0.ch007

Panchenko, V. (2021). Prospects for Energy Supply of the Arctic Zone Objects of Russia Using Frost-Resistant Solar Modules. In P. Vasant, G. Weber, & W. Punurai (Eds.), *Research Advancements in Smart Technology, Optimization, and Renewable Energy* (pp. 149-169). IGI Global. https://doi.org/10.4018/978-1-7998-3970-5.ch008

Panchenko, V. (2021). Photovoltaic Thermal Module With Paraboloid Type Solar Concentrators. *International Journal of Energy Optimization and Engineering*, *10*(2), 1–23. https://doi.org/10.4018/IJEOE.2021040101

Pandey, K., & Datta, S. (2021). Dry Machining of Inconel 825 Superalloys: Performance of Tool Inserts (Carbide, Cermet, and SiAlON). *International Journal of Manufacturing, Materials, and Mechanical Engineering*, *11*(4), 26–39. doi:10.4018/IJMMME.2021100102

Panneer, R. (2017). Effect of Composition of Fibers on Properties of Hybrid Composites. *International Journal of Manufacturing, Materials, and Mechanical Engineering*, *7*(4), 28–43. doi:10.4018/IJMMME.2017100103

Pany, C. (2021). Estimation of Correct Long-Seam Mismatch Using FEA to Compare the Measured Strain in a Non-Destructive Testing of a Pressurant Tank: A Reverse Problem. *International Journal of Smart Vehicles and Smart Transportation*, *4*(1), 16–28. doi:10.4018/IJSVST.2021010102

Paul, S., & Roy, P. (2018). Optimal Design of Power System Stabilizer Using a Novel Evolutionary Algorithm. *International Journal of Energy Optimization and Engineering, 7*(3), 24–46. doi:10.4018/IJEOE.2018070102

Paul, S., & Roy, P. K. (2021). Oppositional Differential Search Algorithm for the Optimal Tuning of Both Single Input and Dual Input Power System Stabilizer. In P. Vasant, G. Weber, & W. Punurai (Eds.), *Research Advancements in Smart Technology, Optimization, and Renewable Energy* (pp. 256-282). IGI Global. https://doi.org/10.4018/978-1-7998-3970-5.ch013

Pavaloiu, A. (2018). Artificial Intelligence Ethics in Biomedical-Engineering-Oriented Problems. In U. Kose, G. Guraksin, & O. Deperlioglu (Eds.), *Nature-Inspired Intelligent Techniques for Solving Biomedical Engineering Problems* (pp. 219–231). Hershey, PA: IGI Global. doi:10.4018/978-1-5225-4769-3.ch010

Pioro, I., Mahdi, M., & Popov, R. (2017). Application of Supercritical Pressures in Power Engineering. In L. Chen & Y. Iwamoto (Eds.), *Advanced Applications of Supercritical Fluids in Energy Systems* (pp. 404–457). Hershey, PA: IGI Global. doi:10.4018/978-1-5225-2047-4.ch013

Plaksina, T., & Gildin, E. (2017). Rigorous Integrated Evolutionary Workflow for Optimal Exploitation of Unconventional Gas Assets. *International Journal of Energy Optimization and Engineering, 6*(1), 101–122. doi:10.4018/IJEOE.2017010106

Popat, J., Kakadiya, H., Tak, L., Singh, N. K., Majeed, M. A., & Mahajan, V. (2021). Reliability of Smart Grid Including Cyber Impact: A Case Study. In R. Singh, A. Singh, A. Dwivedi, & P. Nagabhushan (Eds.), *Computational Methodologies for Electrical and Electronics Engineers* (pp. 163–174). IGI Global. https://doi.org/10.4018/978-1-7998-3327-7.ch013

Quiza, R., La Fé-Perdomo, I., Rivas, M., & Ramtahalsing, V. (2021). Triple Bottom Line-Focused Optimization of Oblique Turning Processes Based on Hybrid Modeling: A Study Case on AISI 1045 Steel Turning. In L. Burstein (Ed.), *Handbook of Research on Advancements in Manufacturing, Materials, and Mechanical Engineering* (pp. 215–241). IGI Global. https://doi.org/10.4018/978-1-7998-4939-1.ch010

Rahmani, M. K. (2022). Blockchain Technology: Principles and Algorithms. In S. Khan, M. Syed, R. Hammad, & A. Bushager (Eds.), *Blockchain Technology and Computational Excellence for Society 5.0* (pp. 16–27). IGI Global. https://doi.org/10.4018/978-1-7998-8382-1.ch002

Ramdani, N., & Azibi, M. (2018). Polymer Composite Materials for Microelectronics Packaging Applications: Composites for Microelectronics Packaging. In K. Kumar & J. Davim (Eds.), *Composites and Advanced Materials for Industrial Applications* (pp. 177–211). Hershey, PA: IGI Global. doi:10.4018/978-1-5225-5216-1.ch009

Ramesh, M., Garg, R., & Subrahmanyam, G. V. (2017). Investigation of Influence of Quenching and Annealing on the Plane Fracture Toughness and Brittle to Ductile Transition Temperature of the Zinc Coated Structural Steel Materials. *International Journal of Surface Engineering and Interdisciplinary Materials Science, 5*(2), 33–42. doi:10.4018/IJSEIMS.2017070103

Robinson, J., & Beneroso, D. (2022). Project-Based Learning in Chemical Engineering: Curriculum and Assessment, Culture and Learning Spaces. In A. Alves & N. van Hattum-Janssen (Eds.), *Training Engineering Students for Modern Technological Advancement* (pp. 1–19). IGI Global. https://doi.org/10.4018/978-1-7998-8816-1.ch001

Rondon, B. (2021). Experimental Characterization of Admittance Meter With Crude Oil Emulsions. *International Journal of Electronics, Communications, and Measurement Engineering, 10*(2), 51–59. https://doi.org/10.4018/IJECME.2021070104

Rudolf, S., Biryuk, V. V., & Volov, V. (2018). Vortex Effect, Vortex Power: Technology of Vortex Power Engineering. In V. Kharchenko & P. Vasant (Eds.), *Handbook of Research on Renewable Energy and Electric Resources for Sustainable Rural Development* (pp. 500–533). Hershey, PA: IGI Global. doi:10.4018/978-1-5225-3867-7.ch021

Sah, A., Bhadula, S. J., Dumka, A., & Rawat, S. (2018). A Software Engineering Perspective for Development of Enterprise Applications. In A. Elçi (Ed.), *Handbook of Research on Contemporary Perspectives on Web-Based Systems* (pp. 1–23). Hershey, PA: IGI Global. doi:10.4018/978-1-5225-5384-7.ch001

Sahli, Y., Zitouni, B., & Hocine, B. M. (2021). Three-Dimensional Numerical Study of Overheating of Two Intermediate Temperature P-AS-SOFC Geometrical Configurations. In G. Badea, R. Felseghi, & I. Aşchilean (Eds.), *Hydrogen Fuel Cell Technology for Stationary Applications* (pp. 186–222). IGI Global. https://doi.org/10.4018/978-1-7998-4945-2.ch008

Sahoo, P., & Roy, S. (2017). Tribological Behavior of Electroless Ni-P, Ni-P-W and Ni-P-Cu Coatings: A Comparison. *International Journal of Surface Engineering and Interdisciplinary Materials Science, 5*(1), 1–15. doi:10.4018/IJSEIMS.2017010101

Sahoo, S. (2018). Laminated Composite Hypar Shells as Roofing Units: Static and Dynamic Behavior. In K. Kumar & J. Davim (Eds.), *Composites and Advanced Materials for Industrial Applications* (pp. 249–269). Hershey, PA: IGI Global. doi:10.4018/978-1-5225-5216-1.ch011

Sahu, H., & Hungyo, M. (2018). Introduction to SDN and NFV. In A. Dumka (Ed.), *Innovations in Software-Defined Networking and Network Functions Virtualization* (pp. 1–25). Hershey, PA: IGI Global. doi:10.4018/978-1-5225-3640-6.ch001

Salem, A. M., & Shmelova, T. (2018). Intelligent Expert Decision Support Systems: Methodologies, Applications, and Challenges. In T. Shmelova, Y. Sikirda, N. Rizun, A. Salem, & Y. Kovalyov (Eds.), *Socio-Technical Decision Support in Air Navigation Systems: Emerging Research and Opportunities* (pp. 215–242). Hershey, PA: IGI Global. doi:10.4018/978-1-5225-3108-1.ch007

Samal, M. (2017). FE Analysis and Experimental Investigation of Cracked and Un-Cracked Thin-Walled Tubular Components to Evaluate Mechanical and Fracture Properties. In P. Samui, S. Chakraborty, & D. Kim (Eds.), *Modeling and Simulation Techniques in Structural Engineering* (pp. 266–293). Hershey, PA: IGI Global. doi:10.4018/978-1-5225-0588-4.ch009

Samal, M., & Balakrishnan, K. (2017). Experiments on a Ring Tension Setup and FE Analysis to Evaluate Transverse Mechanical Properties of Tubular Components. In P. Samui, S. Chakraborty, & D. Kim (Eds.), *Modeling and Simulation Techniques in Structural Engineering* (pp. 91–115). Hershey, PA: IGI Global. doi:10.4018/978-1-5225-0588-4.ch004

Samarasinghe, D. A., & Wood, E. (2021). Innovative Digital Technologies. In J. Underwood & M. Shelbourn (Eds.), *Handbook of Research on Driving Transformational Change in the Digital Built Environment* (pp. 142–163). IGI Global. https://doi.org/10.4018/978-1-7998-6600-8.ch006

Sawant, S. (2018). Deep Learning and Biomedical Engineering. In U. Kose, G. Guraksin, & O. Deperlioglu (Eds.), *Nature-Inspired Intelligent Techniques for Solving Biomedical Engineering Problems* (pp. 283–296). Hershey, PA: IGI Global. doi:10.4018/978-1-5225-4769-3.ch014

Schulenberg, T. (2021). Energy Conversion Using the Supercritical Steam Cycle. In L. Chen (Ed.), *Handbook of Research on Advancements in Supercritical Fluids Applications for Sustainable Energy Systems* (pp. 659–681). IGI Global. doi:10.4018/978-1-7998-5796-9.ch018

Sezgin, H., & Berkalp, O. B. (2018). Textile-Reinforced Composites for the Automotive Industry. In K. Kumar & J. Davim (Eds.), *Composites and Advanced Materials for Industrial Applications* (pp. 129–156). Hershey, PA: IGI Global. doi:10.4018/978-1-5225-5216-1.ch007

Shaaban, A. A., & Shehata, O. M. (2021). Combining Response Surface Method and Metaheuristic Algorithms for Optimizing SPIF Process. *International Journal of Manufacturing, Materials, and Mechanical Engineering, 11*(4), 1–25. https://doi.org/10.4018/IJMMME.2021100101

Shafaati Shemami, M., & Sefid, M. (2022). Implementation and Demonstration of Electric Vehicle-to-Home (V2H) Application: A Case Study. In M. Alam, R. Pillai, & N. Murugesan (Eds.), *Developing Charging Infrastructure and Technologies for Electric Vehicles* (pp. 268–293). IGI Global. https://doi.org/10.4018/978-1-7998-6858-3.ch015

Shah, M. Z., Gazder, U., Bhatti, M. S., & Hussain, M. (2018). Comparative Performance Evaluation of Effects of Modifier in Asphaltic Concrete Mix. *International Journal of Strategic Engineering, 1*(2), 13–25. doi:10.4018/IJoSE.2018070102

Sharma, N., & Kumar, K. (2018). Fabrication of Porous NiTi Alloy Using Organic Binders. In K. Kumar & J. Davim (Eds.), *Composites and Advanced Materials for Industrial Applications* (pp. 38–62). Hershey, PA: IGI Global. doi:10.4018/978-1-5225-5216-1.ch003

Shivach, P., Nautiyal, L., & Ram, M. (2018). Applying Multi-Objective Optimization Algorithms to Mechanical Engineering. In M. Ram & J. Davim (Eds.), *Soft Computing Techniques and Applications in Mechanical Engineering* (pp. 287–301). Hershey, PA: IGI Global. doi:10.4018/978-1-5225-3035-0.ch014

Shmelova, T. (2018). Stochastic Methods for Estimation and Problem Solving in Engineering: Stochastic Methods of Decision Making in Aviation. In S. Kadry (Ed.), *Stochastic Methods for Estimation and Problem Solving in Engineering* (pp. 139–160). Hershey, PA: IGI Global. doi:10.4018/978-1-5225-5045-7.ch006

Siero González, L. R., & Romo Vázquez, A. (2017). Didactic Sequences Teaching Mathematics for Engineers With Focus on Differential Equations. In M. Ramírez-Montoya (Ed.), *Handbook of Research on Driving STEM Learning With Educational Technologies* (pp. 129–151). Hershey, PA: IGI Global. doi:10.4018/978-1-5225-2026-9.ch007

Sim, M. S., You, K. Y., Esa, F., & Chan, Y. L. (2021). Nanostructured Electromagnetic Metamaterials for Sensing Applications. In M. Bhat, I. Wani, & S. Ashraf (Eds.), *Applications of Nanomaterials in Agriculture, Food Science, and Medicine* (pp. 141–164). IGI Global. https://doi.org/10.4018/978-1-7998-5563-7.ch009

Singh, R., & Dutta, S. (2018). Visible Light Active Nanocomposites for Photocatalytic Applications. In K. Kumar & J. Davim (Eds.), *Composites and Advanced Materials for Industrial Applications* (pp. 270–296). Hershey, PA: IGI Global. doi:10.4018/978-1-5225-5216-1.ch012

Skripov, P. V., Yampol'skiy, A. D., & Rutin, S. B. (2021). High-Power Heat Transfer in Supercritical Fluids: Microscale Times and Sizes. In L. Chen (Ed.), *Handbook of Research on Advancements in Supercritical Fluids Applications for Sustainable Energy Systems* (pp. 424–450). IGI Global. https://doi.org/10.4018/978-1-7998-5796-9.ch012

Sözbilir, H., Özkaymak, Ç., Uzel, B., & Sümer, Ö. (2018). Criteria for Surface Rupture Microzonation of Active Faults for Earthquake Hazards in Urban Areas. In N. Ceryan (Ed.), *Handbook of Research on Trends and Digital Advances in Engineering Geology* (pp. 187–230). Hershey, PA: IGI Global. doi:10.4018/978-1-5225-2709-1.ch005

Stanciu, I. (2018). Stochastic Methods in Microsystems Engineering. In S. Kadry (Ed.), *Stochastic Methods for Estimation and Problem Solving in Engineering* (pp. 161–176). Hershey, PA: IGI Global. doi:10.4018/978-1-5225-5045-7.ch007

Strebkov, D., Nekrasov, A., Trubnikov, V., & Nekrasov, A. (2018). Single-Wire Resonant Electric Power Systems for Renewable-Based Electric Grid. In V. Kharchenko & P. Vasant (Eds.), *Handbook of Research on Renewable Energy and Electric Resources for Sustainable Rural Development* (pp. 449–474). Hershey, PA: IGI Global. doi:10.4018/978-1-5225-3867-7.ch019

Sukhyy, K., Belyanovskaya, E., & Sukhyy, M. (2021). *Basic Principles for Substantiation of Working Pair Choice*. IGI Global. doi:10.4018/978-1-7998-4432-7.ch002

Suri, M. S., & Kaliyaperumal, D. (2022). Extension of Aspiration Level Model for Optimal Planning of Fast Charging Stations. In A. Fekik & N. Benamrouche (Eds.), *Modeling and Control of Static Converters for Hybrid Storage Systems* (pp. 91–106). IGI Global. https://doi.org/10.4018/978-1-7998-7447-8.ch004

Tallet, E., Gledson, B., Rogage, K., Thompson, A., & Wiggett, D. (2021). Digitally-Enabled Design Management. In J. Underwood & M. Shelbourn (Eds.), *Handbook of Research on Driving Transformational Change in the Digital Built Environment* (pp. 63–89). IGI Global. https://doi.org/10.4018/978-1-7998-6600-8.ch003

Terki, A., & Boubertakh, H. (2021). A New Hybrid Binary-Real Coded Cuckoo Search and Tabu Search Algorithm for Solving the Unit-Commitment Problem. *International Journal of Energy Optimization and Engineering*, *10*(2), 104–119. https://doi.org/10.4018/IJEOE.2021040105

Tüdeş, Ş., Kumlu, K. B., & Ceryan, S. (2018). Integration Between Urban Planning and Natural Hazards For Resilient City. In N. Ceryan (Ed.), *Handbook of Research on Trends and Digital Advances in Engineering Geology* (pp. 591–630). Hershey, PA: IGI Global. doi:10.4018/978-1-5225-2709-1.ch017

Ulamis, K. (2018). Soil Liquefaction Assessment by Anisotropic Cyclic Triaxial Test. In N. Ceryan (Ed.), *Handbook of Research on Trends and Digital Advances in Engineering Geology* (pp. 631–664). Hershey, PA: IGI Global. doi:10.4018/978-1-5225-2709-1.ch018

Valente, M., & Milani, G. (2017). Seismic Assessment and Retrofitting of an Under-Designed RC Frame Through a Displacement-Based Approach. In V. Plevris, G. Kremmyda, & Y. Fahjan (Eds.), *Performance-Based Seismic Design of Concrete Structures and Infrastructures* (pp. 36–58). Hershey, PA: IGI Global. doi:10.4018/978-1-5225-2089-4.ch002

Vargas-Bernal, R. (2021). Advances in Electromagnetic Environmental Shielding for Aeronautics and Space Applications. In C. Nikolopoulos (Ed.), *Recent Trends on Electromagnetic Environmental Effects for Aeronautics and Space Applications* (pp. 80–96). IGI Global. https://doi.org/10.4018/978-1-7998-4879-0.ch003

Vasant, P. (2018). A General Medical Diagnosis System Formed by Artificial Neural Networks and Swarm Intelligence Techniques. In U. Kose, G. Guraksin, & O. Deperlioglu (Eds.), *Nature-Inspired Intelligent Techniques for Solving Biomedical Engineering Problems* (pp. 130–145). Hershey, PA: IGI Global. doi:10.4018/978-1-5225-4769-3.ch006

Verner, C. M., & Sarwar, D. (2021). Avoiding Project Failure and Achieving Project Success in NHS IT System Projects in the United Kingdom. *International Journal of Strategic Engineering*, 4(1), 33–54. https://doi.org/10.4018/IJoSE.2021010103

Verrollot, J., Tolonen, A., Harkonen, J., & Haapasalo, H. J. (2018). Challenges and Enablers for Rapid Product Development. *International Journal of Applied Industrial Engineering*, 5(1), 25–49. doi:10.4018/IJAIE.2018010102

Wan, A. C., Zulu, S. L., & Khosrow-Shahi, F. (2021). Industry Views on BIM for Site Safety in Hong Kong. In J. Underwood & M. Shelbourn (Eds.), *Handbook of Research on Driving Transformational Change in the Digital Built Environment* (pp. 120–140). IGI Global. https://doi.org/10.4018/978-1-7998-6600-8.ch005

Yardimci, A. G., & Karpuz, C. (2018). Fuzzy Rock Mass Rating: Soft-Computing-Aided Preliminary Stability Analysis of Weak Rock Slopes. In N. Ceryan (Ed.), *Handbook of Research on Trends and Digital Advances in Engineering Geology* (pp. 97–131). Hershey, PA: IGI Global. doi:10.4018/978-1-5225-2709-1.ch003

You, K. Y. (2021). Development Electronic Design Automation for RF/Microwave Antenna Using MATLAB GUI. In A. Nwajana & I. Ihianle (Eds.), *Handbook of Research on 5G Networks and Advancements in Computing, Electronics, and Electrical Engineering* (pp. 70–148). IGI Global. https://doi.org/10.4018/978-1-7998-6992-4.ch004

Yousefi, Y., Gratton, P., & Sarwar, D. (2021). Investigating the Opportunities to Improve the Thermal Performance of a Case Study Building in London. *International Journal of Strategic Engineering*, 4(1), 1–18. https://doi.org/10.4018/IJoSE.2021010101

Zindani, D., & Kumar, K. (2018). Industrial Applications of Polymer Composite Materials. In K. Kumar & J. Davim (Eds.), *Composites and Advanced Materials for Industrial Applications* (pp. 1–15). Hershey, PA: IGI Global. doi:10.4018/978-1-5225-5216-1.ch001

Zindani, D., Maity, S. R., & Bhowmik, S. (2018). A Decision-Making Approach for Material Selection of Polymeric Composite Bumper Beam. In K. Kumar & J. Davim (Eds.), *Composites and Advanced Materials for Industrial Applications* (pp. 112–128). Hershey, PA: IGI Global. doi:10.4018/978-1-5225-5216-1.ch006

About the Contributors

Tanupriya Choudhury completed his undergraduate studies in Computer Science and Engineering at the West Bengal University of Technology in Kolkata (2004-2008), India, followed by a Master's Degree in the same field from Dr. M.G.R University in Chennai, India (2008-2010). In 2016, he successfully obtained his PhD degree from Jagannath University Jaipur. With a total of 14 years of experience in both teaching and research, Dr. Choudhury holds the position of Professor at CSE Department,Symbiosis Institute of Technology, Symbiosis International University, Pune, Maharashtra, 412115, India and also he is holding Visiting Professor at Daffodil International University Bangladesh and Director Research (Honorary) at AI University, Montana US. Prior to this role, he served Graphic Era Hill University Dehradun (Research Professor), UPES Dehradun (Professor), Amity University Noida (Assistant Professor), and other prestigious academic institutions (Dronacharya College of Engineering Gurgaon,Lingaya's University Faridabad, Babu Banarsi Das Institute of Technology Ghaziabad, Syscon Solutions Pvt. Ltd. Kolkata etc.).Recently recognized for his outstanding contributions to education with the Global Outreach Education Award for Excellence in Best Young Researcher Award at GOECA 2018. His areas of expertise encompass Human Computing, Soft Computing, Cloud Computing, Data Mining among others. Notably accomplished within his field thus far is filing 25 patents and securing copyrights for 16 software programs from MHRD (Ministry of Human Resource Development). He has actively participated as an attendee or speaker at numerous National and International conferences across India and abroad. With over hundred plus quality research papers (Scopus) authored to date on record; Dr. Choudhury has also been invited as a guest lecturer or keynote speaker at esteemed institutions such as Jamia Millia Islamia University India, Maharaja Agersen College (Delhi University), Duy Tan University Vietnam etc.He has also contributed significantly to various National/ International conferences throughout India and abroad serving roles like TPC chair/ member and session chairperson. As an active professional within the technical community; Dr.Choudhury holds lifetime membership with IETA (International Engineering & Technology Association) along with being affiliated with IEEE (Institute of Electrical and Electronics Engineers), IET(UK) (Institution of Engineering & Technology UK),and other reputable technical societies.Additionally, he is associated with corporate entities and serves as a Technical Adviser for Deetya Soft Pvt. Ltd., Noida, IVRGURU, and Mydigital360.He is also serving a Editor's in reputed Journals. He currently serves as the Honorary Secretary in IETA (Indian Engineering Teacher's Association-India), alongside his role as the Senior Advisor Position in INDO-UK Confederation of Science, Technology and Research Ltd., London, UK and International Association of Professional and Fellow Engineers-Delaware-USA.

Anitha Mary X completed her B.E.Electonics and Instrumentation Engineering from Bharathiar University in the year 2001, M.E VLSI Design from Anna University in the year 2009, and Ph.D from Karunya University in the year 2015. She is working as an Associate Professor in the Department of Robotics Engineering, Karunya Institute of Technology and Sciences, Coimbatore. Her academic record holds fifteen years of teaching experience. She has 30 Scopus Indexed Publications to her credit. She works in Multidisciplinary research areas in the field of Embedded Systems and sensor interfacing with experts from countries like Israel and Canada. The areas of her expertise are Sensor design, embedded system control algorithms, and Machine Learning Techniques. She is the author of the book "A Beginners Guide for Machine Learning Models with Python Environment" published by LAP LAMBERT Academic Publishing

Subrata Chowdhury is working in the Department of the Computer Science of Engineering of Sreenivasa Institute of Technology And Management as a Associate Professor. He is been working in the IT Industry for more than 5 years in the R&D developments, he has handled many projects in the industry with much dedications and perfect time limits. He has been handling projects related to AI, Blockchains and the Cloud Computing for the companies from various National and Internationals Clients. He had published (4) books from 2014 - 2019 at the domestic market and Internationally Publishers CRC, River . And he been the editor for the 2 books for the CRC& River publisher. He has participated in the Organizing committee, Technical Programmed Committee and Guest Speaker for more than 10 conference and the webinars. He also Reviewed and evaluated more than 50 papers from the conferences and

Karthik Chandran (Member, ACM, Senior Member, IEEE) was born in Madurai, Tamil Nadu, India in 1986. He received the Bachelor of Engineering in Electronics and Instrumentation Engineering at Kamaraj College of Engineering and Technology, India in 2007, the Master's Degree and Ph.D. Degree in Control and Instrumentation Engineering from Kalasalingam Academy of Research and Education (KARE), in 2011 and 2017. In 2011, he joined the Department of Instrumentation and Control Engineering of KARE, India as Assistant Professor. After that, He served as a Lecturer in the Department of Electrical and Computer Engineering, University of Woldia, Ethiopia from 2016–2018. Presently, He was served as a Postdoctoral Researcher at Shanghai Jiaotong University, China. He is serving as Associate Professor in Mechatronics Engineering, at Jyothi Engineering College, Kerala. He is currently involved in research related to Time delay Control problems, Nonlinear system identification, Cascade Control system, and Unmanned vehicle.

C. Suganthi Evangeline currently working as Assistant Professor in the department of Electronics and Communication Engineering at Sri Eshwar College of Engineering, Coimbatore.

A. Jainulafdeen is a dedicated researcher currently pursuing a Ph.D. in Soft Robotics with a focus on Design, Development, and Control using Artificial Intelligence at Anna University, Chennai. His educational journey began with a Bachelor's in Electrical and Electronics Engineering from C.S.I College of Engineering, Ooty, and continued with a Master's in Power Electronics and Drives from Anna University's Regional Centre, Coimbatore. With a strong academic background Jainulafdeen embarked on a career in academia, starting as a Lecturer in EEE and progressing to become the Head of the Department at Sri Ramakrishna Mission Vidyalaya Polytechnic College, a government-aided autonomous institution in Coimbatore. This was followed by a position as Assistant Professor at VSB Engineering College, Karur. His current role is as an Assistant Professor at K. Ramakrishnan College of Engineering, Trichy, where he imparts knowledge and fosters the development of young engineering minds. His areas of interest encompass Power Electronics, Microprocessor and Microcontrollers, Electrical Circuits and Machines, and the exciting domain of Soft Robotics and Artificial Intelligence. His objective is to advance research in Soft Robotics while contributing to academia through teaching and research activities. Jainulafdeen is driven by a passion for innovation and the pursuit of knowledge, making him a promising researcher and educator in the field of engineering.

Sampath Boopathi is an accomplished individual with a strong academic background and extensive research experience. He completed his undergraduate studies in Mechanical Engineering and pursued his postgraduate studies in the field of Computer-Aided Design. Dr. Boopathi obtained his Ph.D. from Anna University, focusing his research on Manufacturing and optimization. Throughout his career, Dr. Boopathi has made significant contributions to the field of engineering. He has authored and published 200 more research articles in internationally peer-reviewed journals, highlighting his expertise and dedication to advancing knowledge in his area of specialization. His research output demonstrates his commitment to conducting rigorous and impactful research. This indicates his innovative thinking and ability to develop practical solutions. With 17 years of academic and research experience, Dr. Boopathi has enriched the engineering community through his teaching and mentorship roles.

Rvea Judie Dolly is an enthusiastic and dedicated professional educator, committed to fostering the social and academic growth of the students. Possessing a strong passion for research, her interests lie in image processing, video compression, machine learning, biomedical signal processing, and pattern recognition. She has successfully published articles in esteemed journals and secured two funded projects from the Indian Council of Medical Research (ICMR) to conduct impactful research benefiting society.

Prabhakar Gunasekaran is currently working as an Assistant Professor in the Department of Electronics and Communication Engineering, Thiagarajar College of Engineering, Madurai – 15 (A Govt. Aided Autonomous Institution Affiliated to Anna University) Tamilnadu, India. He obtained his B.E degree in Electronics & Communication Engineering from Arulmigu Kalasalingam College of Engineering, Krishnankoil, under Anna University, Chennai in the year of 2009, and his M.Tech. Degree in the specialization of Embedded Systems from Hindustan University, Chennai in the year 2011. He obtained his Ph.D. degree in the year 2018 under the faculty of Electrical Engineering, at Anna University, Chennai. He is a recognized Ph. D Supervisor of Anna University, Chennai, under the Faculty of Electrical Engineering, and also guiding 5 Ph.D. scholars. He has published more than 35 research articles around the world including reputed journal transactions like IET, Springer, Taylor & Francis, and Elsevier.

J inesh Peter is currently working as Professor, Department of Computer Science and Engineering at Karunya Institute of Technology and Sciences. He holds the positions include heading the office of international affairs and IAESTE at Karunya from 2017. His recent activities include sending students abroad for semester abroad programs and international internships through IAESTE. Prior to this, he was a full-time research scholar at National Institute of Technology, Calicut, India, from where he received his PhD in computer science and engineering. His research focus includes Big-data, cloud computing, image processing, computer vision, artificial intelligence, machine learning and medicinal plants. He has several publications in various reputed international journals and conference paper which are widely referred to. He is a member of IEEE, CSI & IEI and has served as session chairs and delivered plenary speeches for various international conference and workshops. He has conducted many international conferences and been as editor for springer proceedings and many special issues in journals.

D J. Jagannath, a doctorate from the Faculty of Engineering, specialization in Signal Processing, is currently working as Assistant Professor, Department of Electronics and Communication Engineering at Karunya Institute of Technology and Sciences. He is an experienced researcher in the field of Vision or Pattern Recognition, Bio-inspired Systems, Signal Processing, Fuzzy Logic, Neural Networks, Evolutionary Computing, Machine learning, IoT & Cyber Physical Human Systems. He has worked in R & D research projects funded by DST and ICMR, Indian Government and other funding agencies. He has several publications in various reputed international journals, conference publications and book chapters. He has chaired in several internal conferences and has also delivered plenary speeches for various international conference and workshops. He has also conducted IEEE sponsored international conferences. He is a member of IAENG, ISTE, ISHNE and MISTE.

Anupama Jawale holds a Master's degree in Computer Applications (MCA), a Master's degree in Computer Management (MCM), and an MPhil. She started her career in 2004 as a lecturer. Currently she is Head of the Department and Academic Coordinator for B.Sc, IT program at Narsee Monjee College of Commerce & Economics, Vile Parle. Her research interests lie in cutting-edge areas such as the Internet of Things (IoT), Time Series Analysis, and Data Science.

Jsret Kaur is currently working as an Assistant Professor in University Business School,Chandigarh University,Mohali,Punjab.She is a post graduate (MBA-H.R) from Panjab University,Chandigarh.She has also qualified UGC NET JRF in Human Resource Management/Labour and Social Welfare and has pursued PhD in Business Management from Chandigarh University,Mohali. She has over 8 years of experience in academic and administrative assignments. She also received "Best Teacher of the Department Award " in the year 2019 and 2021 in the field of imparting quality education. Her research interests include Employee Engagement, Management of Organizational Change and Organization Development. She has published several research papers and articles in reputed international and national journals and has presented papers in various national and international conferences. She also contributed one edited book and 10 book chapters on various topics.

T adiarajan completed his UG degree in the field of Computer Science Engineering in the year 2007 and postgraduate in 2010 in field of computer science. He has more than 13 years of teaching experience. His area of interest includes Machine Learning and datamining, data science. He has published research papers in various international journals. Currently, he is pursuing his PhD in field of deep learning.

Anshit Mukherjee is pursuing his BTech degree in computer science from the Abacus Institute of Engineering and Management. He has published many papers in journals, conferences and book chapters to his own credit.

Rjalakshmi Murugesan was born in Madurai, Tamil Nadu, India in 1988. She graduated from Electronics and Instrumentation Engineering of Kamaraj College of Engineering and Technology in 2010. She completed post-graduation in Degree in the Faculty of Instrumentation and Control Engineering from Kalasalingam Academy of Research and Education (KARE), in 2012 and completed her Ph.D. in the faculty of Electrical Engineering from Anna University, Chennai, 2020. She is currently employed as an Assistant Professor in the Thiagarajar College of Engineering, Mechatronics Department, Madurai. She has academic background, with Ten years of teaching experience as an Assistant/Associate professor at various institutions. Besides a research background, she has published several international journals (SCI/Scopus) and conferences (Scopus) from 2012 to till date. Her professional interests focus on Machine learning, Artificial Intelligence, linear and nonlinear control systems, system identification, and her current projects include modeling and controlling nonlinear processes (machine learning algorithms for Biomedical & Robotics).

N. Ayyanar received the B.E. degree in electronics and communication from the Narasu's Sarathy Institute of Technology, Salem, India, in 2013, the M.E. degree in optical communication from the Alagappa Chettiar Government College of Engineering and Technology, Karaikudi, India, in 2015, and the Ph.D. degree in electronics and communication engineering from the National Institute of Technology, Tiruchirappalli, India, in 2020. He is currently working as an Assistant Professor with the Department of Electronics and Communication Engineering, Thiagarajar College of Engineering, Madurai, Tamil Nadu, India. He has published 35 articles in refereed international journals and over 21 papers in conferences. His research interests include PCF-based optical fiber sensor, few mode fibers, fiber laser, plasmonics, and few mode amplifier system designs.

RjrmVssudev Pai Kuchelkar did his graduation in Mechanical Engineering from Goa Engineering College-Goa University (India) in 1994. He began his career in 1994 and has been working in the Automotive Engineering domain in a private organisation. As a part of his interest in the field of computers and information technology, he pursued a PG Diploma in Software Technology from National Center for Software Technology, Mumbai (India) in 2001, PG Diploma in Software Development (Full Stack Development) from upGrad (India)-IIIT Bengaluru (India) in 2021 followed by MS in Computer Science from upGrad (India)-Liverpool John Moores University, UK in 2022.

S enakshi is currently doing Ph.D in the Department of Electronics and Communication Engineering, Thiagarajar College of Engineering, Madurai – 15 (A Govt. Aided Autonomous Institution Affiliated to Anna University) Tamilnadu, India. She obtained her B.E degree in Instrumentation and control Engineering from Sethu Institute of Technology, Kariapatti, under Anna University, Chennai in the year of2009, and her M.Tech. Degree in the specialization of Control and Instrumentation Engineering from Kalasalingam University, Krishnankoil in the year 2012.

S Vijayalakshmi is presently working as Assistant Professor of Computer Science and Technology department at SNS COLLEGE OF ENGINEERING, COIMBATORE since July 2023. Earlier she has worked in PTR COLLEGE OF ENGINEERING AND TECHNOLOGY,MADURAI. She obtained her Master's degree M.E.,CSE in the year 2010 from Anna University Tirunelveli. She possess a vast experience of 13 years of teaching undergraduate and postgraduate engineering students.Her major areas of interest including software testing and Artificial Intelligence and ML.She guided many undergraduate and postgraduate projects.

R. Sharmila had completed her Doctoral Degree in Computer Applications from Manonmaniam Sundaranar University, Tirunelveli. She has the teaching experience of 19 years and presently she is working as Professor and Head in the Department of Computer Applications, Karpagam Academy of Higher Education, Coimbatore. Her area of interest is Data mining, Bigdata Analytics, and Networks. She had published more than 15 Research articles and two books on Opinion mining and Data mining.

Piyanga Subbiah received the B.Tech degree in Information Technology from New Prince Shri Bhavani College of Engineering and Technology, Chennai, India, in 2015 and the M.E. degree in Computer Science and Engineering from Thiagarajar College of Engineering, Madurai, in 2020. He is currently pursuing the Ph.D. degree in Computer Science and Engineering at SRM Institute of Science and Technology, Chengalpattu, Tamil Nadu, India. From 2022, she was a Research Scholar with the Computer Science and Engineering. His research interest includes the processing of images and detection of disease in the plant using Artificial Intelligence.

Priyanga Subbiah received the B.Tech degree in Information Technology from New Prince Shri Bhavani College of Engineering and Technology, Chennai, India, in 2015 and the M.E. degree in Computer Science and Engineering from Thiagarajar College of Engineering, Madurai, in 2020. He is currently pursuing the Ph.D. degree in Computer Science and Engineering at SRM Institute of Science and Technology, Chengalpattu, Tamil Nadu, India. From 2022, she was a Research Scholar with the Computer Science and Engineering. His research interest includes the processing of images and detection of disease in the plant using Artificial Intelligence.

Krthikeyan Subramanian working as a Senior Lecturer in the Automobile Engineering Department at Birmingham City University, Ras Al Khaimah, UAE. He previously worked as an Associate Professor in the Mechanical Engineering Department at Kalasalingam University, India. He has been in the teaching profession for more than 13 years. He started his academic journey with a Bachelor's degree in Automobile Engineering from Sriram Engineering College, Anna University, Chennai. He pursued a Master's degree in Production Engineering from PSG College of Technology, Coimbatore. This educational experience provided me with a solid foundation in automobile and production engineering principles and practices. He earned a Ph.D. in Mechanical Engineering from Kalasalingam University. Additionally, he got experience as a Post-Doctoral Researcher at Szent Istvan University, Godollo, Hungary, where he contributed to cutting-edge research in a dynamic international environment. His academic and research background reflects my dedication to the field of Mechanical and Automobile Engineering.

Preethiya Thandapani received her B.E. degree from Anna University,Chennai in the year 2007 and M.E. degree from Anna University,Thiruchirapalli, Tamil Nadu, India in the year 2009. She has completed Ph.D from Kalasalingam Academy of Research and Education in the field of Mobile Wireless Sensor Network in the year 2020. Her research primarily centered on improving the energy efficiency of mobile unmanned vehicles engaged in communication, with a specific focus on factors related to their speed while in motion. After completing her Ph.D., her curiosity extended to Data Science, and she seamlessly merged it with her WSN expertise, charting a new research trajectory. With over 11 years of teaching experience, she has authored numerous research papers in the field of WSN and Data Science, particularly in addressing environmental monitoring healthcare challenges.

Preethiya Thandapani received her B.E. degree from Anna University,Chennai in the year 2007 and M.E. degree from Anna University,Thiruchirapalli, Tamil Nadu, India in the year 2009. She has completed Ph.D from Kalasalingam Academy of Research and Education in the field of Mobile Wireless Sensor Network in the year 2020. Her research primarily centered on improving the energy efficiency of mobile unmanned vehicles engaged in communication, with a specific focus on factors related to their speed while in motion. After completing her Ph.D., her curiosity extended to Data Science, and she seamlessly merged it with her WSN expertise, charting a new research trajectory. With over 11 years of teaching experience, she has authored numerous research papers in the field of WSN and Data Science, particularly in addressing environmental monitoring healthcare challenges.

Index

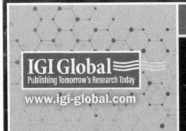

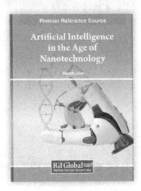
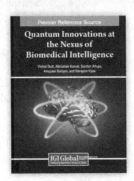
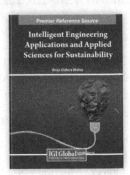
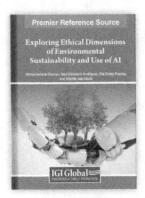
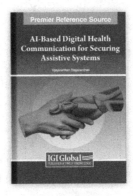
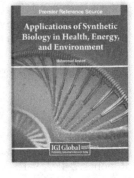

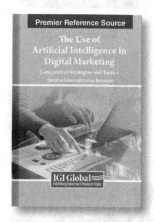 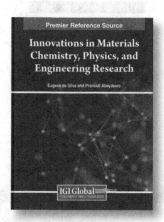 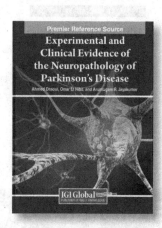 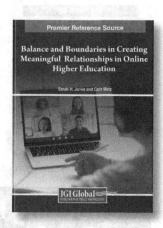

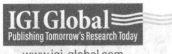
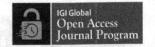
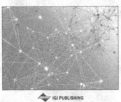
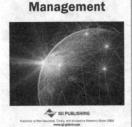
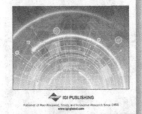
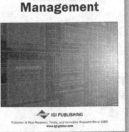
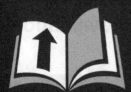

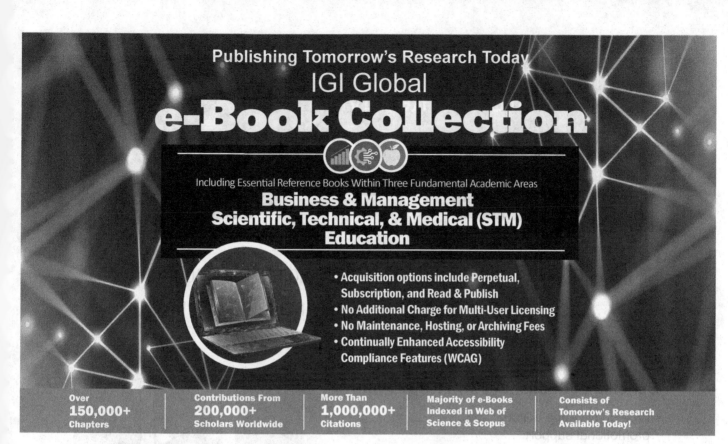
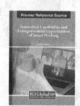
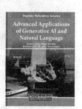
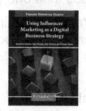
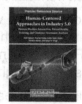
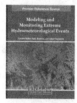
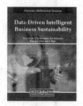
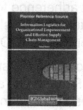
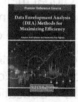

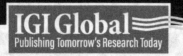

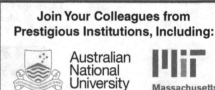
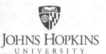

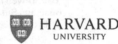

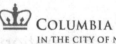

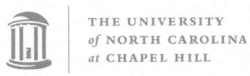

Printed in the United States
by Baker & Taylor Publisher Services